Clinical Physiology
in Obstetrics

We dedicate this volume to the memory of

DR ANGUS MACDONALD
MD FRCP(ED) FRCS(E)

1834–1886

who, in Edinburgh, was Physician and Clinical Lecturer in
Diseases of Women at the Royal Infirmary, Physician to the
Royal Maternal Hospital and Lecturer at Surgeon's Hall in
Midwifery and Diseases of Women. He was the first man to
link the subjects of medicine and obstetrics in his book,
*The Bearings of Chronic Disease of the Heart upon Pregnancy,
Parturition and Childbed* in 1878.

THIRD EDITION

Clinical Physiology in Obstetrics

EDITED BY

GEOFFREY CHAMBERLAIN

MD, FRCS, FRCOG, FACOG, FFFP
Department of Obstetrics and Gynaecology
Singleton Hospital
Swansea

AND

FIONA BROUGHTON PIPKIN

MA, DPhil, FRCOG
Department of Obstetrics and Gynaecology
Queen's Medical Centre
Nottingham

FOREWORD BY

FRANK HYTTEN

b

**Blackwell
Science**

© 1980, 1991, 1998 by
Blackwell Science Ltd
Editorial Offices:
Osney Mead, Oxford OX2 0EL
25 John Street, London WC1N 2BL
23 Ainslie Place, Edinburgh EH3 6AJ
350 Main Street, Malden, MA 02148 5018, USA
54 University Street, Carlton, Victoria 3053, Australia
10, rue Casimir Delavigne 75006 Paris, France

Other Editorial Offices:
Blackwell Wissenschafts-Verlag GmbH
Kurfürstendamm 57, 10707 Berlin, Germany

Blackwell Science KK
MG Kodenmacho Building
7–10 Kodenmacho Nihombashi
Chuo-ku, Tokyo 104, Japan

The right of the Authors to be identified as the
Authors of this Work has been asserted in accordance
with the Copyright, Designs and Patents Act 1988.

First published 1980
Second edition 1991
Reprinted 1995
Third edition 1998

Set by Excel Typesetters Co., Hong Kong
Printed and Bound in Great Britain by
MPG Books Ltd, Bodmin, Cornwall

The Blackwell Science logo is a trade mark of Blackwell
Science Ltd, registered at the United Kingdom Trade Marks
Registry

i 13647660

DISTRIBUTORS

Marston Book Services Ltd
PO Box 269, Abingdon, Oxon OX14 4YN
(*Orders*: Tel: 01235 465500
          Fax: 01235 465555)

USA
Blackwell Science Inc, Commerce Place
350 Main Street, Malden, MA 02148 5018
(*Orders*: Tel: 800 759 6102
               617 388 8250
          Fax: 617 388 8255)

Canada
Login Brothers Book Company
324 Saulteaux Crescent
Winnipeg, Manitoba R3J 3T2
(*Orders*: Tel: 204 224-4068)

Australia
Blackwell Science Pty Ltd
54 University Street, Carlton, Victoria 3053
(*Orders*: Tel: 3 9347 0300
          Fax: 3 9347 5001)

A catalogue record for this title is available
from the British Library

ISBN 0-86542-948-0

Library of Congress
Cataloging-in-publication Data

Clinical physiology in obstetrics /
   [edited by] Geoffrey Chamberlain,
   Fiona Broughton Pipkin;
   foreword by Frank Hytten.—3rd ed.
          p.   cm.
   Includes bibliographical references and index.
      ISBN 0-86542-948-0
      1. Pregnancy—Physiological aspects.
   I. Chamberlain, Geoffrey, 1930– .
   II. Broughton Pipkin, Fiona.
      [DNLM: 1. Pregnancy—physiology.
   WQ 200 C641 1998]
      RG558.C55   1998
      618.2—dc21
      DNLM/DLC
   for Library of Congress   97-42723
                                                         CIP

Contents

Contributors

PROFESSOR CHRISTINE BAYLIS, PhD,
*Professor of Physiology, Robert C. Byrd Health
Sciences Center, West Virginia University,
Morgantown, WV 26506-9229, USA*

PROFESSOR FIONA BROUGHTON
PIPKIN, MA, DPhil, FRCOG, *Professor of
Perinatal Physiology, Department of Obstetrics and
Gynaecology, Queen's Medical Centre, Nottingham,
NG7 2UH*

DR MARY CAMPBELL-BROWN, MBChB,
D(Obst)RCOG, DTM&T (Eng), *Honorary Senior
Research Fellow, Department of Obstetrics and
Gynaecology, Royal Infirmary, 10 Alexander Parade,
Glasgow, G31 2ER*

PROFESSOR G.V.P. CHAMBERLAIN,
MD, FRCS, FRCOG, FACOG, FFFP, *Department of
Obstetrics and Gynaecology, Singleton Hospital,
Sketty, Swansea, SA2 8QA*

PROFESSOR T. CHARD, FRCOG,
*Department of Obstetrics and Gynaecology, St
Bartholomew's Hospital Medical College, London,
EC1A 7BE*

DR G. COTICCHIO, BSc, M.Med.Sci, PhD,
*Academic Division of Obstetrics and Gynaecology,
School of Human Development, University of
Nottingham, Queen's Medical Centre, Nottingham,
NG7 2UH*

PROFESSOR J.M. DAVISON, BSc, MD,
MSc, FRCOG, *Professor in Obstetric Medicine,
Department of Obstetrics and Gynaecology,
Royal Victoria Infirmary, Newcastle upon Tyne,
NE1 4LP*

DR RINA M. DAVISON, MA, MB, BCh,
MRCP (UK), *Department of Endocrinology, The
Cobbold Laboratories, The Middlesex Hospital,
Mortimer Street, London, WIN 8AA*

DR J.J. DUVEKOT, MD, PhD, *Department of
Obstetrics and Gynaecology, St Clara Hospital,
Olympiaweg 350, 3078 HT Rotterdam, The
Netherlands*

DR S. FISHEL, BSc (Hons), PhD (Cantab),
FCPS (Cantab), *Director, CARE (Centres for
Assisted Reproduction), The Park Hospital,
Sherwood Lodge Drive, Arnold, Nottingham,
NG5 8RX*

PROFESSOR MARY L. FORSLING, BSc,
PhD, DSc, *Department of Physiology and Obstetrics
UMDS, St Thomas' Campus, Lambeth Palace Road,
London, SE1 7EH*

DR DIANA HAMILTON-FAIRLEY, MD,
MRCOG, *Consultant Obstetrician and
Gynaecologist, Guy's and St Thomas' Hospital Trust,
St Thomas' Hospital, Lambeth Palace Road, London,
SE1 7EH*

PROFESSOR D.J. HOSKING, MD, FRCP,
*Professor of Mineral Metabolism, Department of
Biochemistry, University of Nottingham and
Consultant Physician, City Hospital, Hucknall Road,
Nottingham, NG5 1PB*

PROFESSOR F.E. HYTTEN, MD, PhD,
FRCOG, *Blossoms, Cobblers Hill, Great Missenden,
Bucks., HP16 9PW*

PROFESSOR D.K. JAMES, MA, MD, FRCOG, DCH, *Professor of Fetomaternal Medicine, Department of Obstetrics and Gynaecology, Queen's Medical Centre, Nottingham, NG7 2UH*

DR M.R. JOHNSON, MB, BS, PhD, MRCP, MRCOG, *Senior Lecturer in Reproductive Medicine, Division of Obstetrics and Gynaecology, Imperial College School of Medicine, Chelsea and Westminster Hospital, 369 Fulham Road, London, SW10 9NH*

DR ELIZABETH A. LETSKY, MB, BS, FRCPath, FRCOG, FRCPCH, *Consultant Perinatal Haematologist, Queen Charlotte's and Chelsea Hospital, Goldhawk Road, London, W6 0XG*

DR I.T. MANYONDA, BSc, PhD, MRCOG, *Consultant Obstetrician and Gynaecologist, Honorary Senior Lecturer in Immunology, St George's Hospital, Blackshaw Road,London, SW17 0QT*

DR J.P. O'HARE, MD, FRCP, *Reader in Medicine and Consultant Physician in Diabetes and Endocrinology, Medical Research Institute, University of Warwick, Coventry, CV 7AL*

DR L.L.H. PEETERS, MD, PhD, *Associated Professor of Obstetrics, Department of Obstetrics and Gynaecology, Academic Hospital Maastricht, PO Box 1918, 6201 AZ, Maastricht, The Netherlands*

DR I.D. RAMSAY, MD, FRCP, FRCPE, *Consultant Endocrinologist, The Cromwell Hospital, Cromwell Road, London, SW5 0TU*

PROFESSOR FELICITY REYNOLDS, MBBS, MD, FRCA, FRCOG, *Emeritus Professor of Obstetric Anaesthesia (UMDS), Department of Anaesthetics, St Thomas' Hospital, London, SE1 7EH*

PROFESSOR P.J. STEER, BSc, MD, FRCOG, *Section of Obstetrics and Gynaecology at Chelsea and Westminster Hospital, Imperial College School of Medicine, 369 Fulham Road, London, SW10 9NH*

PROFESSOR T. STEPHENSON, BSc (Hons), BM, BCh, DM, FRCP (London), FRCPCH, *Professor of Child Health, The University of Nottingham, Honorary Consultant Paediatrician, Nottingham University Hospital, Academic Division of Child Health, School of Human Development, Queen's Medical Centre, Nottingham, NG7 2UH*

DR M. DE SWIET, MD, FRCP, FRCOG, *Consultant Physician, Queen Charlotte's and Chelsea Hospital, Goldhawk Road, London, W6 0XG*

Foreword

Up to the 1950s, pregnancy was generally regarded as a disease by Western obstetricians whose daily experience was of life-threatening complications. As a medical student in the 1940s, I can remember no suggestion that the pregnant woman was in an altered physiological state. When such people as Barcroft in Cambridge were beginning to unravel the complexities of fetal physiology, the mother was certainly not considered to be of comparable interest.

Sir Dugald Baird in Aberdeen was then editing the sixth edition of the *Combined Textbook of Obstetrics and Gynaecology*. With his characteristic long vision and belief that maternal nutrition was likely to play an important part in the success of a pregnancy, he considered that physiology deserved a chapter. I was then a research fellow in the Medical Research Council's Obstetric Medicine Research Unit embedded in the Aberdeen Maternity Hospital and at that time embarked on studies of the changing maternal body composition and other aspects of physiology. The chapter was entrusted to me and to Dr Isabella Leitch, a notable nutritionist at the Rowett Institute. We began an extensive literature search, beginning with the premise that pregnancy was essentially a nutritional exercise: the acquisition of nutrients as fetal building blocks by the mother, their transport to the placental site, their uptake and transfer to the fetus, and, in reverse, the elimination by the mother of fetal waste products, including gases and heat. The amount of information buried in the literature surprised us, and when the textbook chapter was published in 1957, we were left with a considerable pile of papers, abstracts and references, and a growing realization that the physiology of pregnancy was something of a goldmine. Moreover, it presaged a major conceptual shift from the beliefs of those brought up in the age of pathology. They had to be led to understand that the many changes in pregnancy which mimic abnormality (such as the falling concentration of haemoglobin in the blood, the massive gain in body fat, and widespread oedema) were universal in healthy women and presumably beneficial to the pregnancy.

The obvious next step was to assemble these accumulated data as a book, which could include an interpretation of their physiological meaning and suggestions for further research; *The Physiology of Human Pregnancy* by Hytten and Leitch was published in 1964. That first edition was received with some enthusiasm and was translated into Spanish and Czech. By 1971, when I had to prepare the second edition alone, there had been a burgeoning of information, perhaps in part due to the stimulus of that first book, and physiological aspects of pregnancy had become a major feature of obstetric research.

Thereafter, it became obvious that no individual could reasonably do justice to the subject. Professor Geoffrey Chamberlain, with characteristic optimism, persuaded me that we could edit a third edition, put together by friends who were experts in particular aspects of the field, and *Clinical Physiology in Obstetrics* appeared in 1980. It too enjoyed a further edition in 1991, but by now I had begun to lose the energy for keeping abreast, and I am very happy to see a further edition—what I like to think of as a fifth edition of the original book—in the very capable hands of two old friends, Geoffrey Chamberlain and Fiona Broughton Pipkin.

PROFESSOR FRANK HYTTEN

Preface to Third Edition

In 1980 we published the first edition of this book as successor to *The Physiology of Human Pregnancy* by Hytten and Leitch; Professor Frank Hytten in his foreword traces the evolution of the current volume. He has now passed the editorship to a clinician and a physiologist who have gathered an expanded team of scientific writers. The book is aimed at all in obstetrics who want to learn more about the physiological background of their work than the standard textbooks offer. We hope it will also be helpful to other physicians who deal with pregnant women for so many normal physiological changes of pregnancy can compound the findings in the rest of medicine. We hope that by choosing writers who bridge the divide of clinical medicine and scientific work, we will have enabled this book to provide medical insight to basic science research workers.

In the 1980 edition our team members came from the MacDonald Club of physicians and obstetricians. This is named after the Edinburgh physician who was the first to write on medical conditions in pregnancy and we have dedicated the book to him for this reason. Now the team has been broadened and we thank the authors who have produced their careful work, often on time, and for the way they accepted our editorial questioning of their ideas.

We are grateful not just to our authors but to the publishers, particularly Stuart Taylor and Alice Nelson who helped us produce this volume. Much of its clarity is owed to the layout and diagrams. We are also grateful to all those who allowed us to reproduce their material from publications and to the many physiologists and obstetricians whose work we quote.

GEOFFREY CHAMBERLAIN
FIONA BROUGHTON PIPKIN
Swansea and Nottingham 1998

PART 1

The Cardiovascular and Respiratory Systems

Very Early Changes in Cardiovascular Physiology

J.J. DUVEKOT & L.L.H. PEETERS

Introduction

The most important haemodynamic changes in the maternal circulation during pregnancy are the increase in cardiac output and blood volume, and the decrease in peripheral vascular resistance. Pregnancies complicated by fetal growth restriction, pregnancy-induced hypertension and/or pre-eclampsia are associated with relatively lower maternal cardiac output [1,2] and relatively higher total peripheral resistance than are pregnancies without these complications. It is, however, still not clear whether these are primary phenomena (i.e. that the normal adaptations have never taken place) or whether they are secondary responses, initial adaptation having taken place as normal. Whether primary or secondary, the association of phenomena indicates that the normal changes in maternal haemodynamics represent adaptations important for the well-being of the fetus.

It is one of the enigmas of pregnancy that so many changes in maternal physiology are initiated before there is any obvious physiological need for them. Indeed, some are foreshadowed in each ovulatory menstrual cycle, and are simply maintained and amplified should conception occur. The menstrual cycle is thus concerned with much more than the simple provision of a fresh egg each month. It is a proactive process, preparing for pregnancy at many levels. The currently available evidence suggests that hormonal and immunological alterations act together very early to begin the process of haemodynamic adaptation. After this, the increases in cardiac function and blood volume are mainly orchestrated by stimuli from the growing uterus and feto-placental unit, particularly from the vascular endothelium. Nevertheless, it has become increasingly clear that the largest changes in cardiovascular adaptation, volume homeostasis and the immunoregulatory system take place during the first 8 weeks of gestation. This period will be referred to as early pregnancy throughout this chapter.

This chapter begins with an overview of currently available techniques for the measurement of cardiovascular variables. This is followed by

3

4 an introduction to the potential circulatory effects of those vasoactive substances currently considered as being potential mediators of the haemodynamic changes of early pregnancy. We then attempt to arrive at a better understanding of how the early changes occur by putting our current fragmentary knowledge of haemodynamic and volume changes during the menstrual cycle and early pregnancy in chronological order, and within the context of changes in these endocrine systems.

Measurement of cardiovascular parameters

Until the 1980s, radioisotope and X-ray angiography were the methods of choice to evaluate left cardiac function. In the 1990s, the combination of cardiac ultrasound imaging, quantitative Doppler echocardiography and calibrated external pulse recordings was introduced as a powerful set of tools for the clinical assessment of left ventricular performance. At present, the most frequently used methods to study cardiovascular function in humans are either combined cross-sectional and Doppler echocardiography or impedance cardiography. The invasive technique of Swan–Ganz pulmonary artery monitoring is used less frequently, and almost exclusively in critically ill patients.

Combined cross-sectional and Doppler echocardiography

After initial experiments in dogs [3], the validity of non-invasive cardiac output measurement by echocardiography, combined with continuous- or pulsed-wave range-gated Doppler, was demonstrated for non-pregnant humans [4–6]. In this method, stroke volume is calculated as the product of Doppler flow velocity integral, represented by the area under the velocity integral, represented by the area under the velocity curve, and the cross-sectional area (CSA) of the vessel at the site of the flow velocity measurement. The measurement error in stroke volume calculation by this method depends primarily on the echographic method used and the site of measurement of the CSA through which the blood flow is measured. Small differences in diameter have a

disproportionally large impact on CSA, which is itself difficult to measure precisely. Consequently, the measurement error can be as high as 15% [7]. A-mode, M-mode and 2-dimensional imaging have all been used to measure the CSA of the aorta [7–9], but M-mode ultrasound is now probably the most widely used method. Although in the non-pregnant state the aortic CSA does not increase appreciably with increasing flow rates [10], the altered structure, and possibly with it, compliance of connective tissue associated with the increased oestrogen levels in pregnancy, could result in a distension of the aortic valve annulus [11]. Conversely, the lower blood pressure in pregnancy could lead to a smaller aortic diameter. Consequently, it is not surprising that an increase by 10–30% [12–15] as well as no appreciable change [16–19] in aortic valve orifice area have been reported. This still unsettled controversy is probably the most important drawback of the Doppler flow derived cardiac output measurements.

Pulsed- and continuous-wave Doppler echocardiography were originally considered to be equally accurate for velocity measurements in the ascending aorta, both in the non-pregnant and pregnant state [7,19]. However, the pulsed Doppler technique has the advantage that it can be combined with direct imaging. This allows visualization of the beam:vessel intercept angle, which should be as close to tangential as possible. It also allows precise measurement of the valve:vessel area because the exact depth of the vessel can be determined.

The within-subject intra-observer and temporal coefficients of variation during pregnancy for the combined method have been determined by Robson and are less than 5% [20]. A combination of pulsed- and continuous-wave Doppler has been validated against the Fick principle in pregnant patients [20]. There was good agreement between the two methods (correlation coefficient: 0.87–0.93; no intercept differing significantly from zero; none of the slopes differing significantly from unity) at all three insonation gates (aortic root, mitral valve and pulmonary artery). Since the aorta and pulmonary artery are the easiest to visualize in pregnancy, these are probably the insonation sites of choice. Flows measured over the aortic, pulmonary and mitral valves were found to correlate well, both in the pregnant and the non-pregnant state [21]. Since measurement at the level of the aortic valve is technically easier [10,20], permitting adequate and reproducible measurement of the CSA, this site is considered the most appropriate for the measurement of cardiac output [7,9]. In addition, the shape of the aortic valve orifice was found not to differ between diastole and peak-systole [7].

The non-invasive technique has also been validated in human pregnancy using invasive indicator dilution techniques as a reference [22–24]. Although data obtained by both continuous-wave and pulsed Doppler ultrasound imaging correlated well with thermodilution data (correlation coefficient: 0.93–0.98), the study population consisted only of critically ill patients suffering from severe pre-eclampsia.

Stroke volume can also be derived from the difference in left ventricular volume between the diastolic and systolic phases of the cardiac cycle as measured by M-mode echocardiography. In this method, the left ventricular volume is usually calculated using the Teichholz formula [25], which assumes the left ventricle to be ellipsoid, with the long axis having twice the length of the short axis. The temporal coefficients of variation for M-mode measurements of chamber size and ventricular contractility are only approximately 2% and 5%, respectively [26]. Validation studies show this method to be reasonably accurate ($r = 0.81$), but a prerequisite is that the left ventricle contraction is symmetrical or almost symmetrical [25,27]. It follows that abnormal or rapidly changing left ventricular dimensions will lead to erroneous values for stroke volume [28]. Two longitudinal studies have been reported in human pregnancy using this technique [29,30] but it has not been formally validated in pregnancy, a dynamic condition characterized by profound changes in cardiac form and position. M-mode recordings may, however, have an important place in the study of structural changes in the cardiovascular system, because of their precise timing of cardiac events and the excellent axial resolution.

Impedance cardiography

In this technique, stroke volume is calculated from the changes in electrical impedance in the thoracic cavity during the cardiac cycle. The technique is simple to use, since it only requires the application of four circumferential electrodes to the neck and thorax. The outer electrodes apply a small interrogating voltage along the long axis of the thorax, which is detected by the inner electrodes. Changes in the detected voltage relate to the changes in volume of blood in the chest (assumed to be pulmonary blood volume), which in turn relates to the stroke volume. However, the relation is not consistent at all stages of pregnancy, possibly because of changes in pulmonary blood volume and in the elasticity of the blood vessels [31]. One of the major assumptions of the method is a constant ejection flow rate throughout systole. The flow/time profile is likely to alter with pregnancy since the ejection time is substantially reduced in advanced gestation [31]. Doubts have therefore been cast on its accuracy for prospective studies in pregnancy and even in the non-pregnant state there is some ambiguity concerning the accuracy of this technique [32,33].

In spite of these concerns, cardiac output has been measured in late pregnancy by a modified technique of impedance cardiography and was reported to be consistently lower than that simultaneously measured by thermodilution [34,35]. The underestimation of stroke volume during pregnancy was also noted when the technique was employed longitudinally [36,37]. Cardiac output appeared not to increase throughout most of pregnancy and at term actually to decrease to below non-pregnant levels. Serial measurement of stroke volume in pregnancy by the impedance technique would have to take into account the influence of variables such as intrathoracic fluid volume, thorax configuration and hematological characteristics, all of which change with pregnancy and are assumed to be constant in the mathematical formula [34]. It follows that impedance cardiography is probably unsuitable for longitudinal studies of the cardiovascular system in pregnancy.

Swan–Ganz pulmonary artery thermodilution catheter monitoring

Since its introduction into clinical medicine in the 1970s, the pulmonary artery catheter has become an important instrument in the surveillance of critically ill patients. Indications for invasive haemodynamic monitoring in obstetric patients include severe pre-eclamptic hypertension, non-responsive to conventional antihypertensive therapy, pulmonary oedema and oliguria [38]. Because of the invasive character of this method, data on central haemodynamic changes determined with this technique during uneventful pregnancy are scarce [39,40].

Haemodynamic effects of vasoactive endocrine and paracrine substances

The influence of hormones and other vasoactive substances on the cardiovascular system has been the subject of many studies. These substances can exert their largest effect on the heart, volume regulation or on the blood vessels. An additional categorization can be made into endothelium-dependent and endothelium-independent vascular changes. This is particularly important in pregnancy since the generalized vasorelaxation appears likely to be endothelium-dependent. Plasma-borne agents may be responsible for the reduced vascular contractility in pregnancy. In experiments conducted on rat aortic rings, incubation with serum of normotensive pregnant women reduced the contractile responses to phenylephrine [41,42]. This effect was abolished after removal of the endothelial lining of the aortic rings. It is not clear whether the decreased vascular responsiveness or vascular reactivity to constrictor substances is coincidental or even causally related to the vascular relaxation observed already in early pregnancy. According to the classical study by Gant this decreased pressor responsiveness is already present by the 10th week of gestation [43]. There certainly appears to be an endothelium-dependent alteration of the function of the smooth muscle cells in the resistance vessels [44]. In the following section the most important vasoactive substances likely to be involved in the cardiovascular adaptation to pregnancy are reviewed.

Oestrogen

The three major oestrogens in pregnancy, oestrone, oestriol and oestradiol, show different patterns during pregnancy [45]. Oestrone and oestriol excretion are increased about 100 times over non-pregnant levels, while oestradiol levels increase about 1000-fold. In early pregnancy, oestrone and oestradiol show a gradual rise that reaches levels above those during the menstrual cycle by the 10th and 8th week, respectively. Oestradiol concentrations are significantly higher in conception cycles than in non-conception cycles by the 6th day after the luteinizing hormone (LH) surge [46] but oestriol levels remain below the detection threshold until the 9th week of pregnancy, when the fetal adrenal gland secretion of precursor begins [47]. The circulating oestrogen concentrations continue to increase until term.

The effects of exogenously administered oestrogen, usually 17β-oestradiol, on the cardiovascular system have been investigated by several authors. In animal studies, oestrogen administration leads to an increase in cardiac output, merely as a result of an increase in stroke volume, and a decrease in vascular resistance [48–50]. Early longitudinal studies using administration of combined oral contraceptives to healthy women showed similar cardiovascular effects [51,52]. The oestrogen component in these pills turned out to be responsible for these cardiovascular effects [52]. Heart rate seems to vary independently of oestrogen. Induction of a hypo-oestrogenic state results in a fall in cardiac output [53].

The haemodynamic effect of oestrogens seems time-dependent. Initially the aortic flow velocity integral accelerates after the administration of oestrogen, but this response attenuates with ongoing oestrogen exposure [54]. This suggests that at least the vasodilating effect of oestrogen in the human may be only transient [55]. In contrast, the possible inotropic action of oestrogens may be more long-lasting. The lack of increase in cardiac contractility during ovulation induction is probably due to a combination of a cross-sectional study design, a lower oestrogen dose and/or a relatively short treatment interval [56–58]. The apparent positive effect on cardiac muscle may be related to the oestrogen-mediated stimulation of actomyosin production [59,60]. A second mechanism that could explain the oestrogen-mediated increase in stroke volume is an increase in preload secondary to a rise in blood volume. Various human studies have reported plasma volume expansion in response to exogenous oestrogens, both in males and females [52,61]. Similar effects are also observed in animal studies (for review, see [62]). This effect is thought to be mediated by the stimulation of the renin–angiotensin–aldosterone system [63].

So far, there is only indirect support for a role of oestrogens in establishing the overall systemic vasodilation of pregnancy. Several studies in the human as well as in animals reported a fall in vascular resistance and rise in blood flow velocity in response to systemically and locally administered oestrogens [64]. Venous distensibility is also increased by oestrogens [65]. Although this oestrogen-induced vasodilation occurs mainly in reproductive tissues, increases in blood flow to several non-reproductive tissues have also been observed [66]. The dilating effect of exogenous oestrogens on the uterine vascular bed is dose- and agent-dependent [67]. In postmenopausal women endothelium-dependent, flow-mediated vasodilation occurs in response to short-term administration of oestrogens [68] but subsides as delineated above [55]. The mechanism responsible for this phenomenon is still obscure.

The pathway by which oestrogens lead to vasodilation is probably complex. Oestrogens have been found to stimulate endothelium-dependent vasodilation by either increasing synthesis and release of nitric oxide or inhibiting its degradation. Oestrogens may also reduce vasomotor tone by modifying the nitric oxide response to vasodilator stimuli and by suppressing the release of endothelin-1, a potent vasoconstrictor [69]. Furthermore, oestrogens also stimulate the production of vasodilator prostaglandins and alter the balance of vasodilator and vasoconstrictor prostaglandins [68,70], and the cell membrane ionic channels [71]. Finally, oestrogens may indirectly alter vascular tone by modulating the influence of catecholamines [72].

Besides having these functional effects on the vasculature, oestrogens also induce structural changes in the vessel wall by changing the distribution of collagen in the tunica media. Aortic smooth muscle cells cultured in the presence of 17β-oestradiol were shown to produce an altered ratio of type I to type III collagen [11]. A change in this ratio leads to a production of a more soluble collagen, which may be involved in the remodelling of the vasculature during pregnancy. This is confirmed clinically, since treatment with gonadotrophins inducing high endogenous oestrogen levels results in an increased aortic compliance [73].

Progesterone

Conception is not associated with higher luteal progesterone concentrations [46]. The mean plasma level of progesterone changes little between the 5th and the 10th week of gestation. After the 10th week of pregnancy the progesterone level begins to increase progressively, reaching levels of 50% above those in the 5th week of pregnancy by the 13th week. Progesterone levels increase up to threefold by term [47].

To our knowledge, information on the haemodynamic effects of progesterone is scarce. In non-pregnant humans and animals, exogenous progesterone was found to have no appreciable effects on haemodynamic function [49,52]. Since progesterone is known to accelerate endometrial growth and differentiation or decidualization, and to inhibit myometrial contractility, it is conceivable that possible haemodynamic effects of progesterone may be confined to the uterus.

It is uncertain whether progesterone influences blood volume. Theoretically, progesterone may reduce plasma volume by its natriuretic effect, which is due to its affinity to the aldosterone receptor in the distal tubule [74] and its inhibitory effect on sodium reabsorption in the proximal tubule [75]. Accelerated natri-uresis in response to progesterone does not result in volume depletion because of a concomitantly raised activity of the renin–angiotensin–aldosterone system [63]. On the other hand, progesterone and its precursor pregnenolone may act as precursors of dehy-

8 droepiandosterone, which may increase plasma volume indirectly.

Natural progesterone has been reported to reduce blood pressure in hypertensive subjects [76]. In in-vitro studies of the placenta, progesterone proved to induce vascular relaxation [77]. Whether the fall in blood pressure in response to progesterone is secondary to this relaxing effect on the vasculature is obscure. At any rate, finger skin flow did not alter in response to progesterone administration to healthy women [78]. In studies reporting the effects of oral contraception on venous tone, venous distensibility was felt to be increased by progesterone [65]. Vasodilation induced by oestrogens is opposed by progesterone in human and animal studies [64]. During the oestrous cycle in sheep, an inverse relationship exists between uterine blood flow and progesterone levels [79].

Inhibin, relaxin, chorionic gonadotrophin

Among the substances that increase during early pregnancy and disappear after the first trimester are the luteal hormones, inhibin and relaxin. To the best of our knowledge, the haemodynamic effect of these hormones has never been studied in the human. In rat pregnancy, relaxin induces vasodilation and reduces blood pressure [80,81]. In addition, relaxin has a strong chronotropic and inotropic effect on the rat heart, probably mediated through a direct action on relaxin receptors. However, administration of human relaxin to pregnant animals does not exert these cardiovascular effects [82].

Various other hormones which circulate in the first weeks of pregnancy are highly unlikely to have an appreciable direct effect on the cardiovascular function. The resetting of the osmoreceptors in early pregnancy has been proposed to be influenced by human chorionic gonadotrophin. In non-pregnant women, human chorionic gonadotrophin injections were found to decrease their osmotic threshold by 5 mosmol/kg [83], but in males no significant effect was observed [84]. Erythropoiesis is stimulated by several hormones (for a review, see [62]).

The renin–angiotensin system

Angiotensin II (A II), the end product of the renin–angiotensin system, varies as a function of diastolic blood pressure in normotensive pregnancies [85]. Recent studies demonstrated the direct important role of A II in the maintenance of blood pressure during pregnancy [86]. It also has a direct effect on renal function by accelerating tubular sodium reabsorption and influencing renal haemodynamics [87]. During pregnancy, the peripheral concentrations of both precursors and hormones involved in the renin–angiotensin system are markedly elevated. This rise may be, at least in part, related to the marked change in the steroid environment or to the increased prostaglandin production in gestation [88,89]. There is a cyclical pattern in the precursors and hormones of the renin–angiotensin system during the normal menstrual cycle, with most of them peaking during or shortly after ovulation [74,90]. Should conception occur, this peak does not return to basal levels [91]. The renin–angiotensin system is thus one of the earliest hormone systems to recognize pregnancy.

The changes during pregnancy are as follows. Total renin concentration, subdivided into an inactive and an active fraction, decreases after an initial peak in early pregnancy [18]. Meanwhile, the concentration of active renin in the peripheral blood continues to increase until the 30th week [92–94], in concert with angiotensinogen and A II [95]. Afterwards, active plasma renin declines gradually until term [94,96,97]. In spite of the higher basal activity of the renin–angiotensin system during pregnancy, its response to external stimuli remains unaffected [98,99]. Apparently, pregnancy induces a resetting of this system, comparable to that of the baroreceptor [100] and osmoregulatory systems [101]. The effect of the resetting consists of a lower threshold of serum sodium levels for the activation of the renin–angiotensin system [102]. On the other hand, neither the mechanism responsible for the resetting nor the interrelation between the changes in the renin–angiotensin system and volume homeostasis during pregnancy has been elucidated.

The renin–angiotensin system regulates aldosterone release. Both aldosterone concentration and turnover rate are raised in pregnancy to levels as high as those in primary aldosteronism [103]. However, even in the first trimester, the strong aldosterone dependence on renin, as seen in the non-pregnant state, begins to weaken. This is suggested by the increase in aldosterone preceding that in renin [104]. The possible superimposed effect of the increasing progesterone levels has never been substantiated [96,105,106]. It is conceivable that the rapid rise in effective renal plasma flow facilitates the release of renin in the kidneys [95,106]. Other potential contributors are the abruptly developing haemodilution [101], and the change in steroid environment. Although the preserved response of aldosterone to changes in serum sodium and vascular filling supports a simple reset to a lower sodium setpoint, it does not exclude that part of the hyperaldosteronism in pregnancy is caused by suboptimal expansion of the extracellular volume.

Angiotensin II is primarily a vasoconstrictor and is involved in the control of arterial blood pressure. Its vasoconstrictor effects act also on renal flow and result in a decrease in glomerular filtration rate. These vasoconstrictory effects are blunted in human pregnancy [43]. The various effects of this substance suggest an important role in cardiovascular homeostasis [107].

Cytokines

Cytokines are soluble polypeptides that play an important role in the intercellular communication within a biological system. They are released by certain cells and exert their effect after binding to specific receptors on adjacent or otherwise related cells such as the decidua, trophoblast and endothelium in the first instance or latterly the immune and haematopoietic cells. During implantation and early development they provide the intercellular communication network essential for the regulation and coordination of trophoblast invasion and differentiation [108]. Among others, the group of cytokines consists of lymphokines (released by T cells), interleukins, colony-stimulating factors, and interferons. Cytokines that are pro-duced by the trophoblast or fetus have been shown to exert also immunoregulatory activity. The most important cytokines involved in the regulation of local and systemic adaptations in pregnancy are interleukin-1, tumour necrosis factor-α, interferon-γ, granulocyte–macrophage colony-stimulating factor, and colony-stimulating factor [109]. Throughout gestation all these cytokines are detectable in the uterus.

Possible vasoactive effects may be accomplished indirectly. The production of the cytokines interleukin-1β, interleukin-4, interleukin-6, and tumour necrosis factor-α in the uterus are closely linked with uteroplacental prostaglandin synthesis and especially prostaglandin E_2, a known vasodilator [110,111]. Cytokines are also linked with induction of Ca^{2+}-dependent and Ca^{2+}-independent nitric oxide synthetases [112].

Nitric oxide

Nitric oxide, derived from L-arginine by the action of nitric oxide synthase, is a powerful inhibitor of platelet aggregation and a potent vasodilator of the resistance vessels [113]. Nitric oxide synthase exists in a variety of forms. A constitutive, calcium-dependent enzyme is found in endothelial cells and brain, and an inducible, calcium-independent form is seen in macrophages, neutrophils and also in endothelium [112]. Nitric oxide is, in terms of biological activity, stability, and susceptibility to inhibitors and to potentiators, identical to endothelium-derived relaxing factor (EDRF) and is considered to be at least one form of EDRF [114,115]. Its release is stimulated by different physical and chemical stimuli. These include agents released during platelet activation and thrombosis, cytokines, and a large number of hormones and neurotransmitters (e.g. acetylcholine, calcitonin gene-related peptide, substance P, noradrenaline, bradykinin and histamine) [116]. The most important physical stimulus is flow rate, with pulsatile flow showing an increase in EDRF release [117]. Inhibition of nitric oxide synthase can be caused by a limited supply of one of its precursors or cofactors by way of a negative feedback mechanism.

The activity of nitric oxide synthase in the brain and in a variety of peripheral tissues is substantially increased during pregnancy [112]. The neurotransmitter calcitonin gene-related peptide, capable of induction of EDRF and which is distributed in the perivascular nerves, is increased in plasma throughout pregnancy [118].

Prostaglandins

The endometrial concentration of prostaglandins varies with the menstrual cycle, suggesting a relationship with the steroid hormones [110]. Prostaglandins, particularly of the E series, are known to induce the vascular changes that precede decidualization and implantation. The source of synthesis is probably the endometrium, but the stimulus is provided by the blastocyst [119]. In early pregnancy, the decidua produces prostaglandin E_2. The further course of prostaglandin production during pregnancy is not clear but it seems certain that prostaglandin synthesis is enhanced. The half-life of prostaglandins is short and their rate of synthesis is probably determined by their metabolites. Prostaglandins have in the first place a local effect. There is general agreement about elevated levels of circulating vasodilator prostaglandins during the second and third trimesters of pregnancy as is indicated by the elevated levels of the metabolites of prostaglandin E_2 and prostacyclin [88,89,120–123]. However, the higher urinary excretion rate of these metabolites may be secondary to increased renal medullary production [124].

The vasodilator prostanoids prostaglandin E_2 and prostacyclin have strong vasodilatory effects [125]. These substances are likely candidates for involvement in the generalized pregnancy-induced vasodilation. However, cyclo-oxygenase inhibitors have been shown to be unable to neutralize the rise in glomerular filtration rate in midpregnancy in rats and rabbits [88,124]. Administration of indomethacin to healthy pregnant women had no effect on blood pressure and had only a mild lowering effect on stroke volume [126]. Conversely, the decreased pressor responsiveness in pregnancy, which is also thought to be related to prostaglandins, can be diminished by inhibition of prostaglandin synthesis [127].

Haemodynamic changes during early pregnancy

Cardiac output, stroke volume and heart rate

Vasomotor tone [128–130], plasma volume [131] and interstitial fluid volume [130,132] vary with the menstrual cycle. In the luteal phase, peripheral blood flow and foot-swelling rate [130,132–134] are increased relative to the menstrual or follicular phase of the cycle, the latter most likely secondary to a rise in capillary permeability. It is not yet established whether cardiac output varies during an ovulatory, but non-conception, menstrual cycle. Some studies, employing older and less accurate measurement methods, were unable to discern a difference in cardiac output between the follicular and luteal phase [135–137]. In a more recent study, employing impedance cardiography, baseline cardiac output varied little and inconsistently during the menstrual cycle [138]. However, the power of these observations was probably low since measurements were performed only once during the early follicular and late luteal phase. From a teleological point of view, the amplitude of possible cyclic variations can be expected to be modest. Such minor changes are likely to remain undetected, because of the relatively large coefficient of variations inherent in the measurement techniques employed. As mentioned earlier in this chapter, measurable cardiovascular effects are only observed in response to supra-physiologic hormone levels.

Two cardiovascular studies were performed during cycles manipulated by multiple follicular stimulation using gonadotrophins [57,58]. In both studies, stroke volume and cardiac index had increased in the early follicular phase and midcycle as a result of a selective rise in stroke volume. The rise in stroke volume was a result of a 3–5% increase in left ventricular end-diastolic dimension together with a 6–15% fall in vascular resistance index. The changes in these indices are consistent with the effects seen in volume-loading experiments [139] and correlated with the rise in serum oestradiol [57]. All indices returned to baseline levels in the late luteal phase, when no pregnancy was achieved [58]. If pregnancy was established, the rise in cardiac output by 8–15%, as compared to baseline levels and achieved during the pre-ovulatory phase, is maintained throughout the luteal phase [57,58]. However, this effect is probably entirely artificial, associated with the excessive hormonal pattern in these cycles.

Several studies describe the variation in heart rate during the normal menstrual cycle. During the midluteal phase, heart rate is 3–4% higher than in the follicular phase [130,140]. The differences between morning and evening pulse rates [140–142] and those induced by mental stress [143,144] were significantly greater in the luteal phase. Since there is also a diurnal variation in heart rate, with the lowest rate during the night [145], it is difficult to evaluate in its relation to the menstrual cycle. In order to avoid most of these errors, we performed a study using the basal heart rate overnight during sleep (E. Korten, personal communication). By using this measurement technique the coefficient of variation was only 3%. Heart rate increased from a mean of 60 beats per minute during the early and late follicular phase to 66 beats per minute during the late luteal phase, a rise of 10% (Fig. 1.1). Interestingly, the most consistent rise occurred between the early and late luteal phase.

Although the gestational increase in cardiac output was first described more than 80 years

ago [146], it is only in the last decade that it has become technically feasible to determine onset and magnitude from serial measurements within individual subjects. However, there was a wide variation in the magnitude of the rise in cardiac output observed in different studies. This can probably be explained by differences in measurement techniques, by the study designs used and by the size and characteristics of the population studied. The large interindividual differences in cardiac output support the view that the pattern and magnitude of change in cardiac output requires a longitudinal study design. Another problem in this respect is the lack of pre-pregnancy reference in most studies. In all but two studies [14,147] cardiac output measurements in pregnancy were compared with those obtained postpartum. Fortunately, this problem refers to only a limited number of variables since most postpartum and pre-pregnancy values within the same subjects differ little [148,149]. The reported changes in CSA in early pregnancy are small [18]. To circumvent a possible confounding effect of such changes (see above), two longitudinal studies measured stroke and minute distance [150,151]. These parameters are linear analogues of stroke volume and cardiac output, respectively, only calculated from the velocity integral. With respect to the course in early pregnancy, the data in these studies were consistent with other longitudinal studies. In spite of all these drawbacks, it is now generally agreed that most of the increase in cardiac output occurs in the first trimester of pregnancy [36,152], probably starting in the very first weeks [14,18,147,151] (Fig. 1.2).

By 8 weeks, the cardiac output has already increased by 13% above the 5-week reference [14,18]. In mid- and late pregnancy, increases in both stroke volume and heart rate lead to a further rise in cardiac output.

After an initial period of little change, stroke volume begins to increase gradually by the 5th week, the rise being accompanied by an increasing fractional contribution of stroke volume to the concomitantly increasing cardiac output [14,18,153]. The rise in stroke volume merges to a plateau by midpregnancy [14,18,58,147]. In the 5th week, 90% of the change in cardiac output

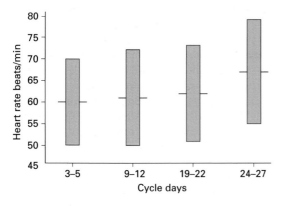

Fig. 1.1. Changes in heart rate in 10 healthy ovulatory women during spontaneous menstrual cycles (E. Korten, personal communication).

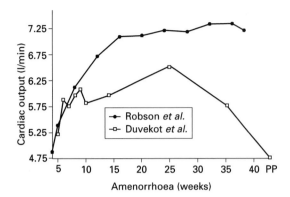

Fig. 1.2. Changes in cardiac output during pregnancy as found by Robson *et al.* [14] and Duvekot *et al.* [18]. PP: postpartum.

can be explained by heart rate variation. This could indicate that the increase in stroke volume is preceded by a period of elevated heart rate [18]. There is no direct information on the changes in heart rate pattern over the 2 weeks following implantation. Indirect information using the 3-months postpartum value as a non-pregnant reference suggests that, in this period, heart rate may already have increased by approximately 15% (from 66 to 76 beats per minute), a large rise that needs to be confirmed using pre-pregnancy reference values. Between 5 and 8 weeks, heart rate changes little, but resumes its increase afterwards, to a maximum of approximately 85 beats per minute in the 35th week [12,14,147,151,153]. The possibly biphasic rise in heart rate in early pregnancy was also noticeable, although not emphasized, in a study by Robson [14]. The consecutive rise in heart rate and stroke volume before, and after the 5th week, respectively, may be related to a very early fall in the vascular filling state, which requires a number of weeks to be balanced again.

Cardiovascular adaptation in multiple pregnancies provides an interesting area of investigation. Two cross-sectional and one longitudinal study have compared cardiovascular haemodynamics in singleton and twin pregnancies [154–156]. Three of these studies reported a 15% larger increase in cardiac output in twin pregnancy. The pattern of change in cardiac output

was similar to that in singleton pregnancy. Although data in early pregnancy are scarce, there is some evidence for a larger initial rise in heart rate in twin pregnancies than in singleton pregnancies. The concomitant increase in stroke volume did not differ from those in singleton pregnancy.

Data from animal studies indicate that where an early rise in cardiac output in pregnancy exists, this is usually driven by a rise in stroke volume, without a significant increase in heart rate [49,157]. Thus, exploration of the mechanisms that underlie the physiological changes in human pregnancy in comparison with animal models have to be made with caution.

Oxygen consumption

The haemodynamic changes in early human pregnancy are paralleled by a fall in total body oxygen extraction. Using the Cournand catheterization technique, it was shown 50 years ago that the arterial–venous oxygen content difference diminished rapidly early in pregnancy to a nadir in the first trimester, followed by a gradual return to non-pregnant levels near term [158–160]. The sharp decrease of the arterial–venous oxygen difference in the first weeks of pregnancy coincides with an increase in minute ventilation and changes in P_{CO_2} [161]. During the first 7 weeks of gestation an increase in minute ventilation by 30% was observed, which rises steadily to nearly 50% at term [153,161,162]. These respiratory changes are not accompanied by changes in respiratory frequency [162].

Progesterone has been proposed to induce the hyperventilation that develops in early pregnancy and is already present in the luteal phase of the menstrual cycle by resetting of the superficial medullary chemoreceptors [163,164]. It is still to be assessed whether the overall more negative pressure in the thorax associated with these early respiratory adaptations and the increase in stroke volume in this period of pregnancy are causally related.

The early-pregnancy rise in systemic blood flow while oxygen consumption remains essentially unchanged, has been attributed to the uterine circulation acting as an arteriovenous shunt [165]. Abrupt closure of the uterine circulation in pregnant rabbits led to haemodynamic changes comparable to those observed after closure of an arteriovenous shunt [166]. Until 20 weeks' amenorrhoea, however, the fractional distribution of cardiac output to the uterus is less than 5%, and it is thus unlikely to act as a potentially important arteriovenous shunt [167].

Blood pressure

Data reported on blood pressure changes during the menstrual cycle are conflicting. In most studies, systolic blood pressure is reported to be slightly higher during the luteal phase than in the follicular phase [142,144,168,169]. Systolic blood pressure increases during the late luteal phase and reaches its peak at the onset of menstruation [130,140,142,170]. Systolic blood pressure decreases rapidly thereafter to its lowest level [140,142,170]. Diastolic blood pressure is 5% lower during the luteal than during the follicular phase [143,169,170]. It follows that pulse pressure is highest during the luteal phase [134,140]. Towards the menstrual period the diastolic blood pressure rises together with the systolic blood pressure [140]. Consequently, mean arterial pressure is unaffected or slightly lower during the midluteal phase.

During pregnancy, the largest change in blood pressure occurs before the 8th week [14,18], when 80–90% of the total pregnancy-related decrease in mean arterial pressure ($\approx$10 mmHg) is accomplished [14,18,153,171,172]. After the 8th week, mean arterial blood pressure continues to decrease to reach its lowest level by approximately the 24th week of pregnancy [14,171,173,174]. The pregnancy-related decrease in mean arterial pressure is almost entirely due to a fall in diastolic blood pressure initiated in the luteal phase of the conception cycle. These data suggest that the so-called midpregnancy drop has already developed in the first few weeks after implantation. It is also probably relevant that subjective complaints which could be related to hypotension, such as fatigue, headache and dizziness, were seen twice as frequently in early pregnancy as during late pregnancy [175].

Blood pressure measurements may be influenced by many external factors [176]. For this reason, recommendations have been made by the American Heart Association to obtain reliable and reproducible blood pressure measurements [177]. In pregnancy, special precautions have to be taken with respect to the posture of the subject and the choice of the Korotkoff sound to measure diastolic blood pressure [176]. Blood pressures measured from the brachial artery are highest in the upright and sitting positions, intermediate in the supine position and lowest when the patient is lying on one side [178–180]. For practical reasons, most studies measure blood pressure in the sitting position, with the cuff at the level of the heart.

It is still unclear whether the diastolic blood pressure is best represented by the value obtained at the phase of muffling of Korotkoff sounds (phase IV) or at their final disappearance (phase V) [181]. The problem is magnified in pregnancy since the difference between phases IV and V is increased in that state. This is probably associated with the hyperdynamic state of the circulation [176]. Studies in which intra-arterial measurements are compared with those obtained by a sphygmomanometer show conflicting results in pregnancy [180,181]. The large measurement error associated with the use of phase IV is undoubtedly an important disadvantage of the latter approach [181]. To overcome this problem, the recent consensus report by the Working Group on High Blood Pressure in Pregnancy advocated the recording of both Korotkoff phases IV and V, to help ensure that no information is lost and that the development of a rise in blood pressure during pregnancy will be noticed. A recent, carefully validated comparative study supports the view that measurement of Korotkoff sound V may be the most reliable in pregnancy [182].

Blood volume

There is indirect evidence for fluctuations in sodium homeostasis and probably with it, blood volume with the menstrual cycle. This is suggested by the reported cycle-dependent changes in the natriuretic and antinatriuretic hormones [74,183,184], renal function [101] and

14 haematocrit [143]. Only two studies so far have measured plasma volume directly during the menstrual cycle [131,185]. In the later study, the daily hematocrit measurement was combined with two plasma volume measurements during the menstrual cycle. In this study, plasma volume was highest in the periovulatory phase and prior to the onset of menstruation, and lowest during menstruation and midluteal. The amplitude of these cyclical changes amounts to 15%. Serial measurements of haematocrit [143] and of α-atrial natriuretic peptide [183,184] support this cyclical pattern in blood volume. The cyclic changes in hematocrit are not accompanied by changes in erythropoietin [186].

Plasma volume and red-cell mass increase at different rates in the course of human pregnancy. The data on the magnitude of the rise in blood and plasma volume during pregnancy reported in the period before 1972 varied widely [187]. Careful analysis of these data suggested that a large proportion of this variation was related to cross-sectional study designs, to differences in methodology and to heterogeneity of the study populations. By correcting as much as possible for these confounding factors, Chesley calculated an average increase in plasma volume by 42% and an average increase in total red-cell mass by 24% [187]. During the first 30 weeks of pregnancy, plasma volume increases gradually by approximately 1250 ml and is maintained at this level until term [188,189]. By direct measurement using Evans' blue dye, the gestational rise in plasma volume becomes detectable between 7 and 12 weeks [189], an observation already reported 25 years ago [190]. Both by this direct method and by indirect estimations from the decrease in haematocrit, the magnitude of this early plasma volume rise amounts to approximately 10% [153,189]. The magnitude of this increase would then be comparable to the fluctuations during the normal menstrual cycle [131]. It follows that most of the pregnancy-related increase in blood volume is accomplished after the first trimester. The phenomenon of the gestational increase in blood volume apparently occurring almost *after* completion of the changes in cardiovascular haemodynamics, has also been found in the baboon [157]. Figures 1.3 and 1.4 illustrate that blood

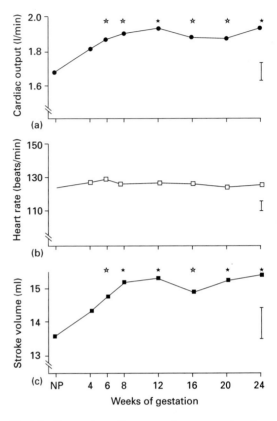

Fig. 1.3. Changes in cardiac output, heart rate and stroke volume during pregnancy in the baboon. The mean values ($n = 8$) at each gestation are shown, with non-pregnancy mean values on the left. Significant differences to the non-pregnant mean are indicated by symbols ($\star P < 0.05$, $\bigstar P < 0.01$). Standard error derived from the pooled variance for all 64 measurements of each parameter is indicated by the bar on the right [157]. NP: non-pregnant.

volume in this primate only begins to increase by the 8th week, when cardiac output has already increased to its maximum at the 6th week.

The gestational increase in total red-cell mass found in various studies ranges from 17% to 40%, with a mean of 24% [187,191]. Iron supplementation may influence this increase in red-cell mass. Cross-sectional studies in the second and third trimester of human pregnancy suggest that red-cell mass increases in concert with plasma volume [190]. Some studies report an initial decrease in red-cell volume during the first weeks or months of pregnancy [192–194].

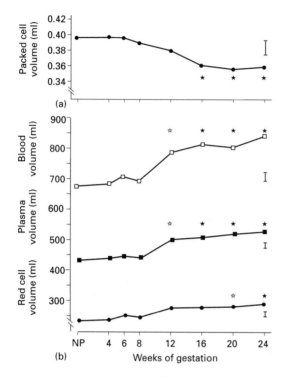

(a)

(b)

Weeks of gestation

Fig. 1.4. Gestational changes in blood volumes in the baboon. Significant differences to the non-pregnant mean are indicated by symbols (☆$P < 0.05$, ★$P < 0.01$) [157]. NP: non-pregnant.

The physiological haemodilution and associated relative anaemia in the first trimester of pregnancy is likely to provide the stimulus for an accelerated red-cell production. Elevated erythropoietin levels in pregnancy tend to support this concept [186,195–197], although erythropoietin levels and reticulocyte counts [198] had only increased by the 10th to 12th week of gestation. It is not likely that this increase in erythropoietin is triggered by hypoxemia or anaemia, the normal circumstances inducing endogenous erythropoietin production. The correlation with human placental lactogen suggests a regulating role of the latter [186]. During late pregnancy the lower life span of erythrocytes [199] and the increase in human placental lactogen may be responsible for the higher erythropoietin levels [200]. Increased erythropoiesis may be responsible for this lower erythrocyte life span, hereby counteracting its own effect [199].

Theoretically, the physiological decline in arterial–venous oxygen difference and the higher renal blood flow [201] in early pregnancy may interfere with erythropoiesis in this period. A reduced red-cell production may be paralleled by a higher rate of mechanical red-cell loss in the hyperdynamic circulation of pregnancy, both phenomena contributing to a decrease in red-cell mass by the end of the first trimester. The pattern of change in haematocrit during pregnancy is characterized by a gradual fall until the 30th week, followed by a gradual rise afterwards [202,203]. Obviously, this pattern is the resultant of the concomitant changes in plasma and red-cell volume. Since red-cell volume does not change or even decreases in early pregnancy, the physiological haemodilution may therefore be used as an indirect indicator for the increase in plasma volume and thus whole blood volume in this period of pregnancy [153].

Peripheral blood flow

Skin flow in women has been reported to be as much as 50% lower than in men only during the reproductive period [204–206]. This gender difference in the perfusion of a non-reproductive tissue is thought to result from a higher basal sympathetic tone in these women, and supports the concept that sex hormones are also involved in the regulation of the perfusion of non-reproductive tissues.

Arterial vascular tone can be assessed by such indirect methods as laser Doppler flux [207]. So far, there is only little information on vascular tone measured with this method during the menstrual cycle. Peripheral finger skin circulation and forearm blood flow were observed to vary with the menstrual cycle [129,134]. During the pre-ovulatory and midluteal phase, forearm blood flow was 30% higher than during the menstrual phase. Some investigators did not find differences during the cycle but by chance their measurements were only performed during the periods of maximal flow, the pre-ovulatory and midluteal phase [208]. No clear correlations were found with the plasma concentrations of oestrogen and/or progesterone [134]. The same is true for the blood supply to the 'target' organs, the ovarian and uterine arteries [209], although

16 clinical observations show a decrease in resistance from the early follicular phase towards ovulation followed by an increase during the luteal phase [209–212].

Arterial vascular tone during pregnancy has been studied frequently recently. Most important in this respect is that cardiac output is redistributed on the basis of different changes in vascular resistance in the various organs. Experimental data on how fractional distribution of cardiac output changes in the first weeks of pregnancy are only fragmentary. The early increase in both cardiac output fraction and blood flow to the kidneys is well documented [213]. The flow increase to other organs, with exception of the skin, follows a much slower increase [214]. Surprisingly, also, the uterine blood flow does not increase appreciably during the first trimester [167]. Blood flow to the extremities even follows a different course during pregnancy [215]. Forearm blood flow does not increase above levels found during the normal menstrual cycle before the third trimester [65,215].

In early pregnancy, skin flow increases while oxygen extraction decreases and oxygen consumption remains essentially unchanged. This combination of changes supports the view that a large fraction of the extra cardiac output is directed towards arteriovenous shunts. At present, the physiological meaning of the accelerated systemic shunting in early pregnancy is obscure. It is possible that the early-pregnancy fall in peripheral vascular resistance is primarily caused by an improved compliance of the arterial tree, a concept supported by the lack of concomitant increase in peripheral oxygen demands and, with it, nutritional flow demands. Improved arterial compliance reduces the resistance to flow encountered by the contracting heart during systole. This enables the ejection of a larger stroke volume and thus a higher cardiac output. The resulting systemic hyperperfusion is counterbalanced by increased arteriovenous shunting so as to protect the microcirculation.

The resting tone of the venous bed is low and its magnitude and importance are unknown [216]. In most studies evaluating the changes during the menstrual cycle, peripheral venous distensibility is greatest during the midluteal phase [65,128,129,132]. Venous distensibility follows closely the progesterone levels in these experiments [128].

Clinically, it is obvious that pregnancy affects venous tone, considering the increased incidence of varicose veins, venous thrombosis and thromboembolism [217–219]. The pattern of venous distensibility during pregnancy has been described using graded venous plethysmography. After the first trimester, venous distensibility increases progressively to levels two to three times those in the non-pregnant state [65,217,220]. The exact pattern in venous tone in early pregnancy has not been elucidated. Since the rise in blood volume during early pregnancy is relatively small, it is unlikely that the generalized vasodilation in this period includes an important fall in venous tone [18].

Functional and structural changes in the heart

To our knowledge, there is little information on structural and functional changes in the heart during the menstrual cycle. During the late follicular phase of stimulated cycles, left ventricular end-diastolic dimension (LVEDD) measured by M-mode echocardiography increases as a function of peripheral oestrogen levels [57,58]. In the course of pregnancy, there is general agreement that the ventricular dimensions change. LVEDD, as measured by M-mode echocardiography, increases between the 10th [14,147] and 20th week of amenorrhoea [12,18,29,221], to a plateau which is approximately 5% higher than in the non-pregnant state. A higher LVEDD is associated with a rise in preload [139,222,223]. Therefore, it is not surprising that the pattern of the increase in LVEDD closely follows that in whole blood volume [188,189].

Left ventricular end-systolic dimension (LVESD) may have decreased to just below the non-pregnant value in the first trimester [12,14,18,29,224,225] to stay at that level until late pregnancy [18,29,221]. In the last weeks of pregnancy, LVESD may increase again slightly to return to the pre-pregnant value [12,14, 224–226]. The observed fall in LVESD in early pregnancy may be secondary to the early-pregnancy rise in heart rate and myocardial contractility.

Changes in atrial diameter could provide an

indirect estimate for changes in blood volume that may occur during the menstrual cycle [139]. However, there seem to be no data on serial measurements of left atrial diameter during the menstrual cycle. Therefore, it remains uncertain whether the reported cyclic changes in α-atrial natriuretic peptide [183,184] which is released in response to atrial wall stretch or pressure [227] will be paralleled by measurable fluctuations in the atrial diameter.

Nearly all data on changes in the atrial dimensions during pregnancy have been based on ultrasonic measurements of the left atrium. The left atrial dimension measurements by ultrasound have been validated using cineangiocardiograms as the gold standard [228]. In early pregnancy, left atrial diameter begins to increase gradually by a total of 15%, which is reached by the 30th week [12,14,15,18]. The gradual increase in left atrial diameter is parallelled by the rise in blood volume during pregnancy [188,189,229]. The diameter of the left atrium has been demonstrated to correlate better with vascular filling state than the LVEDD [139,230–32]. Interestingly, the increase in left atrial diameter does not begin before the 6th week of gestation [14,18] and is possibly preceded by a brief period during which the diameter is even smaller relative to the non-pregnant state [12,18]. The substantially reduced levels of α-atrial natriuretic peptide in this period agree with this observation [18].

Mean circulatory filling pressure, compliance and vascular capacity

The increase in left atrial diameter during the first weeks of pregnancy suggests an early rise in both preload and circulating blood volume [139]. Indirect information on the relative changes in blood and circulatory volumes can also be derived from the mean circulatory filling pressure. Mean circulatory filling pressure is defined as the pressure measured in the circulatory system when the heart is suddenly stopped and the blood rapidly distributed between the arterial and venous beds so that the pressure equalizes throughout the cardiovascular system [233]. The fraction of the blood volume which is responsible for this filling pressure is called

stressed volume. If this stressed volume falls to zero, for example as a result of bleeding, mean circulatory filling pressure also falls to zero. The residual blood volume in the vasculature is then called the unstressed volume. The vascular capacity of the body at a given moment is the sum of the unstressed volume plus the product of the mean circulatory filling pressure and overall vascular compliance [234]. Mean circulatory filling pressure minus right atrial pressure represents the pressure gradient for venous return [235]. Any disproportionate change in blood and vessel volumes can be expected to alter mean circulatory filling pressure.

Right atrial pressure and central venous pressure are unchanged during pregnancy [39,160] while cardiac output and thus also venous return have increased. It follows that mean circulatory filling pressure can be expected to have increased during human pregnancy. Whether vascular compliance increases also in human pregnancy, is still unsettled. So far, only one study reported a threefold increase in aortic compliance during the first trimester [236]. It is likely that, if compliance increases, it will also do so during early pregnancy. In a study that examined the basic mechanical properties of resistance blood vessels in the rat, vascular wall compliance was highest in early pregnancy and diminished with advancing pregnancy, but even at term was higher than in the non-pregnant animals [237]. The results of studies using sympathetic blockade in pregnant rabbits and guinea pigs indicate that this improvement in vascular compliance was not secondary to a lower sympathetic tone [238,239].

Changes in the vascular capacity provide useful information on changes in the pressure-volume characteristics of the vascular bed in pregnancy. The increase in vascular capacity during pregnancy is caused by growth of the vascular (uterine) bed and the increase in vascular compliance. The rise in compliance during rabbit pregnancy enables the accommodation of approximately 60% of the increase in blood volume without raising the mean circulatory filling pressure [239]. The growth of the vascular bed is not sufficient to accommodate the remainder of the extra blood volume resulting in the rise in mean circulatory filling pressure.

Since in early pregnancy the vascular bed is not enlarged the increase in compliance may be sufficient for the accommodation of the blood volume increase in this phase of pregnancy. It is therefore possible that mean circulatory filling pressure only increases in the second half of pregnancy. It is interesting to speculate on the advantages of an increased compliance and capacitance in pregnancy. An increase in unstressed volume would provide a reserve in blood volume that is not haemodynamically active, while increased compliance may serve to buffer blood pressure changes in response to rapid volume changes [238].

Inferior vena cava diameter

The ultrasonic dimensions of the inferior vena cava have been proposed as possible indirect estimates of vascular filling state [240,241]. Although the measurement of the inferior vena cava depends on a healthy right-sided heart function [242,243], its use in early pregnancy seems promising, especially if one wishes to explore the early changes in maternal vascular filling state. In late pregnancy, aortocaval compression by the pregnant uterus is likely to lower its potential value as an indirect estimate for vascular filling state [244,245].

There is no information on the inferior vena cava dimension during the menstrual cycle. In only one study has the diameter of the inferior vena cava been measured longitudinally throughout pregnancy [18] and in that study no appreciable difference was found between the early-pregnancy and postpartum value. By the end of the first trimester the caval diameter decreased. These changes are consistent with a lower filling state of the vascular bed in late pregnancy.

Cardiac contractility

It is difficult to determine whether cardiac contractility increases during pregnancy, as the latter is strongly influenced by changes in heart rate, preload and afterload [221]. As a parameter for myometrial contractility, the mean velocity of circumferential fibre shortening (mean Vcf) has been introduced. Mean Vcf increases in early pregnancy, in concert with the rise in heart rate [14,29]. This increase is more pronounced than might be expected from the concomitant rise in heart rate alone [14,29]. Mean Vcf is strongly influenced by changes in afterload. The interdependence between the adaptation in vascular filling state and that in circulatory function in early pregnancy was explored by assessing in consecutive weeks the covariation between heart rate, stroke volume, and cardiac output changes, on the one hand, and those in various other cardiovascular variables, on the other [18].

As shown in Table 1.1, the changes in cardiac contractility do not correlate positively with the

Table 1.1. Results of multiple linear regression analysis of the relationship between the weekly changes during early pregnancy in cardiac output, stroke volume, and heart rate as dependent variables and the potentially related and concomitantly determined haemodynamic variables left atrial diameter, left ventricular mass, velocity of circumferential fibre shortening, and MAP.

Week of pregnancy	Change in cardiac output	Change in stroke volume	Change in heart rate
5–6	—	—	—
6–7	—	–1.6 change in left atrial diameter (0.4)	—
7–8	+0.2 change in left atrial diameter (0.1)	+1.6 change in left atrial diameter (0.5)	—
8–9	+0.16 change in left atrial diameter (0.04)	+1.1 change in left atrial diameter (0.4)	—
9–10	+0.16 change in left atrial diameter (0.06)	+23 change in velocity of circumferential fibre shortening (8) –0.5 change in MAP (0.2)	—

Only regression coefficients that have P values < 0.05 are quoted. Standard errors for the slope are given in parentheses.

changes in stroke volume until the 9th to 10th week of gestation. Studying systolic time intervals, the estimated period of ventricular contraction before the aortic valves open, may also be used to assess contractility during pregnancy. Reduced systolic time intervals have been reported in early, mid- or late pregnancy [246–248]. Discrepancies in the results of these studies can be explained from the rather wide time-interval (several weeks) during which the measurements were obtained.

Systemic vascular resistance

Systemic vascular resistance is represented by the ratio of mean arterial pressure and cardiac output. Its pattern in pregnancy resembles that of blood pressure with the exception that there is a faster decrease in early pregnancy than observed in the blood pressure, which results from the rapid rise in cardiac output occurring at this time. By the 5th week of pregnancy, systemic vascular resistance has decreased relative to the non-pregnant state [14,18,147]. This suggests that a fall in the systemic vascular resistance may be one of the earliest maternal adjustments to pregnancy. After the 5th week the systemic vascular resistance continues to decrease gradually to its nadir in midpregnancy which is followed by a gradual rise afterwards. Since cardiac output remains elevated until term, systemic vascular resistance is also

decreased until term [14,152,160,249,250] (Fig. 1.5). The mechanism for the fall in systemic vascular resistance, so very early in pregnancy, is still poorly understood.

Pulmonary circulation and pulmonary arterial pressure

Data on the early-pregnancy adaptation of the pulmonary circulation are limited. Using a Cournand right heart catheter, mean pulmonary arterial pressure changed little in a longitudinal study during pregnancy [160]. Similar findings came from a longitudinal study in pregnancy on pulmonary pressure and flow measured by the non-invasive method of Doppler echocardiography [251]. In that study, mean pulmonary artery pressure was calculated from pulsed Doppler velocity trace. These observations have been confirmed recently for the third trimester by Swan–Ganz pulmonary artery catheter monitoring [1,40]. The apparently consistent observation of unchanged pulmonary artery pressure in pregnancy implies a large decrease in pulmonary vascular resistance which mirrors the gestational pattern in cardiac output. Cardiac output may increase by four to six times before pulmonary arterial pressure becomes elevated. The necessary reduction in pulmonary resistance is achieved by pulmonary arteriolar vasodilation, capillary recruitment and possibly also by enhanced arteriovenous shunting [252]. The latter is suggested by the concomitant decrease in arteriovenous oxygen difference in pregnancy.

Early haemodynamic changes during pathological pregnancies

Manifest symptomatology in pregnancies complicated by pre-eclampsia and/or intra-uterine growth retardation (IUGR) is preceded by a long subclinical period. The onset for these disorders is thought to lie much earlier in pregnancy than its clinical presentation. The spiral arteries of the uterus are converted into uteroplacental arteries in early pregnancy. These are physiological changes [253]. This vascular phenomenon is thought to evolve in two stages: first, the conversion of the decidual segments of the spiral arteries by a wave of endovascular trophoblast

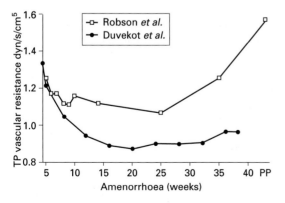

Fig. 1.5. Changes in total peripheral (TP) vascular resistance during pregnancy as found by Robson *et al.* [14] and Duvekot *et al.* [18]. PP: postpartum.

migration in the first 3 weeks after implantation and, after a period of no demonstrable change, a second wave, involving the myometrial segments of the spiral arteries between the 14th and 18th weeks [254]. In complicated pregnancies, the second wave of the endovascular trophoblast invasion shows a defective development [253,254]. Nevertheless, these changes in the spiral arteries of the placental bed are not pathognomonic for pre-eclampsia or IUGR, since they are not present in all cases [255].

Since these histopathological abnormalities have been detected in the beginning of the second trimester, it seems worthwhile to investigate whether this disturbance is preceded by abnormal maternal haemodynamic adaptation in the earlier stages of pregnancy. Results from such studies could be used for two purposes: early detection of abnormalities and, if possible, causal treatment of pregnancy disorders.

Studies of the latent phase of pre-eclampsia and/or IUGR are scarce, and most of these reports are limited to the description of the pattern of change in blood pressure. A rise in blood pressure or an elevated mean arterial pressure in the second trimester have been identified as early signs of impending pre-eclampsia [171,174]. However, the screening value of first and midtrimester blood pressure measurement is limited by its low predictive value. Recently, this method has been assessed to be a predictor of at most transient hypertension, rather than pre-eclampsia [256]. However, blood pressure shows distinct differences in pre-eclamptic pregnancies. In a longitudinal study by Easterling, a group of initially healthy nulliparous women were followed from the 10th week of gestation to the 6th week postpartum [250]. Nine women eventually became pre-eclamptic. These women had a consistently higher mean arterial pressure throughout their entire pregnancy as compared to 89 subjects with uncomplicated pregnancies. This observation was consistent with that in other longitudinal studies on blood pressure in pre-eclamptic subjects [171,172,257]. Postpartum, the difference in mean arterial pressure between the two groups disappears rapidly. Unfortunately, in this study the demographic characteristics of the subjects differed between the two groups with respect to weight. The pre-eclamptic subjects were heavier and therefore had a larger body surface area. Another shortcoming in this study was the large number of missing data, especially in the first and second trimesters.

The other haemodynamic parameters measured in this study [250] show remarkable differences in the subclinical period prior to manifest pre-eclampsia. Cardiac output and cardiac index, which compensated for the demographic differences between the two groups, were consistently higher in the pre-eclamptic group, as a result of an elevated heart rate. This finding contrasts with another study, which reported a decreased heart rate in pre-eclamptic patients during the third trimester [225]. However, the power of the latter observation was low, since in the study the heart rate from all the measurements made during the third trimester prior to analysis was averaged, the gestation at the time of study was much later and the disease process more advanced. The persistent tachycardia in Easterling's pre-eclamptic patients can be explained as the direct effect of a chronically raised sympathetic tone and the indirect effect of a relative vascular underfill. Neither stroke volume nor total peripheral resistance differed between the two groups, not even during the period of clinical disease. Six weeks postpartum, cardiac output was still higher and total peripheral resistance lower in the pre-eclamptic group [250]. The findings in Easterling's study are in agreement with the so-called hyperdynamic disease model [258]. According to this model, endothelial injury, giving rise to the clinical manifestations of pre-eclampsia, is the result of accelerated flow in the entire cardiovascular system.

The concomitantly disturbed volume homeostasis in pregnancies complicated by fetal growth retardation [202,259–262] is likely to have an impact on the maternal cardiovascular status. Only one study so far reported maternal haemodynamics in the latent phase of fetal growth retardation [225,263]. In this study the early-pregnancy patterns of changes in a number of relevant haemodynamic variables were compared between normal pregnancies and pregnancies complicated by fetal growth retardation.

Despite the limited group sizes, it was possible to discern differences between the two groups by measuring a large number of independent variables with some indirect relationship with volume homeostasis. Between the 5th and 8th weeks of pregnancy, the IUGR group differed from the normal group by a failure of the cardiac output and left atrial diameter to increase. Furthermore, left atrial diameter was consistently smaller in the IUGR group in early pregnancy, while the demographic variables of both groups were matched (Fig. 1.6).

These observations provide evidence of a defective maternal haemodynamic adaptation in the first weeks of these complicated pregnancies. This initial vascular underperfusion does not seem to trigger a proper compensatory volume response in these abnormal pregnancies. It can be concluded from this study that the physiological volume increment may already be disturbed from the beginning of pregnancy, long before the clinical manifestations. This is in contrast with the assumptions in pre-eclamptic pregnancies where there is strong evidence that plasma volume contracts after an initially normal increase during the first and second trimesters [264,265].

The initiation of cardiovascular changes in pregnancy

The mechanisms responsible for the circulatory changes in human pregnancy have been subject to research and discussion since the first study on this subject was reported in 1915 [146]. Because of the recent increase in methodological possibilities, it has become feasible to explore non-invasively haemodynamic adaption in human pregnancy. However, these techniques do not provide information about the in-vivo events at the trophoblast–decidual interface, the site where the very first local modulations at the cellular level are likely to initiate a cascade of changes that eventually culminate in the systemic cardiovascular changes primarily described in this chapter. Over the years, the following hypotheses have been postulated to explain the establishment of a high flow, low resistance circulation in pregnancy.

1 A rise in metabolic demands during pregnancy, especially by the uterus and chorioplacental bed, raises cardiac output and decreases peripheral vascular resistance. This concept seems highly unlikely, as oxygen uptake does not increase in concert with haemodynamics [266].

2 A primary hypervolaemia in early pregnancy is responsible for the accelerated cardiovascular function. The observation that the early increase in cardiac output and stroke volume precedes the blood volume expansion is incompatible with this idea.

3 The uteroplacental circulation acts as an arteriovenous shunt, thus accelerating the circulation [160,165,267]. The modest size of the intervillous perfusion in early pregnancy [167], at the time of the cardiac output increase, contradicts this mechanism. Moreover, recent

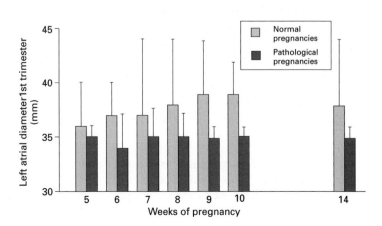

Fig. 1.6. Left atrial diameter during first trimester in 10 normal and 4 pathological pregnancies. Error bars = upper range (Duvekot *et al.* [225]).

evidence suggests that blood flow through the intervillous space does not commence until 12 weeks' gestation [268].

Experimental data recently obtained in early human and baboon pregnancy provide some evidence for the following alternative hypothesis. The first systemic haemodynamic change consists of a non-specific generalized vascular relaxation which causes the vascular filling state to fall [14,18,157,269]. The vasorelaxation and probable improved vascular compliance is an effect of smooth muscle relaxation which implies a larger impact on arteries than on veins. The following two interrelated cascades are initiated:

1 The concomitant arterial underfill triggers the nonosmotic release of antidiuretic hormone and thus water retention, haemodilution and a fall in viscosity.

2 The simultaneous fall in cardiac afterload gives rise to a fall in blood pressure and, therefore, an increase in heart rate by baroreceptor activation [14,18]. It also enables the ejection of a larger stroke volume during systole.

Either pathway results in an accelerated circulation which in turn can be expected to activate volume retention as evidenced by elevated peripheral renin levels [14,18]. In the course of early pregnancy, the accelerated volume retention will raise preload and, with it, stroke volume [14]. The predominant effect of vasorelaxation on the arteriolar tree may explain, on the one hand, the lower blood pressure which induces baroreceptor resetting [100] and, on the other hand, the higher renal blood flow in pregnancy. After restoring the balance in vascular filling by the 8th week of pregnancy [18], the initial vasodilatation is maintained throughout pregnancy. Although the latter hypothesis can explain most of the early-pregnancy changes, the understanding of the exact role of the venous compartment in these changes is still obscure. A rise in venous compliance has only been described as developing in advanced pregnancy [220,270].

Several assumptions have been put forward about the nature of this potent, pregnancy-related vasodilator. This substance should act both systemically and rapidly. Some prostaglandins are potent vasodilators, but it is unlikely that they are directly responsible for this early-pregnancy vasodilation, since cyclooxygenase inhibitors administered to healthy pregnant women had no effect on blood pressure and decreased stroke volume only slightly [126]. Moreover, the circulating levels of prostaglandins are probably too low to cause haemodynamic effects [271]. It is also unlikely that the pregnancy-related hormones oestrogen, progesterone, prolactin, hCG and hPL, alone or in combination, play a direct role in the initial vasorelaxation. In animal studies it was not possible to reproduce a systemic fall in vascular tone resembling that of early pregnancy, with one or any combination of these hormones [272]. A more promising mediator for the vascular effect is an endothelially derived relaxing factor, such as nitric oxide [114,115]. Among other factors its release is stimulated by macrophage cytokines that are present in the uterine environment shortly after implantation as important modulators of the immunoregulatory response [108,273,274]. However, in-vitro experiments on human resistance vessels obtained from pregnant women failed to demonstrate acetylcholine-induced endothelium-dependent relaxation [275]. Acetylcholine-mediated relaxation is predominantly induced by nitric oxide production. However, in this in-vitro study the important flow- and shear stress-mediated release of nitric oxide was excluded. The study of possible links between the processes evolving at the fetal–maternal interface and the enhanced release of factors that stimulate endothelially derived relaxing factors forms the next step in the unravelling of the presumed generalized vasodilatation in early pregnancy.

Conclusions

An important part of the maternal cardiovascular adaptation to pregnancy is accomplished in early pregnancy. Most of the increase in cardiac output is reached before the 8th week of pregnancy, probably by a rise in heart rate before the 5th week, and after this predominantly by an increase in stroke volume. Since most of the pregnancy-dependent fall in blood pressure takes place in the first weeks of pregnancy, the decrease in peripheral vascular resistance represents one of the earliest haemodynamic adaptations to pregnancy. Myocardial contractility does not increase appreciably before the second half of the first trimester, which makes this adaptive change probably a secondary effect. The same may apply to preload and with it blood volume, indirectly represented by the left atrial diameter. Its gradual increase during early pregnancy is likely to reflect the rebalancing of the vascular filling state in response to accelerated volume retention.

References

1 Wallenburg H.C.S. (1988) Hemodynamics in hypertensive pregnancy. In *Hypertension in Pregnancy*. Ed. P.C. Rubin, p. 66. Elsevier Science Publishers, Amsterdam.

2 Belfort M., Uys P., Dommisse J. & Davey D.A. (1989) Haemodynamic changes in proteinuric hypertension: the effects of rapid volume expansion and vasodilator therapy. *British Journal of Obstetrics and Gynaecology* **96**, 643.

3 Colocousis J.S., Huntsman L.L. & Curreri P.W. (1977) Estimation of stroke volume changes by ultrasonic Doppler. *Circulation* **56**, 914.

4 Huntsman L.L., Stewart D.K., Barnes S.R., Franklin S.B., Colocousis J.S. & Hessel E.A. (1983) Noninvasive Doppler determination of cardiac output in man: Clinical validation. *Circulation* **67**, 593.

5 Loeppky J.A., Hoekenga D.E., Greene E.R. & Luft U.C. (1984) Comparison of noninvasive Doppler and Fick measurements of stroke volume in cardiac patients. *American Heart Journal* **107**, 339.

6 Schuster A.H. & Nanda N.C. (1984) Doppler echocardiographic measurement of cardiac output: Comparison with a non-golden standard. *Circulation* **53**, 257.

7 Ihlen H., Amlie J.P., Dale J., Forfang K., Nitter-Hauge S., Otterstad J.E., Simonsen S. & Myhre E. (1984) Determination of cardiac output by Doppler echocardiography. *British Heart Journal* **51**, 54.

8 Gardin J.M., Tobis J.M., Dabestani A., Smith C., Elkayam U., Castleman E., White D., Allfie A. & Henry W.L. (1985) Superiority of 2-D measurement of aortic vessel diameter in Doppler echocardiographic estimates of left ventricular stroke volume. *Journal of the American College of Cardiology* **6**, 66.

9 Bouchard A., Blumlein S., Schiller N.B., Schlitt S., Byrd B.F., Ports T. & Chatterjee K. (1987) Measurement of left ventricular stroke volume using continuous wave Doppler echocardiography of the ascending aorta and M-mode echocardiography of the aortic valve. *Journal of the American College of Cardiology* **9**, 75.

10 Stewart W.J., Jiang L., Mich R., Pandian S., Guerrero J.L. & Weyman A.E. (1985) Variable effects of changes in flow rate through the aortic, pulmonary and mitral valves on valve area and flow velocity: Impact on quantitative Doppler flow calculations. *Journal of the American College of Cardiology* **6**, 653.

11 Beldekas J.C., Smith B., Gerstenfeld L.C., Sonenshein G.E. & Franzblau C. (1981) Effects of 17β-estradiol on the biosynthesis of collagen in cultured bovine aortic smooth muscle cells. *Biochemistry* **20**, 2162.

12 Katz R., Karliner J.S. & Resink R. (1978) Effects of a natural volume overload state (pregnancy) on left ventricular performance in normal human subjects. *Circulation* **58**, 434.

13 Hart M.V., Morton M.J., Hosenpud J.D. & Metcalfe J. (1986) Aortic function during normal human pregnancy. *American Journal of Obstetrics and Gynecology* **154**, 887.

14 Robson S.C., Hunter S., Boys R.J. & Dunlop W. (1989) Serial study of factors influencing changes in cardiac output during human pregnancy. *American Journal of Physiology* **256**, H1060.

15 Vered Z., Poler S.M., Gibson P., Wlody D. & Perez J.E. (1991) Noninvasive detection of the morphologic and hemodynamic changes during normal pregnancy. *Clinics in Cardiology* **14**, 327.

16 Caton D. & Banner T.E. (1987) Doppler estimates of cardiac output during pregnancy. *Bulletin of the New York Academy of Medicine (New York)* **63**, 727.

17 Sadaniantz A., Kocheril A.G., Emaus S.P., Garber C.E. & Parisi A.F. (1992) Cardiovascular changes in pregnancy evaluated by two-dimensional and Doppler echocardiography. *Journal of the American Society of Echocardiography* **5**, 253.

18 Duvekot J.J., Cheriex E.C., Pieters F.A.A., Menheere P.P.C.A. & Peeters L.L.H. (1993) Early-pregnancy changes in hemodynamics and volume homeostasis are consecutive adjustments triggered by a primary fall in systemic vascular tone. *American Journal of Obstetrics and Gynecology* **169**, 1382.

19 Mabie W.C., DiSessa T.G., Crocker L.G., Sibai B.H. & Arheart K.L. (1994) A longitudinal study of cardiac output in normal human pregnancy. *American Journal of Obstetrics and Gynecology* **170**, 849.

20 Robson S.C., Dunlop W., Moore M. & Hunter S. (1987) Combined Doppler and echocardiographic measurement of cardiac output: Theory and application in pregnancy. *British Journal of Obstetrics and Gynaecology* **94**, 1014.

21 Lewis J.F., Kuo L.C., Nelson J.G., Limacher M.C. & Quinones M.A. (1984) Pulsed Doppler echocardiographic determination of stroke volume and cardiac output: clinical validation of two new methods using the apical window. *Circulation* **70**, 425.

22 Easterling T.R., Watts H., Schmucker B.C. & Benedetti T.J. (1987) Measurement of cardiac output during pregnancy: Validation of Doppler technique and clinical observations in preeclampsia. *Obstetrics and Gynecology* **69**, 845.

23 Lee W., Rokey R. & Cotton D.B. (1988) Noninvasive maternal stroke volume and cardiac output determinations by pulsed Doppler echocardiography. *American Journal of Obstetrics and Gynecology* **158**, 505.

24 Easterling T.R., Carlson K.L., Schmucker B.C.,

24

Brateng D.A. & Benedetti T.J. (1990) Measurement of cardiac output in pregnancy by Doppler technique. *American Journal of Perinatology* 7, 220.

25 Kronik G., Slany J. & Mosslacker H. (1979) Comparative value of eight M-mode echocardiographic formulas for determinating left ventricular stroke volume. *Circulation* 60, 1308.

26 Kupari M. (1984) Reproducibility of M-mode echocardiographic assessment of left ventricular function: Significance of the temporal range of measurements. *European Heart Journal* 5, 412.

27 Pombo J.F., Troy B.L. & Russel Jr R.O. (1971) Left ventricular volumes and ejection fraction by echocardiography. *Circulation* 43, 480.

28 Vered Z., Barzilai B. & Perez J.E. (1988) Is M-mode echocardiography still important? *Echocardiography* 5, 229.

29 Rubler S., Damani P.M. & Pinto E.R. (1977) Cardiac size and performance during pregnancy estimated with echocardiography. *American Journal of Cardiology* 40, 534.

30 Bolter C. & Lauckner W. (1990) Echokardiographie während der Schwangerschaft — Verlaufsuntersuchungen bei Primigravidae. *Zentralblatt für Gynäkologie* 112, 1009.

31 de Swiet M. & Talbert D.G. (1986) The measurement of cardiac output by electrical impedance plethysmography: Are the assumptions valid? *British Journal of Obstetrics and Gynaecology* 93, 721.

32 Kubicek W.G., Karnegis J.N., Patterson R.P., Witsoe D.A. & Mattson R.H. (1966) Development and evaluation of an impedance cardiac output system. *Aerospace Medicine* 37, 1208.

33 Gabriel S., Atterhög J.G., Orö L. & Ekelund L.G. (1976) Measurement of cardiac output by impedance cardiography in patients with myocardial infarction. *Scandinavian Journal of Clinical and Laboratory Investigation* 36, 29.

34 Milsom I., Forssman L., Sivertsson R. & Dottori O. (1983) Measurement of cardiac stroke volume by impedance cardiography in the last trimester of pregnancy. *Acta Obstetricia et Gynecologica Scandinavica* 62, 473.

35 Masaki D.I., Greenspoon J.S. & Ouzounian J.G. (1989) Measurement of cardiac output by thoracic electrical bioimpedance and thermodilution. *American Journal of Obstetrics and Gynecology* 161, 680.

36 Atkins A.F., Watt J.M., Milan P., Davies P. & Selwyn Crawford J. (1981) A longitudinal study of cardiovascular dynamic changes throughout pregnancy. *European Journal of Obstetrics, Gynecology and Reproductive Biology (Amsterdam)* 12, 225.

37 Davies P., Francis R.I., Docker M.F., Watt J.M. & Crawford J.S. (1986) Analysis of impedance cardiography longitudinally applied in pregnancy. *British Journal of Obstetrics and Gynaecology* 93, 717.

38 Clark S.L. & Cotton D.B. (1988) Clinical indications for pulmonary artery catheterization in the patient with severe preeclampsia. *American Journal of Obstetrics and Gynecology* 158, 453.

39 Visser W. & Wallenburg H.C.S. (1991) Central hemodynamic observations in untreated preeclamptic patients. *Hypertension* 17, 1072.

40 Clark S.L., Cotton D.B., Lee W., Bishop C., Hill T., Southwick J., Pivarnik J., Spillman T., DeVore G.R., Phelan J., Hankins G.D.V., Benedetti T.J. & Tolley D. (1989) Central hemodynamic assessment of normal term pregnancy. *American Journal of Obstetrics and Gynecology* 161, 1439.

41 Ezimokhai M., Aloamaka C.P., Cherian T., Agarwal M. & Morrison J. (1993) Plasma from normal pregnant women alters the reactivity of rabbit aortic smooth muscle with functional endothelium. *Clinical and Experimental Pharmacology and Physiology (Oxford)* 20, 435.

42 Ezimokhai M., Aloamaka C.P.& Morrison J. (1995) Effect of plasma from preeclamptic subjects on contractions of rat aorta. *Hypertension in Pregnancy* 14, 39.

43 Gant N.F., Daley G.L., Chand S., Whalley P.J. & MacDonald P.C. (1973) A study of angiotensin II pressor response throughout primigravid pregnancy. *Journal of Clinical Investigation* 52, 2682.

44 Aljoamaka C.P., Ezimokhai M., Cherian T. & Morrison J. (1993) Mechanism of pregnancy-induced attenuation of contraction to phenylephrine in rat aorta. *Experimental Physiology* 78, 403.

45 Buster J.E., Sakakini J., Killam A.P. & Scragg W.H. (1975) Serum unconjugated estriol levels in the third trimester and their relationship to gestational age. *American Journal of Obstetrics and Gynecology* 125, 672.

46 Stewart D.R., Overstreet J.W., Nakajima S.T. & Lasley B.L. (1993) Enhanced ovarian steroid secretion before implantation in early human pregnancy. *Journal of Clinical Endocrinology and Metabolism* 76, 1470.

47 Tulchinsky D. & Hobel C.J. (1973) Plasma human chorionic gonadotropin, estrone, estradiol, estriol, progesterone, and 17α-hydroxyprogesterone in human pregnancy. III. Early normal pregnancy. *American Journal of Obstetrics and Gynecology* 117, 884.

48 Ueland K. & Parer J.T. (1966) Effects of estrogens on the cardiovascular system of the ewe. *American Journal of Obstetrics and Gynecology* 96, 400.

49 Hart M.V., Hosenpud J.D., Hohimer R. & Morton M.J. (1985) Hemodynamics during pregnancy and sex steroid administration in guinea pigs. *American Journal of Physiology* 249, R179.

50 Magness R.R. & Rosenfeld C.R. (1989) Local and systemic estradiol-17β: Effects on uterine and systemic vasodilatation. *American Journal of Physiology* 256, E536.

51 Walters W.A.W. & Lim Y.L. (1970) Haemodynamic changes in women taking oral contraceptives. *Journal of Obstetrics and Gynaecology of the British Commonwealth* 77, 1007.

52 Lehtovirta P. (1974) Haemodynamic effects of combined oestrogen/progesterone oral contraceptives. *Journal of Obstetrics and Gynaecology of the British Commonwealth* 81, 517.

53 Eckstein M., Pines A., Fisman E.Z., Fisch B., Limor R., Vagman I., Barnan R. & Ayalon D. (1993) The effect of the hypoestrogenic state, induced by

gonadotropin-releasing hormone agonist, on Doppler-derived parameters of aortic flow. *Journal of Clinical Endocrinology and Metabolism* **77**, 910.

54 Pines A., Fisman E.Z., Ayalon D., Drory Y., Averbuch M. & Levo Y. (1992) Long-term effects of hormone replacement therapy on Doppler-derived parameters of aortic flow in postmenopausal women. *Chest* **102**, 1496.

55 Gilligan D.M., Badar D.M., Panza J.A., Quyyumi A.A. & Cannon R.O. (1995) Effects of estrogen replacement therapy on peripheral vasomotor function in postmenopausal women. *American Journal of Cardiology* **75**, 264.

56 Kessler K.M., Warde D.A.L., Ledis J.E. & Kessler R.M. (1980) Left ventricular size and function in women receiving oral contraceptives. *Obstetrics and Gynecology* **55**, 211.

57 Veille J.C., Morton M.J., Burry K., Nemeth M. & Speroff L. (1986) Estradiol and hemodynamics during ovulation induction. *Journal of Clinical Endocrinology and Metabolism* **63**, 721.

58 La Sala G.B., Gaddi O., Bruno G., Brandi L., Cantarelli M., Salvatore V., Torelli M.G. & Dall'Asta D. (1989) Noninvasive evaluation of cardiovascular hemodynamics during multiple follicular stimulation, late luteal phase and early pregnancy. *Fertility and Sterility* **51**, 796.

59 Csapo A. (1950) Actomyosin formation by estrogen action. *American Journal of Physiology* **162**, 406.

60 King T.M., Whitehorn W.V., Reeves B. & Kubota R. (1959) Effects of estrogen on composition and function of cardiac muscle. *American Journal of Physiology* **196**, 1282.

61 Slater A.J., Gude N., Clarke I.J. & Walters W.A.W. (1986) Haemodynamic changes and left ventricular performance during high dose oestrogen administration to male transsexuals. *British Journal of Obstetrics and Gynaecology* **93**, 532.

62 Longo L.D. & Hardesty J.S. (1984) Maternal blood volume: Measurement, hypothesis of control and clinical considerations. *Reviews in Perinatal Medicine* **5**, 35.

63 Sealey J.E., Itskovits-Eldor J., Rubattu S., James G.D., August P., Thaler I., Levron J. & Laragh J.H. (1994) Estradiol- and progesterone-related increases in the renin–aldosterone system: Studies during ovarian stimulation and early pregnancy. *Journal of Clinical Endocrinology and Metabolism* **79**, 258.

64 Sarrel P.M. (1994) Blood flow. In *Treatment of the Postmenopausal Woman*. Ed. R.A. Lobo, p. 251. Raven Press, New York.

65 Fawer R., Dettling A., Weihs D., Welti H. & Schelling J.L. (1978) Effect of menstrual cycle, oral contraception and pregnancy on forearm blood flow, venous distensibility and clotting factors. *European Journal of Clinical Pharmacology* **13**, 251.

66 Rosenfeld C.R. (1980) Responses of reproductive and nonreproductive tissues to 17β-estradiol during ovine puerperium. *American Journal of Physiology* **239**, E333.

67 Resnik R., Killam A.P., Barton M.D., Battaglia F.C., Makowski E.L. & Meschia G. (1976) The effect of various vasoactive compounds upon the uterine vascular bed. *American Journal of Obstetrics and Gynecology* **125**, 201.

68 Lieberman E.C., Gerhard M.D., Uchata A., Walsh B.W., Selwyn A.P., Ganz P., Yeung A.C. & Creager M.A. (1994) Estrogen improves endothelium-dependent, flow-mediated vasodilation in postmenopausal women. *Annals of Internal Medicine* **121**, 936.

69 Jiang C., Sarrel P.M., Poole-Wilson P.A. & Collins P. (1992) Acute effect of 17β-estradiol on rabbit coronary artery contractile responses to endothelin-1. *American Journal of Physiology* **263**, H271.

70 Miller V.M. & Vanhoutte P.M. (1990) 17β-Estradiol augments endothelium-dependent contractions to arachidonic acid in the rabbit aorta. *American Journal of Physiology* **258**, R1502.

71 McEwen B.S. (1991) Non-genomic and genomic effects of steroids on neural activity. *Trends in Pharmacological Sciences* **12**, 141.

72 Hamlet M.A., Rorie D.K. & Tyce G.M. (1980) Effects of estradiol on release and disposition of norepinephrine from nerve endings. *American Journal of Physiology* **239**, H450.

73 Chelsky R., Wilson R.A., Morton M.J., Burry K.A., Patton P.E., Szumowski J. & Giraud G.D. (1990) Rapid alteration of ascending aortic compliance following treatment with Pergonal. *Circulation (Suppl)* **82**, III,126 (abstract).

74 Brown J.J., Davies D.L., Lever A.F. & Robertson J.I.S. (1964) Variations in plasma renin during the menstrual cycle. *British Medical Journal* **2**, 1114.

75 Oparil S., Ehrlich E.N. & Lindheimer M.D. (1975) Effect of progesterone on renal sodium handling in man: Relation to aldosterone secretion and plasma renin activity. *Clinical Science and Molecular Medicine* **49**, 139.

76 Rylance P.B., Brincat M., Lafferty K., De Trafford J.C., Brincat S., Parsons V. & Studd J.W. (1985) Natural progesterone and antihypertensive action. *British Medical Journal* **290**, 13.

77 Omar H.A., Ramirez R. & Gibson M. (1995) Properties of a progesterone-induced relaxation in human placental arteries and veins. *Journal of Clinical Endocrinology and Metabolism* **80**, 370.

78 Bartelink M.L., Wollersheim H., Vemer H., Thomas C.M.G., De Boo T. & Thien T. (1994) The effects of single oral doses of 17β-oestradiol and progesterone on finger skin circulation in healthy women and in women with primary Raynaud's phenomenon. *European Journal of Clinical Pharmacology* **46**, 557.

79 Roman-Ponce H., Caton D., Thatcher W.W. & Lehrer R. (1983) Uterine blood flow in relation to endogenous hormones during estrous cycle and early pregnancy. *American Journal of Physiology* **245**, R843.

80 Kakouris H., Eddie L.W. & Summers R.J. (1992) Cardiac effects of relaxin in rats. *Lancet* **339**, 1076.

81 Myatt L. (1992) Vaso-active factors in pregnancy. *Fetal Maternal Medical Reviews* **4**, 15.

82 Golub M.S., Working P.K., Cragun J.R., Cannon R.A. & Green J.D. (1994) Effect of short-term infusion of recombinant human relaxin on blood pressure in the late-pregnant rhesus macaque (*Macaca mulatta*). *Obstetrics and Gynecology* **83**, 85.

83 Davison J.M., Shiells E.A., Philips P.R. & Lindheimer

M.D. (1988) Serial evaluation of vasopressin release and thirst in human pregnancy: Role of human chorionic gonadotrophin in the osmoregulatory changes of gestation. *Journal of Clinical Investigation* **81**, 798.

84 Davison J.M., Shiells E.A., Philips P.R. & Lindheimer M.D. (1990) Influence of humoral and volume factors on altered osmoregulation of normal human pregnancy. *American Journal of Physiology* **258**, F900.

85 Symonds E.M. & Broughton Pipkin F. (1978) Pregnancy hypertension, parity and the renin–angiotensin system. *American Journal of Obstetrics and Gynecology* **132**, 473.

86 August P., Mueller F.B., Sealey J.E. & Edersheim T.G. (1995) Role of renin–angiotensin system in blood pressure regulation in pregnancy. *Lancet* **345**, 896.

87 Hollenberg N.K. (1984) The renin–angiotensin system and sodium homeostasis. *Journal of Cardiovascular Pharmacology* **6**, S176.

88 Venuto R. & Donker A.J.M. (1982) Prostaglandin E$_2$, plasma renin activity, and renal function throughout rabbit pregnancy. *Journal of Laboratory and Clinical Medicine (St. Louis)* **99**, 239.

89 Pedersen E.B., Christensen N.J., Christensen P., Johannesen P., Kornerup H.J., Kristensen S., Lauritsen J.G., Leyssac P.P., Rasmussen A. & Wohlert M. (1983) Preeclampsia: A state of prostaglandin deficiency? *Hypertension* **5**, 105.

90 Sealey J.E., Cholst I., Glorioso N., Troffa C., Weintraub I.D., James G. & Laragh J.H. (1987) Sequential changes in plasma LH and plasma prorenin during the menstrual cycle. *Journal of Clinical Endocrinology and Metabolism* **63**, 1.

91 Sundsfjord J.A. & Aakvaag A. (1973) Variations in plasma aldosterone and plasma renin activity throughout the menstrual cycle, with special reference to the pre-ovulatory period. *Acta Endocrinologica (Kobenhavn)* **73**, 499.

92 Weir R.J., Paintin D.B., Brown J.J., Fraser R., Lever A.F., Robertson J.I.S. & Young J. (1971) A serial study in pregnancy of the plasma concentrations of renin, corticosteroids, electrolytes and proteins and of haematocrit and plasma volume. *Journal of Obstetrics and Gynaecology of the British Commonwealth* **78**, 590.

93 Skinner S.L., Lumbers E.R. & Symonds E.M. (1972) Analysis of changes in the renin–angiotensin system during pregnancy. *Clinical Science* **42**, 479.

94 Oats J.N., Broughton Pipkin F., Symonds E.M. & Craven D.J. (1981) A prospective study of plasma angiotensin converting enzyme in normotensive primigravidae and their infants. *British Journal of Obstetrics and Gynaecology* **88**, 1204.

95 Weir R.J., Brown J.J., Fraser R., Lever A.F., Logan R.W., McIlwaind G.M., Morton J.J., Robertson J.I.S. & Tree M. (1975) Relationship between plasma renin, renin-substrate, angiotensin II, aldosterone and electrolytes in normal pregnancy. *Journal of Clinical Endocrinology and Metabolism* **40**, 108.

96 Ledoux F., Genest J., Nowaczynski W., Kuchel O. & Lebel M. (1975) Plasma progesterone and aldosterone in pregnancy. *Canadian Medical Association Journal (Ottawa)* **112**, 943.

97 Karlberg B.E., Ryden G. & Wichman K. (1984) Changes in the renin–angiotensin–aldosterone and kallikrein–kinin systems during normal and hypertensive pregnancy. *Acta Obstetricia et Gynecologica Scandinavica* (Supp.) **118**, 17.

98 Brown M.A., Nicholson E., Ross M.R., Norton H.E. & Gallery E.D.M. (1987) Progressive re-setting of sodium–renin–aldosterone relationships in human pregnancy. *Clinical and Experimental Hypertension* **B5**, 349.

99 Broughton Pipkin F. (1988) The renin–angiotensin system in normal and hypertensive pregnancies. In *Hypertension in Pregnancy*. Ed. P.C. Rubin, p. 118. Elsevier Science Publishers, Amsterdam.

100 Leduc L., Wasserstrum N., Spillman T. & Cotton D.B. (1991) Baroreflex function in normal pregnancy. *American Journal of Obstetrics and Gynecology* **165**, 886.

101 Davison J.M., Valloton M.B. & Lindheimer M.D. (1981) Plasma osmolality and urinary concentration and dilution during and after pregnancy: Evidence that lateral recumbancy inhibits maximal urinary concentrating ability. *British Journal of Obstetrics and Gynaecology* **88**, 472.

102 Gallery E.D.M. & Brown M.A. (1987) Volume homeostasis in normal and hypertensive human pregnancy. *Baillières Clinical Obstetrics and Gynaecology (London)* **1**, 835.

103 Lindheimer M.D. & Katz A.I. (1991) The kidney and hypertension in pregnancy. In *The Kidney*. Eds B.M. Brenner & F.C. Rector Jr, p. 1551. Saunders, Philadelphia.

104 Brown M.A., Broughton Pipkin F. & Symonds E.M. (1988) The effects of intravenous angiotensin II upon sodium and urate excretion in human pregnancy. *Journal of Hypertension* **6**, 457.

105 Smeaton T.C., Andersen G.J. & Fulton I.S. (1977) Study of aldosterone levels in plasma during pregnancy. *Journal of Clinical Endocrinology and Metabolism* **44**, 1.

106 Brown M.A., Sinosich M.J., Saunders D.M. & Gallery E.D.M. (1986) Potassium regulation and progesterone–aldosterone interrelationships in human pregnancy: A prospective study. *American Journal of Obstetrics and Gynecology* **155**, 349.

107 Peach M.J. (1977) Renin–angiotensin system: Biochemistry and mechanisms of action. *Physiological Reviews* **57**, 313.

108 Vinatier D., Tiffet O., Dufour P., Tibergheim, B., Maunoury-Lefebre C. & Monnier J.C. (1992) Cytokines et grossesse: Physiologie. *Journal de Gynécologie Obstétrique et Biologie de la Réproduction (Paris)* **21**, 535.

109 Hill J.A. (1992) Cytokines considered critical in pregnancy. *American Journal of Reproductive Immunology* **28**, 123.

110 Adamson S., Edwin S.S., LaMarche S. & Mitchell M.D. (1993) Actions of interleukin-4 on prostaglandin biosynthesis at the chorion–decidual interface. *American Journal of Obstetrics and Gynecology* **169**, 1442.

111 Hunt J.S. (1992) Prostaglandins, immunoregulation, and macrophage function. In *Immunological Obstet-*

rics. Eds C.B. Coulam W.P. Faulk & J.A. McIntyre p. 73. Norton Medical Books, New York.

112 Knowles R.G. & Moncada S. (1994) Nitric oxide synthase in mammals. *Biochemical Journal* **298**, 249.

113 Palmer R.M.J., Ferrige A.G. & Moncada S. (1987) Nitric oxide release accounts for the biological activity of endothelium-derived relaxing factor. *Nature* **327**, 524.

114 Katz A.M. (1988) Endothelium-derived relaxin factor. *Journal of the American College of Cardiology* **12**, 797.

115 Ramsay B., De Belder A., Campbell S., Moncada S. & Martin J.F. (1994) A nitric oxide donor improves uterine artery diastolic blood flow in normal early pregnancy and in women at high risk of pre-eclampsia. *European Journal of Clinical Investigation* **24**, 76.

116 Henderson A.H. (1991) Endothelium in control. *British Heart Journal* **65**, 116.

117 Pohl U., Busse R., Kuon E. & Bassenge F. (1986) Pulsatile perfusion stimulates the release of endothelial autocoids. *Journal of Applied Cardiology* **1**, 215.

118 Stevenson J.C., MacDonald D.W.R., Warren R.C., Booker M.W. & Whitehead M.J. (1986) Increased concentration of circulating calcitonin gene-related peptide during normal human pregnancy. *British Medical Journal* **294**, 1329.

119 Kennedy T.G. (1983) Embryonic signals and the initiation of blastocyst implantation. *Australian Journal of Biological Sciences (East Melbourne)* **36**, 531.

120 Lewis P.J., Boylan P., Friedman L.A., Hensby C.N. & Dowing I. (1980) Prostacyclin in pregnancy. *British Medical Journal* **280**, 1581.

121 Goodman R.P., Killam A.P., Brash A.R. & Branch R.A. (1982) Prostacyclin production during pregnancy: Comparison of production during normal pregnancy and pregnancy complicated by hypertension. *American Journal of Obstetrics and Gynecology* **142**, 817.

122 Yamaguchi M. Mori N. (1985) 6-Keto prostaglandin $F_1\alpha$ thromboxane B_2 and 13,14-dihydro-15-keto prostaglandin F concentrations in normotensive and pre-eclamptic patients during pregnancy, delivery, and the postpartum period. *American Journal of Obstetrics and Gynecology* **151**, 121.

123 Fitzgerald D.J., Entman S.S., Mulloy K. & Fitzgerald G.A. (1987) Decreased prostacyclin biosynthesis preceding the clinical manifestation of pregnancy-induced hypertension. *Circulation* **75**, 956.

124 Conrad K.P. & Colpoys M.C. (1986) Evidence against the hypothesis that prostaglandins are the vasodepressor agents of pregnancy: Serial studies in chronically instrumented conscious rats. *Journal of Clinical Investigation* **77**, 236.

125 Broughton Pipkin F., Morrison R. & O'Brien P.M.S. (1987) The effect of prostaglandin E1 upon the pressor and hormonal response to exogenous angiotensin II in human pregnancy. *Clinical Science* **72**, 351.

126 Sorensen T.K., Easterling T.R., Carlson K.L., Brateng R.N. & Benedetti T.J. (1992) The maternal hemodynamic effect of indomethacin in normal pregnancy. *Obstetrics and Gynecology* **79**, 661.

127 Gant N.F., Whalley P.J., Everett R.B., Worley R.J. &

MacDonald P.C. (1987) Control of vascular reactivity in pregnancy. *American Journal of Kidney Diseases* **9**, 303.

128 McCausland A.M., Holmes F. & Trotter A.D. (1963) Venous distensibility during the menstrual cycle. *American Journal of Obstetrics and Gynecology* **86**, 640.

129 Keates J.S. & Fitzgerald D.E. (1969) Limb volume and blood flow changes during the menstrual cycle. II. Changes in blood flow and venous distensibility during the menstrual cycle. *Angiology* **20**, 624.

130 Hassan A.A.K., Carter G. & Tooke J.E. (1990) Postural vasoconstriction in women during the normal menstrual cycle. *Clinical Science* **78**, 39.

131 Turner C. & Fortney S. (1984) Daily plasma volume changes during the menstrual cycle. *Federation Proceedings* **43**, 718 (abstract).

132 Keates J.S. & Fitzgerald D.E. (1969) Limb volume and blood flow changes during the menstrual cycle. I. Limb volume changes during the menstrual cycle. *Angiology* **20**, 618.

133 Edwards E.A. & Duntley S.Q. (1949) Cutaneous vascular changes in women in reference to the menstrual cycle and ovariectomy. *American Journal of Obstetrics and Gynecology* **57**, 501.

134 Bartelink M.L., Wollersheim H., Theewes A., Duren D. van & Thien T. (1990) Changes in skin blood flow during the menstrual cycle: influence of the menstrual cycle on the peripheral circulation in healthy female volunteers. *Clinical Science* **78**, 527.

135 Lehtovirta P. (1974) Haemodynamics of the normal menstrual cycle. *Annales Chirurgiae Gynaecologicae Fenniae* **63**, 175.

136 Grollman A. (1931) Physiologic variation in the cardiac output of man. XII. The effect of the menstrual cycle on the cardiac output, pulse rate, blood pressure, and oxygen consumption of a normal woman. *American Journal of Physiology* **96**, 1.

137 Littler W.A., Bojorges-Bueno R. & Banks J. (1974) Cardiovascular dynamics in women during the menstrual cycle and oral contraceptive therapy. *Thorax* **29**, 567.

138 Girdler S.S., Pedersen C.A., Stern R.A. & Light K.C. (1993) Menstrual cycle and premenstrual syndrome: Modifiers of cardiovascular reactivity in women. *Health Psychology* **12**, 180.

139 Duvekot J.J., Cheriex E.C., Tan W.D., Heidendal G.A.K. & Peeters L.L.H. (1994) Volume-dependent echocardiographic parameters are unsuitable for estimating baseline blood volume but are useful for detecting acute changes in vascular filling state. *Basic Research in Cardiology* **189**, 270.

140 Manhem K. & Jern S. (1994) Influence of daily life activation on pulse rate and blood pressure changes during the menstrual cycle. *Journal of Human Hypertension* **8**, 851.

141 Carter Little B. & Zahn T.P. (1975) Changes in mood and autonomic functioning during the menstrual cycle. *Psychophysiology* **11**, 579.

142 Kelleher C., Joyce C., Kelly G. & Ferris J.B. (1986) Blood pressure alters during the normal menstrual

28

cycle. *British Journal of Obstetrics and Gynaecology* **93**, 523.

143 Jern C., Manhem K., Eriksson E., Tengborn L., Risberg B. & Jern S. (1991) Hemostatic responses to mental stress during the menstrual cycle. *Thrombosis and Haemostasis* **66**, 614.

144 Manhem K., Jern C., Pilhall M., Shanks G. & Jern S. (1991) Haemodynamic responses to psychosocial stress during the menstrual cycle. *Clinical Science* **81**, 17.

145 Kool M.J., Wijnen J.A., Derkx F.H., Struijker Boudier H.A. & Van Bortel L.M. (1994) Diurnal variation in prorenin in relation to other humoral factors and hemodynamics. *American Journal of Hypertension* **7**, 723.

146 Lindhard J. (1915) Uber das Minutenvolume des Herzens bei Ruhe und bei Muskelarbeit. *Pflüger's Archiv für Physiologie* **161**, 223.

147 Capeless E.L. & Clapp J.F. (1989) Cardiovascular changes in early phase of pregnancy. *American Journal of Obstetrics and Gynecology* **161**, 1449.

148 Capeless E.L. & Clapp J.F. (1991) When do cardiovascular parameters return to their preconception values? *American Journal of Obstetrics and Gynecology* **165**, 883.

149 Hunter S. & Robson S.C. (1992) Adaptation of the maternal heart in pregnancy. *British Heart Journal* **68**, 540.

150 Campbell D.M., Haites N., MacLennan F. & Rawles J. (1985) Cardiac output in twin pregnancy. *Acta Geneticae Medicae Gemellologiae (Roma)* **34**, 225.

151 McLennan F.M., Haites N.E. & Rawles J.M. (1987) Stroke and minute distance in pregnancy: A longitudinal study using Doppler ultrasound. *British Journal of Obstetrics and Gynaecology* **94**, 499.

152 Walters W.A.W., MacGregor W.G. & Hills M. (1966) Cardiac output at rest during pregnancy and the puerperium. *Clinical Science* **30**, 1.

153 Clapp J.F., Seaward B.L., Sleamaker R.H. & Hiser J. (1988) Maternal physiologic adaptations to early human pregnancy. *American Journal of Obstetrics and Gynecology* **159**, 1456.

154 Rovinsky J.J. & Jaffin H. (1966) Cardiovascular hemodynamics in pregnancy. II. Cardiac output and left ventricular work in multiple pregnancies. *American Journal of Obstetrics and Gynecology* **95**, 781.

155 Veille J.C., Morton M.J. & Burry K.J. (1985) Maternal cardiovascular adaptation to twin pregnancy. *American Journal of Obstetrics and Gynecology* **153**, 261.

156 Robson S.C., Hunter S., Boys R.J. & Dunlop W. (1989) Hemodynamic changes during twin pregnancy: A Doppler and M-mode echocardiographic study. *American Journal of Obstetrics and Gynecology* **161**, 1273.

157 Phippard A.F., Horvath J.S., Glynn E.M., Garner M.G., Fletcher P.J., Duggin G.G. & Tiller D.J. (1986) Circulatory adaptation to pregnancy: Serial studies of haemodynamics, blood volume, renine and aldosterone in the Baboon (*Papio hamadryas*). *Journal of Hypertension* **4**, 773.

158 Hamilton H.F.H. (1949) The cardiac output in normal pregnancy: As determined by the Cournand right heart catheterisation technique. *Journal of Obstetrics and Gynaecology of the British Empire* **56**, 548.

159 Palmer A.J. & Walker A.H.C. (1949) The maternal

circulation in normal pregnancy. *Journal of Obstetrics and Gynaecology of the British Empire* **56**, 537.

160 Bader R.A., Bader M.E., Rose D.J. & Braunwald E. (1955) Hemodynamics at rest and during exercise in normal pregnancy as studied by cardiac catheterization. *Journal of Clinical Investigation* **34**, 1524.

161 Prowse C.M. & Gaensler E.A. (1965) Respiratory and acid-base changes during pregnancy. *Anesthesiology* **26**, 381.

162 Pernoll M.L., Metcalfe J., Kovach P.A., Wachtel R. & Dunham M.J. (1975) Ventilation during rest and exercise in pregnancy and postpartum. *Respiration Physiology* **25**, 295.

163 Novy M.J. & Edwards M.L. (1967) Respiratory problems in pregnancy. *American Journal of Obstetrics and Gynecology* **99**, 1024.

164 Skatrud J.B., Dempsey J.A. & Kaiser D.G. (1978) Ventilatory response to medroxyprogesterone acetate in normal subjects: Time course and mechanism. *Journal of Applied Physiology: Respiratory, Environmental, and Exercise Physiology (Bethesda)* **44**, 939.

165 Longo L.D. (1983) Maternal blood volume and cardiac output during pregnancy: A hypothesis of endocrinological control. *American Journal of Physiology* **245**, R720.

166 Valenzuela G.F., Kim S. & Rauld H.F. (1990) Cardiovascular changes after closure of uterine circulation during pregnancy. *American Journal of Physiology* **258**, R1431.

167 Assali N.S., Rauromo L. & Peltonen T. (1960) Measurement of uterine blood flow and uterine metabolism. *American Journal of Obstetrics and Gynecology* **79**, 86.

168 Von Eiff A.W., Plotz E.J., Beck K.J. & Czernik A. (1971) The effect of estrogens and progestins on blood pressure regulation of normotensive women. *American Journal of Obstetrics and Gynecology* **109**, 887.

169 Greenberg G., Imeson J.D., Thomson S.G. & Meade T.W. (1985) Blood pressure and the menstrual cycle. *British Journal of Obstetrics and Gynaecology* **92**, 1010.

170 Dunne F.P., Barry D.G., Ferriss J.B., Grealy G. & Murphy D. (1991) Changes in blood pressure during the normal menstrual cycle. *Clinical Science* **81**, 515.

171 Moutquin J.M., Rainville C., Giroux L., Raynauld P., Amyot G., Bilodeau R. & Pelland N. (1985) A prospective study of blood pressure in pregnancy: Prediction of preeclampsia. *American Journal of Obstetrics and Gynecology* **151**, 191.

172 Reiss R., O'Shaughnessy R., Quilligan T. & Zuspan F. (1985) Retrospective comparison of blood pressure course during preeclamptic and matched control pregnancies. *American Journal of Obstetrics and Gynecology* **156**, 894.

173 Andros G.J. & Arbor A. (1945) Blood pressure in normal pregnancy. *American Journal of Obstetrics and Gynecology* **50**, 300.

174 Page E.W. & Christianson R. (1976) The impact of mean arterial blood pressure to toxemia of pregnancy in the primigravid patient. *American Journal of Obstetrics and Gynecology* **125**, 740.

175 Hohmann M., Heimann C., Kamali P. & Künzel W.

(1992) Hypotone Symptome und Schwangerschaft. *Zeitschrift für Geburtshilfe und Perinatologie* **196**, 118.

176 Villar J., Repke J., Markush L., Calvert W. & Rhoads G. (1989) The measuring of blood pressure during pregnancy. *American Journal of Obstetrics and Gynecology* **161**, 1019.

177 Frohlich E.D., Grim C., Labarthe D.R., Maxwell M.H., Perloff D. & Weidman W. (1988) Recommendations for human blood pressure determination by sphygmomanometers: Report of a special task force appointed by the steering committee, American Heart Association. *Hypertension* **11**, 209A.

178 MacGillivray I., Rose G.A. & Rowe B. (1969) Blood pressure survey in pregnancy. *Clinical Science* **37**, 395.

179 Eskes T.K.A.B., Weyer A., Kramer N. & Van Elteren P. (1974) Arterial blood pressure and posture during pregnancy. *European Journal of Obstetrics, Gynecology and Reproductive Biology (Amsterdam)* **4**, 87.

180 Wichman K., Ryden G. & Wichman G. (1984) The influence of different positions and Korotkoff sounds on the blood pressure measurements in pregnancy. *Acta Obstetricia et Gynecologica Scandinavica* (Suppl.) **118**, 25.

181 Johenning A.R. & Barron W.M. (1992) Indirect blood pressure measurement in pregnancy: Korotkoff phase 4 versus phase 5. *American Journal of Obstetrics and Gynecology* **167**, 577.

182 de Swiet M. & Shennan A. (1996) Blood pressure measurement in pregnancy. *British Journal of Obstetrics and Gynaecology* **103**, 862.

183 Jensen L.K., Svanegaard J. & Husby H. (1989) Atrial natriuretic peptide during the menstrual cycle. *American Journal of Obstetrics and Gynecology* **161**, 951.

184 Hussain S.Y., O'Brien P.M.S., De Souza V., Okonofua F. & Dandona P. (1990) Reduced atrial natriuretic peptide concentrations in premenstrual syndrome. *British Journal of Obstetrics and Gynaecology* **97**, 397.

185 Cachera R. (1947) Oedèmes et stérols sexuels. *Semaine des Hospitaux de Paris (Paris)* **23**, 2471.

186 Cotes P.M. & Canning C.E. (1983) Changes in serum immunoreactive erythropoietin during the menstrual cycle and normal pregnancy. *British Journal of Obstetrics and Gynaecology* **90**, 304.

187 Chesley L.C. (1972) Plasma and red cell volumes during pregnancy. *American Journal of Obstetrics and Gynecology* **112**, 440.

188 Pirani B.B.K., Campbell D.M. & MacGillivray I. (1973) Plasma volume in normal first pregnancy. *Journal of Obstetrics and Gynaecology of the British Commonwealth* **80**, 884.

189 Whittaker P.G. & Lind T. (1993) The intravascular mass of albumin during human pregnancy: A serial study in normal and diabetic women. *British Journal of Obstetrics and Gynaecology* **100**, 587.

190 Lund C.J. & Donovan J.C. (1967) Blood volume during pregnancy: Significance of plasma and red cell volumes. *American Journal of Obstetrics and Gynecology* **98**, 393.

191 Thomsen J.K., Fogh-Andersen N., Jaszczak P. & Giese J. (1993) Atrial natriuretic peptide decrease during normal pregnancy as related to hemodynamic changes and volume regulation. *Acta Obstetricia et Gynecologica Scandinavica* **72**, 103.

192 Caton W.L., Roby C.C., Reid D.E., Caswell R., Maletskos C.J., Fluharty R.S. & Gibson J.G. (1951) The circulating red cell volume and body haematocrit in normal pregnancy and the puerperium. *American Journal of Obstetrics and Gynecology* **61**, 1207.

193 Berlin N.I., Goetsch C., Hyde G.M. & Parsons R.J. (1953) The blood volume in pregnancy as determined by P32 labeled red blood cells. *Surgery, Gynecology and Obstetrics* **97**, 173.

194 Taylor D.J. & Lind T. (1979) Red cell mass during and after normal pregnancy. *British Journal of Obstetrics and Gynaecology* **86**, 364.

195 Manasc B. & Jepson J. (1969) Erythropoietin in plasma and urine during human pregnancy. *Canadian Medical Association Journal (Ottawa)* **100**, 687.

196 Widness J.A., Clemons G.K., Garcia J.F. & Schwartz R. (1984) Plasma immunoreactive erythropoietin in normal women studied sequentially during and after pregnancy. *American Journal of Obstetrics and Gynecology* **149**, 646.

197 Beguin Y., Lipscei G., Oris R., Thoumsin H. & Fillet G. (1990) Serum immunoreactive erythropoietin during pregnancy and in the early postpartum. *British Journal of Haematology* **76**, 545.

198 Howells M.R., Jones S.E., Napier J.A.F., Saunders K. & Cavill I. (1986) Erythropoiesis in pregnancy. *British Journal of Haematology* **64**, 595.

199 Lurie S. & Danon D. (1992) Life span of erythrocytes in late pregnancy. *Obstetrics and Gynecology* **80**, 123.

200 Jepson J. & Lowenstein L. (1968) Hormonal control of erythropoiesis during pregnancy in the mouse. *British Journal of Haematology* **14**, 555.

201 Davison J.M. & Dunlop W. (1980) Renal hemodynamics and tubular function in normal human pregnancy. *Kidney International* **18**, 152.

202 Koller O. (1982) The clinical significance of hemodilution during pregnancy. *Obstetrical and Gynecological Survey* **37**, 649.

203 Peeters L.L.H. & Buchan P.C. (1989) Blood viscosity in perinatology. *Reviews in Perinatal Medicine* **6**, 53.

204 Bollinger A. & Schlumpf M. (1987) Finger blood flow in healthy subjects of different age and sex and in patients with primary Raynaud's disease. *Acta Chirurgica Scandinavica (Supplement)* **465**, 42.

205 Van de Wal H.J.C.M., Wijn P.F.F., van Lier H.J.J., Kneepkens W.G.H.J. & Skotnicki S.H. (1987) Noninvasive hemodynamic assessment of vasospasm in patients with primary Raynaud's phenomenon. *Angiology* **38**, 315.

206 Cooke J.P., Creager M.A., Osmundson P.J. & Shepherd J.T. (1990) Sex differences in control of cutaneous blood flow. *Circulation* **82**, 1607.

207 Bartelink M.L., De Wit A., Wollersheim H., Theeuwes A. & Thien T. (1993) Skin vascular reactivity in healthy subjects: influence of hormonal status. *Journal of Applied Physiology* **74**, 727.

208 Lehtovirta P. (1982) Forearm blood flow in the

30

normal menstrual cycle. *International Journal of Gynaecology and Obstetrics* **20**, 223.

209 Tinkanen H., Kujansuu E. & Laippala P. (1995) The association between hormone levels and vascular resistance in uterine and ovarian arteries in spontaneous menstrual cycles: A Doppler ultrasound study. *Acta Obstetricia et Gynecologica Scandinavica* **74**, 297.

210 Goswamy R.K. & Steptoe P.C. (1988) Doppler ultrasound studies of the uterine artery in spontaneous ovarian cycles. *Human Reproduction* **3**, 721.

211 Scholtes M.C.W., Wladimiroff J.W., Van Rijen H.J.M. & Hop W.C.J. (1989) Uterine and ovarian flow velocity waveforms in the normal menstrual cycle: A transvaginal Doppler study. *Fertility and Sterility* **52**, 981.

212 Kurjak A., Kupesic-Urek S., Schulman H. & Zalud I. (1991) Transvaginal color flow Doppler in the assessment of ovarian and uterine blood flow in infertile women. *Fertility and Sterility* **56**, 870.

213 Dunlop W. (1980) Serial changes in renal haemodynamics during normal human pregnancy. *British Journal of Obstetrics and Gynaecology* **88**, 1.

214 Katz M. & Sokal M.M. (1980) Skin perfusion in pregnancy. *American Journal of Obstetrics and Gynecology* **137**, 30.

215 Ginsburg J. & Duncan S.L.B. (1967) Peripheral blood flow in normal pregnancy. *Cardiovascular Research* **1**, 132.

216 Rothe C.F. (1983) Reflex control of veins and vascular capacitance. *Physiological Reviews* **63**, 1281.

217 McCausland A.M., Hyman C., Winsor T. & Trotter A.D. (1961) Venous distensibility during pregnancy. *American Journal of Obstetrics and Gynecology* **81**, 472.

218 Goodlin R.C. (1986) Venous reactivity and pregnancy abnormalities. *Acta Obstetricia et Gynecologica Scandinavica* **65**, 345.

219 Stainer K., Morrison R., Pickles C. & Cowley A.J. (1986) Abnormalities of peripheral venous tone in women with pregnancy-induced hypertension. *Clinical Science* **70**, 155.

220 Barwin B.N. & Roddie I.C. (1976) Venous distensibility during pregnancy determined by graded venous congestion. *American Journal of Obstetrics and Gynecology* **125**, 921.

221 Laird-Meeter K., van de Ley G., Bom T.H. & Wladimiroff J.W. (1979) Cardiocirculatory adjustments during pregnancy — an echocardiographic study. *Clinics in Cardiology* **2**, 328.

222 Flessas A.P. & Ryan T.J. (1982) Left ventricular diastolic capacity in man. *Circulation* **65**, 1197.

223 Nixon J.V., Murray R.G., Leonard P.D., Mitchell J.H. & Blomqvist C.G. (1982) Effect of large variations in preload on left ventricular performance characteristics in normal subjects. *Circulation* **65**, 698.

224 Barth J.A. (1990) Echokardiographie während der Schwangerschaft — Verlaufsuntersuchungen bei Primigravidae. *Zentralblatt für Gynäkologie* **112**, 1009.

225 Duvekot J.J., Cheriex E.C., Pieters F.A.A. & Peeters L.L.H. (1995) Severely impaired fetal growth is preceded by maternal hemodynamic maladaptation in very early pregnancy. *Acta Obstetricia et Gynecologica Scandinavica* **74**, 693.

226 Kuzniar J., Piela A. & Sokret A. (1983) Left ventricular function in preeclamptic patients: An echocardiographic study. *American Journal of Obstetrics and Gynecology* **146**, 400.

227 Brenner B.M., Ballermann B.J., Gunning M.E. & Zeidel M.L. (1990) Diverse biological actions of atrial natriuretic peptide. *Physiological Reviews* **70**, 665.

228 Hirata T., Wolfe S.B., Popp R.L., Helman C.H. & Feigenbaun H. (1969) Estimation of left atrial size using ultrasound. *American Heart Journal* **78**, 43.

229 Hytten F.E. & Paintin D.B. (1963) Increase in plasma volume during normal pregnancy. *Journal of Obstetrics and Gynaecology of the British Commonwealth* **70**, 402.

230 Di Donato M., Mori F., Barletta G., Dabizzi R.P. & Fantini F. (1982) Effect of Dextran infusion on left atrial size in normal subjects. *Cardiology* **69**, 257.

231 Cannella G., Albertini A., Assanelli D., Poiesi C., Sandrini M. & Maiorca R. (1988) Effects of changes in intravascular volume on atrial size and plasma levels of immunoreactive atrial natriuretic peptide in uremic man. *Clinics in Nephrology* **30**, 187.

232 Rector W.G., Adair O., Hossack K.F. & Rainguet S. (1990) Atrial volume in cirrhosis: Relationship to blood volume and plasma concentration of atrial natriuretic factor. *Gastroenterology* **99**, 766.

233 Guyton A.C., Jones C.E. & Coleman T.G. (1973) Mean circulatory filling pressure, mean systemic pressure, and mean pulmonary pressure and their effect on venous return. In *Circulatory physiology*. Ed. A.C. Guyton, pp. 205. Saunders, Philadelphia.

234 Rothe C.F. (1986) Physiology of venous return. *Archives of Internal Medicine* **146**, 977.

235 Prather J.W., Taylor A.E. & Guyton A.C. (1969) Effect of blood volume, mean circulatory pressure, and stress relaxation on cardiac output. *American Journal of Physiology* **216**, 467.

236 Hibbard J., Poppas A., Korcarz C., Marcus R., Lindheimer M.D. & Lang R. (1994) Aortic compliance in early pregnancy. *American Journal of Obstetrics and Gynecology* **170**, 286 (abstract).

237 McLauglin M.K. & Reve T.M. (1986) Pregnancy-induced changes in resistance blood vessels. *American Journal of Obstetrics and Gynecology* **155**, 1296.

238 Davis L.E., Hohimer A.R., Giraud G.D., Paul M.S. & Morton M.J. (1989) Vascular pressure–volume relationships in pregnant and estrogen-treated guinea pigs. *American Journal of Physiology* **257**, R1205.

239 Humphreys P.W. & Joels N. (1994) Effect of pregnancy on pressure–volume relationships in circulation of rabbits. *American Journal of Physiology* **267**, R780.

240 Cheriex E.C., Leunissen K.M.L., Janssen J.H.A., Mooy J.M.V. & Van Hooff J.P. (1989) Echography of the inferior vena cava is a simple and reliable tool for estimation of 'dry weight' in haemodialysis patients. *Nephrology, Dialysis, Transplantation (Berlin)* **4**, 563.

241 Duvekot J.J., Cheriex E.C., Heidendal G.A.K., Tan W.D. & Peeters L.L.H. (1994) Measurement of the ultrasonic inferior vena cava anterior–posterior dimensions: A new noninvasive method to assess

acute changes in vascular filling state. *Cardiovascular Research* **28**, 1269.

242 Mintz G.S., Kotler M.N., Parry W.R., Iskandrian A.S. & Kane S.A. (1984) Real-time inferior vena caval ultrasonography: Normal and abnormal findings and its use in assessing right-heart function. *Circulation* **64**, 1018.

243 Kircher B.J., Himelman R.B. & Schiller N.B. (1990) Noninvasive estimation of right atrial pressure from the inspiratory collapse of the inferior vena cava. *American Journal of Cardiology* **66**, 493.

244 Kerr M.G., Scott D.B. & Samuel E. (1964) Studies of the inferior vena cava in late pregnancy. *British Medical Journal* **i**, 532.

245 Milsom I. & Forssman L. (1984) Factors influencing aortocaval compression in late pregnancy. *American Journal of Obstetrics and Gynecology* **148**, 764.

246 Rubler S., Schneebaum R. & Hammer N. (1973) Systolic time intervals in pregnancy and the postpartum period. *American Heart Journal* **86**, 182.

247 Burg J.R., Dodek A., Kloster F.E. & Metcalfe J. (1974) Alterations of systolic time intervals during pregnancy. *Circulation* **49**, 560.

248 Lim Y.L. & Walters W.A.W. (1976) Systolic time intervals in normotensive and hypertensive human pregnancy. *American Journal of Obstetrics and Gynecology* **126**, 26.

249 Mashini I.S., Albazzaz S.J., Fadel H.E., Abdulla A.M., Hadi H.A., Harp R. & Devoe L.D. (1987) Serial noninvasive evaluation of cardiovascular hemodynamics during pregnancy. *American Journal of Obstetrics and Gynecology* **156**, 1208.

250 Easterling T.R., Benedetti T.J., Schmucker B.C. & Millard S.P. (1990) Maternal hemodynamics in normal and preeclamptic pregnancies: A longitudinal study. *Obstetrics and Gynecology* **76**, 1061.

251 Robson S.C., Hunter S., Boys R.J. & Dunlop W. (1990) Serial changes in pulmonary haemodynamics during human pregnancy: A non-invasive study using Doppler echocardiography. *Clinical Science* **80**, 113.

252 Guyton A.C. (1986) The pulmonary circulation. In *Textbook of Medical Physiology*. Ed. A.C. Guyton, p. 287. Saunders, Philadelphia.

253 Brosens I., Robertson W.B. & Dixon H.G. (1967) The physiological response of the vessels of the placental bed to normal pregnancy. *Journal of Pathology and Bacteriology* **93**, 569.

254 Khong T.Y., De Wolf F., Robertson W.B. & Brosens I. (1986) Inadequate maternal vascular response to placentation in pregnancies complicated by preeclampsia and by small-for-gestational age infants. *British Journal of Obstetrics and Gynaecology* **93**, 1049.

255 Pijnenborg R., Anthony J., Davey D.A., Rees A., Tiltman A., Vercruysse L. & Van Assche A. (1991) Placental bed spiral arteries in the hypertensive disorders of pregnancy. *British Journal of Obstetrics and Gynaecology* **98**, 648.

256 Dekker G.A. & Sibai B.M. (1991) Early detection of preeclampsia. *American Journal of Obstetrics and Gynecology* **165**, 160.

257 Gallery E.D.M., Hunyor S.N., Ross M. & Gyory A.A. (1977) Predicting the development of pregnancy-associated hypertension: The place of standardised blood-pressure measurement. *Lancet* **i**, 1273.

258 Easterling T.R. & Benedetti T.J. (1989) Preeclampsia: A hyperdynamic disease model. *American Journal of Obstetrics and Gynecology* **160**, 1447.

259 Gibson H.M. (1973) Plasma volume and glomerular filtration rate in pregnancy and their relation to differences in fetal growth. *Journal of Obstetrics and Gynecology of the British Commonwealth* **80**, 1067.

260 Croall J., Sherrif S. & Matthews J. (1978) Non-pregnant maternal plasma volume and fetal growth retardation. *British Journal of Obstetrics and Gynaecology* **85**, 90.

261 Goodlin R.C., Quaife M.A. & Dirksen J.W. (1981) The significance, diagnosis and treatment of maternal hypovolemia as associated with fetal/maternal illness. *Seminars in Perinatology* **5**, 163.

262 Huisman A. & Aarnoudse J.G. (1986) Increased 2nd trimester hemoglobin concentration in pregnancies later complicated by hypertension and growth retardation. *Acta Obstetricia et Gynecologica Scandinavica* **65**, 605.

263 Duvekot J.J., Cheriex E.C., Pieters F.A.A., Menheere P.P.C.A., Schouten H.J.A. & Peeters L.L.H. (1995) Maternal volume homeostasis in early pregnancy in relation to fetal growth restriction. *Obstetrics and Gynecology* **85**, 361.

264 Gallery E.D.M., Hunyor S.N. & Györy A.Z. (1979) Plasma volume contraction: A significant factor in both pregnancy-associated hypertension (preeclampsia) and chronic hypertension in pregnancy. *Quarterly Journal of Medicine* **48**, 593.

265 Hays P.M., Cruikshank D.P. & Dunn L.J. (1985) Plasma volume determinations in normal and preeclamptic pregnancies. *American Journal of Obstetrics and Gynecology* **151**, 958.

266 Lees M.M., Taylor S.H., Scott D.B. & Kerr M.G. (1967) A study of cardiac output at rest throughout pregnancy. *Journal of Obstetrics and Gynaecology of the British Commonwealth* **74**, 319.

267 Walters W.A.W. & Lim Y.L. (1975) Blood volume and haemodynamics in pregnancy. *Clinics in Obstetrics and Gynaecology* **2**, 301.

268 Hustin J. & Schaaps J.P. (1987) Echographic and anatomic studies of maternotrophoblastic border during the first trimester of pregnancy. *American Journal of Obstetrics and Gynecology* **157**, 162.

269 Schrier R.W. & Briner V.A. (1991) Peripheral arterial vasodilatation hypothesis of sodium and water retention in pregnancy: Implications for pathogenesis of preeclampsia-eclampsia. *Obstetrics and Gynecology* **77**, 632.

270 Goodrich S.M. & Wood J.E. (1964) Peripheral venous distensibility and velocity and venous blood flow during pregnancy or oral contraceptive therapy. *American Journal of Obstetrics and Gynecology* **90**, 740.

271 Friedman S.A. (1988) Preeclampsia: A review of the role of prostaglandins. *Obstetrics and Gynecology* **71**, 122.

272 Barron W.M. (1987) Volume homeostasis during pregnancy in the rat. *American Journal of Kidney Diseases* **9**, 296.

32

273 Fay T.N. & Grudzinskas J.G. (1991) Human endometrial peptides: A review of their potential role in implantation and placentation. *Human Reproduction* **6**, 1311.

274 Daunter B. (1992) Immunology of pregnancy: Towards a unifying hypothesis. *European Journal of Obstetrics, Gynecology and Reproductive Biology (Amsterdam)* **43**, 81.

275 McCarthy A.L., Taylor P., Graves J., Raju S.K. & Poston L. (1994) Endothelium-dependent relaxation of human resistance arteries in pregnancy. *American Journal of Obstetrics and Gynecology* **171**, 1309.

The Cardiovascular System

M. DE SWIET

With few exceptions, measurements in this field are necessarily indirect and the techniques are generally complex and difficult. In addition to the purely technical difficulties of measurement, there are even bigger problems of standardizing conditions. The cardiovascular system, more than any other, is extremely sensitive to changes in such variables as posture, muscular exertion and emotion: large variations in cardiac output, pulse rate, blood pressure and regional blood flow may follow even apparently trivial changes of posture, activity or anxiety.

For these reasons, it is essential to consider all experimental results in terms of how they were obtained; many inconsistencies in the literature are technical and are the result of differences in the standardization of conditions. Technical considerations have already been presented in Chapter 1. Thus, mostly problems of interpretation are included here.

The heart

Position and size

The heart is pushed upwards by the elevation of the diaphragm and rotated forwards so that the apex beat is moved upwards and laterally, appearing in the fourth rather than the fifth intercostal space.

The lateral displacement of the left border of the heart may give a somewhat exaggerated clinical impression of cardiac enlargement, but the heart is indeed a little bigger in pregnancy. By radiological measurement its volume increases by between 70 and 80 ml (about 12%) between early and late pregnancy [1,2]. This degree of cardiac enlargement in pregnancy has been confirmed by echocardiographic studies [3–5], which showed that wall thickness increased very little (and not significantly) so the majority of the increase in heart size is due to an increase in venous filling rather than muscle hypertrophy. The increase in ventricular volume causes dilatation of the valve rings and consequent increase in regurgitant flow velocities as determined by Doppler ultrasound [6].

34 Radiologically, there is straightening of the upper left cardiac border with increased prominence of the pulmonary conus. The lateral view may simulate excessive enlargement of the left atrium and the appearances of early mitral stenosis, with slight backward deviation and indentation of the barium-filled oesophagus [7,8].

The increase in atrial size related to the increase in venous return has been associated by some [9] with an increase in the level of atrial natriuretic peptide (ANP) in pregnancy. Secretion of this hormone which causes natriuresis and a decrease in blood volume is thus appropriate to the increased volume load in pregnancy; it is therefore unlikely that changes in circulating blood volume are caused by a change in ANP concentration. However, reported results for ANP measurement in normal pregnancy are quite variable. Perhaps the most convincing study is that of Steegers *et al.* [10], who found elevated ANP in midpregnancy compared to 6 weeks postpartum, but no significant difference between third trimester and postpartum (presumed non-pregnant) values. At no stage was there a correlation between ANP and any atrial dimension. They postulate that the atrial receptors controlling ANP secretion may be pressure rather than volume sensitive and that they adapt to prolonged stimulus. Voto *et al.* [11] also found no difference in ANP levels at delivery compared to the non-pregnant state. Other studies, however, have shown a persistent and increasing rise in ANP throughout pregnancy [12,13] or no change at all [14–16].

A rise in ANP during the puerperium has also been described [14,15,17], suggesting that ANP may contribute to the well-recognized loss of salt and water that occurs at this time.

Heart sounds

A number of characteristic changes in the pattern of heart sounds occur in a majority of women from early in pregnancy. In a serial phonocardiographic and clinical study of 50 healthy primigravidae, Cutforth and MacDonald [18] made the following observations.

1 *The first sound* became louder before mid-pregnancy and in the majority of women there was an exaggerated splitting of the sound, due to the mitral valve closing earlier than the tricuspid.

2 *The second sound* is not notably affected although the intensity increases, and according to Szekely and Snaith [8] closure of the pulmonary valve may be palpable. In late pregnancy Cutforth and MacDonald noted that the interval between the aortic and pulmonary components of the second sound was less affected by respiration than usual; they attributed the difference to reduced diaphragmatic movement, though this seems unlikely (see Chapter 4).

3 *The third sound* was heard loudly in a majority of women before midpregnancy, and persisted until about 1 week postpartum.

4 *The fourth sound* was detectable by phonocardiography in eight of the 50 patients and was evident in two by auscultation, but it had disappeared by the time of delivery. Similar findings were reported by Breuer [19].

Murmurs

Systolic ejection murmurs developed in most of the women, usually in early systole, although a number were midsystolic. They were best heard along the left sternal edge, although all could be more widely heard and lasted from before midpregnancy until the first week postpartum. Recent Doppler echo studies [5,6] suggest that a proportion of these systolic murmurs may be due to functional tricuspid and other valve regurgitation due to dilatation of the valve annulus in pregnancy. This is of no clinical significance and is not associated with any other clinical or pathological features. Systolic and occasionally more continuous murmurs may arise from the mammary vessels and are commonly heard over the base of the heart [20]; they can be modified by pressure with the chest piece of the stethoscope.

A diastolic murmur occurred, often transiently, in a number of women; it coincided in time with the third heart sound and was best heard along the left sternal border. Cutforth and MacDonald consider it to be a tricuspid flow murmur of no significance.

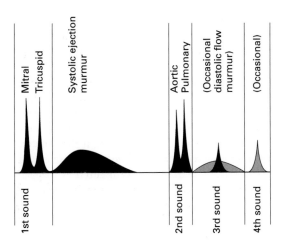

Mitral
Tricuspid
Systolic ejection murmur
Aortic
Pulmonary
(Occasional diastolic flow murmur)
(Occasional)

1st sound
2nd sound
3rd sound
4th sound

Fig. 2.1. Changes in heart sounds and murmurs during normal pregnancy.

The changed sound patterns of the heart described by Cutforth and MacDonald [18] are summarized in Fig. 2.1.

The electrocardiogram

The main changes in the electrocardiogram (ECG) may be attributed to the changed position of the heart; there is a deviation to the left in the electrical axis averaging 15° but as much as 28° in one woman in the study by Hollander and Crawford [7].

Low voltage QRS complexes and deep Q waves have been described, but the Q wave in Lead III may become shallower on deep inspiration and as a rule there is no Q wave in Lead aVF [8].

In many women the T wave becomes flattened or inverted in Lead III [1,7,21–23], with occasional depression of the S–T segment in both chest and limb leads in 14% of patients according to Oram and Holt [24], although this has been denied by Boyle and Lloyd-Jones [25]. Such changes, which are similar to those seen in ischaemic heart disease, occur in healthy women with no detectable structural defect and tend to recur in subsequent pregnancies.

Not surprisingly, about one-third of women subjected to formal exercise testing show significant S–T segment changes at the end of pregnancy [26,27]; and continuous [28] or intermittent [29] electrocardiograph monitoring during and after normal labour has shown similar changes in 15% [28] to 38% of normal women, usually at the time of maximum heart rate. Therefore ECG changes detected during caesarean section under regional anaesthesia do not necessarily indicate ischaemia [30].

Similarly ST–T changes observed during treatment with β-adrenergic drugs (e.g. ritodrine for the suppression of pre-term labour [31] do not necessarily indicate critical myocardial ischaemia.

Atrioventricular and intraventricular conduction are not usually affected but disturbances of cardiac rhythm in the apparently normal heart appear to be commonplace. Atrial or ventricular extrasystoles are frequent and there is an increased susceptibility to supraventricular tachycardia [8].

Myocardial contractility

By the simultaneous use of the ECG, the phonocardiogram and a recording of the external carotid pulse, it is possible to estimate the time during which the left ventricle is contracting before the aortic valve opens, the isovolumetric contraction time or pre-ejection period (PEP), and also the left ventricular ejection time (LVET). The PEP is shortened during most of pregnancy which indicates increased myocardial contractility, probably due to lengthening of the myocardial muscle fibres, and the LVET is, if anything, somewhat lengthened due to the greater stroke volume [32–34]. These altered systolic time intervals are not apparent in late pregnancy when the subjects are lying supine, probably because of reduced venous return and a smaller stroke volume.

The above investigations have been superseded by echocardiographic studies [3] which demonstrated increase in the velocity of circumferential shortening. This, together with increased venous return (increased preload), decreased peripheral resistance (decreased afterload), and increased heart rate, accounts for the observed increase in cardiac output (see below).

Although there is probably a small increase in contractility [35] it is likely that the majority of

36 the increase in cardiac output is derived from the other features mentioned above and which are discussed further below.

Cardiac output

An understanding of the pattern of change in cardiac output has evolved slowly with changes in technique. For many years it was accepted that basal cardiac output rose during pregnancy to a peak at the end of the second trimester, after which it declined towards non-pregnant values at term; this picture was the basis of teaching up to the 1950s [36]. It was largely derived from pioneer work by Burwell with the acetylene method, and subsequent studies by Hamilton [37] with cardiac catheterization and Adams [38] with the dye dilution technique did not appear seriously to contradict these ideas.

Gradually, information accumulated which cast doubt on the slow increase in cardiac output to the traditional 28- to 32-week peak and finally established that the maximum cardiac output is reached quite early in pregnancy. Two of the first catheterization studies were by Hamilton [37] and by Palmer and Walker [39]. They showed remarkable differences in absolute level and in variability, considering that the techniques appeared to be identical, but agreed that cardiac output was close to its maximum from the beginning of the second trimester. A technically superior catheterization study by Bader et al. [40] showed a maximum before 30 weeks. But none of these three studies was entirely satisfactory: all were cross-sectional with few measurements made in early pregnancy. Both Hamilton, and Palmer and Walker assumed an arterial oxygen saturation of 95% and sampled venous blood from the atrium where mixing is known to be incomplete. While Bader et al. [40] measured arterial oxygen saturation directly and sampled mixed venous blood from the pulmonary artery, the relatively high pulse rates of their subjects suggest that they may have paid for their more elaborate technique with a loss of the relaxation and tranquillity necessary for basal measurements. The pattern which seemed to emerge from these three studies was of an early rise in cardiac output to a plateau which did not decline until the last trimester.

The careful serial dye dilution study of 30 normal pregnant women using an ear-piece photoelectric recorder by Walters et al. [41] confirmed that pattern; indeed, the highest mean value recorded was for the period 8–11 weeks as had previously been noted by Werkö [42], although Walters et al. [41] presented suggestive evidence that part of the rise was associated with the natural apprehension of a first measurement. They concluded that cardiac output rose to a plateau at about 1.5 l/min above the mean postpartum level well before the end of the first trimester and did not decline until after 32 weeks. Even so, cardiac output was 1 l/min above the mean postpartum level at 40 weeks.

The next stage in the elucidation of the pattern of change in cardiac output came with the realization that when a woman in late pregnancy lies on her back, as she commonly does for cardiac output measurements, the uterus can seriously impede venous return through the vena cava with a consequent fall in cardiac output. The phenomenon was well described in an important but neglected paper by Vorys et al. [43] and subsequently fully documented by Kerr and his colleagues [44–46]. Cardiac output may also fall in the supine position because of the increased afterload caused by constriction of blood vessels (arterioles and veins) in the uterine vascular bed [47] and because of the partial compression of the aorta [48].

Three invasive studies of cardiac output were made which took account of this phenomenon by having the subjects lie on their sides during the measurement [49–51], and the long-accepted fall in cardiac output in late pregnancy now seems to have been spurious. Pyörälä's study [49] was cross-sectional and referred only to the second half of pregnancy but showed clearly a steadily maintained rise of some 1.7 l/min above the control mean. The study by Lees et al. [50] had the advantage of being a serial investigation and showed almost the same mean cardiac output for each trimester; unfortunately, they provided no control values to judge the rise. Both of these studies demonstrated that the rise maintained in late pregnancy was conditional on the measurements being made with the subjects lying on their sides; in the supine position, the traditional fall was clearly apparent. Of those who made the later studies, only Ueland *et al.* [51] continued in the view that a fall occurs towards the end of pregnancy, greater when the subject is supine.

More recent, non-invasive studies using continuous wave Doppler ultrasound to measure velocity in the aorta (see Chapter 1) indicate that the effect of posture may not be as great as had been thought; the effect of changing from the supine to the lateral position is an increase in cardiac output of not more than 5% in some studies [52–53] although Clark *et al.* [54] showed a 9% difference and Rubler *et al.* [3], in an echocardiographic study of volume changes in the cardiac cycle, still found a 27% increase on changing posture. Part of the discrepancy may come from the marked instability on changing posture. For example, Schneider *et al.* [55] found oscillations in maternal heart rate of amplitude 9–51 beats per minute and cycle length 1–4 seconds when patients not in labour stood up in later pregnancy. This increased variability would also explain why Pyörälä [49] found no significant changes in cardiac output and blood pressure on standing in late pregnancy compared with the anticipated falls in these variables found in midpregnancy. The change in cardiac output on standing is even more marked after delivery [54].

Any consistent decline in cardiac output associated with supine, standing or sitting postures in late pregnancy and due to decreased venous return would be of considerable benefit to those at risk of pulmonary oedema because of heart disease [56].

On standing, noradrenaline levels rise less in pregnancy than in the non-pregnant state. The changes in adrenaline, renin, and angiotensin levels are not affected by pregnancy [57].

The next stage has been the further application of non-invasive techniques to the assessment of changes in cardiac output in pregnancy. These techniques complement measurements of cardiac output, echocardiographic determination of stroke volume, and the use of Doppler velocimetry (see Chapter 1 for details).

Easterling *et al.* [58,59] have reported similar validation data comparing Doppler measurement of cardiac output in the ascending aorta with those derived by thermodilution. Initial

studies were confined to late pregnancy [60] and the puerperium [61]. The study in late pregnancy showed that cardiac output averaged 7 l/min immediately before and 24 hours after labour [60]. Mean cardiac output at 38 weeks was 7.4 l/min, falling to about 5.4 l/min at 2 weeks after delivery [61].

Serial studies are now available using pulsed Doppler which confirm that the rise in cardiac output in the left lateral position is maintained until delivery (Fig. 2.2). Robson *et al.* [4], in an exceptionally thorough study, measured cardiac output in 13 women on two occasions before pregnancy and then monthly until delivery. Cardiac output increased from a mean of 4.9 l/min before conception to a maximum of 7.2 l/min at 32 weeks with no significant change thereafter until labour. The rise in cardiac output was already significant 5 weeks after the last missed period. During the second trimester, heart rate rose while left atrial and left ventricular end-diastolic dimensions increased, suggesting an increase in preload (venous return).

Mabie *et al.* [62] also studied 18 women from early pregnancy, interrogating the aortic valve with pulsed Doppler. They found cardiac output of 6.7 l/min at 8–11 weeks rising to 8.7 l/min at 36–39 weeks before falling to 5.7 l/min 2 weeks after delivery; again, no decrease in cardiac output in late pregnancy.

However, Easterling *et al.* [63] in a study

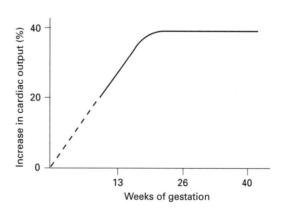

Fig. 2.2. Changes in cardiac output through pregnancy. Note that cardiac output is considerably increased by the end of the first trimester, and the increase is maintained until term [56].

comparing normotensive and pre-eclamptic patients, again using pulsed Doppler, did show a significant small fall of 0.5 l/min in cardiac output between 34 weeks and the last measurement before delivery. This occurred in the normotensive group only and was variable. Cardiac output fell by at least 1 l/min in 29% of subjects but increased by at least 1 l/min in 9%.

Two other studies have looked at the change in cardiac output following delivery in patients where the original pregnancy measurements were made in the left lateral position and where the technique of cardiac output measurement is acceptable. Ueland et al. [51] using dye dilution showed a 12% fall from 5.7 l/min predelivery to 5.0 l/min after delivery. Katz et al. [64], using M mode echocardiography to record chamber dimensions, showed a 37% fall from 8.8 to 5.4 l/min.

In truth, there may be a slight fall in cardiac output at the end of pregnancy but it is likely to be variable and much will depend on patient selection.

A longitudinal study of cardiac output using continuous wave Doppler has been reported by McLennan et al. [65]. The continuous wave interrogated the aortic root and a peak in cardiac output (expressed as minute distance) was observed at 16–24 weeks declining to non-pregnant values at term. However, cross-sectional area of the aorta was not measured and since this may increase by 30% in late pregnancy [66], these results must be viewed with caution.

So too must be the results of a very exhaustive study of the cardiopulmonary adaptation to pregnancy and exercise by Spätling et al. [67]. These authors used the indirect Fick principle and the carbon-dioxide rebreathing technique. However P_{CO_2} was used to calculate CO_2 content in the blood. Since the CO_2 dissociation curve is variably altered by pregnancy [68], this technique is not valid without constructing a CO_2 dissociation curve for each subject.

Earlier studies of cardiac output in women pregnant with twins [69] have been confirmed by Doppler studies [70] which show a 15% greater increase throughout pregnancy. The extra effect of multiple pregnancy is due to the increased heart rate and significantly increased left atrial diameter suggesting increased volume overload [70].

These data refer only to women at complete physical rest, although their mental state and thus their autonomic control of the circulation is likely to have been very variable, accounting for much of the variability within and between the studies cited above. Furthermore, the cardiac output varies greatly depending on a wide range of physical activities. The effect of exercise will be referred to later but the possible effect of uterine contractions deserves mention. No data exist for the effect of contractions prior to labour but in early first stage, when contractions cause a rise of intrauterine pressure little different from that before labour, a contraction can cause a transitory rise in cardiac output of as much as 2 l/min [71]. The rise is partly due to the effect of pain and probably partly due to increased venous return caused by blood expelled from the uterus during contraction. However, there is some evidence to suggest that the intervillous space is distended during a contraction rather than emptied, presumably due to interference with venous outflow [72].

Pulsed Doppler ultrasound is the ideal way to study the effect of contractions since variations in stroke volume can be studied on a beat-to-beat basis. Robson et al. [60] used this technique in a study of 15 patients in labour in the left lateral position and given pethidine and nitrous oxide as analgesics; they showed that basal cardiac output increased from 6.9 l/min in early labour to 7.5 l/min at the end of the first stage (>8 cm dilatation) with further increases brought on by contractions to 8.0 l/min and 10.6 l/min in early labour and at the end of the first stage, respectively. Patients with mitral stenosis do not increase their cardiac output in labour in this way [73].

Even delivery by caesarean section may be associated with an increase in cardiac output as assessed by Doppler ultrasound [74]. But this increase in cardiac output (38%) may have related to general anaesthesia as much as the delivery process.

After delivery, the cardiac output remains elevated for 24 hours and then declines to non-pregnant levels within 2 weeks. Reductions in both heart rate and stroke volume contribute to this decline, although the latter declines significantly over the first 6 months postpartum [4,60,75,76].

Heart rate

The stimulus to increased cardiac output in pregnancy

It was originally thought that cardiac output increased solely to perfuse the uterus (the physiological shunt of pregnancy) [36,77]. But, as indicated above, it was soon apparent that cardiac output was markedly elevated early in pregnancy, when uterine blood flow had not increased significantly. Because oestrogen increases cardiac output [78–79] and oestrogen increases in concentration in early pregnancy, attention then changed to this hormone. However, when transsexuals (admittedly male) are given pharmacological doses of oestrogen, they do not increase cardiac output by nearly as much as occurs in pregnancy [80]. They also only achieve a 9% increase in plasma volume compared to the 50% increase seen in pregnancy. Therefore, other stimuli must be found.

The current hypothesis favours generalized vasodilatation [81] with increased circulating blood volume as a secondary feature, i.e. underfilling of the circulation [82,83]. This is supported by the very early rise in cardiac output [4] at a time when the blood volume has not increased, and by stimulation of the renin–angiotensin system [84], a feature of underfilling.

In recent years, the importance of the regulatory functions of the vascular endothelium for controlling blood vessel tone has become obvious [80] and this has stimulated intense activity with regard to pregnancy. Not only would discovery of the vasodilatory mechanisms be of profound interest concerning the physiology of pregnancy, but also it may reveal the fundamental pathophysiology of pre-eclampsia where failure of vasodilatation appears to be a cardinal feature. The regulatory functions of endothelium are complex [85]. As each new component is discovered, e.g.

prostaglandins [86], calcitonin gene-related peptides [87], endothelin [88], a place is postulated for vascular control in pregnancy and pre-eclampsia. The current favourite is endothelium-derived relaxing factor (EDRF), the nitric-oxide system [89,90], but it is unlikely that this is the sole mediating factor for the vasodilatation of pregnancy.

The increased output of the heart is achieved both by an increase in heart rate and an increased stroke volume. Heart rate is particularly sensitive to many minor stimuli and the variety of published figures indicates the difficulty of achieving standard conditions at rest, but the evidence that heart rate increases in pregnancy is almost unanimous and a detailed review of it appears in Hytten and Leitch [91]. More recent studies are those of Clapp [92], Robson *et al.* [4], Halligan *et al.* [93] and Mabie *et al.* [62].

The increase in rate averages about 15 beats per minute, typically from about 70 to 85, and is present from as early in pregnancy as 4 weeks after the last menstrual period [92]. Women with normal hearts are often more aware of irregularities in heart rate in pregnancy and occasionally persistent atrial tachycardia has been noted [94] without any evidence of cardiac abnormality.

Stroke volume

Stroke volume has been estimated in studies where cardiac output and pulse rate were measured simultaneously and measured directly in studies using Doppler ultrasound [95].

Since the evidence for the increase in cardiac output clearly supports a rise of about 1.5 l/min, from, say, 4.5 to 6.0 l/min, and since equally good evidence shows a rise of pulse rate from about 70 to 85, then stroke volume must rise from about 64 to about 71 ml, a much smaller rise proportionately than that of pulse rate. The proportioning is certainly flexible and no doubt varies considerably from time to time; it is interesting in this context that perfectly normal pregnancy can occur when the mother has an artificial cardiac pacemaker giving a fixed heart rate of about 70 beats per minute [96].

Arteriovenous oxygen difference

The increase in cardiac output in pregnancy is proportionately greater than the increase in oxygen consumption, particularly in early pregnancy when cardiac output has risen considerably and oxygen consumption relatively little (Chapter 4) so that more oxygen is returned to the heart from the venous circulation and the arteriovenous (AV) oxygen difference is smaller.

Palmer and Walker [39] found the AV oxygen difference to be least in early pregnancy, averaging 33 ml/l in the third month and not reaching the average non-pregnant level of about 45 ml/l until the last month. Apart from curiously aberrant findings in the 7th month, all the AV differences before 34 weeks were below the non-pregnant level. The findings of Bader *et al.* [40] are similar: in their series, the AV differences rose from about 34 ml at midpregnancy to 44 ml/l at term.

Hamilton's figures are less striking but similar — the mean AV differences were 42 ml/l in the first trimester, 44 in the second and 48 in the third; the non-pregnant average was 47 [37].

The fact that in pregnancy more oxygen is returned unused to the heart supports the belief that the fall in haemoglobin concentration in the blood is not abnormal. The rise in total haemoglobin — that is, of total oxygen-carrying capacity—is clearly more than sufficient to compensate for the increased oxygen consumption. In such circumstances the term 'physiological anaemia' seems quite inappropriate.

Intravascular pressure

Arterial blood pressure

Arterial blood pressure, blood pressure in the ordinary clinical sense, is generally measured in the brachial artery by indirect means using an inflatable cuff connected to a mercury manometer. Bordley *et al.* [97], in a report of the Scientific Council of the American Heart Association, discussed the errors and inaccuracies of this apparently simple method and made recommendations for the standardization of technique. They began by saying, 'It should be clearly recognized that arterial pressures cannot be measured with precision by means of sphygmomanometers.' This inaccuracy is confounded by poor measurement techniques [98–99].

One aspect of standardization which deserves attention is the size of the cuff. In an elegant study of the effect of cuff size and arm thickness on indicated blood pressure by sphygmomanometry, King [100] found that, for cuffs with a bladder less than 42 cm in length, blood pressure apparently rose with arm girth; with a large cuff there was no relation. But even when cuff size and such variables as the speed of descent of the mercury column are carefully standardized, and the character of the sounds clearly heard, individual differences in the recording of blood pressure can be large. For research purposes, some of the observer error can be eliminated by the use of one of several devices which effectively mask the true level of the mercury column, but they are relatively cumbersome to use and are unlikely to be useful in clinical practice. Most reports in the literature refer to routine clinical measurements and should be viewed in that light.

When compared with the direct measurement of blood pressure, the standard method of sphygmomanometry gives a reading for systolic pressure which is 3–4 mmHg too low and a reading for diastolic pressure which is about 8 mmHg too high. The error in any single measurement is about ±8 mmHg, but Ginsburg and Duncan [101] showed that in pregnancy, sphygmomanometry overestimated both systolic and diastolic pressure in comparison with direct measurements by about 7 and 12 mmHg, respectively.

In the non-pregnant state, the Korotkoff sound phase V, when the sounds disappear, has been recommended for measurement of diastolic blood pressure by conventional sphygmomanometry. Occasionally in hyperdynamic states and, in particular, in pregnancy, there may be no phase V, i.e. the sounds are audible at zero cuff inflation pressure. For this reason, some authorities have recommended the use of the Korotkoff sound phase IV when the sounds become muffled for the measurement of diastolic blood pressure in pregnancy [102]. However, it is now realized that this phenomenon (phase V audible at zero pressure) is much exaggerated [103,104]. It did not occur in any of

85 pregnant women recently studied [105]. Furthermore, two observers could only hear phase IV in 52% of the 340 measurements, and it was in only 19% of the total that *both* observers had noted phase IV [105]. For these reasons, phase V is now recommended for the measurement of diastolic blood pressure in pregnancy [106].

There have been relatively few large systematic studies of healthy pregnant women, and what has been published has been bedevilled by the fact that, as blood pressure rises in pregnancy, it is increasingly associated with pre-eclamptic toxaemia (see, for example, MacGillivray [107]). Thus, women with a blood pressure which exceeds some arbitrary level become abnormal by definition and, while a majority of obstetricians take that level as 140 mmHg systolic and 90 mmHg diastolic, others regard the limit to be as low as 130/80. A classic example of this prejudgement is provided by Andros [108]. In his study, 300 women each had 11 serial readings of blood pressure made during pregnancy and, perhaps uniquely, most of them had at least one record of blood pressure made before pregnancy. The general conclusion that 'systolic blood pressure does not vary at any time during normal pregnancy from the level for a normal and healthy young woman who is not pregnant' is invalidated by the arbitrary condition that 'a systolic pressure of 140 or a diastolic pressure of 90 at any time during the pregnancy eliminated the patient from this study even in the absence of any other sign or symptom of toxaemia'. For the subjects who did not exceed these limits, the mean systolic blood pressure varied little more than 1 mm on either side of about 115 mmHg, but the diastolic pressure was lower in the first two-thirds of pregnancy (about 69 mmHg) than in the final trimester, when it rose to about 72 mmHg, which was the non-pregnant mean. The pulse pressure, the difference between systolic and diastolic pressures, was therefore higher than normal until the last trimester.

This general pattern has been found by all observers: relatively little change in systolic pressure, but a marked fall in diastolic pressure, lowest at midpregnancy, which rises thereafter to approximately non-pregnant levels by term, so that for much of pregnancy there is a notably raised pulse pressure. There is a further rise in blood pressure during labour. In a study of 15 women given pethidine and nitrous oxide as analgesics with measurements made in the left lateral position, Robson *et al.* [60] showed that mean blood pressure rose from 82 to 84 mmHg at the beginning of labour with a further rise in basal mean blood pressure to 91 mmHg at the end of the first stage. Uterine contractions were associated with rises in mean blood pressure of about 10 mmHg paralleling the changes in cardiac output during labour commented on above. That description is representative rather than numerical because the actual readings, which vary considerably from study to study, are probably influenced by the techniques of measuring blood pressure and there would be nothing to gain from attempting any kind of average. Absolute levels are also influenced by other factors, such as age and the time of day; a considerable modification which has been extensively studied is that due to posture. The effect of posture on arterial blood pressure is by no means decided, and differences of opinion are well illustrated by the studies of Schwarz [109] and MacGillivray *et al.* [110]; Schwarz described a fall in both systolic and diastolic pressure when the subject moved from sitting to lying, whereas MacGillivray and his colleagues found a marked rise in systolic pressure but essentially no change in diastolic pressure (Fig. 2.3).

The question has some clinical importance because occasionally there may be a profound fall in blood pressure in a pregnant woman lying on her back: the supine hypotensive syndrome. Howard *et al.* [111] found that 18 of 160 women at term (11.2%) had a fall of at least 30 mmHg in systolic blood pressure after lying on their backs for 3–7 minutes, and describe a woman in whom the fall was so profound as to resemble surgical shock. Fainting in this condition has been shown to relate to reduced cerebral blood flow [112]; the fetus may also be affected [113], presumably by impaired maternal uterine blood flow.

Quilligan and Tyler [114], in a study of 196 women in late pregnancy, found a less striking effect, with a mean drop in pulse pressure of 3 mmHg after 2 minutes in the supine position. Only six of their subjects (3%) showed a fall in

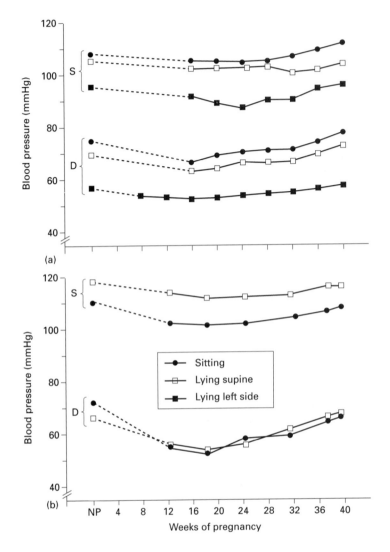

Fig. 2.3. Effect of pregnancy on postural blood pressure, systolic (S), and diastolic (D), as found by (a) Schwarz [109] and (b) MacGillivray *et al.* [110]. Note that MacGillivray finds sitting blood pressure consistently lower than the supine, whereas Schwarz finds the reverse.

systolic blood pressure of 30 mmHg or more when they lay on their backs. Wright [115] studied 100 normal women in late pregnancy and found a fall of 10% or more in systolic blood pressure between sitting up and lying supine in 47 of those, and a fall of 30% or more—sufficient to be distressing—in ten of them.

The phenomenon, due to compression of the vena cava by the uterus, is discussed below. However, the aorta may also be compressed by the term uterus. Bieniarz *et al.* [48] showed that femoral blood pressure was lower than the brachial blood pressure in normotensive women

lying supine and only equalled or exceeded brachial pressure in hypertension. Curiously, Scanlon [116], who also showed a small and not significantly lower femoral blood pressure in normotensive women lying supine, found the femoral blood pressure to be conspicuously lower than the brachial in women with hypertension. The release of the aortic block when the patient turns on her side may explain part of the marked fall in brachial blood pressure shown by Schwarz [109], Trower and Walters [117] and Eskes *et al.* [118]. In Trower and Walters' study, the fall in systolic pressure was variable but of the order of 10% with a diastolic fall of 20–30%. A similar but less obvious fall occurred in non-pregnant subjects.

A very important methodological error contributes to the apparent fall in blood pressure when patients turn from lying supine to lying on their side. In order to measure blood pressure consistently, the sphygmomanometer cuff should be at a constant reference level relative to the heart; usually the level of the left atrium is chosen. When patients turn from lying supine to lying on one side, the arm is usually kept beside the body, and is thus raised about 10 cm relative to the heart if the arm is uppermost. This alone would account for an apparent fall in blood pressure of 10 cm of blood or about 7 mmHg. In several studies [119,120], this factor alone accounted for all the effect of rolling over from supine to the left lateral position. It may also account for some of the variability in the effect of changing posture from sitting to lying already referred to.

In theory, to measure the blood pressure in the lateral position, the arm should be moved so that it is level with the heart. In practice, this is difficult to do but studies have shown that in the lateral position the pressure in the lower arm is similar to that recorded in the supine position [121]. On this basis, measurements made in the lower arm in pregnant patients in the left lateral position are probably acceptable.

In summary, the average normotensive woman in late pregnancy probably has a brachial blood pressure which is highest when she is sitting up, lower when she lies down (a small minority show a massive fall), and somewhat lower still when she lies on one side.

Ambulatory blood pressure measurement

The process of conventional sphygmomanometry is such that only isolated measurements can be made. While such measurements are appropriate for assessment of the circulation at a single point in time (and this, in itself, may be very valuable), they do not give a representative picture of overall blood pressure change during pregnancy; in part because of the inherent variability of blood pressure, both random and diurnal, and also because of extra variability induced by the circumstances of blood pressure measurement.

There have been a few studies of continuous intra-arterial blood pressure measurement in pregnancy [122] but this is such an invasive technique that very few subjects have been studied in this way, certainly not enough to give reliable longitudinal data for the effect of pregnancy on blood pressure.

However, relatively small portable devices are now available which can be programmed to inflate a sphygmomanometer cuff and then use a detection system (either auscultatory or oscillometric) to record blood pressure. The data are usually recorded in machine-readable form and may be down-loaded to a computer for further analysis. These instruments were first applied to the assessment of hypertension in non-pregnant individuals; at least 40 different systems are available. The majority of these instruments have not been adequately validated by the criteria of the Association for the Advancement of Medical Instrumentation (AAMI) [123] or the British Hypertension Society [124] to ensure accuracy and reliability of measurement in the non-pregnant state. But because of the change in haemodynamic pattern of pregnancy and further change in vascular characteristics induced by pre-eclampsia, such instruments should be specifically validated in normal and pre-eclamptic pregnancies [125] if they are to be used in such circumstances.

Clark et al. [126] showed that the Takeda device was accurate for use in pregnancy according to the AAMI criteria. Halligan et al. [93] used the Space-Labs 90207 ambulatory system which has been validated in pregnancy [127] and in pre-eclampsia [128] to study 24 hour ambulatory blood pressure in a cohort of 106 primigravidae. As in the non-pregnant state, ambulatory blood pressures were lower than office blood pressures and this effect was more marked at night (Table 2.1). Ambulatory blood pressures do fall in pregnancy but the effect was not nearly so marked as noted in the study of MacGillivray et al. [110] (see Fig. 2.3) and the nadir was spread over wider gestational ages (9–24 weeks, see Table 2.1). Interestingly, Halligan et al. [93] also found a different pattern of office blood pressure response to pregnancy with nadirs in systolic

44   **Table 2.1.** Ambulatory and office blood pressure (systolic/diastolic)* during pregnancy and postpartum in 100 primigravidae (from [93]).

Ambulatory	Weeks of gestation				
	9–16	18–24	26–32	33–40	6 post-natal
Day	115/70	115/69	116/70	119/74	118/76
Night	100/55	99/54	101/55	106/58	104/59
Office	121/77	124/78	123/78	119/75	117/74

* Values are means.

and diastolic blood pressure occurring at 33–40 weeks.

The application of ambulatory blood pressure monitoring to pregnancy is in its infancy. With regard to the physiology of normal human pregnancy, most studies have considered other variables (e.g. cardiac output) at a single point in time, albeit with repeated single measurements made throughout pregnancy, so it will be a challenge to integrate the date from ambulatory measurements with those data derived from other techniques. The place of ambulatory blood pressure monitoring to study pathophysiology has not been properly evaluated yet, but it is likely to be extensive particularly with regard to the management of pre-eclampsia.

Baroreceptor reflexes

Information concerning baroreceptor reflexes in pregnancy is sparse. However, the reflex appears to be damped as measured by decreased bradycardia following noradrenaline infusion [129], decreased tachycardia following the Valsalva manoeuvre [130], and lower heart rate variability in normal breathing [130].

Peripheral resistance

The peripheral resistance of the circulation is calculated from the mean arterial blood pressure divided by the cardiac output. This variable is therefore usually derived whenever cardiac output is determined. Since cardiac output is raised in pregnancy and arterial blood pressure is not, it follows that the resistance to flow —

the peripheral resistance — must be decreased. Bader et al. [40] calculated from their data that the total peripheral resistance was considerably below normal in midpregnancy, 987 dynes/sec/cm⁵ in the period 14–24 weeks, and rose progressively towards a normal non-pregnant figure of about 1250 at term.

Pyörälä [49] found in his cross-sectional study that peripheral resistance was 979 dynes/sec/cm⁵ in midpregnancy and rose to between 1200 and 1300 later in pregnancy, compared with over 1700 for non-pregnant women. The change is presumed to be due both to the establishment of new vascular beds and to a general relaxation of peripheral vascular tone. A reduction in whole blood viscosity will also contribute [131]. More recent studies using cardiac output measurement derived from Doppler are in agreement [4,13,63].

Venous pressure

Compared to those in arterial blood, changes in venous pressures during pregnancy can be relatively dramatic. It seems established that the pressure in the veins of the arm is not altered by pregnancy [132–134], but pressures in the femoral and other leg veins are high. McLennan [134] reviewed the evidence and presented the results of a large-scale investigation of his own; some of his data are shown in Fig. 2.4.

The femoral veins lead directly to the inferior vena cava and the heart without intervening valves, so that, with the subject horizontal, venous pressures from the legs to the heart are normally similar. The pressure in the right

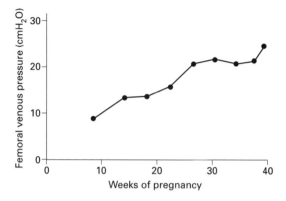

Fig. 2.4. Femoral venous pressure in normal pregnancy.

atrium of the heart is not raised in pregnancy [37–39,135] and central venous pressure has been shown to range between 2.0 and 4.5 cm of water, being about 50% lower in late than early pregnancy with the subject supine [136]. As Ferris and Wilkins [137] pointed out, a rise in femoral venous pressure without a rise in right atrial pressure must indicate venous obstruction between the two points. In pregnancy there are three possible causes for the obstruction.

1   Simple mechanical pressure by the weight of the uterus on both the iliac veins and the inferior vena cava.

2   The pressure of the fetal head on the iliac veins.

3   Hydrodynamic obstruction due to the outflow of blood at relatively high pressure from the uterus.

There is evidence for the action of all these mechanisms. The high pressure in the femoral veins drops abruptly after delivery. McLennan [134], for example, found that at caesarean section femoral venous pressure dropped abruptly when the fetus was removed and before removal of the placenta. He described the change as similar to that seen after removal of a big pelvic tumour and interpreted it as indicating that obstruction in pregnancy is mechanical.

That view has been fully documented by Scott and Kerr and their colleagues [44,46,138]. They showed by direct measurement that, when a woman in late pregnancy lies on her back, pressure in the abdominal vena cava is high, with

radiological evidence of complete flattening above the bifurcation for the length of the uterus; the obstruction was somewhat less marked when the fetal head was fixed in the pelvis and the uterus was less mobile. At caesarean section they confirmed McLennan's observation [134] that delivery of the fetus caused a rapid fall towards normal vena caval pressures. Associated with caval obstruction was a fall in right atrial pressure, cardiac output and arterial blood pressure, the supine hypotensive syndrome. For these women who showed the hypotensive syndrome there was evidence of a lack of any adequate collateral circulation through the vertebral and azygos venous systems.

The height of the obstruction to the vena cava demonstrated by Kerr et al. [44] suggests that the outflow of the renal veins must also often be obstructed and this is further discussed in Chapter 10.

There also is evidence that blood at relatively high pressure does leave the uterus, particularly when it contracts; Palmer and Walker [39] showed a striking rise in right atrial pressure associated with painless uterine contractions in late pregnancy. Bickers [133] measured venous pressure in both femoral veins and showed convincingly that when the pressures were dissimilar, the placenta, which he localized by passing his hand into the uterus after delivery, was always implanted on the side of the high pressure. Where ankle oedema was greater on one side than the other, the greater oedema was on the side of implantation.

As would be expected with a pressure rise due to obstruction, the rate of blood flow in the leg veins is also considerably reduced. Wright et al. [139] injected saline labelled with ^{24}Na into a vein on the dorsum of the foot and timed its appearance at the groin with a counter. The increased time taken is parallel to the rise in pressure shown by McLennan (Fig. 2.4); the speed of flow is approximately halved and the venous pressure doubled by the end of the pregnancy. While it seems likely that both obstruction by the weight of the uterus and the return of the uterine blood each play a part in raising venous pressure in the legs, the weight effect is probably the more important.

46 Both varicose veins of the legs and vulva, and haemorrhoids, may appear in pregnancy or are usually accentuated if present beforehand. It would be reasonable to assume that the heightened venous pressure would contribute to their development. While some women develop huge tortuous veins in pregnancy, the majority of women have no visible varices, which suggests that other influences may be at least as important. McCausland et al. [140] described an ingenious finger plethysmographic method and demonstrated that the distensibility of veins (their degree of dilatation for a given pressure) increased by about half during pregnancy and returned quickly to non-pregnant levels in the puerperium. In women with varicose veins of the legs, the increase in distensibility of the finger veins was much greater than in women who had none. This increase of venous distensibility was confirmed by Goodrich and Wood [141]. Reading from their published graphs, the distensibility of forearm and calf veins increased by about a third or a quarter respectively from the non-pregnant levels. A similar change was brought about in women taking oestrogenic contraceptive pills. Sakai et al. [142] also found increased venous distensibility in pregnancy, an effect that was significantly reduced in patients with pre-eclampsia.

On the other hand, Duncan [143], using a different technique, could find no difference in forearm venous tone between healthy pregnant and non-pregnant women; and Sandström could find no difference between pregnant and non-pregnant women either in vein diameters by ascending phlebography [144] or in vein distensibility by occlusion plethysmography [145]. It is not possible to reconcile these diametrically opposed views on the characteristics of the veins in pregnancy.

Another difference in women with varicose veins was found by Veal and Hussey [146]. Pressure in the popliteal vein of a standing woman was measured before and after the exercise of rising on tiptoe 20–30 times a minute. In women with varicose veins, but not in others, there was a rise in pressure after exercise.

Oedema

Oedema of the lower limbs is commonly seen at routine clinical examination in late pregnancy. An epidemiological study of 24 000 pregnancies by Thomson et al. [147] found almost 40% of normotensive women to have oedema and the majority of these had oedema of the legs. When pregnancy was complicated by hypertension, the incidence was considerably higher. A more intensive prospective study by Robertson [148] suggested that a majority of healthy pregnant women exhibit oedema.

Since the amount by which leg volume increases is only about 500–600 ml even in women with clinical oedema [148,149], gravitational oedema can represent only a small proportion of the total extracellular fluid increases characteristic of pregnancy. This fits with the classic concept of Starling [150] of fluid which has escaped from capillaries to the extravascular space occurring in relatively large collections which can be moved easily by finger pressure (pitting); characteristically, this is lessened when the effect of gravity is reduced by going to bed. Water drunk by a standing pregnant woman appears as increased volume in the legs [151] and the expected diuresis is delayed until she lies down, and contributes to the common aggravation of nocturia.

The Starling relation in pregnancy

The nett capillary filtration of fluid (outwards from the capillary values positive), F, can be written

$$F = L_p \cdot A \left[\left(P_c - P_i \right) - r \left(COP_p - COP_i \right) \right]$$

where L_p = membrane hydraulic conductivity per unit area, A = exchanging surface area, P_c = capillary hydrostatic pressure, P_i = interstitial hydrostatic pressure, COP_p = colloid osmotic pressure of plasma, COP_i = colloid osmotic pressure of interstitial fluid, r = capillary reflection coefficient for plasma proteins [152,153].

In an attempt to account for the frequency of oedema formation in normal pregnancy, Øian et al. [152] performed highly original studies to measure P_i, COP_p and COP_i in the subcutaneous tissue of the thorax and the ankle of patients in the first and third trimesters. Since oedema is uncommon in the first trimester and common in the third, it was assumed that some change in the above variables between the first and third trimesters might indicate the cause of oedema formation; this is not so, for although COP_p fell between first and third trimesters from 23 to 21 mmHg (3.1 to 2.8 kPa), the other variables, P_i and COP_i, changed in directions to offset this effect. Therefore, oedema formation in the systemic circulation must relate to either an increase in membrane hydraulic conductivity or to an increase in the capillary pressure. Since membrane hydraulic conductivity does not change [154], an increase in capillary pressure is more likely to be the cause [152]. Five days after delivery the colloid osmotic pressure has risen either because of increased albumin synthesis or, more likely, because of transport of interstitial proteins back into the vascular compartment [155].

Hunyor et al. [156] believed that capillary permeability increased in pregnancy on the basis of a greater increase in limb size for a given occlusion pressure using venous occlusion plethysmography, although they only considered the relation:

$$F = CFC \times driving\ pressure$$

where F was defined as above, CFC was the capillary permeability and the driving pressure was considered to be constant, making no allowance for changes in interstitial hydrostatic pressure or the changes in osmotic pressure of plasma or interstitial fluid. That is clearly not an expression of the whole Starling relation.

The analysis of Øian et al. [152] discussed above only applies to oedema in the systemic circulation. The tendency of pregnant women to form pulmonary oedema has also been described by MacLennan [153] using the Starling formula. Unfortunately, even fewer of the variables can be measured in the pulmonary circuit, but a rise in pulmonary wedge pressure ($\approx$ pulmonary capillary pressure), and which is equivalent to capillary hydrostatic pressure, has been documented in labour in patients with mitral stenosis [73] and this coupled with the fall in osmotic

pressure of pregnancy could account for the high risk of pulmonary oedema at this time. Furthermore, Gonik and colleagues [157–159] have demonstrated falls in colloid osmotic pressure from about 22 mmHg at the onset of labour to a nadir with a mean of about 16 mmHg 6 hours after delivery. These falls occur in women delivered vaginally or abdominally, under epidural or general anaesthesia, but seem particularly marked in those women given excessive quantities of crystalloid intravenously at delivery. This fall in colloid osmotic pressure, if it does not also occur in pulmonary interstitial fluid, plus the rise in pulmonary capillary pressure, should produce pulmonary oedema more often than occurs clinically. Typically, non-cardiogenic pulmonary oedema occurs at colloid osmotic pressures of 13 to 16 mmHg [160,161]. It is, therefore, surprising that the modern management of labour with liberal use of crystalloid does not cause symptoms more frequently than it does.

Pulmonary blood pressure

Angelino et al. [162] and Bader et al. [40] showed that pressure in the right ventricle, the pulmonary artery and the pulmonary capillaries remained at the normal non-pregnant level throughout pregnancy as would be expected since the pulmonary circulation is known to have a great capacity for absorbing high rates of blood flow without pressure change. It can do this only by decreasing resistance to flow, probably by dilatation of the vascular bed, so that when cardiac output is increased, the volume of the pulmonary circuit also increases. The characteristic radiographic appearance of increased vascularity and enlarged pulmonary vessels supports this view.

Pulsed Doppler pulmonary blood velocities may be used to calculate pulmonary artery pressure. Robson et al. [163] used this technique with simultaneous Doppler measurement of pulmonary blood flow to show that pulmonary resistance fell from 2.85 resistance units before pregnancy to 2.17 resistance units at 8 weeks' gestation. There were no significant changes thereafter. The pulmonary artery resistance was normal by 6 months after delivery.

Conditions where the pulmonary vascular resistance is elevated and fixed have a poor maternal prognosis [164]. This is most frequently seen in Eisenmenger's syndrome where — after what was originally (in childhood) a large left to right shunt at any level from atrial septal defect to patent ductus — the pulmonary vascular resistance rises until it may equal or exceed systemic resistance [165]. The ratio of blood perfusing the pulmonary to systemic circulations is then inversely proportional to the pulmonary resistance divided by the systemic resistance. When the systemic resistance falls in pregnancy, more blood goes to the systemic circulation, and less perfuses the pulmonary circulation [36]. The blood therefore becomes increasingly desaturated with oxygen, an effect which is worsened by the increased oxygen demands of pregnancy. This change is most frequently seen late in pregnancy and the puerperium [164,166]. Eventually, insufficient oxygen is delivered to the myocardium and cardiac output falls with a further decrease in pulmonary blood flow. These patients die following a progressive decrease in cardiac output, most frequently in the puerperium [164,166]. Pre-eclamptic toxaemia is an exacerbating feature, possibly because this condition will further increase pulmonary vascular resistance [167].

Unfortunately, no satisfactory method of measuring pulmonary blood volume has been published. Adams [38] found the central blood volume (which he calculated from his dye indicator curves) to be increased in pregnancy, but he sampled his arterial blood from the femoral artery after injecting dye into an arm vein and the volume measured therefore included all the blood between injection and collection, much more than pulmonary blood volume. On the other hand, Lagerlöf et al. [168], in a dye dilution study, found the mean pulmonary blood volume in eight pregnant women to be below the non-pregnant average.

In the study by Pyörälä [49], where central blood volume extended from a vein in the arm to the capillaries in the ear, there was no significant difference between the controls and pregnant subjects, and Gazioglu et al. [169] estimated that there was no increase in pulmonary capillary blood volume in pregnancy.

Circulation time

Flow in the lower limbs is slowed in late pregnancy, but there is no convincing evidence of a change in the speed of blood flow elsewhere in the body. Speed of blood flow is generally expressed as circulation time — the shortest time a particle of blood takes to go from one point to another — and in practice this is measured between the arm and either the lung or the tongue. If a substance such as saccharin or Decholin is injected into an arm vein, its arrival at the tongue, indicated by a sweet or bitter taste, can be timed. The arm–lung time can be similarly estimated with paraldehyde or ether which is detected when it reaches the breath. More modern methods depend on radioactive tracers or dyes which can be detected objectively.

Theoretically, if a small labelled section of blood travels directly from the point of entry to the point of detection, circulation time is equal to the volume of the vessels between the two points divided by the flow. In fact, the labelling substance inevitably spreads by mixing and if there are big differences in vessel bore en route, not all the blood will travel at the same speed as the label. The measurement is therefore only semi-quantitative and changes are difficult to interpret since they may be due to either a volume change, a change of flow, or both. A big change in blood flow with a parallel change in the volume of the vascular system would result in no alteration in circulation time.

The measurements of circulation time which have been made in pregnancy are contradictory. Spitzer [170] and Landt and Benjamin [21], who measured the arm–tongue circulation time with Decholin, found no change in pregnancy and all values were within the normal non-pregnant range. Greenstein and Clahr [171] used saccharin for arm–tongue times and ether for arm–lung times. They found 13 pregnant subjects to have times which were within the normal non-pregnant range, but claimed that the average times increased during pregnancy, from 11 seconds at 18 weeks to 15 seconds at the end of pregnancy for arm–tongue time and from 4 to 5.5 seconds for arm–lung time. There was considerable individual variation and several exceptions to the average trend. Manchester and Loube [172] made a similar investigation of 48 women, with calcium gluconate and paraldehyde, and came to the opposite conclusion. The mean arm–tongue time fell from 12.4 seconds in the first trimester to 10.2 seconds in the third, and the mean arm–lung time fell from 6.6 to 5.0 seconds.

Pyörälä [49] found the median time taken for a bolus of dye injected into an antecubital vein to reach a photoelectric detector on the ear to fall from about 23 seconds in a non-pregnant control group to about 17 seconds in all pregnant groups. The ranges of times were similar in pregnant and non-pregnant women and the difference was not significant.

It seems reasonable to conclude that, if the circulation time does change, the change is trivial. Since a great increase in blood flow through the lungs is undoubted, that conclusion strengthens the indirect evidence of a parallel increase in pulmonary blood volume.

Regional distribution of increased blood flow

The uterus

The uterus can be regarded as the central target of the increased circulation of pregnancy, but the measurement of uterine blood flow is particularly difficult. Relatively few determinations have been made of absolute uterine blood flow. By contrast, there is a plethora of work relating to uterine artery blood velocity and vascular resistance (see below).

Techniques of measurement

Ideally, what is wanted is a direct measure of uterine blood flow, but, even in animals where direct-reading flowmeters can be introduced into vessels, measurement is by no means easy. The uterus is supplied by a number of arterial channels and it is not possible to know how much of the total supply is destined for the placenta.

An electromagnetic flowmeter was used by Assali *et al.* [173] to measure uterine blood flow in a few women in early pregnancy but in late pregnancy no flowmeters have been used and estimates are all based on indirect methods. Two groups of American workers have used techniques based on an application of the Fick principle with nitrous oxide, a method originally developed by Kety and Schmidt [174] for cerebral blood flow. Techniques of applying this principle to the human uterus have been described by Assali *et al.* [175] and Romney *et al.* [176]. Only one term in the equation can be found with confidence, the arterial concentration, for this can be measured in samples from any convenient artery such as the brachial. By contrast, it is difficult to sample uterine venous blood at all and it may be impossible to get a representative sample. The plexus of veins which drains the uterus drains also the vagina and other structures, and blood predominantly from the placental site is unlikely to be the same as blood from elsewhere in the uterus. A vein can be cannulated directly — at caesarean section, for example — and both teams have done this, although the veins tear easily and it is not as simple as it might first seem. Moreover, the subject must be kept under anaesthesia with the abdomen open and the fetus undelivered for as long as it takes the nitrous oxide to equilibrate with the uterine contents—at least half an hour, possibly much longer.

Assali used a second method of sampling the uterine venous blood, by passing a long Cournand catheter through the basilic vein to the heart, through the right atrium, the inferior vena cava and the iliac veins to the uterine venous plexus under prolonged X-ray fluoroscopy. Not only is this technique unsuccessful in many cases, it is difficult to justify on ethical grounds.

The next difficulty is the estimation of the amount of the nitrous oxide in the uterus and its contents. Romney *et al.* [176] assume that the myometrium is in equilibrium with maternal arterial blood after 30 minutes and assume an average weight of 1 kg for the uterus. They assume also that the fetus and placenta are in equilibrium with umbilical arterial blood although, as Assali recognized, the body fat of the fetus (which may be a considerable though variable quantity at term) dissolves proportionately much more nitrous oxide than the rest of the fetus. The concentration in amniotic fluid can be measured; its volume has to be assumed but errors in assessing the volume would have a relatively small effect on the final sum.

Huckabee [177] criticized the use of nitrous oxide because of its prolonged equilibration time. Instead he injected 4-amino antipyrine in an application of the Fick principle of uterine blood flow and claimed that it diffused quickly into the uterus and fetus, reaching equilibrium in 15–20 minutes.

It must be clear from this brief summary that estimates of uterine blood flow rest on elaborate and difficult techniques which involve a number of assumptions, some of which may lead to substantial errors and which, furthermore, involve hazards which most clinicians would regard as unjustifiable.

One other method of estimating blood flow in the placental site itself has been applied intermittently for 40 years. It is based on the simple principle of injecting a tracer substance into the intervillous space and calculating flow from the speed with which the tracer is washed away. The first tracer to be commonly tried was ^{24}Na (by, for example, Browne and Veall [178]); among other isotopes used there was more recently a vogue for ^{133}Xe (by, for example, Lysgaard and Lefèvre [179], Clavero et al. [180] and Forssman [181]) for which many advantages were claimed. Quantification of these techniques depends on an assumption about the size of the space into which the tracer is injected, but the intervillous space is certainly not homogeneous [182], and there is no means of estimating its size. The technique has no place in physiology and it is doubtful how helpful it is even in a comparison between clinical groups.

A technique of similar principle with similar problems involves the use of a thermoelectric probe; here heat is passed into the intervillous blood and its rate of disappearance is measured [183]. Although this variation allows a continuous measurement and can therefore (at least in principle) record short-term changes in blood flow [184], it cannot be calibrated and enthusiasm for its use has diminished.

Many studies have been performed using Doppler ultrasound to measure blood velocity indices in the maternal uterine artery circulation and its branches during pregnancy. The aim has been to test fetal well-being and the response of the uterine circulation to pregnancy rather than to obtain absolute measurements of uterine blood flow: only one of the four main vessels supplying the uterus is interrogated and that may only be interrogated at a distal branch. For example, Palmer et al. [185] found that uterine artery diameter doubled in pregnancy and that uterine blood flow increased eightfold. This allowed them to calculate blood flow in one uterine artery to be 312 ml/min. Thoresen and Wesche [186] estimated a fivefold increase in uterine artery blood flow between 15 and 38 weeks. This is in keeping with Thaler et al. [187], who calculated an increase in uterine blood flow from 3.5% of the cardiac output in early pregnancy to 12% at term on the basis of transvaginal duplex ultrasonography.

Estimates of blood flow

For early pregnancy we have only the few observations of Assali et al. [173]. They measured the uterine blood flow in 12 women at operation for hysterotomy, both by the electromagnetic flowmeter and by the nitrous oxide method. The flow could be estimated by flowmeter in only the one uterine artery. The resultant value was doubled to give an estimate of blood flow to the uterus and the estimates were similar to those calculated from the nitrous oxide method. The subjects were from 10 to 28 weeks' pregnant (Fig. 2.5). Considering the technical difficulties of the procedure, the curve is astonishingly smooth.

Estimates at term were made by the Boston group [176] using the nitrous oxide method, and these are much more widely scattered; mean blood flow = 12.4 ml/100 g/min; SD = 4.45; range = 6.4–22.0 ml/100 g/min (Fig. 2.5). Faced with this spread, we can do no more than agree with the authors that 'the uterine blood flow is in the order of magnitude of 500 cm³/min'. The figures

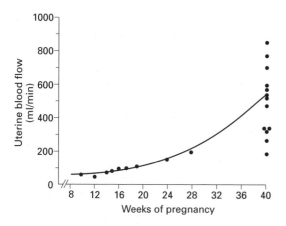

Fig. 2.5. Uterine blood flow in pregnancy. Figures before 30 weeks are from Assali *et al.* [173]; those at term are from Romney *et al.* [176].

are discussed again in relation to oxygen transport in Chapter 4.

Huckabee's [177] technique with 4-amino antipyrine has been applied mostly to studies in ruminants, but he quotes, without any detail, the finding that blood flow through the human uterus at term is 700–800 ml/min.

The uterus is inaccessible and its blood supply is complex. We can only be pessimistic about the possibility of ever achieving precise quantitative estimates of blood flow to the placental site in an intact woman. For physiological calculations we must be satisfied with the data of Fig. 2.5, and comparison with more extensive and more direct measurements in animals suggests that these data are at least in the right range. For clinical purposes, the use of Doppler ultrasound to measure relative if not absolute change in blood velocity, vascular resistance and blood flow is likely to be very valuable.

Mechanics of uterine blood flow

For obvious reasons, there is little experimental evidence about the mechanics of blood flow in the human pregnant uterus and most of what we know rests on the exceedingly elegant experiments, mostly with the monkey, by Ramsey (for example, [188]) as a guide to what happens. The picture is well described by Ramsey *et al.* [189]:

Arterial blood enters the placenta (*intervillous space*) from the endometrial arteries under a head of maternal pressure sufficiently higher than that prevailing in the vast, amorphous lake of the intervillous space so that the incoming stream is driven high up toward the chorionic plate. Gradually this force is spent and lateral dispersion occurs, aided by the villi which, acting as baffles, promote mixing and slowing and, by their own pulsation, effect a mild stirring. Eventually the blood in the intervillous space falls back upon the orifices in the basal plate which connect with maternal veins, and, since there is an additional fall in blood pressure between the intervillous space and the endometrial veins, drainage is accomplished. The pressure differential is further enhanced by the intermittent myometrial contractions (*Braxton Hicks' contractions*) which compress the thin-walled veins, temporarily preventing escape of blood from the placenta (*intervillous space*) and raising the intervillous pressure. When the myometrium relaxes, the elevated intervillous pressure produces rapid drainage.

The details of Ramsey's findings are well discussed by Freese [190].

The best evidence for what happens in the human uterus comes from a large series of radiographs taken after injecting radiopaque dye into the aorta between $6^1/2$ weeks of pregnancy and term, described by Burchell [191]. The intervillous space is visible soon after implantation and, in early pregnancy, puffs of dye appear from numerous entry sites and disappear in 4 or 5 seconds. By the end of pregnancy Burchell was impressed by the size of the arcuate arteries, some as wide as the iliacs, and the considerable non-homogeneity of the intervillous space with rapid diffusion in some areas and stasis in others; time of disappearance of the dye had risen to about half a minute.

The mean uterine arteriolar pressure is probably not much less than the mean peripheral arterial pressure, between 80 and 100 mmHg. Pressure in the intervillous space is probably

52 about 15 mmHg in the relaxed uterus [192] some 5 mmHg above the pressure in the amniotic fluid. In measurements on two subjects not in labour, Prystowsky [193] recorded intervillous space pressure of 3.2 and 5.7 mmHg but, in two resting uteri during the second stage of labour, pressures were 10.5 and 19.8 mmHg. Hellman *et al.* [194] found a mean pressure of about 13 mmHg in eight women at laparotomy, with a range of from about 10 to 20 mm. During uterine contractions the pressure is much greater, and remains above the pressure of the amniotic fluid. For five of Prystowsky's subjects in the second stage of labour, the mean pressure was 38.2 mmHg and in one subject after a pitocin-induced contraction Hellman *et al.* [194] found a pressure of about 35 mmHg.

The amount of blood trapped in the placental intervillous space during a contraction, when the veins are compressed and arterial blood continues to flow in, is not known. On the mistaken assumption that blood was being squeezed from the intervillous space during a contraction, Hendricks [195] calculated from changes in cardiac output that the amount was about 250–300 ml. But the rise in cardiac output, also shown, for example, by Lees *et al.* [196], may be due to other changes, perhaps the relief of large vessel occlusion when the uterus lifts itself forward during contraction.

Arteriovenous shunts

There is some evidence of direct arteriovenous anastomoses in the uterus. Heckel and Tobin [197] injected glass spheres of about 200 μm diameter into the arterial system of pregnant and non-pregnant uteri which had their vascular system washed out after removal at operation. In 12 of the 21 non-pregnant uteri, and in each of the four pregnant uteri, the spheres were found in the veins, suggesting that there are connecting channels of at least 200 μm diameter — the size of a moderate sized arteriole. Nothing is known of these shunts or of any mechanism which might control them, although they could obviously divert a great deal of blood from the placental site if they were open. They might, for example, short circuit the uterine blood flow after the placenta is delivered.

Much has been made in the past of Burwell's suggestion [77] that the intervillous circulation is similar in its effects to an arteriovenous fistula. Among suggested similarities are the increased cardiac output and pulse rate with a low diastolic blood pressure, a bruit over the site of the fistula, and a relatively high oxygen content of blood leaving the area of high blood flow. But uterine venous blood does not have a particularly high content of oxygen and the other signs common to pregnancy and an arteriovenous fistula cannot be attributed to flow through the placental site. Cardiac output and pulse rate increase most rapidly in early pregnancy when uterine blood flow is trivial. It might more convincingly be argued that the sudden increase in renal blood flow in early pregnancy simulates an arteriovenous shunt.

Control of blood flow in the arterial tree is normally dependent on vasomotor activity in the arterioles. But, in the pregnant uterus, the spiral arterioles have their walls destroyed by trophoblast [198] and become merely passive channels. There appears to be no autoregulation in placental blood flow at least in the sheep [199], where flow is almost wholly pressure dependent, but there are both α- and β-adrenergic receptors in the myometrial blood vessels [200].

It may well be that more proximal uterine arteries have specific local control mechanisms. For example, depending on their size, uterine arteries specifically bind human chorionic gonadotrophin which can regulate the formation of vascular eicosanoids [201] and the nerves supplying uterine arteries bind specifically with certain peptides such as vasoactive intestinal peptide and neuropeptide [202] which, with endothelin, activate or modulate vasoconstriction [203,204].

The kidneys

Renal blood flow is highly discussed in Chapter 10. It rises in early pregnancy to about 400 ml/min above non-pregnant levels by the beginning of the second trimester but present information suggests a terminal decline in blood flow.

The skin

There is abundant clinical evidence that blood flow in the skin, particularly in the hands and feet, is greatly increased in pregnancy. The skin is characteristically warm and the hands clammy. The women themselves feel warm and they often complain of the heat and feel more than usually comfortable in cold weather. But in spite of the clear-cut clinical picture, the published measurements are confusing and discrepant.

Many measurements of blood flow in the extremities have been made with a water-filled plethysmograph which records the change in volume caused by the inflow of blood over a given time, when the venous outflow is obstructed. The method is simple in principle but the temperature of the water has a considerable influence on the results. Ideally, the conditions of an ordinarily clothed limb should be simulated. Barcroft and Edholm [205] showed that, for the forearm in non-pregnant subjects, a water temperature of 35°C maintained the deep muscle temperature but caused skin temperature to rise so that blood flow was overestimated. At a water temperature of 33°C, skin temperature remained constant but the temperature of the deeper tissue fell so that blood flow in the forearm was underestimated. They concluded that the best temperature was probably about 34°C.

This temperature has seldom been used for measurements in pregnancy and it is therefore difficult to interpret the published investigations which have been made with widely different temperatures. More recent studies have used strain gauges around the limb rather than the traditional plethysmograph. From the uneven array of published data, some tentative conclusions can be drawn.

Blood flow in the hand is undoubtedly raised, probably six- or sevenfold [206–208] and, in consequence, skin temperature in the fingers is also raised [209–211] to what must approach the physiological maximum, similar to that reached by reactive hyperaemia in non-pregnant women. About forearm blood flow there is no agreement: measurements suggesting no change [206–208], a slight rise [207,210,212,213], and a conspicu-

ous rise [214–215] have all been taken. On balance, a small increase seems probable, attributed by Spetz and Jansson [215] exclusively to forearm skin blood flow, muscle flow remaining constant.

Blood flow in the foot presents a confused picture. Ginsburg and Duncan [208] found a threefold increase, but the study by Ashton [211], which contrasted cigarette smokers with non-smokers, found that, while there was a substantial rise in foot blood flow in the smokers, non-smokers had no increase; the combined data resembled those of Ginsburg and Duncan. Toe temperature followed a similar course — rising throughout pregnancy only in cigarette smokers.

The pattern of blood flow in the leg is even more contentious than that in the forearm. Several studies have shown either no change [206,216] or a slight increase [208,210], but Drummond et al. [213] demonstrated that, when measured in the left lateral position, there was a rise and, in the supine position, a fall. Ashton [211] also showed a reduced blood flow in the legs, more pronounced in the smokers, but her subjects were measured semi-reclining in a supine position, and posture may have contributed to the fall.

An alternative measurement technique is to use a laser Doppler flowmeter. With this instrument, Tur et al. [217] showed that pregnant women do not vasoconstrict in response to isometric exercise or cognitive tasks in the same way as do non-pregnant subjects; i.e. they have relatively fixed vasodilatation.

In summary, Fig. 2.6 shows that blood flow in the hands and feet (generally regarded as a measure of peripheral skin blood flow) is substantially increased, particularly in the hands, and that finger and toe temperature are correspondingly raised. In the forearm and leg, where blood flow is traditionally regarded as indicating muscle blood flow, the changes are relatively insignificant, perhaps marginally raised at least in the forearm skin. Recent recognition of the effect of posture, and of a pronounced unexplained effect of smoking, effectively prevents interpretation of the earlier literature.

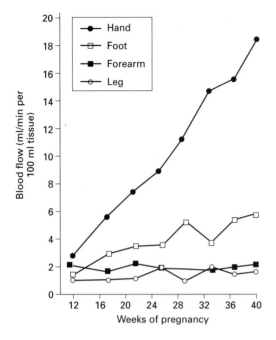

Fig. 2.6. Resting blood flow in the skin of hand, foot, forearm and leg in pregnancy [208].

Peripheral vasodilatation

Melbard [218] examined microscopically the capillaries of the nail bed in 58 pregnant women and found capillary dilatation in two-thirds of them. At term there was an average increase of about 16% in the number of capillaries. Bean *et al.* [219] observed vascular spiders and palmar erythema in about 60% of white women at an antenatal clinic and Barter *et al.* [220] showed that existing haemangiomas may increase in size and new ones may form, particularly on the hands and face.

The vasodilatation in pregnancy apparently obliterates any tendency to arteriolar spasm and Raynaud [221] noticed the effect when he originally described the syndrome which bears his name. The following extract from a contemporary translation of Raynaud's thesis is taken from his description of a case:

> Mme. X, aet. 26 years, has never been ill; but she has been the subject since childhood of an infirmity which makes her an object of curiosity to her acquaintances.

Under the influence of a very moderate cold, and even at the height of summer, she sees her fingers become ex-sanguine, completely insensible, and of a whitish yellow colour. This phenomenon happens often without reason, lasts a variable time, and terminates by a period of very painful reaction, during which the circulation is re-established little by little and recurs to the normal state. Mme. X has no better remedy than shaking her hands strongly or soaking them in lukewarm water. The index of the left hand presents a susceptibility greater than all the other fingers, and is often affected alone. The feet, more impressionable even than the hands, are regularly attacked at meal times and whilst digestion is going on.

Menstruation does not appear to have any influence upon the appearance of the phenomenon, but it is a remarkable fact that the complete disappearance of attacks of local syncope has always been noted by this lady as the first index of a commencing pregnancy.

The increased blood flow to the hands may explain the phenomenon of increased fingernail growth observed by Hillman [222].

Rate of hair growth does not appear to be increased [223] but it changes its character somewhat. In the normal person at any time some 85% of hairs are actively growing; the rest are at a resting stage prior to falling out. In pregnancy, Lynfield [224] found the proportion of growing hairs to rise to about 95%, with fewer at the point of depilation. The pregnant woman therefore reaches the end of pregnancy with many overaged hairs and these fall out in the puerperium leading to the common anxiety about hair coming out 'in handfuls'.

Another area where blood flow is apparently increased during pregnancy is the nasal mucous membrane. Congestion of the mucosa over the turbinates occurs in association with the menstrual cycle, with sexual excitement, and in pregnancy [225]. If we assume, as seems reasonable, that the peripheral vasodilatation is for the purpose of dissipating heat from the fetus, then one would expect the nose to participate, since it apparently serves this purpose in many mammals [226]. In human pregnancy the vasodilatation does little more than provoke nose bleedings, and where the nasal passages are narrow, an irritating blockage; husbands often complain that their wives snore during pregnancy.

The liver

Whether blood flow to the liver changes during pregnancy is not entirely clear. Munnell and Taylor [227], using a continuous infusion of bromosuphthalein (BSP) and hepatic vein catheterization found no difference between pregnant and non-pregnant women; both were between 1400 and 1500 ml/min/1.73 m². Laakso *et al.* [228], who examined the clearance from the blood of labelled colloidal albumin, found no difference between a small number of pregnant and of non-pregnant women; the individual variation was, however, very great and their conclusion was that the method was probably unsuitable.

But a serial study using indocyanine green clearance also found no change in pregnancy [229]. Tindall [230] reported personal data using BSP clearance which indicated a rise from a non-hepatic blood flow of about 800 ml/min to about 1400 ml/min in normal pregnancy. However, there are doubts about the validity of BSP for measurement of hepatic flow in pregnancy since a varying fraction is excreted by extrasplanchnic mechanisms and since the metabolism of BSP is altered by pregnancy. Nevertheless, because of the central role played by the liver in metabolism, it would be reasonable to expect an increase in its activity and in blood flow during pregnancy. The definitive demonstration of this remains to be made.

Other sites

McCall [231] measured cerebral blood flow by the Fick principle with nitrous oxide and found no difference in rate between pregnant women and men. Once again Doppler is being used to monitor changes in blood flow indices (though not absolute blood flow) by insonating the middle cerebral artery [232].

It is possible that spleen size increases during pregnancy but the evidence is fragmentary. Sheehan and Falkiner [233] found spleen size above average in 40% of 163 'unselected routine obstetric necropsies', and stated that the average spleen size increased with length of gestation. It is arguable whether any pregnant women coming to necropsy can be taken as normal and spleen weights were correlated with hyperplasia of marrow in the femur and conditions such as anaemia, accidental ante-partum haemorrhage and gross puerperal infection. Rupture of the spleen, although rare, seems to be somewhat more frequent in pregnancy and has been described in apparently healthy women following slight exertion or quite trivial trauma [234]. At present it is uncertain whether or not splenic enlargement is usual in normal pregnancy.

There are other possible sites of increased vascularity. The breasts are certainly engorged in early pregnancy, and changes which are probably vascular, a sudden enlargement and a sensation of heat and tingling, may be one of the first signs of pregnancy. Dilated veins on the surface of the breast suggest a greatly increased blood supply throughout pregnancy. Blood velocities in the mammary arteries increase 2.5-fold from the 12th to 25th week of pregnancy [186].

The gut may function with more than usual efficiency in pregnancy. It is possible that it too has an increased blood supply.

Summary

It should now be possible to describe the increased cardiac output of pregnancy in terms of regional increases in flow. In Fig. 2.7 we have attempted to do so. The uterine and renal blood flows can be put in with moderate confidence; the rest is tentative.

We can do no more than guess at the total increase in blood flow to the skin, but a figure of 500 ml/min is likely to be realistic; it may be higher in the warm hospital atmosphere where cardiac output is measured.

The distribution of the rest of the cardiac output is even less certain; some undoubtedly goes to the breasts and some to the liver and gut; there may be other areas of increased flow.

Two points are worth making: first, that many

56

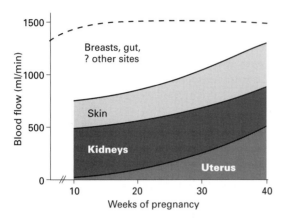

Fig. 2.7. Distribution of increased cardiac output during pregnancy.

of the regional increases in blood flow start early in pregnancy — uterine blood flow is an exception; secondly, that two of the major increases (those to the kidneys and to the skin) serve purposes of elimination — the kidneys of waste material, the skin of heat. Both processes require plasma rather than whole blood which gives point to the *disproportionate* increase of plasma in the expansion of the blood volume.

Control of vascular changes

The mechanisms controlling the regional changes in blood flow in pregnancy are unknown, but the situation is complex. Increasing blood flow to enlarging organs such as the uterus and the breasts is part of their growth and the stimulus to increased vascularity is presumably determined in some way by local demand.

The situation with peripheral blood flow is both more complex and to some extent more important, since changes in peripheral vascular tone have a profound effect on blood pressure. Because of this general effect and because peripheral sites are more readily accessible, their reactions have been the subject of a number of studies.

The overriding influence is vasodilator, well illustrated by the study of Doležal and Figar [235]. When normal non-pregnant women are subject to a variety of stresses, from having to do mental arithmetic to noise and pin pricks,

peripheral vasoconstriction occurs in about 70% of cases. In early pregnancy, more than 60% of responses are vasodilator with a gradual return to a constrictor pattern of response in later pregnancy. Indeed, animal studies [81] indicate that the primary haemodynamic alteration in pregnancy is vasodilatation followed by increases in circulating blood volume and cardiac output.

Several mechanisms may be involved in the tendency to dilatation but there is at present no means of judging their importance. A number of studies [236,237] have shown that the pregnant woman has a lesser pressor response than a non-pregnant woman to a given dose of angiotensin, due to an altered arteriolar responsiveness [238]. This response may be modified as it is in the rat by progesterone [239]. Lloyd and Pickford [240] found evidence in the rat that oestrogens depress sympathetic nervous activity, and Tacchi [241] showed that local instillation of oestrone dilated small conjunctival vessels.

The studies by Assali's group on ganglion-blocking agents is of considerable interest [242]. An intravenous injection of 400 mg of tetraethyl ammonium chloride, a drug which blocks the autonomic system at the ganglia, was given to normal non-pregnant and pregnant women. In the non-pregnant subjects there was little effect on blood pressure; the systolic pressure fell on the average by 8%, the diastolic by 4%. In pregnant women the effect was striking and increased throughout pregnancy until, in the third trimester, the mean fall of systolic blood pressure was 40% and of diastolic 37%. Two or three days after delivery the effect had disappeared.

Assali *et al.* were interested primarily in the fact that this did not occur in women with pre-eclampsia, or indeed in women who did not develop clinical pre-eclampsia until some weeks later, and they suggest that the vessel tone in pre-eclampsia is therefore maintained by a humoral agent. It is possible that the humoral agent may be angiotensin II (A II), since Gant *et al.* [237] have demonstrated that in sharp distinction to normal pregnant women who are relatively unresponsive to A II, the pre-eclamptic woman becomes more than usually responsive (see p. 59). That vessel tone in normal pregnancy is so much more dependent on sympathetic control than before pregnancy, suggests that the autonomic nervous system is correcting for the effect of an active vasodilator substance, perhaps the agent responsible for increasing blood flow in the skin and abolishing Raynaud's disease, reducing the blood pressure and causing the characteristic tendency of pregnant women to faint.

Physiological response to exercise
(see also Chapter 4)

So far this chapter has dealt with cardiovascular adaptations in pregnancy in the basal state, or at least at rest and lying down. The very variable effects of posture have been considered above.

Subjectively, the average pregnant woman becomes progressively less able to perform physical exercise. The ordinary daily round of housework and shopping becomes more tiring; she finds herself cumbersome and awkward, in that climbing stairs and boarding buses, for example, is more difficult. This is hardly surprising since her weight is much increased and the distribution of added weight alters her normal balance. Yet the evidence is that women in good physical condition are unaffected by pregnancy, at least during the first half, and of the 26 female Soviet medal winners in the 1956 Olympic Games, ten were pregnant at the time [243].

The effect of pregnancy on physical work capacity has been reviewed by Erkkola [244], who has himself contributed considerably to the subject. The interpretation of exercise tolerance tests in a population of pregnant women who represent the usual wide range of physical fitness and who are unused to the tests is not straightforward, but in general terms it can be said that when body weight does not have to be lifted, as in sitting exercise, pregnancy appears to make no appreciable difference to the cost of exertion. This view is supported by a considerable body of evidence on the rise in pulse rate, or the rise in oxygen consumption, following standardized work on a bicycle ergometer [1,245]. Where body weight influences the cost of the exercise, as in treadmill walking, then the increased cost in pregnancy is proportional to the increase in body weight.

Bader et al. [40], in their classical haemodynamic study in normal pregnant subjects, found that cardiac output increased normally with exercise (bicycle ergometer) at all stages of pregnancy. This was confirmed by Ueland et al. [246] in normal patients using the dye dilution technique; in contrast, these authors found that patients with valvular heart disease in general, and mitral stenosis in particular, were not able to increase their cardiac output in the same way as normal controls, even though the patients had only mild heart disease (New York Heart Association Classification grades I and II). This supports the observations of Szekely and Snaith [8] that exercise is often a precipitating factor for pulmonary oedema in pregnant patients with mitral stenosis. Presumably these patients have already increased their cardiac outputs to a maximum because of the effect of pregnancy alone. Any further increase in pulmonary blood flow associated with exercise cannot be accommodated by the narrowed mitral valve, and results in pulmonary oedema.

More recently Morton et al. [247] used impedance plethysmography to study the short-term effects of exercising in the sitting position. They found no change in the resting or exercise cardiac outputs between studies at the end of pregnancy and those made in the postpartum period (although because of doubt about suitability of the impedance technique for longitudinal measurements (see Chapter 1) it would have been better to compare the absolute changes induced by exercise in pregnancy with those postpartum). However, in pregnancy the increase in cardiac output was achieved by an increase in heart rate, whereas postpartum the increase was also achieved by an increase in stroke volume, suggesting that reduction in venous return is a limiting factor to the increase in cardiac output induced by exercise in the sitting position in late pregnancy.

By contrast, Van Hook et al. [248], using Doppler, found no change in cardiac output relating to isometric exercise in late normal pregnancy. Blood pressure was elevated by increasing peripheral resistance.

Isometric exercise causes a smaller rise in noradrenaline in pregnancy than postpartum. The responses for adrenaline, renin and angiotensin are not affected by exercise [57].

While pregnancy clearly has no substantial effect on the ability to perform physical work, a more important clinical question is whether physical work affects the pregnancy. Published evidence reviewed by Erkkola [244] suggests that the reproductive performance of athletes in training may be somewhat better than that of non-athletes in terms of length of labour and the proportion of operative deliveries. Pijpers et al. [249] studied the effect of moderate exercise (30–40% maximum oxygen consumption) on a bicycle ergometer. Heart rate, systolic and diastolic blood pressures rose but in these healthy women the cardiac output of the fetus, as assessed by Doppler studies of flow in the descending aorta, did not change.

However, Pomerance et al. [250], who measured the degree of physical fitness in a group of healthy young pregnant women as maximum oxygen uptake (maximum aerobic capacity) in a bicycle ergometer study, found no relation between fitness so measured and length of gestation, length or type of labour, birthweight or any complication of childbearing. On the other hand, there was suggestion in the data [251] that when the fetal heart rate deviated in either direction by more than 16 beats per minute from the pre-exercise rate during the exercise test, then there was a high risk of fetal distress developing in labour. Further, measurements of uteroplacental blood velocity indicate that the vascular resistance increases during exercise on a bicycle. This effect was particularly marked in patients with pregnancies complicated by hypertension or intra-uterine growth retardation [252]. This supports a body of published evidence both on women and animals that severe exercise may constitute a stress test and where the blood supply to the uterus, or oxygen supply to the fetus, may be marginal, then exercise may reduce that margin and threaten the fetus.

Erkkola [244] measured the maximum voluntary work capacity on a bicycle ergometer in two groups of healthy young Finnish primigravidae, half of whom underwent a systematic course of moderately hard physical training during the pregnancy. In early pregnancy the mean for both groups was below the average non-pregnant mean, and in the untrained women it rose to normal by the end of pregnancy. Those who underwent training had a much greater work capacity by late pregnancy and they had somewhat shorter labours when the onset was spontaneous and slightly larger babies and placentae, although there was no statistically convincing evidence of benefit to the reproductive performance.

In summary, it seems that for healthy women with normal pregnancies there is no contraindication to hard physical training, and training can even be undertaken for the first time in pregnancy. Indeed, it is probably true, in general, that the better the physical work capacity of the woman, the more successful the reproductive performance, although the effect is small. It may also be that in some clinical situations where the fetus is compromised in utero, strenuous exercise may be positively harmful, but more information is needed to define these situations.

The haemodynamics of pre-eclampsia

Although Hamilton [253] suggested that cardiac output was raised in the hypertensive pregnancy compared with the normotensive, other workers, such as Assali et al. [254] and Werkö [42] have found cardiac output unchanged or reduced [255]. More recent studies using Swan–Ganz catheterization in patients who are acutely ill with preeclampsia have also been confusing. The cardiac output and peripheral resistance have varied from low to high. Part of the problem has been the effect of therapy, i.e. patients have been given vasodilator antihypertensive drugs such as hydralazine and have been given fluid before they have been studied [256]. Certainly reports such as those of Wallenburg [257] and Belfort et al. [256], who studied patients before they were treated, are more consistent. The peripheral resistance is either normal (for pregnancy) or elevated. But even so, Easterling [63] in a prospective study using Doppler found that patients who developed pre-eclampsia not only had high cardiac output but also had high cardiac output from 10 to 15 weeks' gestation before they developed any clinical manifestations of pre-eclampsia. The peripheral resistance was also consistently lower in those who develop pre-eclampsia, quite at variance with other studies and with current concepts for pathophysiology. But we realize that pre-eclampsia is extraordinarily variable in its clinical presentation and in the time course over which the disease runs; maybe Easterling was studying an atypical group of patients.

The current concept of failure to expand the circulation and vasodilate can be demonstrated very early in pregnancy. The veins share in this vasoconstriction [142]. Gant *et al.* [237] have shown that patients who are destined to demonstrate the clinical manifestations of pre-eclampsia later in pregnancy are very sensitive to infusions of angiotensin from as early as 14 weeks in pregnancy. In contrast, the normal woman vasodilates at this time and is resistant to angiotensin infusion in comparison to the non-pregnant state (see above). The gold standard of the angiotensin infusion test to predict those at risk from pre-eclampsia has been challenged [258]; other workers (reviewed by Kyle *et al.* [258]) have found much lower predictive power of the angiotensin infusion test. It may be that Gant's seminal observations [237] only relate to the young, black primigravidae whom he was studying.

Pulmonary blood flow is also reduced [259] but patients do not become hypoxic even though there is also evidence of additional ventilation/perfusion imbalance [260].

Associated with the low cardiac output are a decreased blood volume [261,262] and high haematocrit, which are also evident in early pregnancy [263]. These are present despite peripheral oedema which is at least in part due to an increase in capillary permeability [262]. Thus, although total body water may be increased, there is a relative and absolute reduction in circulating blood volume, a fact which the clinician faced with a bloated, oedematous patient finds difficult to realize. Changes in blood viscosity do not contribute to the rise in blood pressure seen in mild hypertension [264], although Engelmann [265] showed marked increases in viscosity in five patients with eclampsia.

Intense activity relates to the fundamental cause of these haemodynamic changes. With increasing awareness of the importance of endothelial control mechanisms and the implication of these mechanisms in the vasodilata-

tion of normal pregnancy, it is not surprising that interest has focused on endothelium as the site of the abnormality in pre-eclampsia where there is a failure of vasodilatation. For example, reduction in NO synthase [266] and in platelet activation factor [267] in pre-eclampsia could contribute to vasoconstriction. There do not seem to be significant differences in endothelin [268].

Epidural analgesia and cardiovascular dynamics

Epidural analgesia is increasingly used for pain relief and instrumental delivery, and it is therefore particularly important to consider the profound cardiovascular alterations caused by this procedure. The cardiovascular pharmacology of epidural analgesia has been well described by Bromage [269]. The primary abnormalities are an increase in the venous capacitance and a decrease in peripheral resistance in the lower limbs caused by a partial block of the sympathetic outflow to the veins and arterioles respectively. The increase in venous capacitance causes pooling of blood [270] in the lower limbs with a decrease in effective circulating blood volume, a decrease in venous return and a decreased cardiac output. A careful Doppler study [75] suggests that this effect may be reversed, perhaps completely, by adequate preloading of the circulation — that is, giving 1–2 litres of fluid, usually crystalloid, to increase circulating volume and counteract the decrease in venous return that would otherwise be caused by increased venous capacitance. Ueland *et al.* [271], in a study of 12 patients using dye dilution, found that epidural analgesia was associated with a fall in cardiac output from 5400 to 3560 ml/min. Even if the peripheral resistance were to remain constant, the fall in cardiac output alone would cause a fall in systemic arterial pressure which exceeded 46% in both systolic and diastolic pressures in Ueland's studies. However, the decrease in peripheral resistance exacerbates the effect of the decreasing circulating blood volume and causes a further fall in systemic blood pressure. Spinal anaesthesia is also associated with a decrease in cardiac output, whatever the degree of preloading [272].

60   The effective blood volume is further decreased by compression of the inferior vena cava by the gravid uterus, when the patient is lying supine [271]. As Selwyn Crawford [273] has emphasized, 'there is no excuse for allowing parturient patients to be flat on their backs during labour. In the past, most obstetrical units have been at fault in this respect, and most of us have shared in the guilt' [269]. Cardiac output may be further decreased by the negative inotropic effect of absorbed drugs acting on the heart [274]. The situation is somewhat confused by the possibility of compression of the aorta by the gravid uterus acting to increase peripheral resistance. As previously indicated, Bieniarz *et al.* [275] in elegant arteriographic studies have shown that, during uterine contractions, one or both iliac arteries may be occluded as the uterus is tipped round a fulcrum formed by the sacral promentary. Thus, although the blood pressure may be higher during contractions, uterine perfusion is decreased. This is the syndrome of concealed caval occlusion [276] and its effect too is exacerbated by posture [71]—being more marked in the supine position than the left lateral position.

The clinical application of epidural analgesia is for pain relief, permitting obstetric procedures which would otherwise require other forms of analgesia. Impaired uteroplacental perfusion, with or without hypotension (concealed caval occlusion), is the chief haemodynamic side-effect and this can be controlled by ensuring that patients are nursed in the left lateral position. If this does not succeed, expansion of the circulating blood volume to increase venous return is usually effective and may be performed prophylactically [277], but even so vasopressors are occasionally necessary. Ephedrine is the agent most frequently used because of evidence, at least in sheep, that it does not reduce uterine blood flow [278].

The hypotensive effect of epidural analgesia is used electively in labour complicated by hypertension, although the decreased circulating blood volume of pre-eclamptic toxaemia [261] makes these patients particularly susceptible to hypotension after epidural analgesia [255]. Efficient pain relief associated with epidural analgesia may contribute as much as hypovolaemia to the reduction in blood pressure.

Fig. 2.8. Exercise induced increase in cardiac output at various stages in normal pregnancy, and in pregnancy complicated by heart disease, including mitral stenosis. Note that patients with heart disease in general, and those with mitral stenosis in particular, have a much lower reserve capacity for increasing cardiac output during pregnancy. PP: Postpartum. (Data from Ueland *et al.* [246].)

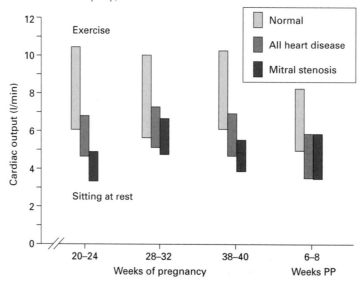

Epidural analgesia is also valuable in the management of labour complicated by heart disease. Again, effective pain relief probably contributes much by reducing cardiac output, but the reduction in venous return is a valuable manoeuvre in reducing the risk of pulmonary oedema. In these cases it is important to beware of the additional risk of profound hypotension [271]. Since peripheral resistance decreases with epidural analgesia, cardiac output must increase to maintain systemic blood pressure. But patients with heart disease, particularly with mitral stenosis, are unable to increase cardiac output further in pregnancy [246] and therefore the blood pressure may fall (Fig. 2.8).

Conclusions

Few aspects of cardiovascular function remain unmodified by pregnancy.

Cardiac output rises quickly in the first trimester to a level some 1.5 l/min above the non-pregnant level, which is maintained for the rest of the pregnancy. It is reduced in late pregnancy when the woman lies supine, due to compression of the inferior vena cava by the uterus. The increase in cardiac output is associated both with an increased stroke volume and a heart rate raised by about 15 beats per minute.

Arterial blood pressure is relatively unaffected, the systolic pressure showing little change, diastolic pressure falling in midpregnancy by something of the order of 10 mmHg and rising again to non-pregnant levels in late pregnancy. But posture, particularly in the final weeks of pregnancy, can have a major effect on blood pressure; it is lower when lying supine than when sitting upright and lower again in the left lateral position.

As would be expected from a raised cardiac output and a relatively unchanged blood pressure, *peripheral resistance* is considerably reduced, and that largely reflects a tendency to peripheral vasodilatation; increased blood flow to the skin, particularly in the hands and feet but to some extent generally, gives a woman a feeling of warmth and a tolerance of cold which is characteristic of pregnancy. The peripheral vasodilatation abolishes the phenomenon of Raynaud's disease and may be responsible for palmar erythema which is common and the increased evidence of vascular spiders and haemangiomata of the skin. It also increases the congestion of the nasal mucous membrane leading to the common complaints of nasal obstruction and nose bleeds.

The mechanisms involved in the tendency to vasodilatation are not fully understood. They are likely to involve the endothelium.

Other targets of the increased cardiac output are the *uterus*, which has a rising blood flow throughout pregnancy reaching about 500 ml/min at term, the *kidneys*, which have an increased flow of about 400 ml/min (declining at the end of pregnancy), and probably the *alimentary tract*.

Venous blood pressure changes only in the lower limbs, where there is a rise as pregnancy progresses, due to mechanical and hydrostatic pressures in the pelvis, particularly when standing. One effect is to increase the distension of veins and exacerbate varicosities (although whether there is a true change in vein distensibility is debatable); another effect is oedema of the lower limbs. Central venous pressure is unaffected by normal pregnancy but may be reduced to half when lying supine in late pregnancy.

The *heart* itself presents a characteristically changed picture in pregnancy; it is raised by the elevated diaphragm and rotated forward so that the apex beat is moved upwards and laterally and a false clinical impression of enlargement may be given, although it is likely that some degree of enlargement does also occur. Radiologically, the upper border is straightened, there is increased prominence of the pulmonary conus, and indentation of the oesophagus by the left atrium may simulate mitral stenosis. There are characteristic changes in the heart sounds: the first sound is frequently split and a third sound is common. A systolic ejection murmur is usual.

Increased myocardial contractility occurs, due to lengthening of the muscle fibres, which results in a shortened pre-ejection period; the left ventricular ejection time is somewhat increased.

The electrocardiogram is also likely to show a number of changes, some of which may simulate ischaemic heart disease. Left axis deviation is the rule, and flattened or inverted T waves, sometimes with a depressed S–T segment, may occur. Disturbances of rhythm are commonplace, with atrial or ventricular extrasystoles and an increased tendency to supraventricular tachycardia.

The effects of exercise in pregnancy are variable. Subjectively, the average pregnant woman may tire more easily and find physical exertion progressively more taxing, although the measured cost of exercise appears to be related only to the need to raise the increased body weight. But in trained athletes, pregnancy — at least in the first half—does not appear to impede athletic performance and there is some evidence to suggest that a healthy woman in physical training may enjoy a more successful pregnancy and an easier labour than her more sedentary counterpart. On the other hand, if the pregnancy is compromised by placental insufficiency, hard exercise may further reduce the uterine blood supply and imperil the fetus.

References

1 Gemzell C.A., Robbe H. & Ström G. (1957) Total amount of haemoglobin and physical working capacity in normal pregnancy and pueperium (with iron medication). *Acta Obstetricia et Gynaecologica Scandinavica* **36**, 93.

2 Ihrman K. (1960) A clinical and physiological study of pregnancy in a material from Northern Sweden. III. Vital capacity and maximal breathing capacity during and after pregnancy. *Acta Societats Medicorum Upsaliensis* **65**, 147.

3 Rubler S., Damani P. & Pinto E.R. (1977) Cardiac size and performance during pregnancy estimated with echocardiography. *The American Journal of Cardiology* **40**, 534.

4 Robson S.C., Hunter S., Boys R.J. & Dunlop W. (1989) Serial study of factors influencing changes in cardiac output during human pregnancy. *American Journal of Physiology* **112**, 1060.

5 Limacher M.C., Ware J.A., O'Meara M.E., Fernandez G.C. & Young J.B. (1985) Tricuspid regurgitation during pregnancy: Two-dimensional and pulsed Doppler echocardiographic observations. *American Journal of Physiology* **155**, 1059.

6 Robson S.C., Richley D., Boys R.J. & Hunter S (1992) Incidence of Doppler regurgitant flow velocities during normal pregnancy. *European Heart Journal* **13**, 84.

7 Hollander A.G. & Crawford J.H. (1943) Roentgenologic and electrocardiographic changes in the normal heart during pregnancy. *American Heart Journal* **26**, 364.

8 Szekely P. & Snaith L. (1974) *Heart Disease and Pregnancy*. Churchill Livingstone, Edinburgh.

9 Cusson J.R., Gutkowska J., Rey E., Michon N., Boucher M. & Larochelle P. (1985) Plasma concentration of atrial natriuretic factor in normal pregnancy. *New England Journal of Medicine* **313**, 1230.

10 Steegers E.A.P., Van Lakwijk H.P.J.M., Fast J.H., Godschalx A.W.H.J., Jongsma H.W., Eskes T.K.A.B., Symonds E.M. & Hein P.R. (1991) Atrial natriuretic peptide and atrial size during normal pregnancy. *British Journal of Obstetrics and Gynaecology* **98**, 202.

11 Voto L.S., Hetmanski D.J. & Broughton Pipkin F. (1990) Determinants of fetal and maternal atrial natriuretic peptide concentrations at delivery in man. *British Journal of Obstetrics and Gynaecology* **97**, 1123.

12 Milsom I., Hedner J. & Hedner T. (1988) Plasma atrial natriuretic peptide (ANP) and maternal haemodynamic changes during pregnancy. *Acta Obstetricia et Gynaecologia Scandinavica* **67**, 717.

13 Sala C., Campise M., Ambroso G., Motta T., Zanchetti A. & Morganti A. (1995) Atrial natriuretic peptide and hemodynamic changes during normal human pregnancy. *Hypertension* **25**, 631.

14 Rutherford A.J., Anderson J.V., Elder M.G. & Bloom S.R. (1987) Release of atrial natriuretic peptide during pregnancy and immediate puerperium. *Lancet* **i**, 928.

15 Grace A.A., D'Souza V., Menon R.K., O'Brien S. & Dandona P. (1987) Atrial natriuretic peptide concentrations during pregnancy. *Lancet* **i**, 1267.

16 Malatino L.S., Strancanelli B. & Greco G. (1988) Atrial natriuretic peptide levels in normal pregnancy and the puerperium. *Medical Science Research* **16**, 1113.

17 Steegers E.A.P., Hein P.R., Groeneveld E.A.M., Jongsma H.W., Tan A.C.I.T.L. & Benraad Th.J. (1987) Atrial natriuretic peptide concentrations during pregnancy. *Lancet* **i**, 1267.

18 Cutforth R. & MacDonald C.B. (1966) Heart sounds and murmurs in pregnancy. *American Heart Journal* **71**, 741.

19 Breuer H.W. (1981) Auscultation of the heart in pregnancy. *Münchner Medizinische Wochenschrift* **123**, 1705.

20 Tabatznik B., Randall T.W. & Hearsch C. (1960) The mammary souffle in pregnancy and lactation. *Circulation* **22**, 1069.

21 Landt H. & Benjamin J.E. (1936) Cardiodynamic and electrocardiographic changes in normal pregnancy. *American Heart Journal* **12**, 592.

22 Zatuchni J. (1951) The electrocardiogram in pregnancy and the puerperium. *American Heart Journal* **42**, 11.

23 de Bettencourt J.M. & Fragoso J.C.B. (1952) L'électrocardiogramme de la femme enceinte. *Acta cardiologica* **7**, 123.

24 Oram S. & Holt M. (1961) Innocent depression of the S–T segment and flattening of the T-wave during pregnancy. *Journal of Obstetrics and Gynaecology of the British Commonwealth* **68**, 765.

25 Boyle D.McC. & Lloyd-Jones R.L. (1966) The electrocardiographic S–T segment in pregnancy. *Journal of Obstetrics and Gynaecology of the British Commonwealth* **73**, 986.

26 Van Doorn M.B., Lotgering F.K., Struijk P.C., Pool J. & Wallenburg H.C. (1992) Maternal and fetal cardiovascular responses to strenuous bicycle exercise. *American Journal of Obstetrics and Gynecology* **166**, 854.

27 Asher U.A., Ben-Shlomo I., Said M. & Nabil H. (1993) The effects of exercise induced tachycardia on the maternal electrocardiogram. *British Journal of Obstetrics and Gynaecology* **100**, 41.

28 Palmer C.M. (1994) Maternal electrocardiographic changes in the peripartum period. *International Journal of Obstetric Anesthesia* **3**, 63.

29 Upshaw C.B.J. (1970) A study of maternal electrocardiograms recorded during labor and delivery. *American Journal of Obstetrics and Gynecology* **107**, 17.

30 McLintic A.J., Lilley S., Pringle S.D., Houston A.B. & Thorburn J. (1991) Electrocardiographic changes during Caesarean Section under regional anaesthesia. *International Journal of Obstetric Anesthesia* **1**, 55.

31 Hendricks S.K., Keroes J. & Katz M. (1986) Electrocardiographic changes associated with ritodrine-induced maternal tachycardia and hypokalaemia. *American Journal of Obstetrics and Gynecology* **154**, 921.

32 Rubler S., Schneebaum R. & Hammer N. (1973) Systolic time intervals in pregnancy and the postpartum period. *American Heart Journal* **86**, 182.

33 Burg J.R., Dodek A., Kloster F.E. & Metcalfe J. (1974) Alterations of systolic time intervals during pregnancy. *Circulation* **49**, 560.

34 Walters W.A.W. & Lim Y.L. (1975) Blood volume and haemodynamics in pregnancy. *Clinics in Obstetrics and Gynaecology* **2**, 310.

35 Hunter S. & Robson S.C. (1992) Adaptation of the maternal heart in pregnancy. *British Heart Journal* **68**, 540.

36 Burwell C.S. & Metcalfe J. (1958) *Heart Disease in Pregnancy: Physiology and Management.* J. & A. Churchill, London.

37 Hamilton H.F.H. (1949) The cardiac output in normal pregnancy: As determined by the Cournand right heart catheterisation technique. *Journal of Obstetrics and Gynaecology of the British Empire* **56**, 548.

38 Adams J.Q. (1954) Cardiovascular physiology in normal pregnancy: Studies with the dye dilution technique. *American Journal of Obstetrics and Gynecology* **67**, 741.

39 Palmer A.J. & Walker A.H.C. (1949) The maternal circulation in normal pregnancy. *Journal of Obstetrics and Gynaecology of the British Empire* **56**, 537.

40 Bader R.A., Bader M.E., Rose D.J. & Braunwald E. (1955) Haemodynamics at rest and during exercise in normal pregnancy as studied by cardiac catheterisation. *Journal of Clinical Investigation* **34**, 1524.

41 Walters W.A.W., MacGregor W.G. & Hills M. (1966) Cardiac output at rest during pregnancy and the puerperium. *Clinical Science* **30**, 1.

42 Werkö L. (1950) In *Studies in the Problems of Circulation in Pregnancy.* Eds J. Hammond, F.J. Browne & G.E.W. Wolstenholme, p. 155. Blakiston, Philadelphia.

43 Vorys N., Ullery J.C. & Hanusek G.E. (1961) The cardiac output changes in various positions in pregnancy. *American Journal of Obstetrics and Gynecology* **82**, 1312.

44 Kerr M.G., Scott D.B. & Samuel E. (1964) Studies of the inferior vena cava in late pregnancy. *British Medical Journal* **i**, 532.

45 Kerr M.G. (1965) The mechanical effects of the gravid uterus in late pregnancy. *Journal of Obstetrics and Gynaecology of the British Commonwealth* **72**, 513.

46 Lees M.M., Scott D.B., Kerr M.G. & Taylor S.H. (1967) The circulatory effects of recumbent postural change in late pregnancy. *Clinical Science* **32**, 453.

47 Blake S., Bonar F., Mecarrthy C. & McDonald D. (1983) The effect of posture on cardiac output in late pregnancy complicated by pericardial constriction. *American Journal of Obstetrics and Gynecology* **146**, 865.

48 Bieniarz J., Maqueda E. & Caldeyro-Barcia R. (1966) Compression of aorta by the uterus in late human pregnancy. I. Variations between femoral and brachial artery pressure with changes from hypertension to hypotension. *American Journal of Obstetrics and Gynecology* **95**, 795.

49 Pyörälä T. (1966) Cardiovascular response to the upright position during pregnancy. *Acta Obstetricia et Gynaecologia Scandinavica* **45** (suppl 5), 1.

50 Lees M.M., Taylor S.H., Scott D.B. & Kerr M.G. (1967) A study of cardiac output at rest throughout pregnancy. *Journal of Obstetrics and Gynaecology of the British Commonwealth* **74**, 319.

51 Ueland K., Novy M.J., Peterson E.N. & Metcalfe J. (1969) Maternal cardiovascular dynamics. IV. The influence of gestational age on the maternal cardiovascular response to posture and exercise. *American Journal of Obstetrics and Gynecology* **104**, 856.

52 Newman B., Derrington C. & Sore C. (1983) Cardiac output and the recumbent position in late pregnancy. *Anaesthesia* **38**, 332.

53 Rawles J.M., Schneider K.T.M., Huch R. & Huch A. (1987) The effect of position and delay on stroke and minute distance in late pregnancy. *British Journal of Obstetrics and Gynaecology* **94**, 507.

54 Clark S.L., Cotton D.B., Pivarnick J., Lee W., Hankins G.D., Benedetti T.J. & Phelan J.P. (1991) Position change and central hemodynamic profile during normal third-trimester pregnancy and post partum. *American Journal of Obstetrics and Gynecology* **164**, 883.

55 Schneider K.T.M., Bollinger A., Huch A. & Huch R. (1984) The oscillating 'vena cava syndrome' during quiet standing: An unexpected observation in late pregnancy. *British Journal of Obstetrics and Gynaecology* **91**, 766.

56 Blake S., O'Neill H. & MacDonald D. (1982) Haemodynamic effects of pregnancy in patients with heart failure. *British Heart Journal* **77**, 495.

57 Barron W.M., Mujais S.K., Zinaman M., Bravo E.L. & Lindheimer M. (1986) Plasma catecholamine responses to physiologic stimuli in normal human pregnancy. *American Journal of Obstetrics and Gynecology* **154**, 80.

58 Easterling T.R., Watts H., Schmucker B.C. & Benedetti T.J. (1987) Measurement of cardiac output during pregnancy: Validation of Doppler technique and clinical observations in preeclampsia. *Obstetrics and Gynecology* **69**, 845.

59 Easterling T.R., Carlson K.L., Schmucker B.C.,

64

Brateng D.A. & Benedetti T.J. (1990) Measurement of cardiac output in pregnancy by doppler technique. *American Journal of Perinatology* **7**, 220.

60 Robson S.C., Dunlop W., Boys R.J. & Hunter S. (1987) Cardiac output during labour. *British Medical Journal* **295**, 1169.

61 Robson S.C., Hunter S., Moore M. & Dunlop W. (1987) Haemodynamic changes during the puerperium: A Doppler and M-mode echocardiographic study. *British Journal of Obstetrics and Gynaecology* **94**, 1028.

62 Mabie W.C., DiSessa T.G., Crocker L.G., Sibai B.M. & Arheart K.L. (1994) A longitudinal study of cardiac output in normal human pregnancy. *American Journal of Obstetrics and Gynecology* **170**, 849.

63 Easterling T.R., Benedetti T.J., Schmucker B.C. & Millard S.P. (1990) Maternal hemodynamics in normal and preeclamptic pregnancies: A longitudinal study. *Obstetrics and Gynecology* **76**, 1061.

64 Katz R., Karliner J.S. & Resnik R. (1978) Effects of a natural volume overload state (pregnancy) on left ventricular performance in normal human subjects. *Circulation* **58**, 434.

65 McLennan F.M., Haites W.E. & Rawles J.M. (1987) Stroke and minute distance in pregnancy: A longtitudinal study using Doppler ultrasound. *British Journal of Obstetrics and Gynaecology* **94**, 499.

66 Hart M.V., Morton M.J., Hosenpud J.D. & Metcalfe J. (1986) Aortic function during normal pregnancy. *American Journal of Obstetrics and Gynecology* **154**, 887.

67 Spätling L., Fallenstein F., Huch A., Huch R. & Rooth G. (1992) The variability of cardio-pulmonary adaptation to pregnancy at rest and during exercise. *British Journal of Obstetrics and Gynaecology* **99** (Suppl. 8), 1.

68 Ward S.J. & Broughton Pipkin F. (1993) The variability of cardiopulmonary adaptation to pregnancy at rest and during exercise. *British Journal of Obstetrics and Gynaecology* **100**, 398.

69 Rovinsky J.J. & Jaffin H. (1966) Cardiovascular hemodynamics in pregnancy. II. Cardiac output and left ventricular work in multiple pregnancy. *American Journal of Obstetrics and Gynecology* **95**, 781.

70 Robson S.C., Hunter S., Boys R.J. & Dunlop W. (1989) Hemodynamic changes during twin pregnancy: A Doppler and M-mode echocardiographic study. *American Journal of Obstetrics and Gynecology* **161**, 1273.

71 Ueland K. & Hansen J.M. (1969) Maternal cardiovascular dynamics. II. Posture and uterine contractions. *American Journal of Obstetrics and Gynecology* **103**, 1.

72 Bleker O.P., Kloosterman G.J., Mieras D.J., Oosting J. & Sallé H.J.A. (1975) Intervillous space during uterine contractions in human subjects: an ultrasonic study. *American Journal of Obstetrics and Gynecology* **123**, 697.

73 Clark S.L., Phelan J.P., Greenspoon J., Aldahl D. & Hortenstein J. (1985) Labor and delivery in the presence of mitral stenosis: Central hemodynamic observations. *American Journal of Obstetrics and Gynecology* **8**, 984.

74 Newman B. (1982) Cardiac output changes during Caesarean section. *Anaesthesia* **37**, 270.

75 Robson S.C., Dunlop W., Hunter S., Boys R.J. & Bryson M. (1989) Haemodynamic changes associated with caesarean section under epidural anaesthesia. *British Journal of Obstetrics and Gynaecology* **96**, 642.

76 Robson S.C., Boys R.J., Hunter S. & Dunlop W. (1989) Maternal hemodynamics after normal delivery and delivery complicated by postpartum hemorrhage. *Obstetrics and Gynecology* **74**, 234.

77 Burwell C.S. (1938) The placenta as a modified arteriovenous fistula considered in relation to the circulatory adjustments to pregnancy. *American Journal of the Medical Sciences* **195**, 1.

78 Walters W.A.W. & Lim Y.L. (1970) Haemodynamic changes in women taking oral contraceptives. *Journal of Obstetrics and Gynaecology of the British Commonwealth* **77**, 1007.

79 Lehtovirta P. (1974) Haemodynamic effects of combined oestrogen/progestogen oral contraceptives. *Journal of Obstetrics and Gynaecology of the British Commonwealth* **81**, 517.

80 Slater A.J., Gude N., Clarke I.J. & Walters W.A.W. (1986) Haemodynamic changes in left ventricular performance during high-dose oestrogen administration in transsexuals. *British Journal of Obstetrics and Gynaecology* **93**, 532.

81 Phippard A.F., Horvath J.S., Glynn E.M., Garner M.G., Fletcher P.J., Duggin G.G. & Tiller D.J. (1986) Circulatory adaptation to pregnancy: Serial studies of haemodynamics, blood volume, renin and aldosterone in the baboon (*Papio hamadryas*). *Journal of Hypertension* **4**, 773.

82 Schrier R.W. (1992) A unifying hypothesis of body fluid volume regulation. *Journal of Royal College of Physicians of London* **26**, 295.

83 Schrier R.W. & Briner V.A. (1991) Peripheral arterial vasodilation hypothesis of sodium and water retention in pregnancy: Implications for pathogenesis of pre-eclampsia/eclampsia. *Obstetrics and Gynecology* **77**, 632.

84 Broughton Pipkin F. (1988) The renin angiotensin system in normal and hypertensive pregnancies. In *Hypertension in Pregnancy*. Ed. P.C. Rubin, p. 118. Elsevier, Amsterdam.

85 Vane J.R., Anggard E.E. & Botting R.M. (1990) Regulatory functions of the vascular endothelium. *New England Journal of Medicine* **323**, 27.

86 Broughton Pipkin F., Morrison R. & O'Brien P.M.S. (1987) The effect of prostaglandin E_1 upon the pressor and hormonal response to exogenous angiotensin II in human pregnancy. *Clinical Science* **72**, 351.

87 Stevenson J.C., MacDonald D.W.R., Warren R.C., Booker M.W. & Whitehead M.I. (1986) Increased concentration of circulating calcitonin gene related peptide during normal human pregnancy. *British Medical Journal* **294**, 1329.

88 Ware Branch D., Dudley D.J. & Mitchell M.D. (1991) Preliminary evidence for homoestatic mechanism regulating endothelin production in pre-eclampsia. *Lancet* **337**, 943.

89 Moncada S. & Higgs A. (1993) The L-arginine-nitric oxide pathway. *New England Journal of Medicine* **329**, 2002.

90 Morris N.H., Eaton B.M. & Dekker G. (1996) Nitric

oxide, the endothelium, pregnancy and pre-eclampsia. *British Journal of Obstetrics and Gynaecology* **103**, 4.

91 Hytten F.E. & Leitch I. (1971) *The Physiology of Human Pregnancy*, 2nd edn. Blackwell Scientific Publications, Oxford.

92 Clapp J.F. III (1985) Maternal heart rate in pregnancy. *American Journal of Obstetrics and Gynecology* **152**, 659.

93 Halligan A., O'Brien E., O'Malley K., Mee F., Atkins N., Conroy R., Walshe J. & Darling M. (1993) Twenty-four-hour ambulatory blood pressure measurement in a primigravid population. *Journal of Hypertension* **11**, 869.

94 Hubbard W.N., Jenkins B.A.G. & Ward D.E. (1983) Persistent atrial tachycardia in pregnancy. *British Medical Journal* **287**, 327.

95 Robson S.C., Dunlop W., Moore W. & Hunter S. (1987) Combined doppler and echocardiographic measurement of cardiac output: Theory and application in pregnancy. *British Journal of Obstetrics and Gynaecology* **94**, 1014.

96 Shouse E.E. & Acker J.E. (1964) Pregnancy and delivery in a patient with external–internal cardiac pacemaker. *Obstetrics and Gynecology* **24**, 817.

97 Bordley J., Connor C.A.R., Hamilton W.F., Kerr W.J. & Wiggers C.J. (1951) Recommendations for human blood pressure determinations by sphygmomanometer. *Circulation* **4**, 503.

98 Perry I.J., Wilkinson L.S., Shinton R.A. & Beevers D.G. (1991) Conflicting views on the measurement of blood pressure in pregnancy. *British Journal of Obstetrics and Gynaecology* **98**, 241.

99 Villar J., Repke J., Markush L., Calvert W. & Rhoads G. (1989) The measuring of blood pressure during pregnancy. *American Journal of Obstetrics and Gynecology* **161**, 1019.

100 King G.E. (1967) Errors in clinical measurement of blood pressure in obesity. *Clinical Science* **32**, 223.

101 Ginsburg J. & Duncan S. (1969) Direct and indirect blood pressure measurements in pregnancy. *Journal of Obstetrics and Gynaecology of the British Commonwealth* **76**, 705.

102 de Swiet M. (1991) Blood pressure measurement in pregnancy. *British Journal of Obstetrics and Gynaecology* **82**, 239.

103 Brown M.A. & Whitworth J.A. (1991) Recording diastolic blood pressure in pregnancy (letter). *British Medical Journal* **303**, 120.

104 Perry I.J., Stewart B.A., Brockwell J., Khan M., Davies P., Beevers D.G. & Luesley D.M. (1990) Recording diastolic blood pressure in pregnancy. *British Medical Journal* **301**, 1198.

105 Shennan A., Gupta M., Halligan A., Taylor D.J. & de Swiet M. (1996) Lack of reproducibility in pregnancy of Korotkoff phase IV as measured by mercury sphygmomanometry. *Lancet* **347**, 139.

106 de Swiet M. & Shennan A. (1996) Blood pressure measurement in pregnancy (Editorial). *British Journal of Obstetrics and Gynaecology* **103**, 862.

107 MacGillivray I. (1961) Hypertension in pregnancy and its consequences. *Journal of Obstetrics and Gynaecology of the British Commonwealth* **68**, 557.

108 Andros G.I. (1943) Blood pressure in normal pregnancy. *American Journal of Obstetrics and Gynecology* **50**, 300.

109 Schwarz R. (1964) Das Verhalten des Kreislaufs in der normalen Schwangershaft. I. Der arterielle Blutdruck. *Archiv für Gvnäkologie* **199**, 549.

110 MacGillivray I., Rose G.A. & Rowe B. (1969) Blood pressure survey in pregnancy. *Clinical Science* **37**, 395.

111 Howard B.K., Goodson J.H. & Mengert W.F. (1953) Supine hypotensive syndrome in late pregnancy. *Obstetrics and Gynecology* **1**, 371.

112 Serra Serra V., Chandran R. & Redman C.W.G. (1991) Abnormal transcranial doppler pattern in pregnant woman during orthostatic hypotension. *Lancet* **337**, 1296.

113 Pirhonen J.P. & Erkkola R.U. (1990) Uterine and umbilical flow velocity waveforms in the supine hypotensive syndrome. *Obstetrics and Gynecology* **76**, 176.

114 Quilligan E.J. & Tyler C. (1959) Postural effects on the cardiovascular status in pregnancy: A comparison of the lateral and supine postures. *American Journal of Obstetrics and Gynecology* **78**, 465.

115 Wright L. (1962) Postural hypotension in late pregnancy: 'The supine hypotensive syndrome'. *British Medical Journal* **i**, 760.

116 Scanlon M.F. (1974) Hypertension in pregnancy. *Journal of Obstetrics and Gynaecology of the British Commonwealth* **81**, 539.

117 Trower R. & Walters W.A.W. (1968) Brachial arterial blood pressure in the lateral recumbent position during pregnancy. *Australian and New Zealand Journal of Obstetrics and Gynaecology* **8**, 146.

118 Eskes T.K.A.B., Weyer A., Kramer N. & Van Elteren P. (1974) Arterial blood pressure and posture during pregnancy. *European Journal of Obstetrics, Gynaecology and Reproductive Biology* **4**, 87.

119 Naftalin A.A., Hart W.G. & Walters W.A.W. (1978) Blood pressure in the arm and leg in late pregnancy. *British Journal of Obstetrics and Gynaecology* **85**, 748.

120 Fleming S.E., Horvath J.S. & Korda A. (1983) Errors in the management of blood pressure. *Australian and New Zealand Journal of Obstetrics and Gynaecology* **23**, 136.

121 Kinsella S.M. & Spencer J.A.D. (1989) Blood pressure measurement in the lateral position. *British Journal of Obstetrics and Gynaecology* **96**, 1110.

122 Dame W.R., Bachour G., Bottcher H.D. & Beller F.K. (1977) Continuous monitoring of direct intra-arterial blood pressure in normal and preeclamptic pregnancies. *Geburtshilfe und Frauenheilkunde* **37**, 708.

123 Association for the Advancement of Medical Instrumentation (1987) *American National Standard for Electronic or Automated Sphygmomanometers.* Arlington, Virginia: American National Standard for Electronic or Automated Sphygmomanometers.

124 O'Brien E., Petrie J., Littler W.A., de Swiet M., Padfield P., Altman D., Atkins N., Bland A. & Coats A. (1993) First revision of the British Hypertension Society protocol for the evaluation of automated and semi-automated blood pressure measuring devices with special references to ambulatory systems. *Journal of Hypertension* (Suppl.), 543.

66

125 Quinn M. (1994) Automated blood pressure measurement devices: A potential source of morbidity in preeclampsia? *American Journal of Obstetrics and Gynecology* **170**, 1303.

126 Clark S.L., Justus Hofmeyr G., Coats A.J.S. & Redman C.W.G. (1991) Ambulatory blood pressure monitoring during pregnancy: Validation of the TM-2420. *Obstetrics and Gynecology* **77**, 152.

127 Shennan A., Kissane J. & de Swiet M. (1993) Validation of the SpaceLabs 90207 ambulatory blood pressure monitor for use in pregnancy. *British Journal of Obstetrics and Gynaecology* **100**, 904.

128 Shennan A., Halligan A., Gupta M., Taylor D.J. & de Swiet M. (1996) Oscillometric blood pressure measurements in severe pre-eclampsia: validation of the SpaceLabs 90207. *British Journal of Obstetrics and Gynaecology* **103**, 171.

129 Ramsay M.M., Broughton Pipkin F. & Rubin P.C. (1993) Pressor, heart rate and plasma catecholamine responses to noradrenaline in pregnant and non-pregnant women. *British Journal of Obstetrics and Gynaecology* **100**, 170.

130 Ekholm E.M.K., Piha S.J., Antila K.J. & Erkkola R.U. (1993) Cardiovascular autonomic reflexes in mid-pregnancy. *British Journal of Obstetrics and Gynaecology* **100**, 177.

131 Sakai K., Maeda H., Tsukimori K. & Nagata H. (1992) How blood viscosity influences changes in circulation during pregnancy? *Fukuoka Igaku Zasshi* **83**, 328.

132 Thomson K.J., Hirsheimer A., Gibson J.G. & Evans W.A. (1938) Studies on the circulation in pregnancy. III. Blood volume changes in normal pregnant women. *American Journal of Obstetrics and Gynecology* **36**, 48.

133 Bickers W. (1942) The placenta: a modified arteriovenous fistula. *Southern Medical Journal* **35**, 593.

134 McLennan C.E. (1943) Antecubital and femoral venous pressure in normal and toxemic pregnancy. *American Journal of Obstetrics and Gynecology* **45**, 568.

135 Clark S.L., Cotton D.B., Lee W., Bishop C., Hill T., Southwick J. & Pivarnick J. (1989) Central hemodynamic assessment of normal term pregnancy. *American Journal of Obstetrics and Gynecology* **161**, 1439.

136 Colditz R.B. & Josey W.E. (1970) Central venous pressure in supine normal position during normal pregnancy. *Obstetrics and Gynecology* **36**, 769.

137 Ferris E.B. & Wilkins R.W. (1937) The clinical value of comparative measurements of the pressure in the femoral and cubital veins. *American Heart Journal* **13**, 431.

138 Scott D.B. & Kerr M.G. (1963) Inferior vena caval pressure in late pregnancy. *Journal of Obstetrics and Gynaecology of the British Commonwealth* **70**, 1044.

139 Wright H.P., Osborn S.B. & Edmonds D.G. (1950) Changes in the rate of flow of venous blood in the leg during pregnancy, measured with radioactive sodium. *Surgery, Gynecology and Obstetrics* **90**, 481.

140 McCausland A.M., Hyman C., Winsor T. & Trotter A.D. (1961) Venous distensibility during pregnancy. *American Journal of Obstetrics and Gynecology* **81**, 472.

141 Goodrich S.M. & Wood J.E. (1964) Peripheral venous distensibility and velocity of venous blood flow during pregnancy or during oral contraceptive therapy. *American Journal of Obstetrics and Gynecology* **90**, 740.

142 Sakai K., Imaizumi T., Maeda H., Tsukimori K., Takeshita A. & Nakano H. (1994) Venous distensibility during pregnancy: Comparisons between normal pregnancy and preeclampsia. *Hypertension* **24**, 461.

143 Duncan S.L.B. (1967) Forearm venous tone in pregnancy. *Journal of Physiology* **191**, 122P.

144 Sandström B. & Löwegren L. (1970) Phlebographic studies of the leg veins in the first half of pregnancy and during oral contraception. *Acta Obstetricia et Gynaecologica Scandinavica* **49**, 375.

145 Sandström B. (1974) Plethsonographic studies of venous volume in the lower legs during normal primipregnancy. *Acta Obstetricia et Gynaecologica Scandinavica* **53**, 97.

146 Veal J.R. & Hussey H.H. (1941) The venous circulation in the lower extremities during pregnancy. *Surgery, Gynecology and Obstetrics* **72**, 841.

147 Thomson A.M., Hytten F.E. & Billewicz W.Z. (1967) The epidemiology of oedema during pregnancy. *Journal of Obstetrics and Gynaecology of the British Commonwealth* **74**, 1.

148 Robertson E.G. (1971) The natural history of oedema during pregnancy. *Journal of Obstetrics and Gynaecology of the British Commonwealth* **78**, 520.

149 Hytten F.E. & Taggart N. (1967) Limb volumes in pregnancy. *Journal of Obstetrics and Gynaecology of the British Commonwealth* **74**, 663.

150 Starling E.H. (1909) *The Fluids of the Body*. Constable, London.

151 Theobald G.W. & Lundborg R.A. (1963) Changes in limb volume and in venous infusion pressures caused by pregnancy. *Journal of Obstetrics and Gynaecology of the British Commonwealth* **70**, 408.

152 Øian P., Malthau J.M., Noddeland H. & Fadnes H.O. (1985) Oedema-preventing mechanisms in subcutaneous tissue of normal pregnant women. *British Journal of Obstetrics and Gynaecology* **92**, 113.

153 Maclennan F.M. (1986) Maternal mortality from Mendelson's syndrome: An explanation. *Lancet* **i**, 587.

154 Spetz S. (1965) Capillary filtration during normal pregnancy. *Acta Obstetricia et Gynaecologica Scandinavica* **44**, 227.

155 Bungum L., Tollan A. & Øian P. (1990) Antepartum to postpartum changes in transcapillary fluid balance. *British Journal of Obstetrics and Gynaecology* **97**, 838.

156 Hunyor S.N., McEniery P.T., Roberts K.A., Bellamy G.R., Roffe D.J., Gallery E.D.M., Gyory A.Z. & Boyce E.S. (1983) Capillary permeability in normal and hypertensive human pregnancy. *Clinical and Experimental Pharmacology and Physiology* **10**, 345.

157 Gonik B., Cotton D., Spillman T., Abouleish E. & Zavisca F. (1985) Peripartum colloid osmotic pressure changes: Effects of controlled fluid management. *American Journal of Obstetrics and Gynecology* **151**, 812.

158 Gonik B. & Cotton D.B. (1982) Peripartum colloid osmotic pressure changes: Influence of intravenous

hydration. *American Journal of Obstetrics and Gynecology* **150**, 99.

159 Cotton D.B., Gonik B., Spillman T. & Dorman K.F. (1984) Intrapartum to postpartum changes in colloid osmotic pressure. *American Journal of Obstetrics and Gynecology* **149**, 174.

160 Stein L., Beraud J.J., Morisette M., Daluz P., Weil M.H. & Shubin H. (1975) Pulmonary edema during volume infusion. *Circulation* **52**, 483.

161 Rackow E.C., Fein A.I. & Lippo J. (1977) Colloid osmotic pressure as a prognostic indicator of pulmonary edema and mortality in the critically ill. *Chest* **72**, 709.

162 Angelino P.F., Actis-Dato A., Levi V., Siliquini P.N. & Revelli E. (1954) Nuovi concetti de emodinamica in gravidanza da indavine con cateterismo angiocardiaco. *Minerva Ginecologica* **6**, 517.

163 Robson S.C., Hunter S., Boys R.J. & Dunlop W. (1991) Serial changes in pulmonary haemodynamics during human pregnancy: A non-invasive study using Doppler echocardiography. *Clinical Science* **80**, 113.

164 Morgan Jones A. (1965) Eisenmenger syndrome in pregnancy. *British Medical Journal* **i**, 1627.

165 Wood P. (1958) The Eisenmenger syndrome or pulmonary hypertension with reversed central shunt. *British Medical Journal* **ii**, 701, 755.

166 Lachelin G.C.L. (1975) The Eisenmenger syndrome and pregnancy. *European Journal of Obstetrics, Gynecology and Reproductive Biology* **5**, 187.

167 Littler W.A., Redman C.W.G., Bonnar J., Beilen L.J. & Lee G. de J. (1973) Reduced pulmonary arterial compliance in hypertensive pregnancy. *Lancet* **i**, 1274.

168 Lagerlöf H., Werkö L., Bucht H. & Holmgren A. (1949) Separate determination of the blood volume of the right and left heart and the lungs in man with the aid of the dye injection method. *Scandinavian Journal of Clinical and Laboratory Investigation* **7**, 114.

169 Gazioglu K., Kaltreider N.L., Rosen M. & Yu P.N. (1970) Pulmonary function during pregnancy in normal women and in patients with cardiopulmonary disease. *Thorax* **25**, 445.

170 Spitzer W. (1933) Die Blutströmungsgeschwindigkeit in normaler und gestörter Schwangershaft, Beitrag zur Funktionsprüfung des Herzens in der Schwangerschaft und vor der Geburt. *Archiv für Gynäkologie* **154**, 449.

171 Greenstein N.M. & Clahr J. (1937) Circulation time studies in pregnant women. *American Journal of Obstetrics and Gynecology* **33**, 414.

172 Manchester B. & Loube S.D. (1946) The velocity of blood flow in normal pregnant women. *American Heart Journal* **32**, 215.

173 Assali N.S., Rauramo L. & Peltonen T. (1960) Uterine and fetal blood flow and oxygen consumption in early human pregnancy. *American Journal of Obstetrics and Gynecology* **79**, 86.

174 Kety S. & Schmidt C.F. (1948) The nitrous oxide method for the quantitative determination of cerebral blood flow in man: Theory, procedure and normal values. *Journal of Clinical Investigation* **27**, 476.

175 Assali N.S., Douglass R.A., Baird W.W., Nicholson D.B. & Suyemoto R. (1953) Measurement of uterine blood flow and uterine metabolism. II. The techniques of catheterisation and cannulation of the uterine veins and sampling of arterial and venous blood in pregnant women. *American Journal of Obstetrics and Gynecology* **66**, 11.

176 Romney S.L., Reid D.E., Metcalfe J. & Burwell C.S. (1955) Oxygen utilisation by the human fetus *in utero*. *American Journal of Obstetrics and Gynecology* **70**, 791.

177 Huckabee W.E. (1962) Uterine blood flow. *American Journal of Obstetrics and Gynecology* **84**, 1623.

178 Browne J.C.M. & Veall N. (1953) The maternal placental blood flow in normotensive and hypertensive women. *Journal of Obstetrics and Gynaecology of the British Empire* **60**, 141.

179 Lysgaard H. & Lefèvre H. (1966) A new method of determining myometrial blood flow in pregnancy with Xenon[133]. *Acta Obstetricia et Gynaecologica Scandinavica* **45** (suppl 9), 84.

180 Clavero J.A., Negueruela J., Oritz L., De Los Heros J.A. & Modrego S.P. (1973) Blood flow in the intervillous space and fetal blood flow. I. Normal values in human pregnancies at term. *American Journal of Obstetrics and Gynecology* **116**, 340.

181 Forssman L. (1975) Methods of calculating uterine blood flow from the wash-out curves of intra-arterial and local injections of 133Xenon. *Acta Obstetricia et Gynaecologica Scandinavica* **54**, 479.

182 Fuchs F., Spackman T. & Assali N.S. (1963) Complexity and non-homogeneity of the intervillous space. *American Journal of Obstetrics and Gynecology* **86**, 226.

183 Prill H.J. & Götz F. (1961) Blood flow in the myometrium and endometrium of the uterus. *American Journal of Obstetrics and Gynecology* **82**, 102.

184 Brotánek V., Kazda S. & Roth L. (1962) A method for studying uterine blood flow in pregnant women. *Physiologia Bohemoslovenica* **11**, 358.

185 Palmer S.K., Zamudio S., Coffin C., Parker S., Stamm E. & Moore L.G. (1992) Quantitative estimation of human uterine artery blood flow and pelvic blood flow redistribution in pregnancy. *Obstetrics and Gynecology* **80**, 1000.

186 Thoresen M. & Wesche J. (1988) Doppler measurements of changes in human mammary and uterine blood flow during pregnancy and lactation. *Acta Obstretricia et Gynaecologica Scandinavica* **67**, 741.

187 Thaler I., Manor D., Itskovitz J., Rottem S., Levit N., Timor-Tritsch I. & Brandes J.M. (1990) Changes in uterine blood flow during human pregnancy. *American Journal of Obstetrics and Gynecology* **162**, 121.

188 Ramsey E.M. (1959) Vascular anatomy of the uteroplacental and foetal circulation. In *Oxygen Supply to the Human Foetus*. Eds J. Walker & A.C. Turnbull, Blackwell Scientific Publications, Oxford.

189 Ramsey E.M., Corner G.W., Long W.N. & Stran N.M. (1959) Studies of amniotic fluid and intervillous space pressures in the rhesus monkey. *American Journal of Obstetrics and Gynecology* **77**, 1016.

190 Freese V.E. (1972) Vascular relations of placental exchange areas in primates and man. In *Respiratory Gas Exchange and Blood Flow in the Placenta*. Eds L.D. Longo and H. Bortels, p. 73. U.S. Department of

68

Health Education and Welfare Publication No. NIH, Washington, D.C.

191 Burchell R.C. (1967) Arterial blood flow into the human intervillous space. *American Journal of Obstetrics and Gynecology* **98**, 303.

192 Alvarez H. & Caldeyro-Barcia R. (1954) Fisiopatologia de la contraccion uterina y sus aplicaciones en la clinica obstetrica. *Segundo Congreso Latino Americano de Obstetrica y Ginecologia, Facultad de Medicina de Montevideo.*

193 Prystowsky H. (1958) Fetal blood studies. VIII. Some observations on the transient fetal bradycardia accompanying uterine contractions in the human. *Bulletin of the Johns Hopkins Hospital* **102**, 1.

194 Hellman L.M., Tricomi V. & Gupta O. (1957) Pressures in the human amniotic fluid and intervillous space. *American Journal of Obstetrics and Gynecology* **74**, 1018.

195 Hendricks C.H. (1958) The hemodynamics of a uterine contraction. *American Journal of Obstetrics and Gynecology* **76**, 969.

196 Lees M.M., Scott D.B. & Kerr M.G. (1970) Haemodynamic changes associated with labour. *Journal of Obstetrics and Gynaecology of the British Commonwealth* **77**, 29.

197 Heckel G.P. & Tobin C.E. (1956) Arteriovenous shunts in the myometrium. *American Journal of Obstetrics and Gynecology* **71**, 199.

198 Brosens I., Robertson W.B. & Dixon H.G. (1967) The physiological response of the vessels of the placental bed to normal pregnancy. *Journal of Pathology and Bacteriology* **93**, 569.

199 Greiss F.C. (1966) Pressure–flow relationships in the gravid uterine vascular bed. *American Journal of Obstetrics and Gynecology* **96**, 41.

200 Greiss F.C. (1972) Differential reactivity of the myometrial and placental vasculatures: Adrenergic responses. *American Journal of Obstetrics and Gynecology* **112**, 20.

201 Toth P., Li X., Rao C.V., Lincoln S.R., Sanfilippo J.S., Spinnato J.A. & Yussman M.A. (1994) Expression of functional human chorionic gondatrophin/human luteinizing hormone receptor gene in human uterine arteries. *Journal of Clinical Endocrinology and Metabolism* **79**, 307.

202 Ekesbo R., Alm P., Ekstrom P., Lundberg L.M. & Akerlund, M. (1991) Innervation of the human uterine artery and contractile responses to neuropeptides. *Gynecologic and Obstetric Investigation* **31**, 30.

203 Fried G. & Samuelson U. (1991) Endothelin and neuropeptide Y are vasoconstrictors in human uterine blood vessels. *American Journal of Obstetrics and Gynecology* **164**, 1330.

204 Ekstrom P., Alm P. & Akerlund M. (1991) Differences in vasomotor responses between main stem and smaller branches of the human uterine artery. *Acta Obstetricia et Gynecologica Scandinavica* **70**, 429.

205 Barcroft H. & Edholm O.G. (1945) Temperature and blood flow in the human forearm. *Journal of Physiology* **104**, 366.

206 Abramson D.I., Flachs K. & Fierst S.M. (1943) Peripheral blood flow during gestation. *American Journal of Obstetrics and Gynecology* **45**, 666.

207 Burt C.C. (1950) The peripheral circulation in pregnancy. *Edinburgh Medical Journal* **57**, Trans 18.

208 Ginsburg J. & Duncan S.L.B. (1967) Peripheral blood flow in normal pregnancy. *Cardiovascular Research* **1**, 132.

209 Burt C.C. (1949) Peripheral skin temperature in normal pregnancy. *Lancet* **ii**, 787.

210 Herbert C.M., Banner E.A. & Wakim K.G. (1958) Variations in the peripheral circulation during pregnancy. *American Journal of Obstetrics and Gynecology* **76**, 742.

211 Ashton H. (1975) Cigarette smoking in pregnancy: Differences in peripheral circulation between smokers and nonsmokers. *British Journal of Obstetrics and Gynaecology* **82**, 868.

212 MacGregor W.G. & Snodgrass C.A. (1970) Measurement of forearm blood flow in pregnancy and the puerperium. *International Journal of Gynaecology and Obstetrics* **8**, 257.

213 Drummond G.B., Scott S.E.H., Lees M.M. & Scott D.B. (1974) Effects of posture on limb blood flow in late pregnancy. *British Medical Journal* **ii**, 587.

214 Spetz S. (1964) Peripheral circulation during normal pregnancy. *Acta Obstetricia et Gynaecologica Scandinavica* **43**, 309.

215 Spetz S. & Jansson I. (1969) Forearm blood flow during normal pregnancy studied by venous occlusion plethysmography and [133]Xenon muscle clearance. *Acta Obstetricia et Gynaecologica Scandinavica* **48**, 285.

216 Sandström B. (1973) Calf blood flow during normal primipregnancy. *Acta Obstetricia et Gynaecologica Scandinavica* **52**, 199.

217 Tur E., Tamir A. & Guy R.H. (1992) Cutaneous blood flow in gestational hypertension and normal pregnancy. *Journal of Investigative Dermatology* **99**, 310.

218 Melbard S.M. (1938) Valeur diagnostique de la capillaroscopie dans la grossesse et dans la sepsie puerpérale. *Gynécologie et Obstétrique* **37**, 200.

219 Bean W.G., Dexter M.W. & Cogswell R.C. (1947) Vascular spiders and palmar erythema in pregnancy. *Journal of Clinical Investigation* **26**, 1173.

220 Barter R.H., Letterman G.S. & Schurter M. (1963) Hemangiomas in pregnancy. *American Journal of Obstetrics and Gynecology* **87**, 625.

221 Raynaud M. (1862) *On Local Asphyxia and Symmetrical Gangrene of the Extremities* (Trans. T. Barlow), p. 1888. New Sydenham Society, London.

222 Hillman R.W. (1960) Fingernail growth in pregnancy: Relations to some common parameters of the reproductive process. *Human Biology* **32**, 119.

223 Trotter M. (1935) Activity of hair follicles with reference to pregnancy. *Surgery, Gynecology and Obstetrics* **60**, 1092.

224 Lynfield Y.L. (1960) Effect of pregnancy on the human hair cycle. *Journal of Investigative Dermatology* **35**, 323.

225 Fabricant N.D. (1960) Sexual functions and the nose. *American Journal of the Medical Sciences* **239**, 498.

226 Scott J.H. (1954) Heat-regulating function of the nasal mucous membrane. *Journal of Laryangology and Otology* **65**, 308.

227 Munnell E.W. & Taylor H.C. (1947) Liver blood flow

in pregnancy: Hepatic vein catheterization. *Journal of Clinical Investigation* **26**, 952.

228 Laakso L., Ruotsalainen P., Punnonen R. & Maatela J. (1971) Hepatic blood flow in late pregnancy. *Acta Obstetricia et Gynaecologica Scandinavica* **50**, 175.

229 Robson S.C., Mutch E., Boys R.J. & Woodhouse K.W. (1990) Apparent liver blood flow during pregnancy: A serial study using indocyanine green clearance. *British Journal of Obstetrics and Gynaecology* **97**, 720.

230 Tindall V.R. (1975) The liver in pregnancy. *Clinics in Obstetrics and Gynaecology* **2**, 441.

231 McCall M.L. (1949) Cerebral blood flow and metabolism in toxemias of pregnancy. *Surgery, Gynecology and Obstetrics* **89**, 715.

232 Kyle P.M., de Swiet M., Buckley D., Serra Serra V. & Redman C.W.G. (1993) Noninvasive assessment of the maternal cerebral circulation by transcranial Doppler ultrasound during angiotensin II infusion. *British Journal of Obstetrics and Gynaecology* **100**, 85.

233 Sheehan H.L. & Falkiner N.M. (1948) Splenic aneurysm and splenic enlargement in pregnancy. *British Medical Journal* **ii**, 1105.

234 Sparkman R.S. (1958) Rupture of the spleen in pregnancy. *American Journal of Obstetrics and Gynecology* **76**, 587.

235 Doležal A. & Figar S. (1965) The phenomenon of reactive vasodilation in pregnancy. *American Journal of Obstetrics and Gynecology* **93**, 1137.

236 Schwartz R. & Retzke U. (1968) Untersuchungen über die Kreislaufwirkung von Angiotensin II in der normalen Schwangershaft. *Zeitschrift für Kreislaufforschung* **57**, 1015.

237 Gant N.F., Daley G.L., Chand S., Whalley P.J. & MacDonald P.C. (1973) A study of angiotensin II pressor response throughout primigravid pregnancy. *Journal of Clinical Investigation* **52**, 2682.

238 Gant N.F., Chand S., Whalley P.J. & MacDonald P.C. (1974) The nature of pressor responsiveness to angiotensin II in human pregnancy. *Obstetrics and Gynecology* **43**, 854.

239 Hettiaratchi E.S.C. & Pickford M. (1968) The effect of oestrogen and progesterone on the pressor action of angiotensin in the rat. *Journal of Physiology* **196**, 447.

240 Lloyd S. & Pickford M. (1961) The action of posterior pituitary hormones and oestrogens on the vascular system of the rat. *Journal of Physiology* **155**, 161.

241 Tacchi D. (1960) The response of the bulbar conjuctival vascular bed to humoral stimuli. *Journal of Obstetrics and Gynaecology of the British Commonwealth* **67**, 966.

242 Assali N.S., Vergon J.M., Tada Y. & Garber S.T. (1952) Studies on autonomic blockade VI. The mechanisms regulating the hemodynamic changes in the pregnant woman and their relation to the hypertension of toxemia of pregnancy. *American Journal of Obstetrics and Gynecology* **63**, 978.

243 Zakharieva E.K. & Sigler J.J.G. (1963) Maternidad y deporte. *Toko-ginecologia práctica* **22**, 144.

244 Erkkola R. (1976) The influence of physical training during pregnancy on physical work capacity and circulatory parameters. *Scandinavian Journal of Clinical and Laboratory Investigation* **36**, 747.

245 Guzman C.A. & Caplan R. (1970) Cardiorespiratory response to exercise during pregnancy. *American Journal of Obstetrics and Gynecology* **108**, 600.

246 Ueland K., Novy M.J. & Metcalfe S. (1972) Hemodynamic responses of patients with heart disease to pregnancy and exercise. *American Journal of Obstetrics and Gynecology* **113**, 47.

247 Morton M.J., Paul M.S., Campos G.R., Hart M.V. & Metcalfe J. (1985) Exercise dynamics in late gestation: Effects of physical training. *American Journal of Obstetrics and Gynecology* **152**, 91.

248 Van Hook J.W., Gill P., Easterling T.R., Schmucker B., Carlson K. & Benedetti T.J. (1993) The hemodynamic effects of isometric exercise during late normal pregnancy. *American Journal of Obstetrics and Gynecology* **169**, 870.

249 Pijpers L., Wladimiroff J.W. & McGhie J. (1984) Effect of short-term maternal exercise on maternal and fetal cardiovascualr dynamics. *British Journal of Obstetrics and Gynaecology* **91**, 1081.

250 Pomerance J.J., Gluck L. & Lynch V.A. (1974) Maternal exercise as a screening test for uteroplacental insufficiency. *Obstetrics and Gynecology* **44**, 383.

251 Pomerance J.J., Gluck L. & Lynch V.A. (1974) Physical fitness in pregnancy: Its effect on pregnancy outcome. *American Journal of Obstetrics and Gynecology* **119**, 867.

252 Hackett G.A., Cohen-Overbeek T. & Campbell S. (1992) The effect of exercise on uteroplacental Doppler waveforms in normal and complicated pregnancies. *Obstetrics and Gynecology* **79**, 919.

253 Hamilton H.F.H. (1951) Cardiac output in hypertensive toxaemias of pregnancy. *Journal of Obstetrics and Gynaecology of the British Empire* **58**, 977.

254 Assali N.S., Holm L.W. & Parker H.R. (1964) Systemic and regional hemodynamic alterations in toxemia. *Circulation* **30** (Suppl. 2), 53.

255 Freund K., French W., Carlson R.W., Weil M.H. & Shubin H. (1977) Hemodynamic and metabolic studies of a case of toxemia of pregnancy. *American Journal of Obstetrics and Gynecology* **127**, 206.

256 Belfort M., Uys P., Dommisse J. & Davey D.A. (1989) Haemodynamic changes in gestational proteinuric hypertension: The effects of rapid volume expansion and vasodilator therapy. *British Journal of Obstetrics and Gynaecology* **96**, 634.

257 Wallenburg H.C.S. (1988) Hemodynamics in hypertensive pregnancy. In *Handbook of Hypertension.* Ed. P.C. Rubin, p. 66. Amsterdam, Elsevier.

258 Kyle P.M., Buckley D., Kissane J., de Swiet M. & Redman C.W.G. (1995) The angiotensin sensitivity test and low-dose aspirin are ineffective methods to predict and prevent hypertensive disorders in nulliparous pregnancy. *American Journal of Obstetrics and Gynecology* **173**, 865.

259 Littler W.A., Redman C.W.G., Bonnar J., Berkin L.S. & Lee G. de J. (1973) Reduced pulmonary arterial compliance in hypertensive pregnancy. *Lancet* **i**, 1274.

260 Templeton A.A. & Kelman G.R. (1977) Arterial blood gases in pre-eclampsia. *British Journal of Obstetrics and Gynaecology* **84**, 290.

70

261 Arias F. (1975) Expansion of intravascular volume and fetal outcome in patients with chronic hypertension and pregnancy. *American Journal of Obstetrics and Gynecology* **123**, 610.

262 Brown M.A., Zammit V.C. and Lowe S.A. (1989) Capillary permeability and extracellular fluid volumes in pregnancy-induced hypertension. *Clinical Science* **77**, 599.

263 Murphy J.F., O'Riordan J., Newcombe R.G., Coles E.C. & Pearson J.F. (1986) Relation of haemoglobin levels in first and second trimesters to outcome of pregnancy. *Lancet* **i**, 992.

264 Hamilton H.F.H. (1950) Blood viscosity in pregnancy. *Journal of Obstetrics and Gynaecology of the British Empire* **57**, 530.

265 Engelmann F. (1916) Über weitere Erfahrungen mit der 'Therapie der mittleren Linie' bei der Eklampsiebehandlung. *Zentralblatt für Gynäkologie* **40**, 617. Cited by Chesley, L.C. (1978) in *Hypertensive Disorders in Pregnancy*. Appleton-Century-Crofts, New York.

266 Delacretaz E., de Quay N., Waeber B., Vial Y., Schulz P.E., Burnier M., Brunner H.R., Bossart H. & Schaad N.C. (1995) Differential nitric oxide synthase activity in human platelets during normal pregnancy and pre-eclampsia. *Clinical Science* **88**, 607.

267 Beilin L.J., Croft K.D., Michael C.A., Ritchie J., Schmidt L., Vandongen R. & Walters B.N.J. (1993) Neutrophil platelet-activating factor in normal and hypertensive pregnancy and in pregnancy-induced hypertension. *Clinical Science* **85**, 63.

268 Benigni A., Orisio S. & Gaspari F. (1992) Evidence against a pathogenetic role for endothelin in pre-eclampsia. *British Journal of Obstetrics and Gynaecology* **99**, 798.

269 Bromage P.R. (1978) *Epidural Analgesia*. W.B. Saunders, Philadelphia.

270 Wiederman M.P. (1963) Dimensions of blood vessels from distributing artery to collecting vein. *Circulation Research* **12**, 375.

271 Ueland K., Gills R. & Hansen J.M. (1968) Maternal cardiovascular dynamics. I. Cesarean section under subarachnoid block anaethesia. *American Journal of Obstetrics and Gynecology* **100**, 42.

272 Robson S.C., Boys R.J., Rodeck C. & Morgan B. (1991) Haemodynamic changes during epidural and spinal anaesthesia for elective caesarean section: correlation with umbilical artery pH. *Journal of Obstetrics and Gynaecology* **11**, 301.

273 Crawford J.S. (1972) *Principles and Practice of Obstetric Anaesthesia*, 3rd edn, p. 179. Blackwell Scientific Publications, Oxford.

274 Morales-Aguilerá A. & Vaughan Williams E.M. (1965) The effects on cardiac muscle of beta-receptor antagonists in relation to their activity as local anaesthetics. *British Journal of Pharmacology* **24**, 332.

275 Bieniarz J., Crottogini J.J., Curuchet E., Romero-Salinas G., Yoshida T., Poseiro J.J. & Caldeyro-Barcia R. (1968) Aortocaval compression by the uterus in late human pregnancy. II. An arteriographic study. *American Journal of Obstetrics and Gynecology* **100**, 203.

276 Crawford J.S., Burton M. & Davies P. (1972) Time and lateral tilt at Caesarean section. *British Journal of Anaesthesia* **44**, 477.

277 Woolman S.B. & Marx G.F. (1968) Acute hydration for prevention of hypotension of spinal anaesthesia in parturients. *Anaesthesiology* **29**, 374.

278 Ralston D.H., Shnider S.M. & Lorimer A.A. (1974) Effects of equipotent ephedrine, Metaraminol, Mephentermine and Methoxamine on uterine blood flow in the pregnant ewe. *Anesthesiology* **40**, 354.

The Haematological System

ELIZABETH A. LETSKY

The physiological changes in the circulating blood during pregnancy and the puerperium are marked and show wide variations. It is not possible to assess accurately the haematological status of pregnant women by criteria used for males and non-pregnant females.

The dramatic changes in whole blood volume which affect haemoglobin, red-cell indices and the metabolism of haematinics are considered in Chapter 2. The haemostatic mechanisms show profound alterations compared with the non-pregnant state.

Blood volume

Plasma volume and total red-cell mass are under separate control and bear no fixed relation to one another. Changes in pregnancy provide a dramatic illustration of this point [1].

Both the major components of blood, the red cells and the plasma may be measured by methods based on the dilution principle. Without doubt the best estimate of total blood volume is obtained when plasma volume and red-cell mass are measured simultaneously, but the two measurements are rarely made together. The majority of published reports of blood vol-

ume in pregnancy are based either on measured plasma volume or red-cell volume, the fraction not directly estimated then being calculated from the haematocrit. It is essential that physiological conditions and methods are standardized if measurements from different subjects and from different times in the same subject are to be comparable [2]. The subject is considered in Chapter 2.

In summary, healthy women in a normal first pregnancy increase their plasma volume from a non-pregnant level of about 2600 ml by about 1250 ml. In subsequent pregnancies the increase is greater and may be about 1500 ml. Most of the rise takes place before 32–34 weeks' gestation, and thereafter there is relatively little change. The increase is related to the size of the fetus, and there are particularly large increases in plasma volume associated with multiple pregnancy.

Red-cell mass

The red-cell mass expressed in units of volume is a confusing term which represents the total volume of red cells in the circulation. The more logical alternative of red-cell volume is not used

72 because of its specific meaning in haematology of the volume of a single erythrocyte.

There is less published information on red-cell mass than plasma volume and the results are more variable. The earliest method of measuring erythrocyte mass was by labelling haemoglobin with carbon monoxide (CO), which also attaches itself to myoglobin and other body pigments and crosses the placenta so that measurement overestimates maternal red-cell mass by 12–16%. Radioactive labels suitable for red cells became available in the 1940s and the use of CO as a label has disappeared.

Radioactive isotopes of iron, ^{55}Fe and ^{59}Fe, are unsuitable for use in pregnancy both because donor cells must be labelled *in vivo* and because of the hazard of a long-lived source of radiation (^{55}Fe has a half-life of nearly 3 years, ^{59}Fe of 45 days, and they will be transferred to the fetus). The most popular technique is the in-vitro labelling of a sample of the subject's own cells with ^{51}Cr [3–5], or, less frequently, with ^{32}P [6].

There is still disagreement as to how much the red-cell mass increases in normal pregnancy. The extent of the increase is considerably influenced by iron medication which will cause the red-cell mass to rise further in apparently healthy women with no clinical evidence of iron deficiency. The published data are so unsatisfactory that it is not possible to single out any study as a firm basis for discussion—a summary of the earlier literature is set out in detail by Hytten and Leitch [7]. More recent studies continue to add to the controversies and confusion mainly because of the extrapolation of haemoglobin concentrations to reflect red-cell mass. In iron-replete pregnancy, the haemoglobin concentration is dependent largely on the plasma volume increase which is under separate control and directly reflects healthy reproduction. This had led to high haemoglobin concentrations being associated with poor outcome [8,9].

If one accepts, from those studies where direct estimates were made with labelled red cells, a figure of about 1400 ml for the quantity of red cells in the average healthy woman before pregnancy, then in round figures the rise in pregnancy for women not given iron medication is about 240 ml (18%) and for those given iron about 400 ml (30%). It is not possible from the available data to determine the shape of the curve of increase, but it is probably linear from about the end of the first trimester to term. As with plasma volume, the extent of the increase is likely to be related to the size of the conceptus. The mean red-cell mass in eight women with twins at 37–40 weeks was 2127 ml, 902 ml above the control volume [10]. A woman with quadruplets [11] had a red-cell mass at 34 weeks of 2795 ml — 1005 ml above her non-pregnant value (see Fig. 3.1).

Nothing is known about the effects of such variables as age, parity and other maternal char-

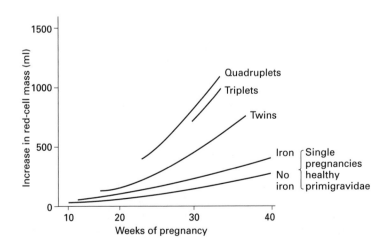

Fig. 3.1. Red-cell mass in single and multiple pregnancies.

acteristics on the increase in red-cell mass and large scope remains for careful research in this field, particularly with relation to iron status.

Changes in blood volume at parturition and during the puerperium

Dramatic changes in maternal blood volume occur at delivery whether *per vaginam* or by caesarean section due to the acute blood loss. If the blood loss at vaginal delivery is meticulously measured, it proves to be slightly more than 500 ml of blood associated with the delivery of one infant and almost 1000 ml on delivery of twins. Caesarean section is associated with an average loss of 1000 ml of whole blood if performed under general anaesthetic but there is anecdotal evidence that the blood loss is considerably less if performed under epidural anaesthesia [12].

The response of the mother to this acute blood loss differs from that of non-pregnant women, in whom a rapid blood loss is accompanied by a drop in blood volume compensated for by vasoconstriction. Within a few days, the blood volume expands to near normal values because of an increase in plasma volume. This leads to a considerable fall in the haematocrit which is proportional to the amount of blood lost in the non-parturient woman.

In the normal pregnant woman at term, the hypervolaemia modifies the response to blood loss considerably. The blood volume drops following the acute loss at delivery but remains relatively stable unless the blood loss exceeds 25% of the pre-delivery volume. There is no compensatory increase in blood volume and there is a gradual fall in plasma volume, due primarily to diuresis. The red-cell mass increase during pregnancy is not totally lost at delivery but slowly reduced as the remaining red cells come to the end of their lifespan. The overall result is that the haematocrit gradually increases and the blood volume returns to non-pregnant levels [13].

In the first few days following delivery, there are fluctuations in plasma volume and haematocrit following individual responses to dehydration, pregnancy hypervolaemia, and the rapidity of blood loss. The average blood loss which can be tolerated without causing a significant fall in haemoglobin concentration is around 1000 ml, but this depends in turn on a healthy increase in blood volume prior to delivery. Almost all the blood loss occurs within the first hour following delivery under normal circumstances. In the following 72 hours only approximately 80 ml are lost *per vaginam*. Patients with uterine atony, extended episiotomy or lacerations will, of course, lose much more. If the haematocrit or haemoglobin concentration at 5–7 days postdelivery proves to be significantly less than predelivery levels, either there was pathological blood loss at delivery, or there was a poor increase in blood volume during pregnancy, or both [14,15].

Red-cell production

There is evidence of a more rapid red-cell production in pregnancy. In one study, labelled iron given by injection was incorporated into cells more rapidly than in the non-pregnant state and more of the red cells near term appeared to be young. Red-cell survival was unchanged and there were more reticulocytes and a higher glycolytic and cholinesterase activity [5]. In an Australian study [16], a mean reticulocyte count of between 1 and 2% was found in the last trimester in healthy women of Anglo-Saxon descent; a very much higher count, between 2 and 3%, was found in women of Greek or Italian descent. This was even when thalassaemia, haemoglobin variants and glucose 6-phosphate dehydrogenase deficiency were excluded. This difference is unexplained.

The red-cell mass is reduced immediately at delivery as a result of blood loss [13], and this is followed by a temporary erythroid hyperplasia until non-pregnant blood volumes are reached around 3 weeks after delivery [14,15].

The nature of the stimulus to red-cell production is not known, but erythropoietin (Epo) is known to be involved. There is a threefold increase in the concentration of Epo in plasma by the second trimester and a marked increase in the urine at 20 weeks' gestation corresponding with maximal Epo activity in the plasma [17]. More recent studies have confirmed the significant increase of Epo concentration in normal pregnancy [18–22]. These studies have also shown that in the presence of anaemia or iron deficiency during pregnancy there was a further statistically significant increase in the serum Epo. Other hormones are raised and may exert an effect on erythropoiesis in pregnancy and it has been shown that human placental lactogen augments the effect of Epo in mice [23].

Together with the increase in erythropoiesis, there appears to be a reactivation of fetal haemoglobin (HbF) production. HbF is largely replaced by adult haemoglobin (HbA) during the first year of life. The 1–2% of HbF which persists in the blood of normal adults is confined to a small number of red cells called F cells. The only physiological state in adult life where there appears to be reactivation of HbF is pregnancy. However, the rise in HbF is slight and, in earlier studies, it was impossible to determine whether this happens in all pregnancies, or to time the onset or duration of the increased HbF production [24].

The introduction of sensitive immunological techniques to demonstrate HbF in individual red cells has shown that there is a significant increase in F cells in all pregnancies. The number of F cells reaches a peak at 18–22 weeks and usually returns to normal by 8 weeks postpartum. The increase in HbF is of maternal origin and not derived from the fetus by transplacental bleeding [25]. Recent evidence in this and other similar situations indicates that the stimulus for HbF synthesis is related to an increased rate of production of red cells.

Total haemoglobin

The haemoglobin concentration, haematocrit and red-cell count decline during pregnancy because the expansion of plasma volume is greater than that of the red-cell mass, in spite of the rise in total circulating haemoglobin related to the increase in red-cell mass. This in turn is dependent partly upon the iron status of the individual. A survey of 4015 pregnant women attending a charity hospital in the US showed a total rise of only 69 g of haemoglobin in those not given iron compared with 152 g in the iron-treated group [26]. Other studies found

a rise of 95 g between the first and third trimesters [27] and a maximum rise of 172 g between the 2nd and 7th month [28]. More direct estimates [29] using carbon monoxide were technically unsatisfactory and more difficult to interpret because of the contribution of HbF and myoglobin. The published evidence for the rise in total haemoglobin is very unsatisfactory and is confused by the iron status of the women studied. It is impossible to give limits for the expected rise in total haemoglobin while controversies covering the optimal physiological iron status for women during pregnancy continue.

Composition of blood

The white cells

Neutrophils

The total white-cell count rises in pregnancy. This is due to an increase in neutrophil polymorphonuclear leucocytes [30]. The neutrophil count rises at the time of oestrogen peak of a normal menstrual cycle and if fertilization has occurred the neutrophils continue to rise [31]. A maximum is reported by the 15th postovulation day followed by a fall [32]. There is a subsequent rise in the neutrophils from the 45th day of pregnancy to reach a peak at 30 weeks [33] and plateau during the third trimester. The mean total white-cell count is around $9.0 \times 10^9/l$, the mean neutrophil count being $6.578 \times 10^9/l$ [30]. There is a further neutrophilia at the onset of labour, the total leucocyte count rising as high as $40.0 \times 10^9/l$ in uncomplicated pregnancies [34]. The count returns to non-pregnant levels by 6 days postpartum. There is a tendency for the total leucocyte count to rise with increasing parity, but this is not statistically significant. Normal pregnant women may have up to 3% myelocytes or metamyelocytes in their circulating blood [35], but these decrease in the last month of pregnancy [30].

The metabolic activity of granulocytes is increased during pregnancy. The leucocyte alkaline phosphatase score rises from the non-pregnant state to reach levels in the third trimester which are usually encountered only during the course of significant infections in the non-pregnant woman [36]. There is a fall in activity a few days before delivery and then a sharp rise during labour. Alkaline phosphatase activity returns to the non-pregnant level by 6 weeks postpartum [37], but breast feeding may prolong the elevation [38].

Hexose monophosphate activity, glucose oxidation and myeloperoxidase activity, important in the phagocytosis and intracellular destruction of bacteria and fungi, are increased during pregnancy [39,40]. Döhle bodies which are usually associated with severe infections are seen in the neutrophils of over 90% of blood films examined from uncomplicated pregnancies [41]. The neutrophilia and the increase in metabolic activity would appear to be the result of oestrogen stimulation [42,43].

Eosinophils, basophils, monocytes

The absolute eosinophil count shows a slight elevation, but the percentage of total leucocytes remains steady or drops a little [44]. There is a sharp fall in circulating eosinophils during labour and at delivery they are virtually absent. They return to non-pregnant levels by the 3rd postpartum day. There has been one report of a reduction in basophils during pregnancy [45]. The monocyte count appears to be unchanged [30].

Lymphocytes

The lymphocyte count does not alter significantly during pregnancy and there is no change in the proportion of circulating T cells and B cells [46]. However, factors in maternal serum suppress in-vitro lymphocyte function and cell-mediated immunity is profoundly depressed [47,48]. The raised oestrogen levels in women taking oral contraceptives and in pregnancy may depress cellular immunity by increasing the concentration of glycoproteins which coat the lymphocyte surface, thus impairing response to stimuli [49].

Other hormones associated with pregnancy, such as human chorionic gonadotrophin and prolactin, are known to suppress lymphocyte function [50,51]. In contrast, there is no evidence of impairment in the production of immunoglobulins or of humoral immunity [52]. The depression of cell-mediated immunity during pregnancy may be relevant to the survival of the fetus [53], but is associated with decreased resistance to viral infections. There are published reports of increased susceptibility to herpes [54], influenza [55], poliomyelitis [56], rubella and hepatitis [57]. Pneumococcal infections, particularly meningitis, are also more common in pregnancy and of greater severity, according to one report from Nigeria [58]. Perhaps the most important results of altered immunity in pregnancy, on a worldwide basis, is the decreased resistance in immune women to malaria, particularly during first pregnancy [59]. The placenta is infected and this results in a high incidence of abortion, prematurity and low birthweight [60].

The success of nature's graft — the placenta — and the survival of the fetus, which is an allograft (since half its genetic endowment is paternally derived), is a complex subject which has excited intense interest in recent years (see Chapter 5).

The platelets

Platelet counts have been shown to decrease slightly but significantly during pregnancy and the decrease may be explained by haemodilution or by an increased consumption. Only a few studies of platelet function in pregnancy have been reported and no convincing evidence of any significant changes in function has been obtained. The platelets will be discussed in more detail in the section which deals with haemostasis.

The red cells

Because the increase in red-cell mass during pregnancy is proportionately less than the increase in plasma volume, the concentration of red cells in the blood falls. The size and haemoglobin content of the cells show only minor changes so that the haemoglobin concentration

76 and haematocrit fall in parallel with the red-cell count.

Red-cell count

Red-cell counts have been accurate since the introduction of electronic counters. A fall from about $4.2 \times 10^{12}/l$ in early pregnancy to a plateau in the last trimester at approximately $3.8 \times 10^{12}/l$ has been observed in one study [61], and a fall to a mean count $3.67 \times 10^{12}/l$ at 240–269 days of gestation in another [32].

Haematocrit packed cell volume

The haematocrit falls in parallel with the red-cell count and haemoglobin concentration, from an average non-pregnant figure of 0.40–0.42 to a minimum of 0.31–0.34. These figures are derived from healthy pregnant women not receiving iron supplements; this reduction is modified in those taking supplementary iron.

Haemoglobin concentration

If the lowest normal haemoglobin in the healthy, adult, non-pregnant woman, living at sea-level, is accepted as 12.0 g/dl, then it can be calculated from the plasma volume and red-cell mass expansion in iron-sufficient subjects that the lowest haemoglobin in normal single pregnancy should be 10.6 g/dl. The lowest haemoglobin observed in a carefully studied, iron-sufficient group was 10.4 g/dl [62]. In most published studies the mean minimum in pregnancy is between 11 and 12 g/dl. This is in close agreement with the World Health Organization (WHO) [63] figure of 11.0 g/dl. The lowest haemoglobin is observed at around 32 weeks' gestation when plasma volume expansion is maximal, after this time there is a rise of approximately 0.5 g/dl [62,64].

Clinical experience shows that many apparently healthy women are able to proceed through pregnancy with haemoglobins lower than 11.0 g/dl without complications. On investigation, however, a fair proportion can be shown to be iron and folate deficient.

Mean cell haemoglobin concentration

The average concentration of haemoglobin in each red cell changes relatively little in pregnancy. There is a slight progressive fall in those women not given iron supplements. The mean corpuscular haemoglobin concentration (MCHC) is very sensitive to small errors in measurement of haemoglobin concentrations or of haematocrit. It was regarded as a useful index of iron deficiency in the past but with the advent of automation, and particularly of accurate reproducible red-cell counts, the MCHC seems likely to disappear in favour of mean corpuscular volume (MCV), which in the non-pregnant state is a more sensitive and helpful haematological index of iron status (Table 3.1).

Mean cell volume

The older literature reviewed by Hytten and Leitch [7] suggested no obvious change in MCV, although the errors involved in deriving the figure from a manual red-cell count and haematocrit were considerable.

A decline of MCV in early pregnancy followed by an increase in the latter half in iron-replete women has been reported [32]. Taylor & Lind [61] showed a rise from about 85 to 88 fl (femtolitres) at the end of the second trimester and a return to about 85 fl at term in women not receiving iron supplements. The terminal fall did not occur when iron was given and the MCV

Table 3.1. Red-cell indices and how they change in iron deficiency.

		Normal range	Iron deficiency
PCV RBC	MCV	75–99 fl	Reduced
Hb RBC	MCH	27–31 pg	Reduced
Hb PCV	MCHC	32–36 g/dl	Reduced

PCV: packed cell volume; RBC: red cell count; Hb: haemoglobin; MCV: mean corpuscular volume; MCH: mean corpuscular haemoglobin; MCHC: mean corpuscular haemoglobin concentration.

continued to rise to a level of about 89 fl at the end of pregnancy. These changes are small and within the normal non-pregnant range. More recently it has become clear that healthy iron-replete pregnancy is associated with a small physiological increase in red-cell size, on average 4 fl, but in some women the increase may be as high as 20 fl [65].

The increased drive to erythropoiesis resulting in a higher proportion of young large red cells appears to mask the effect of iron deficiency on the MCV in pregnancy even when anaemia has become established. Experience has shown that the MCV is a poor indicator of iron deficiency which develops during the course of pregnancy [66]. In a recent study [67] of 160 patients attending the antenatal clinic at Queen Charlotte's Hospital, the mean MCV remained within normal limits (90.7 fl) in the anaemic, iron-depleted patients (mean ferritin, 0.9 µg/l) compared with the non-anaemic, iron-replete patients (mean MCV, 90.6 fl; mean ferritin, 43.3 µg/l). None of the values in either group fell in the accepted microcytic range (Table 3.1) which indicates iron deficiency in the non-pregnant state.

Qualitative changes in the red cell

Red-cell fragility or osmotic resistance is measured by the osmotic strength of a sodium chloride solution which causes the cell to burst, and is expressed as the solution strength required to cause haemolysis of 50% of cells. In non-pregnant subjects, the mean concentration of sodium chloride required to cause 50% haemolysis is about 0.4435 g/l. In pregnancy, in one study the concentration rose to a peak of 0.460 g/l with a slight terminal decline in fragility which may reflect the increase in young and therefore more resistant cells in the circulation [64]. It is suggested that the cells become more spherical because of imbibition of water as would be expected with the fall in plasma colloid osmotic pressure. A dilution of cell contents is confirmed by the fall in red-cell electrolyte concentration.

Maternal respiratory alkalosis (see Chapter 4) enables the fetus to off-load carbon dioxide but would tend to increase maternal haemoglobin oxygen affinity. This is offset by a raised 2,3-diphosphoglycerate (2,3-DPG) in maternal red cells which pushes the oxygen dissociation curve to the right and thus facilitates oxygen release to the fetus and to maternal tissue [68]. Oxygen transfer is further helped by HbF, which has a high affinity for oxygen and a low affinity for 2,3-DPG [69].

However, the differential oxygen affinity across the placenta produced by HbA in the maternal circulation and the higher affinity HbF of the fetus is not essential to ensure adequate oxygen delivery for normal fetal development and growth. Women with genetically determined hereditary persistence of fetal haemoglobin have normal pregnancies and offspring. In a recent study, one woman with hereditary persistence of fetal haemoglobin underwent regular exchange transfusions throughout pregnancy in order to reduce HbF from over 80% to less than 50%. Another woman with virtually 100% HbF had no transfusion before, during or after completion of her pregnancy. Both women delivered a normal healthy baby at term [70].

Activity of various red-cell enzymes appears to be unchanged except for a tendency to greater activity with a younger cell population [5]. However, a decrease in glucose 6-phosphate dehydrogenase and 6-phosphoglucose dehydrogenase has been reported in late pregnancy.

Iron metabolism

Requirements

In pregnancy the demand for iron is increased to meet the needs of the expanded red-cell volume and the requirements of the developing fetus and placenta. The total requirement for iron is of the order of 700–1400 mg [7,62]. By far the greatest single demand for iron is that for the expansion of the red-cell mass, which requires 570 mg. The normal adult insensible loss in skin, stool and urine of 1 mg/day amounts to approximately 250–280 mg over normal gestation. The fetus derives its iron from the maternal serum by active transport across the placenta mainly in the last 4 weeks of pregnancy [71]. The iron transferred to the fetus is of the order of 200–370 mg. The iron content of the placenta and cord is 35–100 mg. Moderate blood loss at delivery of 200–500 ml accounts for 100–250 mg iron, and breast feeding over 6 months could result in the loss of another 100–180 mg. However, the amount of iron conserved during 15 months of amenorrhoea may amount to 240–480 mg. The increased need for iron is relatively small in early pregnancy and is greatest in the third trimester. Overall, the requirement is 4 mg/day but this rises from 2.8 mg/day in the non-pregnant to 6.6 mg/day in the last few weeks of pregnancy. This can be met only by mobilizing iron stores in addition to achieving maximum absorption of dietary iron. It has been suggested that the main physiological role of iron stores is to balance the very high iron requirements in late pregnancy [72]. Many women enter pregnancy with insufficient stores to cover the extra demands, particularly in the third trimester. This may explain why iron supplementation is needed in a physiological state such as pregnancy to maintain iron stores and to prevent the development of true anaemia.

Absorption

A normal mixed diet contains on average about 14 mg of iron each day, of which only 1–2 mg (5–10%) is normally absorbed. On the whole, the overall composition of the diet determines how much iron is available for absorption. There are at least two distinct pathways for iron absorption—one for iron attached to haem and one for inorganic iron. Haem iron is derived from the haemoglobin and myoglobin proteins in foods of animal origin. It is usually absorbed from the food more effectively than non-haem iron and is not affected by the factors interfering with or promoting the absorption of inorganic iron. The availability of food iron is quite variable. In foods derived from grain, iron often forms a stable complex with phytates, and only small amounts can be converted to a soluble form. The iron in eggs is poorly absorbed because of binding with phosphates present in the yolk. Milk, particularly cows' milk, is poor in iron content. In most foods, non-haem iron is in the ferric form and has to be converted to the ferrous form before absorption can take place. It follows that absorption is enhanced by reducing sub-stances such as ascorbic acid, and by hydrochloric acid in gastric juice. The intestinal mucosal control of iron is complex and incompletely understood, but absorption is increased when there is erythroid hyperplasia, rapid iron turnover and a high concentration of unsaturated transferrin—all of which are present in the pregnant woman. There is evidence that absorption of dietary iron is enhanced and rates of up to 40% or higher may be attained in the latter half of pregnancy [73,74]. The amount of iron absorbed will depend very much on the rate of erythropoiesis, the status of the iron stores, the content of the diet and whether or not iron supplements are being given.

In a carefully controlled study in Sweden [75], it was found that absorption rates differed markedly between those pregnant women receiving 100 mg ferrous iron supplements daily and those receiving a placebo. In the placebo group, iron absorption increased continuously throughout pregnancy. In the supplemented group, no increase occurred between the 12th and 24th week of gestation and thereafter the increase in absorption was about 60% of that of the placebo group in late pregnancy. After delivery, the mean absorption in the placebo group was markedly higher—about double that of the iron-treated group. These differences can mainly be explained by the different amount of storage iron in both groups. Oral supplementation of 60–80 mg elemental iron per day from early pregnancy maintains the haemoglobin in the recognized normal range for pregnancy in most subjects on a 'Western' diet, but does not maintain or restore the iron stores [62,76]. The WHO [63] recommends that supplements of 30–60 mg/day be given to those pregnant women with iron stores, and 120–240 mg to those women with none.

The observations that oral iron supplements may reduce the bioavailability of zinc [77] and maternal zinc levels during pregnancy [78] has led to speculation about the relationship of these findings and the association of maternal tissue zinc depletion with fetal growth retardation [79]. A study of serial changes in serum zinc and magnesium concentrations before conception, throughout pregnancy to 12 weeks postpartum, indicates that the decrease in concentrations of both elements is a normal physiological adjustment to pregnancy and that oral iron supplementation does not influence these changes [80].

Serum iron, transferrin and total iron-binding capacity

In health, the serum iron of adult non-pregnant women lies between 13 and 27 μmol/l (60–150 μg/dl), but it shows immense individual diurnal variability and fluctuates even from hour to hour. The processes which determine the changes are not fully understood. Serum iron may be low even when large stores of iron can be demonstrated in the marrow. In general, however, the serum iron is low in iron-deficiency anaemia and can be raised by administration of iron to treat the anaemia.

The total iron-binding capacity (TIBC) in the non-pregnant state lies in the range 45–72 μmol/l (250–400 mg/dl). It is raised in association with iron-deficiency and found to be low in chronic inflammatory states. The specific iron-binding protein transferrin is between 1.2 and 2.0 g/l (120–200 μg/dl). Normally, in the non-anaemic individual, the TIBC is approximately one-third saturated with iron.

In pregnancy, most workers report a fall in the serum iron and percentage saturation of the total iron-binding capacity. At term, the average serum iron concentration is reduced to about 35% below the mean in non-pregnant women. The iron-binding capacity which depends on the β_1 globulin transferrin is raised and so the percentage saturation of iron binding is low. The total serum transferrin concentration rises from 1.2–2.0 g/dl to 4.7 g/l by the second trimester and there is a corresponding increase in the TIBC to around 90 μmol/l. Similar but slightly lower figures have been reported in other studies, possibly because the women included were receiving iron supplements [62,76]. The TIBC cannot be brought down to non-pregnant levels by treatment with iron although it is slightly reduced by iron supplements in those women who are iron deficient. The raised TIBC returns to non-pregnant levels within 3 weeks of delivery; similar increases observed in women receiving oral contraceptives suggest that this is associated with oestrogen levels. The total serum iron

(3.0 mg) does not alter significantly in iron-replete pregnant women. Serum iron of less than 12 μmol/l (70 μg/dl) and a TIBC saturation of less than 15% indicate deficiency of iron during pregnancy.

Ferritin

Serum iron, even in combination with TIBC, is not a reliable indication of iron stores, because it fluctuates widely and is affected by recent ingestion of iron and other factors not directly involved with iron metabolism. The discovery that ferritin, a high molecular weight glycoprotein which was previously thought to be a totally intracellular iron storage compound, circulates in the plasma of healthy adults in a range of 15–300 μg/l [81] has considerably simplified the assessment of iron stores in pregnancy. It is stable, is not affected by recent ingestion of iron, and appears to reflect the iron stores accurately and quantitatively, particularly in the lower range associated with iron deficiency which is so important in pregnancy.

A study of serum ferritin during the course of pregnancy was made in 154 Cardiff women [82] who were divided randomly and one group received oral iron supplements. There was a rapid decrease in ferritin, and by implication in iron stores, during early pregnancy in all women studied, irrespective of iron therapy, but the stores were prevented from reaching iron-deficient levels during the latter half of pregnancy in the supplemented group. This pattern has been previously demonstrated semi-quantitatively in one examination of the stainable iron in the bone marrow at term [62].

It has been suggested that women at risk from iron-deficiency anaemia could be identified by estimating the serum ferritin concentration in the first trimester. A serum ferritin of less than 50 g/l in early pregnancy is an indication for daily iron supplements. Women with serum ferritin concentrations greater than 80 g/l are unlikely to require iron supplements. Unnecessary routine supplementation would thus be avoided in women enjoying good nutrition, and any risk to the pregnancy arising from severe maternal anaemia would be avoided by prophylaxis and prompt treatment [83].

A study at Queen Charlotte's Maternity Hospital, London, is of interest in this respect. Serum ferritin levels were estimated in 669 consecutive women who booked at 16 weeks' gestation or earlier with a haemoglobin concentration of 11.0 g/dl or above; 552 women (82.5%) had serum ferritins of 50 g/l or below, and would therefore qualify for routine daily iron supplements by the above criteria. These women are drawn from a cosmopolitan, largely well-nourished population; 12% had serum ferritins of less than 12 µg/l and were already iron deficient at booking in spite of having a haemoglobin of 11 g/dl or more. Only 51 (7.6%) had ferritins of 80 µg/l or above [84].

A smaller study of 137 pregnant patients attending a New York obstetric unit supports these findings and demonstrates the value of serum ferritin as a screening test for iron deficiency [66].

Free erythrocyte protoporphyrin

Erythroblast protoporphyrin represents the substrate unused for haem synthesis and levels rise when there is defective iron supply to the developing red cell. This test takes 2–3 weeks to become abnormal once iron stores are depleted. Estimation may be of value in patients recently treated with iron because there is also a delay in values returning to normal. However, the use of this estimation is limited in that a misleading rise in free erythrocyte protoporphyrin levels is observed in patients with chronic inflammatory disease, malignancy or infection.

Transferrin receptor

Serum transferrin receptor (TfR) provides a new, allegedly reliable, method for assessing cellular iron status [85]. It is present in all cells as a transmembrane protein which binds transferrin-bound iron and transports it to the cell interior. The extracellular domain comprises 90% of the molecule. Any reduction in iron supply results in an increase of TfR synthesis. Studies using sensitive immunological techniques have shown that TfR circulates in small amounts in the plasma of all individuals and that the concentration is proportional to the total body mass of TfR. The only notable exception is in patients with iron-deficiency anaemia in whom the serum receptor is elevated some threefold. This is accompanied by an increase in the density of surface TfR in iron-deficient cells. There is little or no change in serum receptor concentration during the early stages of storage-iron depletion but as soon as tissue-iron deficiency is established, the serum TfR concentration increases directly proportional to the degree of iron deficiency. This change precedes the reduction in MCV and the rise in erythrocyte protoporphyrin and therefore is a valuable measurement for detection of early tissue-iron lack. This measurement of iron status is particularly helpful in identifying iron deficiency in pregnancy [86]. It will identify the truly iron-deficient women from those who have a low haemoglobin concentration due to haemodilution or those who have low serum ferritin due to storage-iron mobilization. In combination with serum ferritin, TfR will give a complete picture of iron status — the serum ferritin reflecting iron stores and TfR the tissue-iron status [85].

Marrow iron

In experienced hands, a reliable method of assessing iron stores in pregnancy is by examination of an appropriately stained preparation of a bone marrow sample. If properly performed, marrow aspiration need not result in any major discomfort. In skilful hands, the procedure takes no more than 10 minutes. The iliac crest (anterior or posterior) should always be used as the aspiration site in preference to the sternum, for the benefit and comfort of the patient. In the absence of iron supplementation, there is no detectable stainable iron in over 80% of women at term [62]. No stainable iron (haemosiderin) may be visible once the serum ferritin has fallen to below 40 µg/l [87], but other stigmata of iron deficiency in the developing erythroblasts, particularly in the late normoblasts, will confirm that the anaemia is indeed due to iron deficiency in the absence of stainable iron. The effects of frequently accompanying folate deficiency will also be apparent. A block of incorporation of iron into haemoglobin occurs in the course of chronic inflammation, particularly of the urinary tract, even if iron stores are replete. This problem will be revealed by examination of the marrow aspirate stained for iron.

With the development of the new non-invasive tests of iron status described above, bone marrow examination will be reserved for the differential diagnosis of anaemia during pregnancy when the cause cannot be determined by any other means, and for the investigation of other haematological abnormalities which may arise de novo during the index pregnancy.

Non-haematological effects of iron deficiency

Effect on the mother

Overt symptoms of iron deficiency are generally not prominent. Defects in oxygen-carrying capacity are compensated for but the health implications of iron deficiency have recently been examined in a more detailed manner. Of particular interest are effects produced by impairment of the function of iron-dependent tissue enzymes. These are not the ultimate manifestation of severe untreated iron deficiency, but develop hand in hand with the fall in haemoglobin concentration [88].

Tissue enzyme malfunction undoubtedly occurs even in the very first stages of iron deficiency. Treatment with oral or parenteral iron results in improved well-being long before the haemoglobin starts to rise significantly, suggesting a central nervous system (CNS) effect [89]. Effects of iron deficiency on neuromuscular transmission may be responsible for the anecdotal reports of increased blood loss at delivery in anaemic women. The various effects of iron deficiency on cellular function may be responsible for the reported association between anaemia during pregnancy and preterm birth [90–93].

Effect on fetus and newborn

The fetus derives its iron from maternal serum by active transport across the placenta in the last 4 weeks of pregnancy.

Concentrations of ferritin in the cord blood are substantially higher than that in the mother's circulation at term whether she is iron-deficient or not and all fall within the normal adult range. However, babies born to iron-deficient mothers have significantly decreased cord ferritin levels compared to the others. This has an important bearing on iron stores and development of anaemia in the first year of life when iron intake is very poor [20,22,82].

Studies have also suggested behavioural abnormalities in children with iron deficiency related to changes in the concentration of chemical indicators in the brain [94,95]. Iron deficiency in the absence of anaemia is associated with poor performance in the Bayley Mental Developmental Index. Moreover, poor performance of 12- to 18-month-old iron-deficient anaemic infants in mental and motor development can be improved to the level of iron-sufficient infants by treatment with ferrous sulphate [96].

Even more far-reaching effects of maternal iron deficiency during pregnancy have been suggested. A correlation has recently been shown between maternal iron-deficiency anaemia, high placental weight, and an increased ratio of placental to birth weight. This suggests that maternal iron deficiency results in poor fetal growth compared to that of the placenta. High blood pressure in adult life has been linked to lower birth weight and with those whose birth weight was lower than would be expected from the weight of the placenta. Prophylaxis of iron deficiency may therefore have important implications for the prevention of adult hypertension which appears to have its origin in fetal life [97].

Comment

There is still considerable controversy about whether all women need iron supplements during pregnancy. Many authors are not able to accept that the physiological requirements for iron in pregnancy are considerably higher than the usual intake of most healthy women with apparently good diets in industrial countries [9,74]. The arguments about policy among nutritionists wishing to prevent iron deficiency are complicated by the varying problems of applying strategies in countries at different stages of development. The greatest experience in prevention comes from those countries where

82 iron deficiency is least common and least severe [98].

There is no doubt that in poorly developed countries, the incidence of anaemia and iron deficiency is high. Many women enter pregnancy either anaemic or with grossly depleted iron stores. Although there are other interacting factors which contribute to the anaemia, such as malaria, hookworm, HIV and haemoglobinopathies, most reports emphasize the contribution of iron deficiency after these conditions have been allowed for and the fact that iron supplements will maintain or improve haemoglobin levels during pregnancy in these populations [99–102].

One of the earliest large studies in the UK [103] showed that in over 2000 non-anaemic women who did not receive iron supplements during pregnancy, there was a progressive fall in haemoglobin concentration to term and it took more than a year postpartum before the pre-pregnancy haemoglobin was regained. Those women who took iron supplements maintained consistently higher haemoglobin concentrations which rose to pre-pregnancy haemoglobin levels much more rapidly after delivery.

Hemminki and Starfield [104] reviewed controlled clinical trials of iron administration during pregnancy in developed Western countries. Seventeen trials were found which fulfilled their stated criteria. As a result of their analysis, they concluded that there was no beneficial effect in terms of birthweight, length of gestation, maternal and infant morbidity, and mortality in those women receiving iron compared with controls. Nevertheless, the majority of women who do not receive iron supplements have no stores at all at the end of pregnancy [20,62,82]. Also, offspring of non-anaemic women who have not received supplements have lower iron stores than those of iron-replete women [20,82].

Svanberg [75] comments that the suggestion that absence of iron stores in women of fertile age is to be considered as physiological and that the increased iron demand during pregnancy may be met by increased absorption, is not borne out by very careful studies.

From what evidence is available, it would appear that a high proportion of women in reproductive years do lack storage iron. The reasons may be different in different populations. Over thousands of years the human race has changed its way of living and eating, from a society based on hunting and fishing to the present one with a lower intake of iron and a lower intake of meat and fish [88]. Recent dietary changes in industrialized countries have made it difficult for women to build up iron stores so that iron balance can be maintained in pregnancy.

The conclusion is that even with maximum iron content in the diet, the immediate demands of pregnancy cannot be covered by an increased absorption from food intake.

In summary, negative iron balance throughout pregnancy, particularly in the latter half, may lead to iron deficiency anaemia in the third trimester. This hazard, together with the increasing evidence of non-haematological effects of iron deficiency without severe anaemia on exercise tolerance, cerebral function, and fetal, neonatal and infant development, leads to the conclusion that it is safer, more practical, and in the long term less expensive in terms of investigation, hospital admission and treatment, to offer all women iron supplements from 16 weeks' gestation [20,72,88,105,106].

Folate metabolism

Folate together with iron has assumed a central role in the nutrition of pregnancy. This vitamin, widely distributed in nature, was isolated, identified and synthesized in the mid-1940s by various groups studying food factors associated with macrocytic anaemia in primates and the growth of certain microorganisms. At a cellular level, folic acid is reduced first to dihydrofolic acid and then to tetrahydrofolic acid which forms the cornerstone of cellular folate metabolism. It is essential to cell growth and cell division as a supplier of 1-carbon fragments. The more active a tissue is in reproduction and growth, the more dependent it will be on the efficient turnover and supply of folate coenzymes. Bone marrow and epithelial linings are therefore particularly at risk [107].

Requirements for folate are increased in pregnancy to meet the needs of the growing fetus and the placenta, for uterine hypertrophy and the expanded maternal red-cell mass. The placenta transports folate actively to the fetus even in the face of maternal deficiency but maternal folate metabolism is altered early in pregnancy like many other maternal functions, before fetal demands act directly.

Assessment of folate status

The diagnosis of folate deficiency by finding unequivocal megaloblastic haematopoiesis in a bone marrow aspirate can only be made when the deficiency is well established. For this reason, a number of alternative investigations have been developed to assess folate status before the appearance of overt megaloblastic anaemia, and to permit treatment while the deficiency is still subclinical [108]. These include assay of serum and red-cell folate activities, the measurement of formimino-glutamic acid (FIGLU) excretion in the urine after a histidine load, and the clearance from the plasma of intravenously administered folic acid. Logically, there is no reason why the results of these investigations should be identical because they reflect different aspects and stages of a continuous process. In deficiency states, low serum folate levels may precede megaloblastic anaemia by about 4 months and red-cell folate levels will fall more slowly than plasma levels because it will take some time for the erythrocyte population to be replaced by folate-deficient cells [108].

Plasma folate

It is generally agreed that plasma folate falls as pregnancy advances, so that, at term, it is about half the non-pregnant value [109–112].

Plasma clearance of folate by the kidneys is more than doubled as early as the 8th week of gestation [113,114]. The glomerular filtration rate is raised and the marked contrast between the comparatively unchanging plasma levels and the wide variation in urinary loss suggests a change in tubular reabsorption, rather than some alteration in folate metabolism. It is unlikely that this is a major drain on maternal resources and it cannot play more than a marginal role.

There appears to be no change in absorption of either folate monoglutamates or polyglutamates in healthy pregnancy [115,116], but there is invariably a wide scatter of results. The incidence of abnormally low serum folates in late pregnancy varies with the population studied and presumably reflects the local nutritional standards.

Substantial day-to-day variations of plasma folate are possible and postprandial increases have been noted which will limit the diagnostic value of an occasional sample taken at an antenatal clinic.

Red-cell folate

The estimation of red-cell folate may provide more useful information as it does not reflect daily or other short-term variations in plasma folate levels. It is thought to give a better indication of overall tissue levels, but the turnover of red blood cells is slow and there will be a delay before significant reductions are evident in the folate concentration of the red cells, due to folate deficiency [117,118].

There is evidence that patients who have low red-cell folate at the beginning of pregnancy develop megaloblastic anaemia in the third trimester [117].

Excretion of formimino-glutamic acid

A loading dose of histidine leads to increased FIGLU excretion in the urine when there is folate deficiency. As a test for folate deficiency in pregnancy it has little to recommend it, primarily because the metabolism of histidine is altered and this results in increased FIGLU excretion in normal early pregnancy [119].

Postpartum events

In the 6 weeks following delivery there is a tendency for all the indices discussed to return to non-pregnant values. However, should any deficiency of folate have developed and remain untreated in pregnancy, it may present clinically for the first time in the puerperium and its consequences may be detected for many months after delivery. Lactation provides an added folate stress. A folate content of 5 µg per 100 ml of human milk and a yield of 500 ml/day implies a daily loss of 25 µg folate in breast milk. In the Bantu, megaloblastic anaemia commonly appears in the year following pregnancy in association with lactation. Dietary folate intake is poor and it has been shown [120] that, as lactation continues, folate deficiency becomes more apparent, as demonstrated by using FIGLU excretion. In this country, as early as 1919, Osler described the severe anaemias of pregnancy with a high colour index and a striking incidence in the postpartum period [121].

Red-cell folate levels in lactating mothers are significantly lower than those of their infants during the first year of life.

Interpretations of investigations during pregnancy

The blood picture is complex and may be difficult to interpret. There is a physiological increase in red-cell size in healthy, iron-replete pregnancy.

Outside pregnancy, the hallmark of megaloblastic haemopoiesis is macrocytosis, first identified in routine laboratory investigations by a raised MCV. In pregnancy, macrocytosis by non-pregnant standards is the norm and in any event may be masked by iron deficiency. Examination of the blood film may be more helpful. There may be occasional oval macrocytes in a sea of iron-deficient microcytic cells. Hypersegmentation of the neutrophil polymorph nucleus is significant because in normal pregnancy there is a shift to the left. If more than 5% of 100 neutrophils have five or more lobes, hypersegmentation is present, but hypersegmentation is observed in pure iron deficiency, uncomplicated by folate deficiency.

The value of the various investigations described above in predicting megaloblastic anaemia and assessing subclinical folate deficiency has been the subject of numerous reports. Using these various tests, folate 'deficiency' in pregnancy is not invariably accompanied by any significant haematological change.

In the absence of any changes, megaloblastic haemopoiesis should be suspected when the expected response to adequate iron therapy is not achieved.

The diagnosis of folate deficiency in pregnancy then has to be made entirely on morphological grounds and would usually involve examination of a suitably prepared marrow aspirate. In current practice this investigation is not thought to be desirable or necessary.

Megaloblastic anaemia and pregnancy

The cause of megaloblastic anaemia in pregnancy is nearly always folate deficiency. Vitamin B_{12} is only very rarely implicated. A survey of reports from the UK over the past two decades suggests an incidence ranging from 0.2 to 5.0%, but a considerably greater number of women have megaloblastic changes in their marrow which are not suspect on examination of the peripheral blood only [65,122]. The incidence of megaloblastic anaemia in other parts of the world is considerably greater and is thought to reflect the nutritional standards of the population. Several workers have pointed to the poor socio-economic status of their patients as the major aetiological factor contributing to the anaemia, which may be further exacerbated by seasonal changes in the availability of staple foodstuffs. Food folates are only partially available and the amount of folate supplied in the diet is difficult to quantify. In Great Britain, analysis of daily folate intake in foodstuffs showed a range of 129–300 µg. The folate content of 24-hour food collections in various studies in Sweden and Canada proved to be round about 200 µg on average, with a range as large as 70 µg to 600 mg [123].

Foods that are very rich in folate include broccoli, spinach and Brussels sprouts, but up to 90% of their folate content is lost within the first few minutes, by boiling or steaming. These vegetables are unlikely to be eaten raw. Dietary folate-deficiency megaloblastic anaemia occurs in about one-third of all pregnant women in the world, despite the fact that folate is found in nearly all natural foods, because folate is rapidly destroyed by cooking, especially in finely divided foods such as beans and rice [108]. Asparagus, avocados, mushrooms and bananas also have a fairly high folate content, which may delight social class I patients in the UK, but will not help the average working-class mother to improve her folate intake.

The effects of dietary inadequacy may be further amplified by frequent childbirth and multiple pregnancy. Several reports have shown a markedly increased incidence of megaloblastic anaemia in multiple pregnancy. An incidence of 1 in 11 in twin pregnancies compared with the expected incidence of 1 in 80 of singleton pregnancies was noted in one survey of over 1000 patients [110].

The normal dietary folate intake is inadequate to prevent megaloblastic changes in the bone marrow in approximately 25% of pregnant women. The fall in serum and red-cell folate could be a physiological phenomenon in pregnancy, but the incidence of megaloblastic change in the bone marrow is reduced only when the blood folate levels are maintained in a steady state by adequate oral supplements.

The fetus and folate deficiency

There is an increased risk of megaloblastic anaemia occurring in the neonate of a folate-deficient mother, especially if delivery is preterm.

The young infant's requirement for folate has been estimated at 20–50 µg/day (4–10 times the adult requirement on a weight basis). Serum and red-cell folates are consistently higher in cord than in maternal blood, but the premature infant is in severe negative folate balance because of high growth rate and reduced intake. The usual fall in serum and red-cell folate in the term baby is yet greater in the premature baby and even in the absence of other complicating factors may result in megaloblastic anaemia. This can be prevented by giving supplements of 50 µg/day [124,125].

To investigate the alleged association of maternal folate deficiency with neural tube defects [126–128], the Medical Research Councie performed a randomized double-blind study of preconception and early pregnancy folic acid supplements. This trial started in July 1983, was run at 33 centres in seven countries and looked at over 1800 women. Women with a previous neural tube defect pregnancy were allocated to one of four groups which were given folic acid, other vitamins, both folic acid and other vitamins and no supplements respectively. The study was discontinued prematurely in April 1991 because the results were so clear-cut.

The two groups with no folic acid supplements had a significantly higher recurrence rate of CNS abnormalities (3.5 as opposed to 1%) than in the groups given folate [129]. The specific role of folic acid supplements in the prevention of neural tube defects is established. Preconception folic acid supplements should be offered to all women who have had a baby with a previous neural tube defect.

More recently it has also been shown in Hungary, in a large, randomized, controlled trial that periconceptional supplement of 800 µg of folic acid prevented the first occurrence of neural tube defects [130]. What public health measures should be taken to ensure that the diet of a woman in her reproductive years contains adequate folic acid will need careful prospective planning [131].

Prophylaxis of folate deficiency during uncomplicated pregnancy

The case for giving prophylactic folate supplements throughout pregnancy is a strong one and an example of excellent preventative medicine, particularly in countries where overt megaloblastic anaemia is frequent.

The WHO's recommendations for daily folate intake are as high as 800 µg in the antenatal period and 600 µg during lactation and 400 µg in the non-pregnant adult [63].

There is an increased need for about 100 µg folic acid daily during pregnancy which, without supplements, must be found from natural folates in the diet. The WHO's [63] recommended intakes clearly overestimate the needs. The daily amount of folate that has been given prophylactically in pregnancy varies from 30 to 500 µg and even pharmacological doses of 5–15 mg [110], 30 µg/day, were found to be too small to influence folate status appreciably, but supplements of 100 µg or more all reduced the frequency of megaloblastic changes in the marrow and eliminated megaloblastic anaemia as a clinical entity. In order to meet the folate needs of those women with a dietary intake well below average, the daily supplement during pregnancy should be of the order of 200–300 μg/day — still very much below the WHO's recommended daily intake [65]. This should be given in combination with iron supplements and there are several suitable combined preparations available.

Vitamin B_{12}

Muscle, red cell and serum vitamin B_{12} concentrations fall during pregnancy [111,132,133]. Non-pregnant serum levels of 205–1025 μg/l fall to 20–510 μg/l at term, with lower levels in multiple pregnancy. Women who smoke tend to have lower serum B_{12} levels [134], which may account for the positive correlation between birthweight and serum levels in non-deficient mothers.

Vitamin B_{12} absorption is unaltered in pregnancy [135]. It is probable that tissue uptake is increased by the action of oestrogens, as oral contraceptives cause a fall in serum vitamin B_{12} [136]. Cord blood serum vitamin B_{12} is higher than that of maternal blood; the fall in serum vitamin B_{12} in the mother may be related to preferential transfer of absorbed B_{12} to the fetus at the expense of maintaining the maternal serum concentration [110], but the placenta does not transfer vitamin B_{12} with the same efficiency as it does folate. Low serum vitamin B_{12} levels in early pregnancy in vegetarian Hindus do not fall further, while their infants often have subnormal concentrations [137]. The vitamin B_{12}-binding capacity of plasma increases in pregnancy [138], analogous to the rise in transferrin. The rise is confined to the liver-derived transcobalamin II which is concerned with the transport of vitamin B_{12} rather than the leucocyte-derived transcobalamin I (the other vitamin B_{12} binding protein) which is raised in the myeloproliferative conditions [138].

Pregnancy does not make a vast impact on maternal vitamin B_{12} stores: adult stores are of the order of 3000 μg or more and vitamin B_{12} stores in the newborn infant are about 50 μg [110,137].

Addisonian pernicious anaemia does not usually occur during the reproductive years and the associated vitamin B_{12} deficiency is associated with infertility. Pregnancy is likely only if the deficiency is remedied [110], but severe vitamin B_{12} deficiency may be present without morphological changes in haemopoietic and other tissues. Pregnancy in such patients may be followed by death *in utero* or proceed uneventfully [65]. Vitamin B_{12} deficiency in pregnancy may be associated with chronic tropical sprue. The megaloblastic anaemia which develops is due to long-standing vitamin B_{12} and folate deficiency — the result both of pregnancy and poor folate intake. The cord vitamin B_{12} levels remain above the maternal levels in these cases, but the concentration in the breast milk may follow the maternal serum levels [110].

The recommended intake of vitamin B_{12} is 2.0 μg/day in the non-pregnant and 3.0 μg per day during pregnancy [63]. This will be met by almost any diet, however deficient in other essential substances, which contains animal products. However, in these days of processed foods, certain animal products may lose their B_{12} content in preparation. It has been reported [108] that a surprising number of underprivileged young adults were suffering from B_{12} deficiency in Mexico City. Their sole source of dietary B_{12} was in processed milk which on investigation was found to have very little B_{12} content indeed. Strict vegans who will not eat any animal-derived substances may have a deficient intake of vitamin B_{12} and their diet should be supplemented during pregnancy. The animal protein intake of women in poorer parts of the world is very low. In a pilot study of aetiology of anaemia in pregnant women in Malawi whose basic diet consists of maize, a surprising proportion of such women were shown to have very low serum B_{12} associated with megaloblastic changes in the bone marrow [139].

Haemostasis and fibrinolysis

The integrity and patency of the vascular tree is dependent upon a finely controlled interaction between the coagulation system and fibrinolysis. During pregnancy, major changes occur in the components of the haemostatic system, and some of these physiological adaptations are unique to human pregnancy. Their significance and their relation to haemorrhage and thrombosis, which are major hazards for the pregnant woman, can only be appreciated with a knowledge of the haemostatic mechanism in the healthy non-pregnant individual.

Haemostasis

Haemostasis in health has three primary functions:
- To confine the circulating blood to the vascular bed.
- To maintain its fluidity.
- To arrest bleeding from injured vessels.

All these aspects of haemostasis depend on a complex interaction between vasculature, platelets, coagulation factors and fibrinolysis (Fig. 3.2).

Vascular integrity, platelets and prostacyclin

It is not known how vascular integrity is normally maintained but it is clear that platelets have a key role to play since conditions in which their number is depleted or their function is abnormal are characterized by widespread spontaneous capillary haemorrhages. It is thought that the platelets in health are constantly sealing microdefects in the vasculature, by forming mini fibrin clots, the unwanted fibrin being removed by a process of fibrinolysis. Generation of prostacyclin appears to be the physiological mechanism which protects the vessel wall from excess deposition of platelet aggregates and explains the fact that contact of platelets with healthy vascular endothelium is not a stimulus for thrombus formation [140].

The endothelial cell plays a vital part in the maintenance of vascular integrity and blood flow and also in the response to injury. Platelets do not adhere to the intact, undamaged surface of a normal blood vessel and this phenomenon is not yet fully understood, although it is essential to maintain vascular integrity. Platelet adhesion occurs when the endothelial surface is damaged and when a vessel is severed or punctured so that subendothelial collagen components are exposed. The endothelial cell is a source of von Willebrand's factor which will bind to both exposed collagen and glycoprotein receptors on the platelet surface resulting in platelet adhesion.

Prostacyclin is the principal prostanoid synthesized by blood vessels. It is a powerful vasodilator and a potent inhibitor of platelet aggregation. Moncada and Vane [140] have proposed that there is a balance between the production of prostacyclin by the vessel wall, and the production of the vasoconstrictor and powerful aggregating agent thromboxane by the platelet (Fig. 3.3).

When injury is minor, small platelet thrombi form. The extent of the injury is an important determinant of the size of the thrombus — and

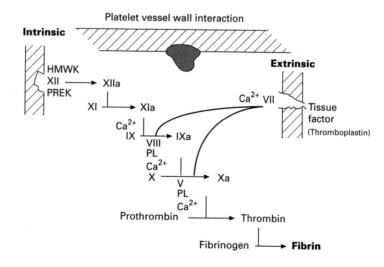

Fig. 3.2. Haemostatic/coagulation pathways. HMWK: high molecular weight kininogen; PREK: prekallikrein.

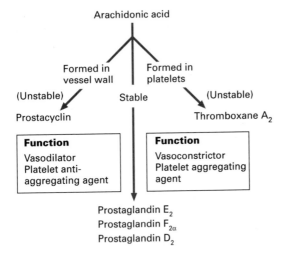

Fig. 3.3. The prostaglandins derived from arachidonic acid metabolism (after Moncada & Vane [140]).

whether or not platelet aggregation is stimulated. Prostacyclin synthetase is abundant in the intima and progressively decreases in concentration from the intima to adventitia, whereas the pro-aggregating elements increase in concentration from the subendothelium to the adventitia. It follows that severe vessel damage or physical detachment of the endothelium will lead to the development of a large thrombus as opposed to simple platelet adherence.

There are several conditions in which production of prostacyclin could be impaired, thereby upsetting the normal balance. Deficiency of prostacyclin production has been suggested in platelet consumption syndromes such as haemolytic uraemic syndrome and thrombotic thrombocytopenic purpura [141]. Prostacyclin production has also been shown to be reduced in fetal and placental tissue from pre-eclamptic pregnancies [142], and the current role of prostacyclin in the pathogenesis of pre-eclampsia is undergoing active investigation.

Platelet production is thought to be regulated by humoral factors. The plasma serum and urine of thrombocytopenic animals and humans do contain megakaryocytopoietic and thrombopoietic activities that are lineage specific and distinct from known cytokines. These activities are referred to as meg-CSF or thrombopoietin

depending on their ability to effect proliferation (meg-CSF) or maturation (thrombopoietin). Attempts to purify these substances, known since the 1960s, have been unsuccessful in the past. Recently, meg-CSF/thrombopoietin-like protein present in the plasma of irradiated pigs has been purified and cloned [143] and the information used to isolate a human complementary DNA. This protein has sequence homology with erythropoietin and has both meg-CSF and thrombopoietin-like activities. The availability of a recombinant protein affecting megakaryocyte and platelet production makes a careful evaluation of its role in regulating thrombopoiesis and its potential to affect other haematopoietic activity possible. Thrombopoietin is being cautiously introduced in the management of some patients with thrombocytopenia as a potential alternative to platelet transfusion [144].

Platelets produced in the bone marrow by the megakaryocytes have a lifespan of only 9–12 days. At the end of their normal lifespan the effete cells are engulfed by cells of the reticuloendothelial system and most damaged platelets are sequestered in the spleen.

There have been conflicting reports concerning the platelet count during normal pregnancy. A review of publications over 25 years [145] revealed a majority consensus (of six), suggesting a small diminution in the platelet count towards term; two publications suggesting that there are no changes; and one early, probably inaccurate, study documenting a rise. However, few of these studies obtained longitudinal data bases and in none of them was a within-patient analysis performed. The most recent studies, many surveying large populations with the use of automated counting equipment, suggest that if mean values for platelet concentration are analysed throughout pregnancy, there is a downward trend [146–148], even though most values may be within the accepted non-pregnant range [147–150]. Furthermore, individual responses are variable. There is conflicting evidence of increased platelet turnover [151,152] and low-grade platelet activation as pregnancy advances, resulting in a large proportion of younger platelets with a greater mean platelet volume [149].

Most investigators agree that low-grade chronic intravascular coagulation within the uteroplacental circulation is a part of the physiological response of all women to pregnancy. This is partially compensated for and it is not surprising that the platelets should be involved, either showing evidence of increased turnover [153] or in some cases a reduction in number. In one study, women with a normal pregnancy compared with non-pregnant controls were shown to have a significantly lower platelet count and an increase in circulating platelet aggregates. *In vitro*, the platelets were shown to be hypoaggregable. This was interpreted as suggesting platelet activation during pregnancy causing platelet aggregation and followed by exhaustion of platelets [146]. Earlier publications suggesting that there was no evidence of changes in platelet function [154] or differences in platelet lifespan [151] between healthy non-pregnant and pregnant women have been reassessed in the face of more recent investigations.

A careful longitudinal study examined platelet behaviour in normal pregnancy and the puerperium using whole blood in the test system [155]. This newer technique is thought to be more valid in physiological terms than in in-vitro examination of platelet rich plasma. Increases in platelet reactivity were demonstrated throughout gestation, starting at 16 weeks and maximal in the third trimester. Platelet activity did not return to non-pregnant state until 12 weeks postpartum. Adrenalin-induced release reaction and platelet aggregation were significantly increased as was arachidonic acid-induced aggregation but not release reaction.

The problem remains in defining completely normal pregnancy. Certain disease states specific to pregnancy have profound effects on platelet consumption, lifespan and function [156, 157]. For example, a decrease in platelet count has been observed in pregnancies with fetal growth retardation [158] and the lifespan of platelets is shortened significantly even in mild pre-eclampsia.

A prospective study of 2263 healthy women delivering during 1 year at a Canadian obstetric centre [147] showed that 112 (8.3%) had mild thrombocytopenia at term (platelet counts, 97–150 × 10^9/l). The frequency of thrombocytopenia in their offspring was no greater than that of those babies born to women with platelet counts in the normal range and none of these infants had a platelet count of less than 100 × 10^9/l. This supports an earlier study [146] showing decreased platelet counts and increase in circulating aggregates in women with normal pregnancies compared with non-pregnant controls.

Burrows and Kelton [148] extended their original prospective study to include 6715 consecutive deliveries over three years. Thrombocytopenia was found in 513 women (7.6%). Of these, the majority (65%) were made up of healthy women where thrombocytopenia was inadvertently detected. The rest had a variety of medical and obstetric conditions ranging from diabetes, idiopathic thrombocytopenic purpura and pregnancy-induced hypertension. There was no direct morbidity or mortality resulting from thrombocytopenia in the mother or her infant.

Arrest of bleeding

An essential requirement of the haemostatic system is a rapid reaction to injury, the effect of which remains confined to the area of damage. This requires control mechanisms which stimulate coagulation after trauma but limit the extent of the response. The substances involved in the formation of the haemostatic plug normally circulate in the blood in an inert form until activated at the site of vascular injury or by some factor released into the circulation which triggers intravascular coagulation.

When a small blood vessel is injured, the first recognizable event is the adherence of the platelets to the collagen in the exposed subendothelium of the vessel wall. This adherence triggers a series of alterations in the platelets which can be shown *in vitro* and include formation of pseudopodia, change of shape and the release of constituents such as adenosine diphosphate (ADP) serotonin, calcium and secreted platelet proteins [159]. Many of the substances released are of obvious haemostatic importance and include thromboxane, β-thromboglobulin, fibrinogen, Factor V and

90 Factor VIII related antigen, but platelets can also modify the functions of other cells, particularly the endothelial cells of the vessel wall by releasing a number of platelet proteins, e.g. growth factors and vascular permeability factor. In this way platelets play a vital role in a number of processes influencing replication of endothelial cells, tissue repair, wound healing and inflammation [160]. ADP release increases the platelet plug by stimulating further aggregation of the platelets at the site of injury. Serotonin release promotes vasoconstriction and also stimulates further aggregation. The coagulation cascade is triggered and the action of thrombin leads to the formation of fibrin which in turn converts the loose platelet plug into a firm stable wound seal. In the repair of small endothelial breakage in the microvasculature, platelets alone are probably enough to prevent haemorrhage. The role of platelets is of less importance in injury involving large vessels because platelet aggregates are of insufficient size and strength to breach the defect. Here the coagulation mechanism is of major importance in conjunction with vascular constriction.

The platelet contractile protein is required not only for the secretion of active principles from the platelet but for the subsequent clot retraction. This helps to bring together injured edges and to clear the vascular lumen so allowing blood flow to continue.

Blood coagulation

The end result of blood coagulation is the formation of an insoluble fibrin clot from the soluble precursor fibrinogen which is in the plasma. This involves a complex interaction of clotting factors and a sequential activation of a series of proenzymes. The original enzyme cascade of the coagulation system proposed by Macfarlane [161] has been modified as a result of the recognition of complexes which form between certain activated factors [162]. Table 3.2 gives a list of the clotting factors using their assigned Roman numeral, their functions and some of the alternative names used, together with the plasma concentrations.

When a blood vessel is injured, blood coagulation is initiated by activation of Factor XII by

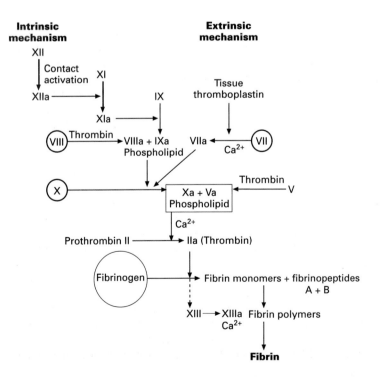

Fig. 3.4. The interaction of factors involved in blood coagulation. Those factors known to be increased in pregnancy are circled.

Table 3.2. Components of blood coagulation, their function and plasma concentration.

Category and name	Haemostatic function	Plasma concentration (μg/ml)
Contact activation factors		
F.XII (Hageman factor)	Activate F.XI and PK	30
HMW kininogen	Bring F.XI and PK to a surface	70
Prekallikrein	Activate F.XII	45
F.XI (PTA)	Activate F.IX	4
Vitamin K-dependent proenzymes		
Prothrombin (F.II)	Precursor of thrombin	150
F.X (Stuart–Prower factor)	Activate prothrombin	8
F.IX (Christmas factor)	Activate F.X	4
F.VII (proconvertin)	Activate F.IX and F.X	0.5
Protein C	Inactivate VIIIa and Va	3.5
Cofactors		
Tissue factor (F.III)	Cofactor for F.VII and VIIa	—
Platelet procoagulant phospholipid (PF 3)	Cofactor for F.IXa and F.Xa	—
F.VIII (antihaemophilic factor)	Cofactor for F.IXa	0.1
F.V (proaccelerin)	Cofactor for F.Xa	7
Protein S	Cofactor for activated protein C	35
Factors of fibrin deposition		
Fibrinogen (F.I)	Precursor of fibrin	2.500
F.XIII (fibrin-stabilizing factor)	Crosslink fibrin	8

F: factor; PK: prekallikrein; HMW: high molecular weight; PTA: plasma thromboplastin antecedent; PF: platelet factor.

collagen (intrinsic mechanism) and activation of Factor VII by thromboplastin release (extrinsic mechanism) from the damaged tissue. Both the intrinsic and extrinsic mechanisms are activated by components of the vessel wall and both are required for normal haemostasis. The two mechanisms are diagrammatically represented in Fig. 3.4.

Strict division between the two pathways does not exist and interaction between activated factors in both pathways has been shown [163]; the system is a biochemical amplifier. Coagulation factors present in picogram amounts stimulate a sequential series of enzyme conversions leading to the conversion of milligrams of fibrinogen to fibrin. The intrinsic and extrinsic systems share a common pathway, following the activation of Factor X. The intrinsic pathway, or contact system, proceeds spontaneously and is relatively slow—requiring from 5 to 20 minutes for visible fibrin formation. All tissues contain a specific lipoprotein, thromboplastin, which markedly increases the rate at which blood clots, but it is particularly concentrated in the lung and brain. The placenta also is very rich in tissue factor and small amounts of placenta added to the blood will produce fibrin formation within 12 seconds. This acceleration of coagulation by the tissue factor system is brought about by bypassing all the reactions involving the contact system [164].

The final steps in the clotting reaction for both systems involve the conversion of prothrombin to thrombin and the action of thrombin on fibrinogen. Fibrinogen is the only clotting factor present in sufficient quantity to allow its measurements in terms of milligrams of protein. Plasma levels in health lie between 2.5 and 4.0 g of fibrinogen per litre. The molecular weight of fibrinogen is approximately 344 000 and the molecule consists of three pairs of polypeptide chains linked by means of disulphide bonds. Thrombin, a proteolytic enzyme, splits off two pairs of small peptides (fibrinopeptide A and B) to produce fibrin monomer (Fig. 3.4). The removal of fibrinopeptides A and B, which carry negative charges, allows polymerization of fibrin monomer. Polymeric fibrin, unlike fibrin monomer, is insoluble and on electron microscopy appears as fibrin strands which have characteristic cross-striations. The fibrin polymer is strengthened by the action of Factor XIII (fibrin-stabilizing factor) which, by linking amino acids of adjacent areas of the polymerized fibrin, confers tensile strength and insolubility to the fibrin and provides a medium suitable for tissue repair. Bleeding after separation of the umbilical cord, delayed bleeding after trauma, defective healing of wounds and the formation of wide scars are characteristic of hereditary deficiency of Factor XIII [163].

The naturally occurring anticoagulants

Mechanisms that limit and localize the clotting process at sites of trauma are critically important to protect against generalized thrombosis, and also to prevent spontaneous activation of those powerful procoagulant factors which circulate in normal plasma.

Recently, investigation of healthy haemostasis has switched emphasis from the factors which promote clotting to those that prevent generalized and spontaneous activation of these factors. An account of the complex interactions and biochemistry of all of these factors is not appropriate here and only those of major importance in haemostasis and their relevance to pregnancy will be mentioned. The balance of procoagulant and inhibitory factors is discussed in a review article [165]. The principle still stands, although obviously the review does not include the recent identification of new factors involved in homeostasis and haemostasis.

Antithrombin III

Antithrombin III (At III) is the main physiological inhibitor of thrombin and Factor Xa and possibly the main inhibitor of Factors IXa, XIa and XIIa [166]. An inherited deficiency of At III is one of the few conditions in which a familial tendency to thrombosis has been described.

Heparin is the oldest anticoagulant drug and remains the most potent available. It has been in clinical use for over 40 years. Heparin markedly accelerates the rate at which At III reacts to thrombin and Factor Xa [167]. The interaction between heparin and At III is of considerable clinical importance in the treatment and prophylaxis of thromboembolism [168]. At least six different types of antithrombin have been described but only the first three have been shown to play any significant role in haemostasis [169]. The activity in plasma which causes progressive destruction of thrombin was originally termed antithrombin III. It is now recognized that at least three proteins contribute towards this activity — two general proteinase inhibitors, α_1-antitrypsin and α_2-macroglobin and an α_2-globulin with more specific antithrombin activity, now known as antithrombin III (At III). Addition of a specific antibody to At III removes all the heparin cofactor activity from plasma and the evidence is overwhelming that these factors are identical. At III, therefore, is not only the major thrombin inhibitor in plasma but also the plasma protein through which heparin exerts its effect [170]. As At III is synthesized in the liver, its activity is low in cirrhosis and other chronic diseases of the liver as well as in protein-losing renal disease, disseminated intravascular coagulation (DIC) and hypercoagulable states.

During uncomplicated pregnancy there is no change in At III levels during the antenatal period [171], but some lowering during delivery and then an increase 1 week postpartum. The authors suggest that At III synthesis must be increased during pregnancy to maintain normal mean levels in the face of increasing plasma volume. The principle of laboratory measurement of biological activity of At III depends on its ability to neutralize thrombin or Factor Xa. Fixed amounts of thrombin or Factor Xa are added to dilutions of the test plasma and the residual enzyme activity measured immunologically using monospecific antisera, but this will give no indication of its biological activity. In clinical laboratories the advent of chromogenic substances for the measurement of thrombin and Factor Xa has had a major impact on the measurement of At III activity [170].

Oral contraception and haemostasis

The commonest association of a small reduction in plasma At III is with the use of oral contraceptives [172–174]. In the past 20 years is has become obvious that there is a causal relation between oral contraceptive steroids and venous thromboembolism, though this role in thrombopathogenesis has not been fully evaluated. It is obvious that the oestrogen content is important and since the introduction of low-dose oestrogen pills the associated incidence of venous thromboembolism has fallen dramatically [175]. A significant fall in At III has been found in women taking combined oral contraceptives, regardless of the oestrogen content, but not in association with progestogen-only pills [176].

The depression of At III activity may be the result of consumption due to increased thrombin generation resulting from increased production of various procoagulants associated with oestrogen-containing oral contraceptives.

In a retrospective analysis of the plasma of 50 women taking combined oral contraception, 6–12 months after an episode of thromboembolism, none had demonstrable At III deficiency but over 30% had defective fibrinolytic activity [177]. In a prospective study of At III (Xa1) activity associated with low-dose oestrogen oral contraceptives, there was a significant reduction in Xa1 activity after one month of oestrogen consumption but no significant difference between those women taking 30 μg and 50 μg in terms of At III levels [178].

Accumulating evidence suggests that suppression of At III is only one of many contributory interacting risk factors associated with venous thromboembolism and oestrogen-containing oral contraceptives.

Until recently, however, the only evidence for differences in the risk of venous thromboembolism between different types of combined oral contraceptives has been related to the oestrogen content. Those preparations containing 50 μg or more of ethinyl oestradiol were associated with greater risks than those containing less than 50 μg [175,178,179]. The low-dose oestrogen-containing pills have become the mainstay of contraceptive practice.

Since July 1995, several studies have shown an unexpected increased risk of thromboembolism related to different progestogens (gestodene and desogestrel) involved in two types of third-generation combined oral contraceptives [180–182].

An increased risk for non-fatal venous thromboembolism associated with third-generation combined oral contraceptives (low-dose oestrogen plus gestodene or desogestrel) compared with second-generation oral contraceptives (<35 μg oestrogen + levonogestrel) was found in a study based on 370 general practices in a cohort of 283 130 otherwise healthy women. The data were taken from the UK General Practice Research Database [182].

Probably the largest study to date [181] describes the risk of venous thromboembolism with current use of combined oral contraceptives among 1143 patients and 2998 age-matched controls from 21 centres in Africa, Asia, Europe and Latin America. Odds ratios for venous thromboembolism associated with the use of combined oral contraceptives containing third-generation progestogens were higher than for those observed with first-generation progestagens (norethandrone type) and second (norgestrel group)-generation [180,181]. In this study, odds ratios for venous thromboembolism were also increased for obesity and, an unexpected finding, for those women with a history of hypertension in pregnancy.

The UK Committee on Safety of Medicines in October 1995 [183] in a press release recommended that all contraceptive pills containing the progestogens gestodene or desogestrel should be restricted to women intolerant of other brands following the premature release of the results of non-completed studies which showed an increased risk of thrombosis with these products. This press release was accompanied by simultaneous mailing of all medical practitioners regarding the possible increased risk of venous thromboembolism associated with the use of these products. The way in which the data were interpreted and dealt with in the UK resulted in a furore at the inexplicable haste and urgency with which action was taken. A coordinator of one of the key studies led the attack against the UK Committee on Safety of

Medicines [184], pointing out that although preliminary results suggest a modest association with third-generation oral contraceptives and deep venous thrombosis and pulmonary embolism, a causal link is unclear. In addition, the fact that these preparations are probably protective for heart attacks and the associated mortality was not appropriately emphasized.

The absolute risk of venous thromboembolism has been calculated to rise from 15 per 100 000 women per year with second-generation oral contraceptives to 30 per 100 000 per yer in those women using oral contraceptives containing desogestrel or gestodene. This is the first time that differences in venous thromboembolism incidence have been found between the newer low-dose oestrogen oral contraceptives and linked to progesterone derivatives. To put this extra risk into perspective, during pregnancy a woman's risk of thrombosis increases to about 60 per 100 000. However, the greatest risk to health comes from smoking while taking the pill — whatever type is used. Young women smokers using oral contraceptives are 10 times more likely to suffer myocardial infarction than users who do not smoke [185]. Venous thromboembolism remains rare among women in the reproductive years but we have to balance the risk of oral contraceptives of any sort against the possible benefits such as protection against myocardial infarction. Women with risk factors for venous thromboembolism (e.g. personal or family history) should be screened for thrombophilia and it would appear sensible not to start them on third-generation oral contraceptives. It is hoped 'that any disproportionate fear of litigation soon gives way to intelligent and well-informed collaborative decision-making' [186]. As this chapter goes to press, active investigation and further epidemiological studies are under way. The US Food and Drug Administration has stated that it 'considers it prudent to treat the data with caution before deciding on the policy implications'. The whole subject has been reviewed recently [187].

Protein C, thrombomodulin, Protein S and activated Protein C cofactor

Protein C inactivates Factors V and VIII in con-junction with its cofactors thrombomodulin and Protein S. To exert its effect, Protein C, a vitamin K-dependent anticoagulant synthesized in the liver, must be activated by an endothelial cell cofactor termed thrombomodulin. The importance of the Protein C–thrombomodulin–Protein S system is exemplified by the absence of thrombomodulin in the brain where the priority for haemostasis is higher than for anticoagulation.

Many kindreds with a deficiency or a functional deficit of Protein C with associated recurrent thromboembolism have been described [188]. Purpura fulminans neonatalis is the homozygous expression of Protein C deficiency with severe thrombosis and neonatal death [189].

Protein S, also a vitamin K-dependent glycoprotein, acts as a cofactor for activated Protein C by promoting its binding to lipid and platelet surface thus localizing the reaction.

Several families have been described with Protein S deficiency and thromboembolic disease.

Data on Protein C and Protein S levels in healthy pregnancy are sparse [190]. One study showed a significant reduction in functional Protein S levels during pregnancy and the puerperium [191]. Fourteen patients followed longitudinally throughout gestation and postpartum showed a rise of Protein C within the normal non-pregnant range during the second trimester. In contrast, free Protein S fell from the second trimester onwards but remained within the confines of the normal range [192].

More recently, a cross-sectional study of 91 normal pregnant women who had plasma concentration of Proteins C and S, measured during the first, second and third trimesters, showed no change in antigenic or functional Protein C but confirmed a significant fall in free Protein S from the first to second trimester with no further fall in the third trimester [193].

Activated Protein C cofactor: a new cofactor in the Protein C anticoagulant pathway

Deficiency of Protein C, Protein S or At III (the first naturally occurring anticoagulant to be identified) can be found in approximately 20%

of patients with a history of thromboembolism under the age of 45 years. These deficiencies are especially frequent in those with a family history. Recently, Dahlbäck and colleagues [194] identified a second cofactor for activated Protein C (APC) in a family with clear-cut thrombophilia. The defect could be corrected by the addition of normal plasma. In a further study to establish the prevalence of activated Protein C resistance (APCR) in patients with venous thrombosis [195], the defect was found in 33% of the patients studied. Precipitating factors for thrombosis such as pregnancy and the use of oral contraceptives were identified in 60% of these patients. The defect was identified in the laboratory using a modified activated partial thromboplastin time (APTT) test performed in the usual way (see below) but with and without the addition of APC. The results were expressed as APC sensitivity ratios defined as APTT (+APC) divided by APTT (−APC). In most laboratories which have adopted the technique, the normal ratio is above 2.0. An abnormal APTT ratio (<2.0) was detected in 64 of 301 (21%) unselected consecutive young patients in Holland on investigation of their first episode of thromboembolism [196].

Dahlbäck and Hildebrand [197] have recently identified the procoagulant Factor V as the factor responsible for hereditary APCR. A single missense mutation in the Factor V gene changing arginine to glutamate has been associated with the vast majority of cases with an abnormal APTT ratio—the so-called Factor V Leiden mutation. It is clear from subsequent studies that this defect is the most important cause of hereditary thrombophilia identified to date. In healthy pregnancy, APC resistance increases and the APC sensitivity ratio decreases, probably due to increased Factor VIIIC production. The *in vitro* values usually remain within normal limits [198,199].

A recent retrospective study of venous thromboembolism associated with pregnancy and the use of oral contraceptives showed that 59% of 34 women during pregnancy and 30% of 28 women using oral contraceptives had APC ratios of less than 2.0 indicating APCR [200].

A 1995 study [201] showed an especially high risk of venous thromboembolism among carriers of Factor V Leiden mutation using oral contraceptives and confirmed the increased risk in users of third-generation combined oral contraceptives even if they lacked the V Leiden mutation and had no family history.

Selem [202] asserted that 'There is little doubt that more components will be recognised in the near future which will allow a better and more thorough understanding of the mechanisms underlying venous and arterial thromboembolism.'

Fibrinolysis

The fibrinolytic enzyme system has four basic components: plasminogen, plasmin, activators and inhibitors (Fig. 3.5).

Fibrin and fibrinogen are digested by plasmin, a proteolytic enzyme derived from an inactive plasma precursor — plasminogen. Plasminogen is a β-globulin and estimates of its molecular weight vary between 81 000 and 143 000 [163]. Synthesis, most probably in the liver, can take place fairly rapidly, and treatment with streptokinase results in an increase in the plasminogen from barely detectable levels (in the presence of freshly formed clot) to normal within 12–24 hours. Plasminogen is stable over a wide range of temperature and pH in plasma and serum. It is a single polypeptide chain which, when converted to plasmin, becomes a

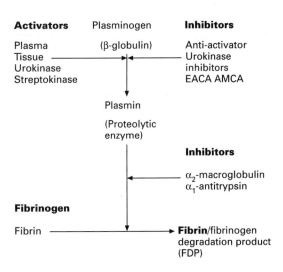

Fig. 3.5. Components of the fibrinolytic enzyme system.

two-chain molecule connected by a single disulphide bond.

Physiological fibrinolytic activity depends on plasminogen activators in the blood. Increased amounts are found in the plasma after strenuous exercise, emotional stress, surgical operations and other trauma. Plasma activator is difficult to assay because it is extremely labile and *in vitro* has a half-life of 15 minutes. During clotting plasma activators are absorbed onto fibrin.

Naturally occurring activators are found in blood, tissue and urine. Tissue activator can be extracted from most human organs with the exception of the placenta. Tissues especially rich in activator include the uterus, ovaries, prostate, heart, lungs, thyroid, adrenal glands and lymph nodes. Activity in tissues is concentrated mainly around blood vessels, veins having greater activity than arteries. Venous occlusion of the limbs will stimulate fibrinolytic activity of the blood and this has been used as a test for evaluating an individual's potential to release activator from the vascular endothelium [203].

Plasmin, the proteolytic enzyme derived from plasminogen, can digest many proteins, including fibrinogen and fibrin. Normally the action of plasmin is confined to the digestion of fibrin because of the presence of plasmin inhibitors in the blood. Other proteins which can be digested by plasmin include prothrombin, Factors V and VIII, glucagon, adrenocorticotrophic hormone and growth hormone.

There are two main inhibitors of the fibrinolytic system: antiactivators, which inhibit plasminogen activation, and antiplasmins, which are inhibitors of formed plasmin. Antiactivators have been separated [204], and identified in human serum and shown to develop during the process of spontaneous blood coagulation [205].

Several aliphatic–amino compounds are competitive inhibitors of plasminogen activation and include epsilon aminocaproic acid (EACA), tranexamic acid and aprotinin (Trasylol), which is commercially prepared from bovine lung.

Both plasma and serum exert a strong inhibitory action on plasmin. Platelets have antiplasmin activity which is probably of importance in stabilizing platelet thrombi. Normally plasma antiplasmin levels exceed the levels of plasminogen and hence the levels of potential plasmin, otherwise the stability of healthy vasculature would be destroyed.

Fibrin and fibrinogen degradation products

When fibrinogen or fibrin is broken down by plasmin, degradation products (FDPs) are formed (Fig. 3.6). Plasmin first splits off fragment X with some smaller fragments A, B and C. Further digestion of fragment X, which is still slowly but completely clottable by thrombin, results in the formation of fragments Y and D, which will not clot under the action of thrombin. Fragment Y is further broken down to fragments D and E, the 'end split products'. Fragments X and Y are termed 'high-molecular-weight split products'.

When a fibrin clot is formed, approximately 70% of fragment X is retained in the clot, fragment Y is retained to a somewhat lesser extent, and D and E are retained to 10% only.

Serum therefore can contain small amounts of fragment X, larger amounts of Y, D and E, as well as complexes of fibrin monomers, fibrinogen and fragment Y and X. All of these components have antigenic determinants in common with fibrinogen, and will be recognized by antifibrinogen antisera.

In recent years, the development of tests to measure specific FDPs such as Fibrinopeptide A and D-dimer using chromogenic assays have aided the laboratory investigation of fibrinolysis considerably.

Menstrual blood contains a high level of plas-

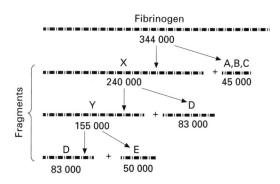

Fig. 3.6. Degradation of fibrinogen by plasmin.

minogen activator which has been correlated with the concentration of activator in the endometrium. Although some workers have been unable to demonstrate fibrinogen or fibrin in menstrual blood [206] and it has been reported that menstrual clots are gels of red-cell aggregates, others have been able to demonstrate fibrin using the electron microscope [207]. The importance of fibrinolysis in menstruation is supported by the decrease in menstrual loss during treatment with the fibrinolytic inhibitor EACA. The haemostatic events involved in normal human menstruation are strikingly different from those that are observed following trauma or surgery and there are still deficiencies in our understanding of the underlying mechanisms. For an account of current knowledge of normal and pathophysiology in relation to the part played by thrombosis and haemostasis in the menstruating endometrium, the reader is referred to a review by Cameron and Smith [208].

Tests of haemostatic function

There are simple rapid screening tests which establish the competence of the haemostatic system. These tests can be performed in any general haematological laboratory and do not require an expert coagulation unit. No attempt is made to give technical details of the tests recommended for they can be found easily elsewhere in pathology texts, but the basic mechanism is outlined for understanding of its relevance and the significance of results reported. Emphasis is laid on easily available investigations, the results of which will help those in obstetric practice to come to a rapid decision concerning the nature of haemostatic failure in their patients.

All the tests referred to are performed on suitably prepared aliquots of specimens of whole blood acquired by venepuncture.

In order to avoid testing artefacts it is essential that the blood is obtained by a quick, efficient, non-traumatic technique, with particular emphasis on the following points.

Thromboplastin contamination Thromboplastin release from damaged tissues may contaminate the specimen and alter the results. This is likely to occur if difficulty is encountered in finding the vein or if the vein is only partly canalized and the flow is slow, or if there is excessive squeezing of tissues and repeated attempts to obtain a specimen with the same needle. In such circumstances the specimen may clot in the tube in spite of the presence of anticoagulant or the coagulation times of the various tests will be altered and not reflect the true situation *in vivo*. The platelets may aggregate in clumps and give a falsely low count, be it automated or manual.

Heparin contamination Heparin characteristically prolongs the partial thromboplastin time and thrombin time out of proportion to the prothrombin time. As little as 0.05 units of heparin per millilitre will prolong the coagulation test times. It is customary, though not desirable, to take blood for coagulation tests from lines which have been washed through with fluids containing heparin to keep them patent. It is almost impossible to overcome the effect on the blood passing through such a line however much blood is taken and discarded before obtaining a sample for investigation. It is strongly recommended that blood be taken from another site not previously contaminated with heparin.

Fibrinolysis in vitro Any blood taken into a glass tube without anticoagulant will clot within a few minutes and natural fibrinolysis will continue *in vitro*. Unless the blood is taken into a fibrinolytic inhibitor such as EACA, a falsely high level of FDPs will be found which bears no relation to fibrinolysis *in vivo*. Similarly, leaving a tourniquet on too long before taking the specimen will stimulate local fibrinolytic activity *in vivo*.

Screening tests for haemostatic function

Tests related to vasculature integrity

Bleeding time The length of time a small skin wound continues to bleed depends largely on the number and function of platelets, i.e. their ability to form plugs at the site of injury. Ivy's

98 method is recommended but the test is unpleasant for the patient and tedious if the bleeding is prolonged (normal range, up to 7–10 minutes; 15–20 minutes, clearly abnormal). It is not of value in assessing haemostatic failure in an obstetric emergency. It may be of value, however, if the anaesthetist is unhappy about placement of an epidural catheter in a patient who may have a low-grade coagulopathy or who has been treated with an antiplatelet agent such as aspirin. It is the only rapidly performed in-vivo test of platelet vascular interaction [209]. Details of in-vitro platelet function tests can be found elsewhere [210].

Platelet count The commonest platelet disorder is thrombocytopenia. It may be an isolated haemostatic defect or part of a generalized consumptive coagulopathy. Examination of the blood film by a competent haematology laboratory worker may provide valuable information concerning the nature of the haemostatic disorders. The platelet count is a valuable rapid screening test in assessing acute obstetric haemostatic failure, particularly in helping the attendants, together with other assessments, to diagnose the presence and severity of disseminated intravascular coagulation.

Coagulation mechanisms (see Dacie and Lewis [210]) Blood for investigation should be taken into trisodium citrate; a measured standard amount of citrate is used so that the dilution factor is constant. It is essential that the exact amount of blood required for laboratory testing is delivered into the citrate-containing bottle or the proportion of anticoagulant to blood will be altered and the results will be unreliable. There are three simple, rapid *in vitro* tests of the integrity of the coagulation cascade:
1 Activated partial thromboplastin time (APTT)—intrinsic system
2 Prothrombin time (PT)—extrinsic system
3 Thrombin time (TT)—final common pathway
For the relation of these tests to the coagulation cascade see Fig. 3.7.

Activated partial thromboplastin time This test is also known as the partial thromboplastin

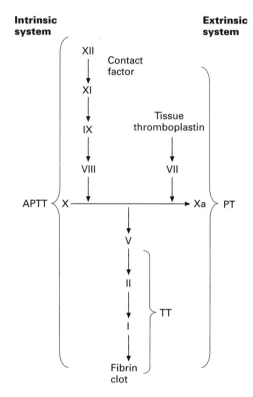

Fig. 3.7. In-vitro screening tests of coagulation and their relationship to the systems involved. PT: prothrombin time; APTT: activated partial thromboplastin time; TT: thrombin time.

time with kaolin and the kaolin cephalin clotting time. It gives a crude assessment of the integrity of the intrinsic coagulation system. The normal range usually lies between 35 and 45 seconds, but all tests must always be compared with a known normal plasma. Prolongation occurs with isolated factor deficiencies of Factors VIII, IX and XI and also in the presence of therapeutic heparin levels.

Prothrombin time This test measures the clotting time of citrated plasma after the addition of an optimal concentration of tissue extract (thromboplastin). It is a measure of the overall efficiency of the extrinsic clotting system. Normal range is approximately 10–14 seconds. It is prolonged in isolated Factor VII deficiency and in liver failure, and it is the test used to monitor dosage of warfarin (INR) in those on oral anticoagulants.

Thrombin time This test is a measure of the final common pathway of the extrinsic and intrinsic coagulation systems (Fig. 3.4). Normal plasma will give a thrombin clotting time of 15–19 seconds. The commonest causes of a delayed TT are the presence of FDPs, depletion of fibrinogen and the presence of heparin.

Both the clotting time and the appearance of the clot are informative.

Fibrinogen estimation (Clauss technique) (see Dacie and Lewis [210]) It should be remembered that in late pregnancy, i.e. after 30 weeks' gestation, the normal non-pregnant range of fibrinogen, 2.0–4.5 g/l, is increased to 4.0–6.0 g/l. Reduction of fibrinogen is seen in severe consumptive coagulopathy and in rare inherited deficiencies of fibrinogen.

Detection of fibrinogen/fibrin degradation products Healthy subjects have FDP concentrations of less than 10 μg/ml. Concentrations between 10 and 40 μg/l are seen in acute inflammatory disorders — in acute, venous and arterial thrombosis and after strenuous exercise or major surgery. High levels of FDPs are seen in association with severe acute disseminated intravascular coagulation and following thrombolytic therapy with streptokinase.

Using the above simple tests in the screening of a patient with an acute or chronic haemostatic disorder, together with a detailed clinical history, it is possible to place them into categories or even to make a provisional diagnosis which indicates how to proceed further in order to confirm the provisional diagnosis, e.g. to platelet function tests or individual coagulation factor assays.

It is essential that these more exacting tests should be carried out in an expert, competent and specialized laboratory and, because of the rapidity with which changes in coagulation factors take place *in vitro*, such units usually prefer to see the patient themselves rather than receiving blood samples taken at other centres, even if they are delivered by car or other rapid transport.

Coagulation and fibrinolysis during normal pregnancy

Coagulation system

Normal pregnancy is accompanied by major changes in the coagulation system [164, 211–213], with increases in the levels of Factors VII, VIII and X and a particularly marked increase in the level of plasma fibrinogen (Fig. 3.4). The increased quantity of fibrinogen in the plasma alters the negative surface charge of the red cells which, on standing, will form aggregates in a pattern described as *rouleaux* which settle in a glass tube more quickly than single erythrocytes. The increase in fibrinogen is probably the chief cause of the accelerated erythrocyte sedimentation rate observed during pregnancy.

The effect of pregnancy on the coagulation factors can be detected from about the third month of gestation. The plasma fibrinogen level increases from non-pregnant levels of about 2.5–4.0 g/l to as high as 6.0 g/l in late pregnancy and labour. If the increase in plasma volume is taken into consideration, the amount of fibrinogen in late pregnancy is at least double that of the non-pregnant state. This marked rise in fibrinogen results from increased synthesis, as has been shown in pregnant monkeys [214]. The elevation of Factor VII in pregnancy may be increased as much as tenfold and an increase in this factor has also been observed in women taking oestrogen/progestogen contraceptives [215].

Factor VIII, antihaemophilic factor, is elevated in late pregnancy, the coagulation activity being approximately twice that in the non-pregnant state. Some workers have found a parallel increase both in the biological activity of Factor VIII and in the Factor VIII-related antigen [216], while others have found an increase in the ratio between the antigenic and coagulant activity [217]. In uncomplicated pregnancies, the ratio remains around 1:1 but it is raised in pregnancies associated with severe pre-eclampsia or septic abortion because of a greater increase in Factor VIII-related antigen and reduction in Factor VIIIC due to thrombin activation [218].

Elevations of Factor IX (Christmas Factor)

during pregnancy have been reported by several authors, as have decreases in Factor XI — with levels down to 60–70% of the non-pregnant value and a gradual fall in fibrin-stabilizing Factor XIII reaching 50% of the normal non-pregnant value at term [219].

Increased concentrations of high molecular weight fibrin/fibrinogen complexes in the plasma have been demonstrated during normal pregnancy and confirmed by comparing the levels in normal pregnancy with those found in non-pregnant age-matched controls [220]. An increase in the level of fibrinopeptide A and a thrombin-like influence on Factor V activity has also been described. There appears to be an increased ability to neutralize heparin in late pregnancy as demonstrated by the need for a moderately increased dose to achieve similar plasma levels in the third trimester in those women receiving prophylactic low-dosage unfractionated heparin [221] and low molecular weight heparin [222,223].

These changes in the coagulation system in normal pregnancy are consistent with a continuing low-grade process of coagulant activity. Using electron microscopy, fibrin deposition can be demonstrated in the intervillous space of the placenta and in the walls of spiral arteries supplying the placenta [224]. As pregnancy advances, the elastic lamina and smooth muscle of these spiral arteries are replaced by a matrix containing fibrin. This allows an expansion of the lumen to accommodate an increasing blood flow and reduces the pressure in arterial blood flowing to the placenta. At placental separation during normal childbirth, a blood flow of 500–800 ml/min has to be staunched within seconds or serious haemorrhage will occur. Myometrial contraction plays a vital role in securing haemostasis by reducing the blood flow to the placental site. At separation of the placenta, rapid closure of the terminal part of the spiral arteries by the unique mechanism of myometrial contraction will be facilitated by the structural changes described. The placental site is rapidly covered by a fibrin mesh following delivery; the amount of fibrinogen deposited represents 5–10% of the total circulating fibrinogen.

The increased levels of fibrinogen and coagulation factors during pregnancy probably represent a compensatory response to local utilization. The resulting hypercoagulability will be advantageous to meet the sudden demand for haemostatic components at placental separation.

Fibrinolysis

Plasma fibrinolytic activity is decreased during pregnancy, remains low during labour and delivery, and returns to normal within one hour of placental delivery. Fibrinolytic activity in the walls of veins is reduced in late pregnancy.

The rapid return of systemic fibrinolytic activity to normal following delivery of the placenta and the fact that the placenta has been shown to contain inhibitors which block fibrinolysis [225] suggested that inhibition of fibrinolysis during pregnancy is mediated through the placenta.

The identification of a placentally derived circulating plasminogen activation inhibitor [226] supports this contention. In addition, the activity of the fibrinolytic system in response to stimulation has been found to be significantly reduced during pregnancy [203]. This physiological impairment of fibrinolysis could contribute to the increased thrombotic risk in pregnancy.

Since fibrinolysis is depressed during pregnancy, the level of FDP will not necessarily reflect the amount of local intravascular coagulation. The increase of FDP in the circulation in labour may originate from the uterus. FDP levels in uterine blood during caesarean section carried out in the course of labour were considerably higher than those during elective caesarean section [227].

Haemostatic problems associated with pregnancy

As has already been outlined, pregnancy is known to induce complex changes in the physiological systems concerned with haemostasis [211,228,229]. The alterations in the coagulation and fibrinolytic systems which take place during pregnancy, together with the increased blood volume and unique phenomenon of myometrial contraction, help to combat the hazard of haemorrhage during and after placental separation; however, they carry the risk of more rapid and increased response to coagulant stimuli. The characteristic tendency to venous stasis in the lower limbs may provide initiating conditions and the incidence of venous thrombosis, though low, is undoubtedly raised in pregnancy. An association has been shown recently between genetic thrombophilia and increased fetal loss, particularly in women with combined defects [230].

The local activation of the clotting system during parturition carries with it a risk not only of thromboembolism but of disseminated intravascular coagulation, consumption of clotting factors and platelets leading to severe generalized — and, in particular, uterine — bleeding. Despite the advances in obstetric care and highly developed blood transfusion services, haemorrhage still constitutes a major factor in maternal mortality and morbidity [231,232].

The most recently published *Report on Confidential Enquiries into Maternal Deaths in the United Kingdom* [232] highlights the hazard of pulmonary embolism which has been second only to hypertension as a direct cause of maternal mortality over many years. However, unexpectedly, the absolute numbers and the incidence of death due to haemorrhage has increased in the last two triennia, bringing haemorrhage into the first three leading direct causes of maternal mortality. Most of the reported deaths were not associated with disseminated intravascular coagulation initially, which only appeared to develop after prolonged shock.

Fibrinolysis is stimulated by disseminated intravascular coagulation and the FDPs resulting from the process interfere with the formation of firm fibrin clots; a vicious circle is thus established which results in further disastrous bleeding. The classic example of this complication is *abruptio placentae*. Tissue thromboplastin is released into the hypercoagulable maternal circulation from the placental site, and it has been shown that severe protracted postpartum bleeding in cases of *abruptio placentae* was associated with high concentrations of FDPs and atony of the uterus. It is possible that high levels of FDP interfere not only with coagu-

lation but also inhibit myometrial contraction [233].

A more subtle low-grade process of intravascular coagulation is thought to occur in pre-eclampsia. Deviations from the levels of normal pregnancy for the platelet count and serum FDP occur around 24 weeks' gestation. The ratio of Factor VIII-related antigen to Factor VIII coagulant activity is markedly increased. Levels of soluble fibrin/fibrinogen complexes are also high in patients with pre-eclampsia compared with levels in normal pregnancy [220]. Although administration of small-dose subcutaneous heparin results in lowering of the FDP levels and the return of the platelet count from thrombocytopenic levels to normal, no apparent change is effected in the clinical course of pre-eclampsia [234]. Pilot studies have suggested that small-dose aspirin may protect women at risk from developing pre-eclampsia and pregnancy-associated hypertension; this mode of therapy is thought to act by selectively inhibiting the production of thromboxane from arachidonic acid by the platelet, thereby enhancing the effect of prostacyclin generation from the endothelium (Fig. 3.3). One such study randomized over 3000 nulliparous normotensive women in the second trimester to receive 60 mg of aspirin per day or placebo [235]. The incidence of pre-eclampsia was lower in the aspirin-treated group (4.6%) than in the placebo group (6.3%). There were no significant differences in infants' birthweights, intrauterine growth retardation (IUGR), neonatal bleeding or postpartum haemorrhage but an increased incidence of *abruptio placenta* was observed in those women who received aspirin (11 women, versus 2 in the placebo group). The results published by the Collaborative Low-dose Aspirin Study in Pregnancy [236] do not support routine prophylaxis or therapeutic administration of antiplatelet therapy in pregnancy to all women at increased risk of pre-eclampsia or IUGR. The multicentre placebo-controlled trial did suggest that low-dose aspirin may be justified in women judged to be at risk of early onset pre-eclampsia severe enough to need very preterm delivery. It is possible that one of the reasons for the disappointing result of this large multicentre trial was that the randomization in some centres excluded those women judged to be at especially increased risk of severe eclampsia. One reassuring spin-off from this large study is that low-dose aspirin 60–75 mg daily did not appear to result in any adverse effects—particularly bleeding in the fetus, neonate or mother. There were no increases in intraventricular bleeds in preterm infants or other neonatal haemorrhages and there were no significant increases in antepartum haemorrhages or excess bleeding with epidural anaesthesia in the mother.

It is not appropriate to discuss pathological coagulation further in a book concerned with normal physiology of pregnancy. For details of inherited and acquired conditions which may compromise haemostasis during pregnancy the reader is referred to monographs devoted entirely to this subject [212,228,229,237,238].

Developmental haemostasis and prenatal diagnosis of coagulation defects

Observations in the 1960s and 1970s on midterm abortions and preterm infants showed that clotting factors were present in fetal life and were independent of maternal blood levels. With the obstetric advances in ultrasound scanning and fetal blood sampling, it has been possible to obtain serial ranges of normal in-utero fetal concentration of platelets and of the important coagulation factors [239].

During the last decade obstetric and laboratory techniques have been successfully applied to the accurate prenatal diagnosis of congenital haematological disorders [240–242]. Fetal blood cannot be obtained easily before 18 weeks' gestation and, if findings indicate, this may result in a midtrimester termination of pregnancy. However, a few conditions remain which cannot be diagnosed by any other method and this technique will continue to have value. In the last decade there has been an explosion of knowledge about human molecular genetics. There has been a change in emphasis in the analysis of human genetic disease from the clinical cellular and biochemical levels to the molecular level. Using recombinant DNA techniques, the new tools of molecular biology, it has been possible to study the structure of human genes directly and how their activity is controlled and their role in protein synthesis.

Table 3.3. Chromosomal localization of genes controlling haemostatic coagulation and fibrinolytic components.

Chromosome no.	Component
1	Tissue factor, At III
2	Protein C
3	Protein S
4	Fibrinogen
6	Factor XIII (a-sub-unit), Factor XII, plasminogen
8	Tissue plasminogen activator
11	Prothrombin
12	von Willebrand factor
13	Factors VII, X and XIII (b-sub-unit)
17	Platelet glycoproteins IIb, IIIa
20	Thrombomodulin
X	Factors VIII and IX

The fetal tissue necessary for DNA analysis can be obtained much earlier in gestation and will therefore result in earlier termination of pregnancy if desired and indicated. The chromosomal site of many of the genes responsible for producing haemostatic factors are now known (Table 3.3). Fetal sexing may be determined at a much earlier stage of pregnancy than was possible from amniotic fluid cells by DNA analysis of chorion biopsy material obtained at 8–10 weeks' gestation and also by the new, more discriminating ultrasound. Cloning of the genes for Factors VIII and IX has facilitated prenatal diagnosis in many but not all cases at risk of haemophilia. The identification of most haemophilia carriers as well as affected fetuses if desired by direct analysis of DNA is now in routine practice.

For a review of the techniques involved and their application to clinical practice in this area and many other conditions, the reader is referred to Weatherall's masterly monograph [243].

With the help of this new discipline of molecular genetics the systems involved in the control of haemostasis continue to be unravelled. The discovery of new procoagulants, anticoagulants and fibrinolytic factors increases our understanding of their complex interactions and allows revisions of the model for physiological initiation, regulation and control [244].

References

1 Hytten F. (1985) Blood volume changes in normal pregnancy. In *Haematological Disorders in Pregnancy: Clinics in Haematology*, vol. 14, p. 601. Saunders, Eastbourne.

2 Overall J.E. & Williams C.M. (1959) A note concerning sources of variance in determination of human plasma volume. *Journal of Laboratory and Clinical Medicine* **54**, 186.

3 Lund C.J. & Donovan J.C. (1967) Blood volume during pregnancy. *American Journal of Obstetrics and Gynecology*, **98**, 394.

4 Paintin D.B. (1962) The size of the total red cell volume in pregnancy. *Journal of Obstetrics and Gynaecology of the British Commonwealth* **69**, 719.

5 Pritchard J.A. & Adams R.H. (1960) Erythrocyte production and destruction during pregnancy. *American Journal of Obstetrics and Gynecology* **79**, 750.

6 Berlin N.I., Goetsch C., Hyde G.M. & Parsons R.J. (1953) The blood volume in pregnancy as determined with P^{32}-labelled red blood cells. *Surgery, Gynecology and Obstetrics* **97**, 173.

7 Hytten F.E. & Leitch I. (1971) The volume and composition of the blood. In *The Physiology of Human Pregnancy*, 2nd edn, p. 1. Blackwell Scientific Publications, Oxford.

8 Murphy J.F., O'Riordan J., Newcombe R.G., Coles E.C. & Pearson J.F. (1986) Relation of haemoglobin levels in first and second trimesters to outcome of pregnancy. *Lancet* **i**, 992.

9 Steer P., Ash Alam M., Wadsworth J. & Welch A. (1995) Relation between maternal haemoglobin concentration and birth weight in different ethinic groups. *British Medical Journal* **310**, 489.

10 Rovinsky J.J. & Jaffin H. (1965) Cardiovascular hemodynamics in pregnancy. I. Blood and plasma volumes in multiple pregnancy. *American Journal of Obstetrics and Gynecology* **93**, 1.

11 Fullerton W.T., Hytten F.E., Klopper A.I. & McKay E. (1965) A case of quadruplet pregnancy. *Journal of Obstetrics and Gynaecology of the British Commonwealth* **72**, 791.

12 Combs C.A., Murphy E.L. & Laros R.K. (1991) Factors associated with hemorrhage in cesarean deliveries. *Obstetrics and Gynecology* **77**, 77.

13 De Leeuw N.K.M., Lowenstein L., Tucker E.C. & Dayal S. (1968) Correlation of red cell loss at delivery with changes in red cell mass. *American Journal of Obstetrics and Gynecology* **100**, 1092.

14 Chesley L.C. (1972) Plasma and red cell volumes during pregnancy. *American Journal of Obstetrics and Gynecology* **112**, 440.

15 Peck T.M. & Arias F. (1979) Hematologic changes associated with pregnancy. *Clinical Obstetrics and Gynecology* **22**, 785.

16 Traill L.M. (1975) Reticulocytes in healthy pregnancy. *Medical Journal of Australia* **2**, 205.

17 Manasc B. & Jepson J. (1960) Erythropoietin in plasma and urine during human pregnancy. *Canadian Medical Association Journal* **100**, 687.

18 Beguin Y., Lipscei G., Oris R., Thoumsin H. & Fillet G. (1990) Serum immunoreactive erythropoietin during pregnancy and in the early postpartum. *British Journal of Haematology* **76**, 545.

19 Riikonen S., Saijonmaa O., Jarvenpaa A.L. & Fyhrquist F. (1994) Serum concentrations of erythropoietin in healthy and anaemic pregnant women. *Scandinavian Journal of Clinical Laboratory Investigation* **54**, 653.

20 Milman N., Agger A.O. & Nielsen O.J. (1994) Iron status markers and serum erythropoietin in 120 mothers and newborn infants: Effect of iron supplementation in normal pregnancy. *Acta Obstetrica et Gynaecologica Scandinavica* **73**, 200.

21 Harstad T.W., Mason R.A. & Cox S.M. (1992) Serum erythropoietin quantitation in pregnancy using an enzyme-linked immunoassay. *American Journal of Perinatology* **9**, 233.

22 Milman N., Agger A.O. & Nielsen O.J. (1991) Iron supplementation during pregnancy: Effect on iron status markers, serum erythropoietin and human placental lactogen — A placebo controlled study in 207 Danish women. *Danish Medical Bulletin* **38**, 471.

23 Jepson J.H. & Friesen H.G. (1968) The mechanism of action of human placental lactogen on erythropoiesis. *British Journal of Haematology* **15**, 465.

24 Pembrey M.E., Weatherall D.J. & Clegg J.B. (1973) Maternal synthesis of haemoglobin F in pregnancy. *Lancet* **i**, 1350.

25 Popat N., Wood W.G., Weatherall D.J. & Turnbull A.C. (1977) Pattern of maternal F-cell production during pregnancy. *Lancet* **ii**, 377.

26 Lund C.J. (1951) Studies on the iron deficiency anemia of pregnancy including plasma volume, total hemoglobin, erythrocyte protoporphyrin in treated and untreated normal and anemic patients. *American Journal of Obstetrics and Gynecology* **62**, 947.

27 Roscoe M.H. & Donaldson G.M.M. (1946) The blood in pregnancy. II. The blood volume, cell volume and haemoglobin mass. *Journal of Obstetrics and Gynaecology of the British Empire* **53**, 527.

28 Tysoe F.W. & Lowenstein L. (1950) Blood volume and hematologic studies in pregnancy and the puerperium. *American Journal of Obstetrics and Gynecology* **60**, 1187.

29 Gemzell C.A., Robbe H. & Sjöstrand T. (1954) Blood volume and total amount of haemoglobin in normal pregnancy and the puerperium. *Acta Obstetricia et Gynaecologica Scandinavica* **33**, 289.

30 Efrati P., Presentey B., Margalith M. & Rozenszajn L. (1964) Leukocytes of normal pregnant women. *Obstetrics and Gynecology* **23**, 429.

31 Cruickshank J.M., Morris R., Butt W.R. & Crooke A.C. (1970) The relationship of total and differential leukocyte counts with urinary oestrogen and plasma cortisol levels. *Journal of Obstetrics and Gynaecology of the British Commonwealth* **77**, 634.

32 Good W., MacDonald H.N., Hancock K.W. & Wood J.E. (1973) Haematological changes in pregnancy following ovulation induction therapy. *Journal of Obstetrics and Gynaecology of the British Commonwealth* **80**, 486.

33 Cruickshank J.M. (1970) The effects of parity on the leucocyte count in pregnant and non-pregnant women. *British Journal of Haematology* **18**, 531.

34 Gibson A. (1937) On leucocyte changes during labour

and the puerperium. *Journal of Obstetrics and Gynaecology of the British Empire* **44**, 500.

35 Kuvin S.F. & Brecher G. (1962) Differential neutrophil counts in pregnancy. *New England Journal of Medicine* **266**, 877.

36 Quigley H.J., Dawson E.A., Hyun B.H. & Custer R.P. (1960) The activity of alkaline phosphatase in granular leukocytes during pregnancy and the puerperium: A preliminary report. *American Journal of Clinical Pathology* **33**, 109.

37 Polishuk W.Z., Diamant Y.Z., Zuckerman H. & Sadovsky E. (1970) Leukocyte alkaline phosphatase in pregnancy and the puerperium. *American Journal of Obstetrics and Gynecology* **107**, 604.

38 Fleming A.F. (1975) Haematological changes in pregnancy. *Clinics in Obstetrics and Gynaecology* **2**, 269.

39 Mitchell G.W., Jacobs A.A., Haddad V., Paul B.B., Strauss R.R. & Sbarra A.J. (1970) The role of the phagocyte in host–parasite interactions. XXV. Metabolic and bactericidal activities of leukocytes from pregnant women. *American Journal of Obstetrics and Gynecology* **108**, 805.

40 Ramsdale E.H. & Mowbray J.F. (1973) Positive N.B.T. tests in pregnancy. *Lancet* **i**, 1246.

41 Abernathy M.R. (1966) Döhle bodies associated with the uncomplicated pregnancy. *Blood* **27**, 380.

42 Elder M.G., Bonello F. & Ellul J. (1971) Neutrophil alkaline phosphatase in pregnancy and its relationship to urinary estrogen excretion and serum heat-stable alkaline phosphatase levels. *American Journal of Obstetrics and Gynecology* **111**, 319.

43 Jacobs A.A., Selvaraj R.J., Strauss R.R., Paul B.B., Mitchell G.W. & Sbarra A.J. (1973) The role of the phagocyte in host–parasite interactions. XXXIX. Stimulation of bactericidal activity of myeloperoxidase-containing leukocyte fractions by estrogens. *American Journal of Obstetrics and Gynecology* **117**, 671.

44 Andrews W.C. & Bonsnes R.W. (1951) The leucocytes during pregnancy. *American Journal of Obstetrics and Gynecology* **61**, 1129.

45 Thonnard-Neumann E. (1961) The influence of hormones on the basophilic leukocytes. *Acta Haematologica (Basel)* **25**, 261.

46 Brain P., Marston R.H. & Gordon J. (1972) Immunological responses in pregnancy. *British Medical Journal* **4**, 488.

47 Hill C.A., Finn R. & Denye V. (1973) Depression of cellular immunity in pregnancy due to a serum factor. *British Medical Journal* **3**, 513.

48 Purtilo D.T., Hallgren H.M. & Yunis E.J. (1972) Depressed maternal response to phytohaemagglutinin in human pregnancy. *Lancet* **i**, 769.

49 Davis J.C. & Hipkin L.J. (1974) Depression of lymphocyte transformation in women taking oral contraceptives. *Lancet* **ii**, 217.

50 Contractor S.F. & Davies H. (1973) Effect of chorionic somatomammotrophin and human chorionic gonadotrophin on phytohaemagglutinin-induced lymphocyte transformation. *Nature New Biology* **243**, 284.

51 Karmali R.A., Lauder I. & Horrobin D.F. (1974) Prolactin and the immune response. *Lancet* **ii**, 106.

52 Studd J.W.W. (1975) The plasma proteins in pregnancy. *Clinics in Obstetrics and Gynecology* **2**, 285.

53 Jones E., Curzen P. & Gaugas J.M. (1973) Suppressive activity of pregnancy on mixed lymphocyte reaction. *Journal of Obstetrics and Gynaecology of the British Commonwealth* **80**, 603.

54 Goyette R.E., Donowho E.M., Hieger L.R. & Plunkett G.D. (1974) Fulminant herpes virus hominis hepatitis during pregnancy. *Obstetrics and Gynecology* **43**, 191.

55 Greenberg M., Jacobziner H., Pakter J. & Weisl B.A.G. (1958) Maternal mortality in the epidemic of Asian influenza, New York City 1957. *American Journal of Obstetrics and Gynaecology* **76**, 897.

56 Rindge M.E. (1957) Poliomyelitis in pregnancy. *New England Journal of Medicine* **256**, 281.

57 Anon. (1974) Nature's transplant. *Lancet* **i**, 345.

58 Lucas A.O. (1964) Pneumococcal meningitis in pregnancy and the puerperium. *British Medical Journal* **1**, 92.

59 Gilles H.M., Lawson J.B., Sibelas M., Voller A. & Allan N. (1969) Malaria, anaemia and pregnancy. *Annals of Tropical Medicine and Parasitology* **63**, 245.

60 MacGregor J.D. & Avery J.G. (1974) Malaria transmission and fetal growth. *British Medical Journal* **3**, 433.

61 Taylor D.J. & Lind T. (1976) Haematological changes during normal pregnancy: Iron-induced macrocytosis. *British Journal of Obstetrics and Gynaecology* **83**, 760.

62 De Leeuw N.K.M., Lowenstein L. & Hsieh Y.S. (1966) Iron deficiency and hydremia in normal pregnancy. *Medicine, Baltimore* **45**, 291.

63 World Health Organization (1972) Nutritional anaemias. *Technical Report Series* No. 503, Geneva.

64 Robertson E.G. & Cheyne G.A. (1972) Plasma biochemistry in relation to oedema of pregnancy. *Journal of Obstetrics and Gynaecology of the British Commonwealth* **79**, 769.

65 Chanarin I. (1985) Folate and cobalamin. In *Haematological Disorders in Pregnancy: Clinics in Haematology*, vol. Ed. E.A. Letsky, 14, p. 629. W.B. Saunders, London.

66 Thompson W.G. (1988) Comparison of tests for diagnosis of iron depletion in pregnancy. *American Journal of Obstetrics and Gynecology* **159**, 1132.

67 Ibidapo D. & Letsky E.A. (1998) Ferritin vs. MCV as an indicator of iron deficiency in pregnancy. *Journal of Laboratory and Clinical Medicine*.

68 Rorth M. & Bille Brahe N.E. (1971) 2,3-diphosphoglycerate and creatinine in the red-cell membrane during human pregnancy. *Scandinavian Journal of Clinical and Laboratory Investigation* **28**, 271.

69 Oski F.A. (1973) The unique fetal red cell and its function. *Pediatrics* **51**, 494.

70 Kaeda J.S., Prasad K., Howard R.J., Mehta A., Vulliamy T. & Luzzatto L. (1994) Management of pregnancy when maternal blood has a very high level of fetal haemoglobin. *British of Journal of Haematology* **88**, 432.

71 Fletcher J. & Suter P.E.N. (1969) The transport of iron by the human placenta. *Clinical Science* **36**, 209.

72 Hallberg L. (1994) Prevention of iron deficiency. *Clinical Haematology* **7**, 805.

73 Hallberg L. (1992) Iron balance in pregnancy and lactation. In *Nutritional Anaemias*, Eds S.J. Forget & S. Zlotkin, p. 13. Raven Press, New York.

74 Barrett J.F.R., Whittaker P.G., Williams J.G. & Lind T. (1994) Absorption of non-haem iron from food during normal pregnancy. *British Medical Journal* **309**, 79.

75 Svanberg B. (1975) Absorption of iron in pregnancy. *Acta Obstetricia et Gynaecologica Scandinavica* (Suppl.) **48**, 1.

76 Fleming A.F., Martin J.D., Hahnel R. & Westlake A.J. (1974) Effects of iron and folic acid antenatal supplements on maternal haematology and fetal well-being. *Medical Journal of Australia* **2**, 429.

77 Meadows N.J., Gainger S.L., Warwick R., Keeling P.W.N. & Thompson R.P.H. (1983) Oral iron and the bioavailability of zinc. *British Medical Journal* **287**, 1013.

78 Hambridge K.M., Krebs N.F., Jacobs M.A., Guyette L. & Ikle D.N. (1983) Zinc nutritional status during pregnancy: A longitudinal study. *American Journal of Clinical Nutrition* **37**, 425.

79 Meadows N.J., Ruse W., Smith M.F., Day J., Keeling P.W.N., Scopes J.W. & Thompson R.P.H. (1981) Zinc and small babies. *Lancet* **ii**, 1135.

80 Sheldon W.L., Aspillaga M.O., Smith P.A. & Lind T. (1985) The effects of oral iron supplementation on zinc and magnesium levels during pregnancy. *British Journal of Obstetrics and Gynaecology* **92**, 892.

81 Jacobs A., Miller F., Worwood M., Beamish M.R. & Wardrop C.A. (1972) Ferritin in serum of normal subjects and patients with iron deficiency and iron overload. *British Medical Journal* **4**, 206.

82 Fenton V., Cavill I. & Fisher J. (1977) Iron stores in pregnancy. *British Journal of Haematology*, **37**, 145.

83 Bentley L.P. (1985) Iron metabolism and anaemia in pregnancy. In *Haematological Disorders in Pregnancy: Clinics in Haematology*, vol. 14, Ed. E.A. Letsky, p. 613. Saunders, Eastbourne.

84 Letsky E.A. (1987) Anaemia in obstetrics. In: *Progress in Obstetrics and Gynaecology*, vol. 6, p. 23. Churchill Livingstone, London.

85 Cook J.D. (1994) Iron deficiency anaemia. *Baillière's Clinical Haematology* **7**, 787.

86 Carriaga M.T., Skikne B.S., Finley B., Cutler B. & Cook J.D. (1991) Serum transferrin receptor for the detection of iron deficiency in pregnancy. *American Journal of Clinical Nutrition* **54**, 1077.

87 Krause J.R. & Stolc V. (1979) Serum ferritin and bone marrow iron stores. I. Correlation with absence of iron in biopsy specimens. *American Journal of Clinical Pathologists* **72**, 817.

88 Finch C.A. & Huebers H. (1982) Perspectives in iron metabolism. *New England Journal of Medicine* **306**, 1520.

89 Addy D.P. (1986) Happiness is: iron. *British Medical Journal* **292**, 969.

90 Allen L.H. (1993) Iron-deficiency anemia increases risk of preterm delivery. *Nutritional Review* **51**, 49.

91 Scholl T.O., Hediger M.L., Fischer R.L. & Shearer J.W. (1992) Anaemia vs. iron deficiency: Increased risk of preterm delivery in a prospective study. *American Journal of Clinical Nutrition* **55**, 985.

92 Kaltreider D.F. & Kohl S. (1980) Epidemiology of preterm delivery. *Clinics in Obstetrics and Gynecology* **23**, 17.

93 Klebanoff M.A., Shiono P.H., Selby J.V., Trachtenberg A.I. & Graubard B.I. (1991) Anemia and spontaneous preterm birth. *American Journal of Obstetrics and Gynecology* **164**, 59.

94 Oski F.A. (1985) Iron deficiency: Facts and fallacies. *Pediatric Clinics of North America* **32**, 493.

95 Walter T. (1994) Effect of iron deficiency anaemia on cognitive skills in infancy and childhood. *Baillière's Clinical Haematology* **7**, 815.

96 Idjradinata P. & Pollitt E. (1993) Reversal of developmental delays in iron-deficient anaemic infants treated with iron. *Lancet* **341**, 1.

97 Godfrey K.M., Redman C.W.G., Barker D.J.P. & Osmond C. (1991) The effect of maternal anaemia and iron deficiency on the ratio of fetal weight to placental weight. *British Journal of Obstetrics and Gynaecology* **98**, 886.

98 Hercberg S. & Galan P. (1992) Nutritional anaemias. *Baillière's Clinical Haematology* **5**, 143.

99 Fleming A.F. (1989) The aetiology of severe anaemia in pregnancy in Ndola, Zambia. *Annals of Tropical Medicine and Parasitology* **83**, 37.

100 Kuizon M.D., Platon T.P., Ancheta L.P., Angeles J.C., Nunez C.B. & Macapinlac M.P. (1979) Iron supplementation among pregnant women. *South East Asian Journal of Tropical Medicine* **10**, 520.

101 Mayet F.G.H. (1985) Anaemia of pregnancy. *South African Medical Journal* **67**, 804.

102 Ogunbode O., Akinyele I.O. & Hussain M.A. (1979) Dietary iron intake of pregnant Nigerian women with anaemia. *International Journal of Gynaecology and Obstetrics* **17**, 290.

103 Magee H.E. & Milligan E.H.M. (1951) Haemoglobin levels before and after labour. *British Medical Journal* **ii**, 1307.

104 Hemminki E. & Starfield B. (1978) Routine administration of iron and vitamins during pregnancy: Review of controlled clinical trials. *British Journal of Obstetrics and Gynaecology* **85**, 404.

105 Kullander S. & Kallen B. (1976) A prospective study of drugs and pregnancy. *Acta Obstetricia et Gynaecologica Scandinavica* **55**, 287.

106 Letsky E.A. (1995) Blood volume, haematinics, anaemia. In *Medical Disorders in Obstetric Practice*, 3rd edn. Ed. M. de Swiet, p. 33. Blackwell Science, Oxford.

107 Herbert V. (1962) Experimental nutritional folate deficiency in man. *Transactions of the Association of American Physicians* **75**, 307.

108 Herbert V. (1985) Biology of disease: Megaloblastic anaemias. *Laboratory Investigations* **52**, 3.

109 Landon M.J. (1975) Folate metabolism in pregnancy. *Clinics in Obstetrics and Gynaecology* **2**, 413.

110 Chanarin I. (1979) Megaloblastic anaemia associated with pregnancy. In *The Megaloblastic Anaemias*, 2nd edn, p. 466. Blackwell Scientific Publications, Oxford.

111 Ball E.W. & Giles C. (1964) Folic acid and vitamin B$_{12}$ levels in pregnancy and their relation to megaloblastic anaemia. *Journal of Clinical Pathology* **17**, 165.

112 Fleming A.F., Martin J.D. & Stenhouse N.S. (1974)

106

Pregnancy anaemia, iron and folate deficiency in Western Australia. *Medical Journal of Australia* **2**, 479.

113 Fleming A.F. (1972) Urinary excretion of folate in pregnancy. *Journal of Obstetrics and Gynaecology of the British Commonwealth* **79**, 916.

114 Landon M.J. & Hytten F.E. (1971) The excretion of folate in pregnancy. *Journal of Obstetrics and Gynaecology of the British Commonwealth* **78**, 769.

115 McLean F.W., Heine M.W., Held B. & Streiff R.B. (1970) Folic acid absorption in pregnancy: Comparison of the pteroylpolyglutamate and pteroylmonoglutamate. *Blood* **36**, 628.

116 Landon N.J. & Hytten F.E. (1972) Plasma folate levels following an oral load of folic acid during pregnancy. *Journal of Obstetrics and Gynaecology of the British Commonwealth* **79**, 577.

117 Chanarin I., Rothman D., Ward A. & Perry J. (1968) Folate status and requirement in pregnancy. *British Medical Journal* **ii**, 390.

118 Avery B. & Ledger W.J. (1970) Folic acid metabolism in well-nourished pregnant women. *Obstetrics and Gynecology* **35**, 616.

119 Stone M.L., Luhby A.L., Feldman R., Gordon M. & Cooperman J.M. (1967) Folic acid metabolism in pregnancy. *American Journal of Gynecology* **90**, 638.

120 Shapiro J., Alberts H.W., Welch P. & Metz J. (1965) Folate and vitamin B_{12} deficiency associated with lactation. *British Journal of Haematology* **11**, 498.

121 Osler W. (1919) Observations on the severe anaemias of pregnancy and the postpartum state. *British Medical Journal* **u**, 1.

122 Lowenstein L., Brunton L. & Hsieh Y.-S. (1966) Nutritional anemia and megaloblastosis in pregnancy. *Canadian Medical Association Journal* **94**, 636.

123 Chanarin I. (1975) The folate content of food-stuffs and the availability of difference folate analogues for absorption. In *Getting the Most out of Food* p. 41. Van den Bergh and Jurgens, London.

124 Haworth C. & Evans D.I.K. (1981) Nutritional aspects of blood disorders in the new-born. *Journal of Human Nutrition* **35**, 323.

125 Oski F.A. (1979) Nutritional anemias. *Seminars in Perinatology* **3**, 381.

126 Elwood J.M. (1983) Can vitamins prevent neural tube defects? *Canadian Medical Association Journal* **129**, 1088.

127 Laurence K.M., James N., Miller M.H., Tennant G.B. & Campbell H. (1981) Double-blind randomised controlled trial of folate treatment before conception to prevent recurrence of neural tube defects. *British Medical Journal* **282**, 1509.

128 Smithells R.W., Nevin N.C., Seller M.J., Sheppard S., Harris R., Read A.P., Fielding D.W. *et al.* (1983) Further experience of vitamin supplementation for prevention of neural tube defect recurrences. *Lancet* **i**, 1027.

129 MRC Vitamin Study Research Group (1991) Prevention of neural tube defects: Results of the Medical Research Council Vitamin Study. *Lancet* **338**, 131.

130 Czeizel, A.E. & Dudás I. (1992) Prevention of the first occurrence of neural-tube defects by periconceptional vitamin supplementation. *New England Journal of Medicine* **327**, 1832.

131 Wald N.J. & Bower C. (1995) Folic acid and the prevention of neural tube defects. *British Medical Journal* **310**, 1019.

132 Edelstein T. & Metz J. (1969) The correlation between vitamin B_{12} concentration in serum and muscle in late pregnancy. *Journal of Obstetrics and Gynaecology of the British Commonwealth* **76**, 545.

133 Temperley I.J., Meehan M.J.M. & Gatenby P.B.B. (1968) Serum vitamin B_{12} levels in pregnant women. *Journal of Obstetrics and Gynaecology of the British Commonwealth* **75**, 511.

134 McGarry J.M. & Andrews J. (1972) Smoking in pregnancy and vitamin B_{12} metabolism. *British Medical Journal* **ii**, 74.

135 Cooper B.A. (1973) Folate and vitamin B_{12} in pregnancy. *Clinics in Haematology* **2**, 461.

136 Briggs M. & Briggs M. (1972) Endocrine effects on serum vitamin B_{12}. *Lancet* **ii**, 1037.

137 Roberts P.D., James H., Petrie A., Morgan J.O. & Hoffbrand A.V. (1973) Vitamin B_{12} status in pregnancy among immigrants to Britain. *British Medical Journal* **iii**, 67.

138 Herbert V. (1968) Diagnostic and prognostic values of measurement of serum vitamin B_{12}-binding proteins. *Blood* **32**, 305.

139 Van den Broek N. & Letsky E.A. (Submitted for publication) Pilot study of aetiology of anaemia of pregnant women in Malawi.

140 Moncada M.D. & Vane J.R. (1979) Arachidonic acid metabolites and the interactions between platelets and blood-vessel walls. *New England Journal of Medicine* **300**, 1142.

141 Lewis P.J., Boylan P., Friedman L.A., Hensby C.N. & Downing I. (1980) Prostacyclin in pregnancy. *British Medical Journal* **280**, 1581.

142 Lewis P.J. (1982) The role of prostacyclin in preeclampsia. *British Journal of Hospital Medicine* **28**, 393.

143 de Sauvage F.J., Hass P.E., Spencer S.D. *et al.* (1994) Stimulation of megakaryocytopoiesis and thrombopoiesis by the c-Mpl ligand. *Nature* **369**, 533.

144 Levin J. (1997) Thrombopoietin: Clinically realized? *New England Journal of Medicine* **336**, 434.

145 Sill P.R., Lind T. & Walker W. (1985) Platelet values during normal pregnancy. *British Journal of Obstetrics and Gynaecology* **92**, 480.

146 O'Brien W.F., Saba H.I., Knuppel R.A., Scerbo J.C. & Cohen G.R. (1986) Alterations in platelet concentration and aggregation in normal pregnancy and preeclampsia. *American Journal of Obstetrics and Gynecology*, **155**, 486.

147 Burrows R.F. & Kelton J.G. (1988) Incidentally detected thrombocytopenia in healthy mothers and their infants. *New England Journal of Medicine* **319**, 142.

148 Burrows R.F. & Kelton J.G. (1990) Thrombocytopenia at delivery: A prospective survey of 6715 deliveries. *American Journal of Obstetrics and Gynecology* **162**, 731.

149 Beal D.W. & de Masi A.D. (1985) Role of the platelet count in the management of the high-risk obstetric

patient. *Journal of the American Osteopathic Association* **85**, 252.

150 Fenton V., Saunders K. & Cavill I. (1977) The platelet count in pregnancy. *Journal of Clinical Pathology* **30**, 68.

151 Rakoczi I., Tallian F., Bagdan Y.S. & Gati I. (1979) Platelet life-span in normal pregnancy and pre-eclampsia as determined by a non-radioisotope technique. *Thrombosis Research* **15**, 553.

152 Wallenberg H.C.T. & Van Kessel P.H. (1978) Platelet lifespan in normal pregnancy as determined by a non-radioisotopic technique. *British Journal of Obstetrics and Gynecology* **85**, 33.

153 Fay R.A., Hughes A.O. & Farron N.T. (1983) Platelets in pregnancy: Hyperdestruction in pregnancy. *Obstetrics and Gynecology* **61**, 238.

154 Romero R. & Duffy T.P. (1980) Platelet disorders in pregnancy. *Clinics in Perinatology* **7**, 327.

155 Louden K.A., Broughton Pipkin F., Heptinstall S., Fox S.C., Mitchell J.R.A. & Symonds E.M. (1990) A longitudinal study of platelet behaviour and thromboxane production in whole blood in normal pregnancy and the puerperium. *British Journal of Obstetrics and Gynaecology* **97**, 1108.

156 Burrows R.F. & Kelton J.G. (1992) Thrombocytopenia during pregnancy. In *Haemostasis and Thrombosis in Obstetrics and Gynaecology*. Eds I.A. Greer, A.G.G. Turpie & C.D. Forbes, p. 407. Chapman & Hall, London.

157 Letsky E.A. & Greaves M. (1996) Guidelines on the investigation and management of thrombocytopenia in pregnancy and neonatal alloimmune thrombocytopenia. *British Journal of Haematology* **95**, 21.

158 Redman C.W.G., Bonnar J. & Bellin C. (1978) Early platelet consumption in pre-eclampsia. *British Medical Journal* **i**, 467.

159 Niewiarowski S. (1994) Secreted platelet proteins. In *Haemostasis and Thrombosis*, 3rd edn. Eds A.L. Bloom, C.D. Forbes, D.P. Thomas & E.G.D. Tuddenham, p. 167. Churchill Livingstone, Edinburgh.

160 Hardisty R.M. (1982) Platelets, blood vessels and haemostasis: Disorders of platelet and vascular function. In *Blood and its Disorders*. Eds R.M. Hardisty & D.J. Weatherall, p. 1031. Blackwell Scientific Publications, Oxford.

161 Macfarlane R.G. (1964) An enzyme cascade in the blood clotting mechanism and its function as a biochemical amplifier. *Nature* **202**, 498.

162 Forbes C.D. & Greer I.A. (1992) Physiology of haemostasis and the effect of pregnancy. In *Haemostasis and Thrombosis in Obstetrics and Gynaecology*. Eds I.A. Greer, A.G.G. Turpie & C.D. Forbes, p. 1. Chapman & Hall, London.

163 Hathaway W.E. & Bonnar J. (1987) Hemostasis: General considerations. In *Hemostatic Disorders of the Pregnant Woman and Newborn Infant*, p. 1. John Wiley and Sons, Chichester.

164 Bonnar J. (1987) Physiology of coagulation in pregnancy. In *Hemostatic Disorders of the Pregnant Woman and Newborn Infant*. p. 39. John Wiley and Sons, Chichester.

165 Lämmle B. & Griffin J.H. (1985) Formation of the fibrin clot: The balance of procoagulant and inhibitory factors. In *Coagulation Disorders: Clinics in Haematology*, vol. 14. Ed. Z.M. Ruggeri, p. 281. W.B. Saunders, London.

166 Abildgaard U. (1981) Antithrombin and related inhibitors of coagulation. In *Recent Advances in Blood Coagulation*, vol. 3. Ed. C. Pollar, p. 151. Churchill Livingstone, Edinburgh.

167 Barrowcliffe T.W., Johnson E.A. & Thomas D. (1987) Antithrombin III and heparin. *British Medical Bulletin* **34**, 143.

168 Lane D.A., Olds R.J. & Thein S.L. (1994) Antithrombin and its deficiency. In *Haemostasis and Thrombosis*. Eds A.L. Bloom, C.D. Forbes, D.P. Thomas & E.G.D. Tuddenham, p. 655. Churchill Livingstone, Edinburgh.

169 Lane J.L. & Biggs R. (1977) The natural inhibitors of coagulation: antithrombin III, heparin cofactor and antifactor Xa. In *Recent Advances in Blood Coagulation*. Ed. L. Poller, p. 123. Churchill Livingstone, Edinburgh.

170 Barrowcliffe T.W. & Thomas D.P. (1994) Heparin and low molecular weight heparin. In *Haemostasis and Thrombosis*, 3rd edn. Eds A.L. Bloom, C.D. Forbes, D.P. Thomas & E.G.D. Tuddenham, p. 1417. Churchill Livingstone, Edinburgh.

171 Hellgren M. & Blomback M. (1981) Blood coagulation and fibrinolysis in pregnancy, during delivery and in the puerperium. *Gynecologic Obstetric Investigation* **12**, 141.

172 Howie P.W., Prentice C.R.M., Mallinson A.C., Horne C.H.W. & McNicol G.P. (1970) Effect of combined oestrogen-progestagen oral contraceptives, oestrogen and protestagen on antiplasmin and antithrombin activity. *Lancet* **ii**, 1329.

173 Fagerhol M.K. & Abildgaard U. (1970) Immunological studies on human antithrombin III. Influence of age, sex and use of oral contraceptives on serum concentration. *Scandinavian Journal of Haematology* **7**, 10.

174 Von Kaulla E. & Von Kaulla K.N. (1970) Oral contraceptives and low antithrombin III activity. *Lancet* **i**, 36.

175 Bottiger L.E., Boman G., Eklund G. & Westerholm B. (1980) Oral contraceptives and thromboembolic disease: Effects of lowering oestrogen content. *Lancet* **i**, 1097.

176 Conard J., Cazenave B., Samama M., Horellou M.H., Zorn J.R. & Neau C. (1980) A III content and antithrombin activity in oestrogen-progestogen and progestogen-only treated women. *Thrombosis Research* **18**, 675.

177 Bergqvist A., Bergqvist D. & Hedner U. (1982) Oral contraceptives and venous thromboembolism. *British Journal of Obstetrics and Gynaecology* **89**, 381.

178 Bergqvist A., Bergqvist D. & Tangen O. (1983) The influence of oral contraceptives on activated factor X inhibitor (Xa1) activity: A prospective study. *British Journal of Obstetrics and Gynaecology* **90**, 953.

179 Thorogood M. (1993) Oral contraceptives and cardiovascular disease: An epidemiologic overview. *Pharmacoepidemiol Drug Safety* **2**, 3.

180 World Health Organization Collaborative Study of Cardiovascular Disease and Steroid Hormone Contraception (1995) Effect of different progestagens

108

in low oestrogen oral contraceptives on venous thromboembolic disease. *Lancet* **346**, 1582.

181 World Health Organization Collaborative Study of Cardiovascular Disease and Steroid Hormone Contraception (1995) Venous thromboembolic disease and combined oral contraceptives: Results of international multicentre case-control study. *Lancet* **346**, 1575.

182 Jick H., Jick S.S., Gurewich V., Myers M.W. & Vasilakis C. (1995) Risk of idiopathic cardiovascular death and non-fatal venous thromboembolism in women using oral contraceptives with differing progestagen components. *Lancet* **346**, 1589.

183 Committee on Safety of Medicines (1995) *Combined Oral Contraceptives and Thromboembolism.* London: CSM.

184 Spitzer W.O. (1995) Data from transnational study of oral contraceptives have been misused. *British Medical Journal* **311**, 1162.

185 Lewis M.A., Spitzer W.O., Heinemann L.A., McRae K.D., Bruppacher R. & Thorogood M. (1996) Third generation oral contraceptives and risk of myocardial infarction: An international case-control study. *British Medical Journal* **312**, 88.

186 McPherson K. (1996) Third generation oral contraception and venous thromboembolism. *British Medical Journal* **312**, 68.

187 Vandenbroucke J.P., Helmerhorst F.M., Bloemenkamp W.M. & Rosendaal F.R. (1997) Third-generation oral contraceptive and deep venous thrombosis: From epidemiologic controversy to new insight in coagulation. *American Journal of Obstetrics & Gynecology* **177**, 887.

188 Bertina R.M., Briet E., Engesser L. & Reitsma P.H. (1988) Protein C deficiency and the risk of venous thrombosis. *New England Journal of Medicine* **318**, 930.

189 Seligsohn U., Berger A., Abend M., Rubin L., Attias D., Zivelin A. & Rapaport S.I. (1984) Homozygous protein C deficiency manifested by massive venous thrombosis in the newborn. *New England Journal of Medicine* **310**, 559.

190 Malm J., Laurell M. & Dahlback B. (1988) Changes in the plasma levels of vitamin K-dependent proteins C and S and of C4b-binding protein during pregnancy and oral contraception. *British Journal of Haematology* **68**, 437.

191 Comp P.C., Thurnau G.R., Welsh J. & Esmon C.T. (1986) Functional and immunologic Protein S levels are decreased during pregnancy. *Blood* **68**, 881.

192 Warwick R., Hutton R.A., Goff L., Letsky E. & Heard M. (1989) Changes in Protein C and free Protein S during pregnancy and following hysterectomy. *Journal of the Royal Society of Medicine* **82**, 591.

193 Faught W., Garner P., Jones G. & Ivey B. (1995) Changes in protein C and protein S levels in normal pregnancy. *American Journal of Obstetrics and Gynecology* **172**, 147.

194 Dahlbäck B., Carlsson M. & Svensson P.J. (1993) Familial thrombophilia due to a previously unrecognized mechanism characterized by poor anticoagulant response to activated protein C: Prediction of a cofactor to activated protein C. *Proceedings of the National Academy of Sciences USA* **90**, 1004.

195 Svensson P.J. & Dahlback B. (1994) Resistance to activated protein C as a basis for venous thrombosis. *New England Journal of Medicine* **330**, 517.

196 Koster T., Rosendaal F.R., de Ronde Hl., Briët E., Vandenbroucke J.P. & Bertina R.M. (1993) Venous thrombosis due to poor anticoagulant response to activated protein C: Leiden Thrombophilia Study. *Lancet* **342**, 1503.

197 Dahlbäck B. & Hildebrand B. (1994) Inherited resistance to activated protein C is corrected by anticoagulant cofactor activity found to be a property of factor V. *Proceedings of the National Academy of Sciences USA* **91**, 1396.

198 Peek M.J., Nelson-Piercy C., Manning R.A., de Swiet M. & Letsky E.A. (1997) Activated protein C resistance in normal pregnancy. *British Journal of Obstetrics and Gynaecology* **104**, 1084.

199 Cumming A.M., Tait R.C., Fildes S., Yoong A., Keeney S. & Hay C.R. (1995) Development of resistance to activated protein C during pregnancy. *British Journal of Haematology* **90**, 725.

200 Hellgren M., Svensson P.J. & Dahlbäck B. (1995) Resistance to activated protein C as a basis for venous thromboembolism associated with pregnancy and oral contraceptives. *American Journal of Obstetrics and Gynceology* **173**, 210.

201 Bloemenkamp K.W.W., Rosendaal F.R., Helmerhorst F.M., Büller H.R. & Vandenbroucke J.P. (1995) Enhancement by factor V Leiden mutation of risk of deep-vein thrombosis associated with oral contraceptives containing third-generation progestagen. *Lancet* **346**, 1593.

202 Selem H.H. (1986) The natural anticoagulants. In *Thrombosis and the Vessel Wall: Clinics in Haematology*, vol. 15, p. 371. W.B. Saunders, London.

203 Ballegeer V., Mombarts, P., Declerk P.J., Spitz B., Van Assche F.A. & Collen D. (1987) Fibrinolytic response to venous occlusion and fibrin fragment D-Dimer levels in normal and complicated pregnancy. *Thrombosis and Haemostasis* **58**, 1030.

204 Aoki N. & Von Kaulla K.V. (1971) Human serum plasminogen antiactivator: Its distinction from antiplasmin. *American Journal of Physiology* **220**, 1137.

205 Bennet N.B. (1970) Further studies on an inhibitor of plasminogen activation in human serum: Release of the inhibitor during coagulation and thrombus formation. *Thrombosis et Diathesis Haemorrhagica* **23**, 553.

206 Beller F.K. (1971) Observations on the clotting of menstrual blood and clot formation. *American Journal of Obstetrics and Gynecology* **111**, 535.

207 Sheppard B.L., Dockeray C.J. & Bonnar J. (1983) An ultrastructural study of menstrual blood in normal menstruation and dysfunctional menstrual bleeding. *British Journal of Obstetrics and Gynaecology* **90**, 259.

208 Cameron I.T. & Smith S.K. (1992) Menorrhagia. In *Haemostasis and Thrombosis in Obstetrics and Gynecology*. Eds I.A. Greer, A.G.G. Turpie & C.D. Forbes, p. 77. Chapman & Hall, London.

209 Vandermeulen E.P.E., Vermylen J. & Van Aken H. (1993) Epidural and spinal anaesthesia in patients receiving anticoagulant therapy. *Baillière's Clinical Anaesthesiology* **7**, 663.

210 Dacie J.V. & Lewis S.M. (1995) Investigation of haemostasis and a bleeding tendency. In *Practical Haematology*, 8th edn, p. 297. Churchill Livingstone, Edinburgh.

211 Greer I.A. (1994) Haemostasis and thrombosis in pregnancy. In *Haemostasis and Thrombosis*, 3rd edn. Eds A.L. Bloom, C.D. Forbes, D.P. Thomas & E.G.D. Tuddenham, p. 987. Churchill Livingstone, Edinburgh.

212 Letsky E.A. (1985) *Coagulation Problems during Pregnancy* (Current Reviews in Obstetrics & Gynaecology, vol. 10). Churchill Livingstone, Edinburgh.

213 Stirling Y., Woolf L., North W.R.S., Seghatchian M.J. & Meade T.W. (1984) Haemostasis in normal pregnancy. *Thrombosis and Haemostasis* **52**, 176.

214 Regoeczi E. & Hobbs K.R. (1969) Fibrinogen turnover in pregnancy. *Scandinavian Journal of Haematology* **6**, 175.

215 Gjonnaess H. (1973) Cold-promoted activation of Factor VII. *Gynecological Investigation* **4**, 61.

216 Bennett B. & Ratnoff O.D. (1972) Changes in AHF procoagulant activity and AHF-like antigen in normal pregnancy and following exercise and pneumoencephalography. *Journal of Laboratory and Clinical Medicine* **80**, 256.

217 Van Royen E.A. & Ten Cate J.W. (1973) Antigen-biological activity ratio for Factor VIII in late pregnancy. *Lancet* **ii**, 449.

218 Caires D., Arocha-Piñango C.L., Rodriguez S. & Linares J. (1984) Factor VIIIR : Aga/factor VIII : C and their ratio in obstetrical cases. *Acta Obstetricia et Gynaecologica Scandinavica* **63**, 411.

219 Coopland A., Alkjaersig N. & Fletcher A.P. (1969) Reduction in plasma Factor XIII (fibrin stabilising factor) concentration during pregnancy. *Journal of Laboratory and Clinical Medicine* **73**, 144.

220 McKillop C., Howie P.W., Forbes C.D. & Prentice C.R.M. (1976) Soluble fibrinogen/fibrin complexes in pre-eclampsia. *Lancet* **i**, 56.

221 Bonnar J. (1976) Long-term self-administered heparin therapy for prevention and treatment of thromboembolic complications in pregnancy. In *Heparin Chemistry and Clinical Usage*. Eds V.J. Kakkar & D.P. Thomas, p. 247. Academic Press, New York.

222 Nelson-Piercy C., Letsky E.A. & de Swiet M. (1997) Low molecular weight heparin for obstetric thromboprophylaxis: Experience of sixty-nine pregnancies in sixty-one women at high risk. *American Journal of Obstetrics and Gynecology* **176**, 1062.

223 Sturridge F., de Swiet M. & Letsky E.A. (1994) The use of low molecular weight heparin for thromboprophylaxis. *British Journal Obstetrics and Gynaecology* **101**, 69.

224 Sheppard B.L. & Bonnar J. (1974) The ultrastructure of the arterial supply of the human placenta in early and late pregnancy. *Journal of Obstetrics and Gynaecology of the British Commonwealth* **81**, 497.

225 Wiman B., Csemiczky G., Marsk L. & Robbe H. (1984) The fast inhibitor of tissue plasminogen activator in plasma during pregnancy. *Thrombosis and Haemostasis* **52**, 124.

226 Booth N., Reith A., Bennett B. (1988) A plasminogen activator inhibitor (PA1-2) circulates in two molecular forms during pregnancy. *Thrombosis and Haemostasis* **59**, 77.

227 Hahn L. (1974) Fibrinogen-fibrin degradation products in uterine and peripheral blood during caesarean section. *Acta Obstetricia et Gynaecologica Scandinavica* **53** (Suppl 28), 19.

228 Greer I.A., Turpie A.G.G. & Forbes C.D. (1992) *Haemostasis and Thrombosis in Obstetrics and Gynaecology*. Chapman & Hall Medical, London.

229 Letsky E.A. & de Swiet M. (1994) Maternal hemostasis: Coagulation problems of pregnancy. In *Thrombosis and Hemorrhage*. Eds A.I. Schafer & J. Loscalzo, p. 965. Blackwell Scientific Publications, Cambridge, MA.

230 Preston F.E., Rosendaal F.R., Walker I.D., Briët E., Berntrop E., Conard J., Fontcuberta J. *et al.* (1996) Increased fetal loss in women with heritable thrombophilia. *The Lancet* **348**, 913.

231 Letsky E.A. (1992) Management of massive haemorrhage: The haematologist's role. In *Maternal Mortality: The Way Forward*. Ed. N. Patel, p. 63. Royal College of Obstetricians and Gynaecologists, London.

232 Department of Health (1996) *Report on Confidential Enquiries into Maternal Deaths in the United Kingdom, 1991–1993*. Her Majesty's Stationery Office, London.

233 Basu H.K. (1969) Fibrinolysis and abruptio placentae. *Journal of Obstetrics and Gynaecology of the British Commonwealth* **76**, 481.

234 Howie P.W., Prentice C.R.M. & Forbes C.D. (1975) Failure of heparin therapy to affect the clinical course of severe pre-eclampsia. *British Journal of Obstetrics and Gynaecology* **82**, 711.

235 Sibai BM., Caritis S.N., Thom E., Klebanoff M., McNellis D., Rocco L., Paul R.H. *et al.* (1993) Prevention of preeclampsia with low-dose aspirin in healthy, nulliparous pregnant women. *New England Journal of Medicine* **329**, 1213.

236 Collaborative Low-dose Aspirin Study in Pregnancy Collaborative Group (1994) CLASP: A randomised trial of low-dose aspirin for the prevention and treatment of pre-eclampsia among 9364 pregnant women. *Lancet* **343**, 619.

237 Letsky E.A. (1995) Coagulation defects. In *Medical Disorders in Obstetric Practice* 3rd edn. Ed. M. de Swiet, p. 71. Blackwell Science, Oxford.

238 Hathaway W.E. & Bonnar J. (1987) *Hemostatic Disorders of the Pregnant Woman and Newborn Infant*. John Wiley and Sons, Chichester.

239 Mibashan R., Peake I. & Nicolaides K. (1990) Prenatal diagnosis of hemostatic disorders. In *Perinatal Hematology: Methods in Haematology*, vol. 21, Ed. B.P. Alter, p. 64. Churchill Livingstone, Edinburgh.

240 Forestier F., Daffos, F., Kaplan C. & Sole Y. (1992) The development of the coagulation system in the human fetus and the prenatal diagnosis and management of bleeding disorders with fetal blood sampling. In *Haemostasis and Thrombosis in Obstetrics and Gynaecology*. Eds I.A. Greer, A.G.G. Turpie & C.D. Forbes, p. 487. Chapman & Hall, London.

241 Letsky E.A. (1995) Haematological disorders. In *Prenatal Diagnosis in Obstetric Practice*, 2nd edn.

110

Eds M. Whittle & M. Connor, p. 68. Blackwell Scientific Publications, Oxford.

242 Nicolaides K.H., Rodeck C.H. & Mibashan R.S. (1985) Obstetric management and diagnosis of haematological disease in the fetus. In *Haematological Disorders in Pregnancy: Clinics in Haematology*, vol. 14, p. 775. W.B. Saunders, London.

243 Weatherall D.J. (1990) *The New Genetics and Clinical Practice*, 3rd edn. Oxford University Press, Oxford.

244 Tuddenham E.G.D. & Cooper D.N. (1993) *The Molecular Genetics of Haemostasis and its Inherited Disorders.* Oxford University Press, Oxford.

The Respiratory System

M. DE SWIET

The main purpose of breathing is to acquire oxygen and to eliminate carbon dioxide in amounts closely related to the needs of the body. To that end the rate and depth of breathing must be exactly controlled. The mixing and effective distribution of gases in the lungs depend on that control. More remotely, tissue respiration and the metabolic activities of the body generally make demands on gas exchange, and the whole is subject to central nervous control. Not all of these aspects of respiratory function have been studied in pregnancy.

There have been major advances in the technology of respiratory function testing, but of the range of tests now available, relatively few have been applied to normal pregnant women. It is likely that this field will be slow to develop because tests of lung function need the co-operation of the patient and are all more or less unpleasant, so that an ethical problem is involved. Cotes [1], for example, believes that, in general, tests should be submaximal, noninvasive and of short duration: 'Procedures which do not meet these criteria, including the measurement of compliance, the arterial blood gas tension and the capacity for exercise, should be reserved for occasions when there is a positive indication for their use.' That very reasonable philosophy raises a dilemma, for it is probable that the results of tests will be modified by pregnancy; when a 'positive indication for their use' should arise, presumably in some disease state, then lack of a normal background will make their interpretation difficult.

Methods of investigation

A detailed discussion of the methods of investigation is not necessary to an understanding of the results which follow and this introduction gives no more than a reminder of the divisions of lung volume and a few definitions. Comroe *et al.* [2] and Hytten and Leitch [3] give clear expositions of this subject.

Four lung volumes and four capacities are recognized and commonly measured in respiratory physiology (Fig. 4.1).

The four volumes, which do not overlap, are:
1 *The tidal volume*, the volume of gas inspired or expired in each respiration. Obviously, tidal volume will vary with need, but when not otherwise defined, the term refers to quiet respiration at rest. The position of the chest at the end of quiet expiration, when the respiratory muscles

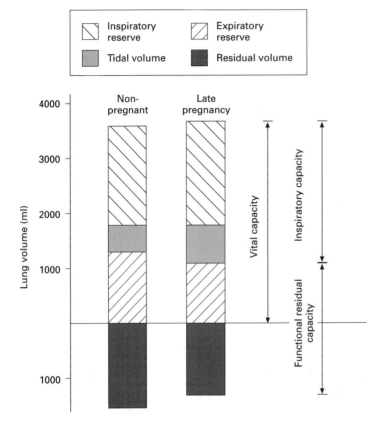

Fig. 4.1. Subdivisions of lung volume and their alterations in pregnancy.

are inactive, is known as the resting end-expiratory position.

2 *Inspiratory reserve volume* is the maximum amount of air which can be inspired, beyond the normal tidal inspiration.

3 *Expiratory reserve volume* is the maximum amount of air which can be expired from the resting end-expiratory position.

4 *Residual volume* is the volume of gas remaining in the lungs, not including the anatomical dead space of the trachea and bronchial tree, at the end of maximal expiration.

The four capacities each include two or more of the volumes defined above:

1 *Total lung capacity* includes them all; it is the total amount of gas in the lung at the end of a maximum inspiration.

2 *Vital capacity* includes all but the residual volume; it is the maximum volume of gas which can be expired after a maximum inspiration.

3 *Inspiratory capacity* is tidal volume plus the inspiratory reserve volume; that is, it is the maximum volume of gas which can be inspired from the resting end-expiratory position.

4 *Functional residual capacity* is expiratory reserve volume plus the residual volume; that is, the amount of gas which remains in the lungs in the resting end-expiratory position, and the volume of gas with which the tidal air must mix.

Except for the residual volume and the lung capacities which contain it, those spaces can readily be measured by direct spirometry. The residual volume must be estimated by a more elaborate gas dilution technique.

Average volumes and capacities for normal healthy women are given in standard physiological texts. Since they vary a little with the technique of measurement and with the population studied, measurements to compare pregnant and non-pregnant women should be made by the same investigators and, ideally, on the same women. Data for normal non-pregnant women will therefore be given when the findings for pregnant women are discussed.

A few more terms must be defined in relation to ventilation. The volume of air breathed and indices derived from it form the basis of many measurements of lung function for which data have been collected in pregnancy. The minute volume is the amount of air inspired in a minute; it is thus the tidal volume multiplied by the rate of respiration. From a functional viewpoint, this simple measure is insufficient. Some of the tidal air merely fills the anatomical dead space and makes no contribution to gas exchange, and the important measure is alveolar ventilation, which is based on the tidal volume less the volume of the physiological dead space. The physiological dead space is the anatomical dead space plus the extra volume of the alveoli that do not contribute to gas exchange. It should be clear, therefore, that, for a given minute volume, a fast respiratory rate with a small tidal volume gives a smaller alveolar ventilation than a slow respiratory rate with a correspondingly bigger tidal volume. The ventilatory equivalent for oxygen is the number of litres of ventilation for each 100 ml of oxygen taken up by the body.

Gas transfer

Gas transfer from inspired gas to the blood is tested with carbon monoxide (CO) and is expressed as the transfer factor for CO. Previously termed the pulmonary diffusing capacity, it measures more than mere diffusion across the alveolar membrane, for it contains in addition a component both of ventilation and gas distribution in the alveoli, and of the amount of pulmonary capillary blood and its haemoglobin content. There are few data on this aspect of gas transfer in pregnancy, but many studies of alveolar gas content, of blood gases and pH.

Tests of ventilation

The classical test — the maximum breathing capacity (MBC), maximum voluntary ventilation, or ventilatory capacity — is the maximum amount of air which can be inspired or expired by forced voluntary breathing over 15 seconds. It measures the maximal ability to move gas in and out of the lung and is a resultant of all the mechanical attributes of the lungs and chest wall. When the test is performed conscientiously, it is extremely exhausting and requires considerable co-operation from the subject. The measurement is also influenced by the characteristics of the measuring equipment, the extent to which the subject has practised the necessary manoeuvres, the time when the measurement is performed and the skill and personality of the operator [1].

In practice ventilation is assessed by two more simple tests:

1 The forced expiratory volume in one second (FEV_1), expressed either as the amount of gas, or the proportion of the vital capacity, which can be forcibly expired from a maximal inspiration in one second. FEV_1 is perhaps the most used, and most useful test of ventilation; it is fairly reproducible, relatively independent of effort, and, with the vital capacity, is the measurement of first choice for routine use [1].

2 The peak expiratory flow rate is measured by simple devices such as the Wright peak flow meter, which indicate the maximum rate of gas flow during forced expiration. It correlates well with FEV_1 but is more dependent on expiratory effort and is less reproducible. These tests estimate the function of the large airways.

A third test of ventilatory function in the small airways is the estimation of closing volume. Towards the end of expiration some small airways begin to close, the first to do so being those to the lung bases. Largely for gravitational reasons the apical regions get most of the inspired gas at the beginning of inspiration and are the last to empty at the end of expiration, so that a bolus of foreign gas inhaled at the beginning of a breath will go mostly to the apices and will reappear during expiration when the basal airways begin to close, and apical areas to empty. The point so estimated is termed the closing volume (or, if all the residual gas in the lung including residual volume is estimated, the closing capacity). It is interpreted as the summation of all the factors which determine the calibre of the small airways. An increase in closing volume—that is, evidence that the basal airways are closing while more gas than normal remains in the lung—is taken as an indication of airway obstruction.

Respiratory function in pregnancy

The literature prior to 1970 has been reviewed in detail by Hytten and Leitch [3]. While more recent work has not questioned the general trends reported there, the absolute figures have changed considerably, presumably because of technical advances in measuring equipment. Other general reviews are those of Weinbergen *et al.* [4] and Fishburne [5].

Vital capacity

The many early studies, taken together, indicated that there was no real change in vital capacity in pregnancy, but the evidence was unsatisfactory. The datailed and careful study of Cugell *et al.* [6] showed no change between late pregnancy and the postpartum period, either in the upright or supine positions in 19 healthy women, but Rubin *et al.* [7] found their group of eight women to have a vital capacity in late pregnancy which as almost 300 ml below that at 7–14 weeks postpartum. Support for those two points of view was divided, and more recent studies are also divided in their conclusions. In a small cross-sectional study, Heidenreich *et al.* [8] found no significant change; neither did Lehmann and Fabel [9] in a serial study of 23 women, nor did Sims *et al.* [10] in a serial study of 27 patients with asthma, and 12 controls. Of the four subjects examined in detail by Woolcock and Read [11], two showed no real change and two a substantial rise, but Gazioglu *et al.* [12] with eight subjects studied serially, and Knuttgen and Emerson [13] with 13, showed a significantly raised vital capacity in late pregnancy, as did Puranik *et al.* [14] in 50 normal women. By contrast, another Indian study showed a significant decrease in vital capacity in the third trimester compared to non-pregnant controls [15].

The truth may be that some, but not all, pregnant women increase or decrease their vital capacity during pregnancy, and the difference may be related to body build since Eng *et al.* [16] showed the vital capacity to be reduced in late pregnancy in 12 obese women. Overall, there is probably an increase of perhaps 100 or 200 ml. It is less easy to decide whether there is a progressive change during the course of pregnancy, but where an increase has been shown it appears to have taken place from about midpregnancy [15–17].

It might be expected that tests relying on maternal effort such as measurement of vital capacity would show impairment immediately after delivery. This was not so in a group of 11 healthy women studied serially for 72 hours after normal delivery: the vital capacity was not different from that at 6–8 weeks postpartum [18].

Inspiratory capacity

The inspiratory capacity (tidal volume plus inspiratory volume) is increased in late pregnancy, although the older literature was divided in its opinion about this. The more recent studies [8,9,12–14] are unanimous and suggest an increase of the order of 300 ml; the change appears to occur progressively throughout pregnancy.

Expiratory reserve volume

The well-established finding of a reduced expiratory reserve volume has been repeatedly confirmed by more modern studies [8,9,12–14,16]. The fall is of the order of 200 ml from about 1300 to 1100 ml and probably occurs progressively from early pregnancy.

Residual volume, functional residual capacity

All published studies agree that the residual volume is conspicuously and progressively reduced in pregnancy but the absolute values have changed considerably with improvements in technique. Thus, while Cugell *et al.* [6] in 1953 described a 20% fall from 965 to 770 ml in late pregnancy, the more modern studies [8,9,12,13,16] show a similar percentage fall but from about 1500 to 1200 ml. The functional residual capacity, comprising two volumes (the residual volume and the expiratory reserve volume) which are both reduced, is itself considerably smaller in pregnancy by about 500 ml.

The changes in lung volumes and capacities are summarized in Fig. 4.1.

Tidal volume, respiratory rate and minute ventilation

Tidal volume rises throughout pregnancy but, compared with the studies of lung capacities, remarkably few data have been collected. The continuous rise reported by Cugell et al. [6] from 487 to 678 ml in late pregnancy is confirmed by the more recent study of Lehmann and Fabel [19] which showed a continuous rise from 548 to 738 ml. Thus there appeared to be an increase of some 200 ml from about 500 to about 700 ml — an increase above the non-pregnant tidal volume of some 40%.

The respiratory rate does not change during pregnancy [13,19,20] from its normal frequency of 14 or 15 per minute or even falls a little [21] so that the minute ventilation rises in parallel with tidal volume.

Most authors have found the rise to be from a non-pregnant average of about 7.5 l/min to about 10.5 l/min in late pregnancy — a rise of 40%. Spätling et al. [21] found higher figures, i.e. 9.4 l/min non-pregnant, 12.6 l/min at term, either because of differences in apparatus or because their subjects were more anxious.

Functional implications

The resting pregnant woman increases her ventilation by breathing more deeply and not more frequently. Although her physiological dead space is somewhat raised by dilatation of the smaller bronchioles (by about 60 ml in the study of Pernoll et al. [20]), alveolar ventilation will be increased even more than overall ventilation, perhaps to more than 50%.

Compared to the increase in resting oxygen uptake (see below) that is a very large rise, and the overbreathing becomes even more impressive when seen against the background of a diminishing functional residual capacity, because the increased tide of fresh air brought in with each inspiration is required to mix with a

much smaller residual quantity of air remaining in the lungs.

Anatomical changes in pregnancy

The major influence in the phenomenon of overbreathing is a change in central respiratory control (to be discussed later) but alterations in the subdivision of lung volumes are largely due to anatomical changes. Alterations in the configuration of the chest during pregnancy (outlined in Fig. 4.2) have been recognized for many years and pregnant women themselves are well aware that their lower ribs flare and do not always fully recover their original position after pregnancy. Thomson and Cohen [17] found the subcostal angle to increase progressively from about 68° in early pregnancy to 103° in late pregnancy. The changes began before there was any possibility that they could be attributed to mechanical pressure. In this series of patients

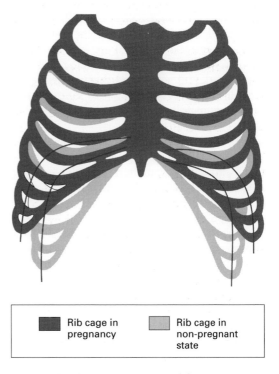

| Rib cage in pregnancy | Rib cage in non-pregnant state |

Fig. 4.2. The rib cage in pregnancy and the non-pregnant state, showing the increased subcostal angle, the increased transverse diameter and the raised diaphragm in pregnancy.

the angle had returned to normal within a few weeks of delivery. Thomson and Cohen also noted, in X-ray studies, that the level of the diaphragm rose in pregnancy by a maximum of about 4 cm and that the transverse diameter of the chest increased by about 2 cm. Similar changes were shown by Klaften and Palugyay [22,23] and by Möbius [24]. McGinty [25] in a comprehensive review of the literature found that the idea of the diaphragm being splinted and its action obstructed by pregnancy had been current since the early nineteenth century, with few dissentients. He made a careful X-ray study of two pregnant women and found the excursion of the diaphragm during breathing, whether sitting or lying down, to be greater in pregnancy than in the puerperium, and he concluded that breathing in pregnancy is more diaphragmatic than costal. The study by Möbius [24] confirmed that finding. He found the excursion of the right and left sides of the diaphragm to be 5.6 and 6.1 cm in late pregnancy compared to 4.7 and 4.6 cm, 8–10 days after delivery. Omatsu [26] quotes the work of a colleague, Takano, who found by electromyography that the abdominal muscles have less tone and are less active in pregnancy. This is confirmed by the work of Gupta et al. [18] who found that women were not able to achieve as great a maximum expiratory pressure following normal delivery as at 6–8 weeks postpartum.

Lung markings are always found to be increased in radiographs taken during pregnancy, partly because of the more collapsed state of the lungs in expiration and partly because of increased filling of pulmonary blood vessels (see Chapter 2).

Earlier suggestions that pleural effusion is a common occurrence immediately after delivery following a normal pregnancy [27] have not been confirmed by others [28] who found that it only occurred following pre-eclampsia [29].

Pregnancy stresses the respiratory system very little compared with its effect on the cardiovascular system. During pregnancy the minute ventilation increases by about 40% from 7.5 to 10.5 l/min and oxygen consumption increases by about 16% from about 220 to 255 ml/min. Yet, in exercise, minute ventilation may increase to 80 l/min [2] — a tenfold or

1000% increase. Cardiac output also rises by approximately one third from 4.5 to 6 l/min in pregnancy (Chapter 1), but, in contrast, the maximum cardiac output achieved in exercise is probably no greater than a threefold increase — 12 l/min. Thus, although cardiac output and minute ventilation increase by approximately 30–40% each in pregnancy, the increase in cardiac output represents a far greater proportion of the normal reserve than does the increase in ventilation. For this reason, patients with respiratory disease are much less likely to deteriorate in pregnancy than those with cardiac disease. Only in patients on the brink of respiratory failure does the extra 30–50 ml/min oxygen consumption of pregnancy make a difference. Examples are acute conditions such as extensive pneumonia or chronic disease such as severe cystic fibrosis.

Tests of pulmonary function

Maximum breathing capacity

As a test of ventilatory capacity, MBC must now be regarded as of no more than historical interest; it is an exhausting and unpleasant test which is heavily dependent both on subject cooperation and on training.

Most studies could find no difference between late pregnancy and postpartum [6,7,19,30]; only one report, by Heidenreich et al. [8], showed values in pregnancy to be significantly below those postpartum, but the data are cross-sectional and do not convincingly contradict the consensus that there is no change.

Forced expiratory volume in 1 second (FEV$_1$), peak expiratory flow rate

FEV$_1$ is not affected by pregnancy. Almost all published studies are agreed that between 80% and 85% of the vital capacity can be forcibly expired in 1 second whether or not the subject is pregnant [6,7,9,10,12,13,16,31–33]. As might be expected from the unchanged FEV$_1$, peak expiratory flow rate is similarly unaffected by normal pregnancy [7,12,13]. The effect of pregnancy on airways' resistance in disease is controversial. Studies of asthma in pregnancy have found either no change [34–35], deterioration [36] or improvement [37]. However, these studies have been retrospective and based on the patients' or physicians' subjective impressions. A prospective study of 27 patients with asthma in pregnancy [10] found no significant changes in FEV_1 between pregnancy and the non-pregnant state as measured at least 6 weeks after delivery. Thus, in patients with asthma as well as in healthy women, FEV_1 is not affected by pregnancy. Alternatively, any small fluctuations in FEV_1 associated with pregnancy are trivial compared to the variable nature of the disease.

By contrast, in asthma, airways responsiveness — the degree to which airways constrict following inhaled metacholine — is reduced in pregnancy [35].

Airways' resistance

The FEV_1 is only an indirect measurement of airflow resistance, since it depends on the compliance of the lungs as well as the resistance of the bronchial tree to airflow. A more specific assessment may be made by simultaneous measurement of driving pressure divided by airflow, the pulmonary resistance. This has been measured by Milne et al. [33] who, in contrast to earlier findings [7,38], found no change in pregnancy.

The lack of change of FEV_1, peak expiratory flow rate and airways resistance is likely to be the net effect of different influences: bronchodilation induced by prostaglandin E and the smooth muscle relaxing effect of progesterone [39] and bronchoconstriction due to the reduction in total lung capacity (see Fig. 4.1) and to prostaglandin $F_2\alpha$ [40]. Fortunately, prostaglandin E is used rather than prostaglandin $F_2\alpha$ for the induction of labour and prostaglandin $F_2\alpha$ (used for severe postpartum haemorrhage) should only be given to asthmatics in the knowledge that it will cause severe bronchoconstriction.

Closing volume

Bevan et al. [41] found an increased closing volume in pregnancy, with closure beginning during normal tidal volume in half their sub-jects. That would suggest that the calibre of small airways is decreased in pregnancy. It is of course possible that the large airways which account for most of the airways' resistance could be dilated in pregnancy, whereas the small airways could be relatively constricted to give no overall change in airways' resistance. However, the data of Bevan et al. [41] were collected from a group of 20 women of whom eight had hypertension. Those with hypertension had the greatest increase in closing volume [42]. Since pregnancy hypertension is associated with abnormal pulmonary capillary blood flow [43], part of the changes found by Bevan et al. may be due to hypertension or the other conditions for which the patients were admitted, rather than pregnancy alone. Furthermore, to infer that closure occurred during normal tidal volume, it was assumed that residual volume is 20% of total lung capacity which is not necessarily so; more detailed data from Garrard et al. [44] and Templeton and Kelman [45] in normal women do not confirm that closing volume intrudes into normal tidal volume in pregnancy. Garrard et al. [44] did observe a small increase in closing volume which may be due to an increase in lung water in pregnancy [46].

Gas distribution in the lungs

As would be expected from the greatly increased alveolar ventilation, mixing and distribution of gas in the lungs is more efficient in pregnant than in non-pregnant women and Cugell et al. [6] found the pulmonary mixing index—the percentage of nitrogen remaining in the lungs after 7 minutes of breathing pure oxygen—to be considerably reduced in pregnancy. The effect may be more dependent on posture in pregnancy, a feature demonstrated by blood gas levels in a study by Ang et al. [47]. These workers found arterialized capillary P_{O_2} to be 85 mmHg (11.4 kPa) when the subjects were lying supine and 98 mmHg (13 kPa) when sitting up, and they suggested that the improvement with sitting might be due to more effective ventilation. However, interpretation of these data is not straightforward and the change could be circulatory rather than respiratory. In any event, blood gas samples should be taken for clinical purposes with the patient sitting rather than lying whenever possible.

Gas transfer (pulmonary diffusing capacity) and alveolar–arterial oxygen gradient

While early studies of pulmonary diffusing capacity with carbon monoxide by Bedell and Adams [48] and Krumholz et al. [31] showed no difference attributable to pregnancy, more recent data demonstrate a clear decrease from before midpregnancy [9,12,49]. The studies are in close agreement, that by Lehmann and Fabel [19] showed a fall from 26.5 ml/min/mmHg in the non-pregnant state to 22.5 ml/min/mmHg in late pregnancy. The reduction in gas transfer may be partly explained by the normally lower haemoglobin concentration in circulating blood, but Gazioglu et al. [12] suggest that the alveolar capillary wall may be altered by the effect of oestrogen on mucopolysaccharides—a phenomenon which has been demonstrated in a male subject by Pecora et al. [50]. However, in pregnancy the alveolar–arterial oxygen gradient increases to a mean of 14 mmHg in patients sitting and 20 mmHg in the supine position [51], probably due to decreased transfer factor, the effect of posture being caused by changes in cardiac output and ventilation/perfusion mismatching. Any added impediment to oxygen diffusion will be offset, at least partly, by the increased efficiency of gas distribution and higher partial pressures in the alveoli.

Gas exchange

Oxygen consumption (V_{O_2})

All work on basal oxygen consumption (basal metabolic rate) has to face the difficulty of ensuring that the subject is in the postabsorptive state and completely relaxed. It is less easy for a woman in late pregnancy to relax, especially since the supine position may be uncomfortable for her and the fetus may be restless. In the past the measuring equipment itself, usually involving the use of a noseclip, was a source of discomfort and considerable training was needed before reproducible measurements were obtained. For these technical reasons, and because no effective

serial study had been made, Hytten and Leitch, who reviewed the subject in 1971, found the published data unsatisfactory [3].

Data published since then are technically much superior and include three serial studies in which non-pregnant measurements were made postpartum in those subjects studied in pregnancy; there are, however, still wide discrepancies and it is clear that the definitive information has yet to be published.

The difficulties are well illustrated by studies from two American groups, those of Emerson and Pernoll. Emerson and his colleagues first published some data [52] on seven healthy women in positive energy balance and describe a rise from a computed pre-pregnancy V_{O_2} of 217 ml/min to a maximum rate of 249 ml/min in late pregnancy, an increase of 32 ml/min. Later [13], they described a measured rise between a value taken at 6 weeks postpartum and late pregnancy in 13 women of from 191 to 249 ml/min, an increase of 58 ml/min.

Pernoll et al. [53] have provided the most complete information on 12 healthy subjects with V_{O_2} measured in resting rather than truly basal conditions. From a (postpartum) mean of 254 ml/min, V_{O_2} rose progressively by 42 ml to a plateau averaging about 296 ml/min throughout most of the last trimester except for a sudden unexplained rise to 331 ml/min in the period 39–42 weeks.

It is clearly difficult to form a conclusion from these data; all that can be said is that the best evidence available suggests an increase of basal oxygen consumption in pregnancy of between 30 and 40 ml/min, which at least has the merits of matching the calculated extra oxygen requirements set out in Table 4.1 and Fig. 4.3.

Table 4.1 and Fig. 4.3 are synthesized from a variety of sources. It is assumed that the fetus, which does not have an external surface and does not need to maintain its own body temperature, has a metabolic rate comparable to that of the mother, and that the placenta and extra maternal tissues have rates of oxygen consumption found in vitro. Direct measurements of oxygen consumption of the pregnant uterus at term are in substantial agreement.

It will be obvious that the major adaptations made by the mother in cardiac, respiratory and

Table 4.1. The extra components of oxygen consumption in pregnancy.

Source of extra energy output	Increment at given weeks of pregnancy				Estimated cost (ml O_2/min)	Increment of O_2 consumption (ml/min) at given weeks of gestation				Reference
	10	20	30	40		10	20	30	40	
Cardiac output (l/min)	1.0	1.5	1.5	1.5	About 20 at 4.5 l/min. Increase pro rata	4.5	6.8	6.8	6.8	Chapter 2
Respiration (l/min)	0.75	1.50	2.25	3.00	1.0 per litre ventilation	0.8	1.5	2.3	3.0	Chapter 4
Kidneys Reabsorption of Na (mEq/min)	7	7	7	7	About 1 per mEq	7	7	7	7	Chapter 10
Uterine muscle (g)	140	320	600	970	3.7 per kg	0.5	1.2	2.2	3.6	Chapter 2
Placenta (g) Wet	20	170	430	650	3.3 per 100 g dry weight	0	0.5	2.2	3.7	Chapter 11
Dry	2	17	65	110						
Fetus (g)	5	300	1500	3400	3.65 per kg	0	1.1	5.5	12.4	Chapter 11
Breasts (g)	45	180	360	410	3.3 per kg	0.1	0.6	1.2	1.4	Chapter 11
					Total ml/min	12.9	18.7	27.2	37.9	

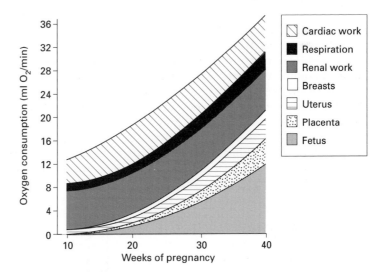

Fig. 4.3. Partition of the increased oxygen consumption of pregnancy amongst the organs concerned.

renal performance account for the bulk of extra oxygen needs in the first two-thirds of pregnancy, and almost half of the needs at term. That total specific increment should probably be reduced a little to take account of an overall reduction in maternal metabolic tempo due to the reduced levels of free thyroid hormone (Chapter 13), but it is not possible to put a figure on this adjustment.

A specific maximum increment for pregnancy of 30–40 ml O_2/min, found both by direct measurement and by computation, is little more than 15% of the average non-pregnant oxygen consumption and is in excellent accord with the increment in oxygen-carrying capacity of the blood estimated at 18%, giving a difference which will account for the reduced arterio-venous oxygen difference at the heart (Chapter 2).

Ventilatory equivalent

With oxygen consumption increasing by less than 20% and minute ventilation increasing by more than 40%, it is clear that there is considerable hyperventilation, all the more pronounced in view of the more effective ventilation of pregnancy. The ventilatory equivalent (respiratory minute volume divided by oxygen consumption) or the number of litres breathed for every 100 ml of oxygen consumed is therefore considerably raised in pregnancy. To take average figures, it rises from about 3.2 l per 100 ml to almost 4.0 l per 100 ml of oxygen consumed.

Carbon dioxide output

Measurement of carbon dioxide production by the body is difficult. While oxygen is taken up from minute to minute in response to needs, the minute-to-minute output of carbon dioxide depends on much more than its rate of production. The body has a considerable capacity for storing CO_2 in the blood, largely as bicarbonate, and the amount breathed out by the lungs in a short interval will be influenced to a large extent by storage, or release of CO_2 from stores, with changes of blood pH. For this reason the ratio of carbon dioxide breathed out to oxygen breathed in — the respiratory quotient (RQ) — cannot be reliably interpreted when estimated from a short observation period such as most investigators have employed for the measurement of oxygen consumption. A valid measure of RQ would require collection of expired gas for some hours under carefully controlled conditions.

Within certain limits it is possible, from a knowledge of the RQ, to estimate not only the energy output of the subject but also the nature of the food mixture from which the energy was derived. For example, an RQ of 0.71 would indicate that pure lipid was being burned, an RQ of 1.0, pure carbohydrate, and intermediate values are associated with varying mixtures of the two. Such RQs are more properly known as non-protein RQs and assume that protein is not also being burned as a metabolic fuel; they require a knowledge of protein combustion from urinary excretion of nitrogen. The older literature, reviewed by Hytten and Leitch [3] was unsatisfactory, and only Emerson and his colleagues [13,52] have provided good serial data of non-protein RQ. They describe a progressive rise from about 0.76 before pregnancy to 0.83 in late pregnancy, which indicates a greater use of carbohydrate as an energy source.

Alveolar and arterial gas tension

P_{CO_2}

Overbreathing in pregnancy causes carbon dioxide to be washed out of the lungs and the alveolar, and arterial, concentration of CO_2 is lower than in the non-pregnant subject.

The phenomenon has been recognized for many years and repeatedly demonstrated, but there is still some argument about the precise pattern of change. It is agreed that, in late pregnancy, the P_{CO_2} is about 30 mmHg (4 kPa), usually slightly above when measured in alveolar air [53–56], and slightly below when measured in arterial blood [16,57,58] compared to non-pregnant levels which are generally between 35 and 40 mmHg (4.7–5.3 kPa). But whilst most studies agree that the lowest level of P_{CO_2} is reached in early pregnancy, usually within the first trimester, Bouterline-Young and Bouterline-Young [55] found the values to decline until the end of the second trimester, and Lucius et al. [57], who calculated a regression for their cross-sectional data, claimed a continuous decline to late pregnancy.

At high altitudes when P_{CO_2} tends to be lower because of increased ventilation, the reduction due to pregnancy is added to the altitude effect. Hellegers et al. [59] studied women living at an altitude of 14 500 ft (4400 m) in Peru and found the mean alveolar P_{CO_2} to be 27.9 mmHg (3.7 kPa) in non-pregnant women and 22.9 mmHg (3.0 kPa) in pregnancy at a similar altitude. Sobrevilla *et al.* [60] found the arterial P_{CO_2} to be 24.5 mmHg (3.3 kPa).

It may be presumed that the fetus, like the newborn infant, is more sensitive to CO_2 than the adult [61] so that the reduced maternal arterial P_{CO_2} allows it to preserve a tolerable level while at the same time having a reasonable gradient across the placenta along which it can dispose of CO_2. If that is the purpose of the maternal change then it is a good illustration of the general truth that adaptations in pregnancy occur in advance of the need for them; the decline in P_{CO_2} is clearly apparent in the luteal phase of each menstrual cycle even before the fertilized ovum embeds [55,62].

The reduction in arterial P_{CO_2} as a result of overbreathing is due to progesterone [63]. Perhaps the first demonstration of that was by Döring *et al.* [64] who also found that oestrogen has a similar but small effect and that the two steroids together were more effective than either alone. Goodland *et al.* [65] reduced alveolar P_{CO_2} in male medical students by about 2.5 mmHg by injecting progesterone and Tyler [66] induced hyperventilation with a dramatic fall in P_{CO_2} in patients with emphysema and hypercapnia. Pa_{CO_2} is inversely related to the progesterone concentration during the menstrual cycle and in pregnancy [63]. Women who are not ovulating (either postmenopausal or amenorrhoeic) have a lower resting ventilatory rate [67]. Tyler also demonstrated that the effect was not common to all progestagens. Progesterone itself had a pronounced effect, but anhydrohydroxyprogesterone, 1,2-dehydroprogesterone and 19-norethinyl testosterone were ineffective. Progesterone may stimulate the respiratory centre directly, but in pregnancy cerebrospinal fluid levels of progesterone are either undetectable, or similar to the plasma level in the non-pregnant state [68].

In addition, progesterone increases the level of carbonic anhydrase B in red cells. A close relation has been shown to exist between the levels of carbonic anhydrase and plasma progesterone in pregnancy, in the menstrual cycle and during oral contraception [69]. An increase in carbonic anhydrase facilitates carbon dioxide transfer and will tend to decrease P_{CO_2} independently of any change in ventilation.

During the menstrual cycle, changes in the base excess exactly parallel changes in P_{CO_2}, maintaining a normal pH. We therefore cannot use blood gas estimation to distinguish whether the progesterone effect is respiratory or metabolic [70]. The effect of injected progesterone is not seen until 3–24 hours after administration, and the maximal hyperventilation does not occur until several days after progesterone levels have peaked in the luteal phase. It is therefore certainly possible that the primary effect of progesterone could be metabolic rather than a direct stimulant to the respiratory centre. Nevertheless, the site of action is presumed to be the respiratory centres and a study by Wilbrand *et al.* [71] showed that, while progesterone lowered the threshold of the respiratory centres to P_{CO_2}, oestrogen increased their sensitivity. Lyons and Antonio [56], on the other hand, claimed that both the reduced threshold and the increased sensitivity could be induced by progesterone alone.

The increased sensitivity of the respiratory centres is impressive. According to Prowse and Gaensler [72], normal subjects increase their ventilation by about 1.5 l/min for each rise of 1 mmHg in P_{CO_2}; in pregnancy the equivalent rise in ventilation is about 6 l/min, an increase which is similar to that of men acclimatized to an altitude of 14 000 ft (4250 m). A similar effect has been shown both by Pernoll *et al.* [20] in normal women (Fig. 4.3) and by Eng *et al.* [16] in obese pregnant women.

The relatively simple process of lowering P_{CO_2} by overbreathing brings a train of physiological consequences. First, it may be extremely uncomfortable for the mother and can lead to dyspnoea and giddiness. Second, if pH is to be maintained, then plasma bicarbonate must be lowered and sodium with it. Thus the mother's plasma osmolality is reduced, requiring further adjustments by altering the response of the osmoreceptors so that a state analogous to diabetes insipidus does not ensue. However this cannot be the whole story, since osmotic pressure of plasma falls very early in pregnancy, before any change in ventilation can be demonstrated.

Po_2

Increasing the alveolar ventilation not only lowers Pco_2, it must reciprocally raise Po_2, but few measurements have been made to demonstrate the point. Lucius et al. [57], with a cross-sectional study of arterial Po_2, showed, by regression, a rise which reflected the fall in Pco_2, from 85 mmHg (11.3 kPa) at 10 weeks to 92 mmHg (12.3 kPa) at term. Templeton and Kelman [45] showed a similar pattern with different values: non-pregnant Po_2 = 93.4 mmHg (12.5 kPa), 12 weeks = 106.4 mmHg (14.2 kPa), term = 101.8 mmHg (13.6 kPa). However, in obese women who showed a relatively small fall in Pco_2, Eng et al. [16] could demonstrate no rise in Po_2.

The change in Po_2 is relatively trivial, and because of the shape of the haemoglobin dissociation curve, will have no real effect on haemoglobin saturation, particularly since the haemoglobin dissociation curve is shifted to the right (lower affinity) in pregnancy, i.e. $P50$ increases from 26.7 mmHg (3.6 kPa) in the non-pregnant state to 30.2 mmHg (4.0 kPa) at term [73]. However, it is possible that in adverse circumstances the pregnancy effect could be of great importance. Sobrevilla et al. [60], in a study at high altitude (13 800 ft, 4200 m), showed that arterial Po_2 was 60.8 mmHg (8.1 kPa) in 12 women at term compared to 47.6 mmHg (6.3 kPa) in healthy men. Hellegers et al.'s [59] smaller study indicated a similar difference: 59.0 mmHg (7.9 kPa) in pregnancy and 50.7 mmHg (6.8 kPa) in the non-pregnant. Moore and colleagues have equivalent data from the Andes [74] and Colorado [75]. Modern aircraft are pressurized to maintain a cabin pressure equivalent to an altitude of 2500 m (8200 ft). Huch et al. [76] studied 12 pregnant women on commercial flights and showed that although transcutaneously measured Po_2 fell to about 65 mmHg (8.7 kPa), there was no change in maternal ventilation or Pco_2 apart from transients at take-off and landing. Similarly, there were only transient changes in the fetal heart rate at take-off and landing, suggesting that normal commercial aircraft travel causes no strain on maternal or fetal respiration and that it is safe in normal pregnancy. By contrast, breathing 12% oxygen,

which is equivalent to breathing air at 13 000 ft (3950 m) above sea level, has been shown to impair fetal habituation patterns [77].

Templeton [78] suggested that unusually low Po_2 levels in a patient with bronchiectasis caused fetal growth retardation in her two pregnancies. However, this has not been confirmed in other studies [79] of bronchiectasis, although patients with severe asthma may also have growth-retarded infants [10].

pH

The fall in Pco_2 is matched by an equivalent fall in plasma bicarbonate concentration and all the evidence suggests that arterial pH is not altered from the normal non-pregnant level of about 7.40. Peripheral venous pH on the other hand is higher: 7.38 compared to a non-pregnant level of 7.35. The reduced arteriovenous difference which appears early in pregnancy is presumably a reflection of the increased peripheral blood flow [80].

The cost of ventilation

The work of breathing becomes proportionately greater with increasing rates of ventilation, and, in pregnancy, the effect is accentuated. Bader et al. [81] had a group of 11 women in late pregnancy breathe at a fixed rate of 20 per minute and vary their minute volume by changing only tidal volume; carbon dioxide was added to the mixture in sufficient quantities to prevent discomfort. The rise of oxygen consumption with ventilation rate was much steeper for the pregnant women than for three non-pregnant controls. For example, at a ventilation rate of 15 l/min, the non-pregnant women used additional oxygen at a rate of between 1.2 and 2.2 ml/l of ventilation, and a typical pregnant woman needed 3.3 ml of O_2/l. Judged from the information given by Bader et al., about 3 ml O_2/l of ventilation would be a reasonable average over the range of resting ventilation found in late pregnancy.

Bader and his group suggest that the cost is likely to be less for more natural, slower rates of ventilation and their figures may be more appropriate for respiration after exercise than for respiration at rest. They are certainly much above the averages found by Campbell *et al.* [82] for young men who used only 0.65 ml of O_2/l of ventilation in the range 9–22 l/min — a level which agrees with most other published studies. Until Bader's study has been repeated and extended, most are unwilling to accept their very high figures. The possibility that ventilation in pregnancy costs more than before pregnancy seems reasonable, but it would be surprising if it were much above about 1 ml O_2/l of ventilation.

The effect of exercise [83,84]

The capacity for exercise, which implies exercising to exhaustion, has not been tested in pregnancy and there would be little point in attempting it. The question of physiological interest is whether or not ordinary exercise costs more, or is performed less efficiently, in pregnancy. For any exercise which involves lifting the body there will be an inevitable extra cost in pregnancy due to increasing body weight, and it may be that all tests of exercise contain some element of body-weight lifting. Step tests, which involve stepping up and down a fixed height of step at varying rates, will be heavily influenced by changing body weight, as will walking on a treadmill. But sitting exercise — as, for example, on a cycle ergometer — should be less affected. Widlund [85], who used a series of graded step tests, found that the pregnant woman incurred a larger oxygen debt for moderately hard exercise (lifting the body 17 m per minute) than the non-pregnant woman and that the difference seemed to be attributable both to increasing body weight and also to an accentuated hyperventilation, since ventilation increased proportionately more than the oxygen debt.

Cugell *et al.* [6], on the other hand, could show no excess ventilation with exercise in pregnancy. Seitchik [86] found no increase in the cost of standard exercise on a cycle ergometer in pregnancy, a conclusion that was confirmed by Knuttgen and Emerson [13]. More recently, Artal *et al.* [87] showed that exercise on a treadmill cost less in pregnancy and was associated with a smaller increase in oxygen consumption and lower ventilatory equivalent. By contrast, Pernoll *et al.* [53] found that mild exercise on a

cycle ergometer was less efficient in pregnancy and the extra cost was more than could be accounted for by increased ventilation and myocardial work. The question therefore remains open and it may be that a great deal depends on the subjects tested and the circumstances of the test. Edwards *et al.* [88] studied the rates of change of ventilation, oxygen absorption is and carbon dioxide elimination by the lungs during exercise on a bicycle ergometer in pregnancy. They found that all these variables increased more rapidly in pregnancy, particularly in the first 10 seconds of exercise; i.e. there is an accelerated respiratory response to exercise in pregnancy which was ascribed to the effect of a larger pool of venous blood entering the lungs and possibly travelling to the respiratory centre.

It is also important to know whether maternal exercise, possibly by diverting blood from the placenta, compromises the normal or abnormal fetus.

Moderate exercise (75 w for 5 minutes on a bicycle ergometer) has no effect on fetal heart rate or cardiac function as assessed by M mode echocardiography [89]. More prolonged exercise (20 minutes' treadmill run) causes fetal tachycardia of about 20 beats per minute at 20 and 32 weeks' gestation but the cause and therefore the significance of the tachycardia are unknown [90]. In another study [91] of treadmill exercise, most patients showed an increased fetal heart rate at all levels of exercise, the degree of tachycardia independent of the severity of exercise.

Labour

For the reasons stated at the outset, it is difficult to perform complicated respiratory function tests in pregnancy and these difficulties are compounded in labour.

It has been suggested that oxygen saturation falls from 95% at the end of pregnancy to 89% at the end of the second stage of labour, rising to 95% by the first day postpartum [92,93]. This may be a genuine phenomenon, associated with pooling of blood in the lungs during labour and increased venous admixture. It may also be due to a sampling error arising from the increased likelihood of sampling relatively desaturated blood that has just been expelled from the uterus after uterine contraction.

Epidural block

Epidural block is being used with increasing frequency for analgesia in labour or anaesthesia for instrumental delivery. In some units up to 70% of women are delivered in this way. The procedure is attractive to patients and staff since consciousness is preserved and since patients breathe spontaneously, in theory reducing the risk of postoperative atelectasis. In addition, the elimination of pain is associated with reduced oxygen consumption [94]. However serial studies of pulmonary function have shown that peak flow rate, FEV_1 and forced vital capacity (FVC) all decrease in patients immediately after a spinal block for caesarean section [95]. There is a further decrease in these variables once the abdomen is open. For example, FVC decreased from 3.0 litres pre-block to 2.25 litres when the abdomen was open [95]. This procedure therefore does not eliminate potential respiratory complications of instrumental delivery.

Dyspnoea

Normally, we are not conscious of the automatic process of breathing, and, even when moderate exercise increases the ventilation rate, the change is usually unnoticed. When the need to breathe becomes a conscious one, there is 'shortness of breath', which is one of the commoner causes of complaint by the pregnant woman. In pregnancy the symptom is not necessarily related to exercise and, paradoxically, it may be present when sitting down but not when walking about. Moreover, it adds confusion in a situation where there may be other misleading signs which are usual in pregnancy but otherwise are regarded as abnormal, such as a low haemoglobin concentration, or equivocal signs of heart disease.

Dyspnoea is common when ventilation is mechanically restricted or when there is airways' resistance. Neither of these accounts for the symptom in pregnancy; on the contrary, resistance to breathing is less. Cugell et al. [6] showed that dyspnoea, which was a complaint

of 13 of their 19 subjects, was not related to maximum breathing capacity, oxygen uptake, ventilation, vital capacity or any of the subdivisions of lung volume. Two of the women with a definite reduction in maximum breathing capacity had no dyspnoea; two others with considerably increased maximum breathing capacity were short of breath even at rest. Eighteen of the 31 women studied by Thomson and Cohen [17] complained of dyspnoea, but its appearance was capricious; it might be present one month and not the next. Its appearance was not related to vital capacity. Milne et al. [96] have documented the dyspnoea felt by 62 women in pregnancy. There was a marked increase in symptoms until about 20 weeks' gestation. After this point there was little change. The authors suggest that the time lapse of the symptoms of dyspnoea fits the time lapse of the fall in $Paco_2$ noted by Bouterline-Young and Bouterline-Young [55].

An ingenious theory has been developed by Campbell and Howell [97] to explain the sensation of dyspnoea: they believe that it arises when the ventilatory response is inappropriate to the demand, which must imply that some centre is continuously relating the demand for ventilation to the actual ventilation. Although Comroe et al. [2] have claimed a number of exceptions to the theory, it appears to cover most situations.

As we have seen, there is overbreathing in pregnancy so that, in one sense, ventilation is inappropriate to demand. A study by Gilbert et al. [98] supports the suggestion that it may be the basis of dyspnoea. They studied ventilatory adjustments of 14 normal pregnant women during mild exercise. Five of the subjects complained of dyspnoea during the exercise and dyspnoea occurred when alveolar Pco_2 was lowest. Moreover, these five women had a higher Pco_2 than the others before pregnancy and the authors suggest that their sensations of breathlessness might be due to their unfamiliarity with low tensions of CO_2. For a woman habituated to breathing with an alveolar Pco_2 of over 35 mmHg (4.7 kPa) the compulsion to breathe in pregnancy with an alveolar Pco_2 of perhaps 30 mmHg (4 kPa) may very well seem, in Campbell's phrase, 'inappropriate'.

More recently, Gilbert and Auchincloss [99]

found other differences between healthy pregnant women who did or did not experience dyspnoea. The dyspnoeic group developed a much lower alveolar P_{CO_2} after mild exercise, sometimes low enough to reduce cerebral blood flow and cause dizziness. Two women who became dizzy also had end-tidal P_{CO_2} levels of only 20 and 12 mmHg (2.7 and 1.6 kPa). In addition, the dyspnoeic group had a much increased sensitivity in their ventilatory response to changes in P_{CO_2}. Gilbert and Auchincloss confirmed that the changes occurred particularly in pregnancy; two of their multiparous subjects recognized dyspnoea as their first indication of pregnancy. These observations would fit the recent suggestion, made from observations on men and non-pregnant women, that the intensity of dyspnoea relates to the level of effective reflex stimulation of the respiratory-related neurones in the medulla [100].

References

1 Cotes J.E. (1975) *Lung Function, Assessment and Application in Medicine*, 3rd edn. Blackwell Scientific Publications, Oxford.

2 Comroe J.J., Forster R.E., Dubois A.B., Briscoe W.A. & Carlsen E. (1962) *The Lung, Clinical Physiology and Pulmonary Function Tests*. Year Book Medical Publishers, Chicago.

3 Hytten F.E. & Leitch I. (1971) *The Physiology of Human Pregnancy*, 2nd edn, chapter 3. Blackwell Scientific Publications, Oxford.

4 Weinbergen S.E., Weiss S.T., Cohen W.R., Weiss J.W. & Johnson T.S. (1980) Pregnancy and the lung. *American Review of Respiratory Diseases* **121**, 559.

5 Fishburne J.I. (1979) Physiology and disease of the respiratory system in pregnancy: a review. *Journal of Reproductive Medicine* **22**, 177.

6 Cugell D.W., Frank N.R., Gaensler E.A. & Badger T.L. (1953) Pulmonary function in pregnancy. I. Serial observations in normal women. *American Review of Tuberculosis and Pulmonary Diseases* **67**, 568.

7 Rubin A., Russo N. & Goucher D. (1956) The effect of pregnancy upon pulmonary function in normal women. *American Jouranl of Obstetrics and Gynecology* **72**, 963.

8 Heidenreich J., Kafarnik D., Westenburger U. & Beck L. (1971) Statische und dynamische Ventilationsgrössen in der Schwangerschaft und im Wochenbett. *Archiv für Gynakologie* **210**, 208.

9 Lehmann V. & Fabel H. (1973) Lungenfunktionsuntersuchungen an Schwangeren, Teil I: Lungenvolumina. *Zeitschrift für Geburtshilfe* und *Perinatologie* **177**, 387.

10 Sims C.D., Chamberlain G.V.P. & de Swiet M. (1976) Lung function tests in bronchial asthma during and after pregnancy. *British Journal of Obstetrics and Gynaecology* **83**, 434.

11 Woolcock A.J. & Read J. (1972) In *Human Reproductive Physiology*. Ed. R.P. Shearman, p. 639. Blackwell Scientific Publications, Oxford.

12 Gazioglu K., Kaltreider N.L., Rosen M. & Yu P.N. (1970) Pulmonary function during· pregnancy in normal women and in patients with cardiopulmonary disease. *Thorax* **25**, 445.

13 Knuttgen H.G. & Emerson K. (1974) Physiological response to pregnancy at rest and during exercise. *Journal of Applied Physiology* **36**, 549.

14 Puranik B.M., Kaore S.B., Kurhade G.A., Agrawal S.D., Patwardhan S.A. & Kher J.R. (1994) A longitudinal study of pulmonary function tests during pregnancy. *Indian Journal of Physiology and Pharmacology* **38**, 129.

15 Mokkapatti R., Prasad E.C., Venkatraman S. & Fatima K. (1991) Ventilatory functions in pregnancy. *Indian Journal of Physiology and Pharmacology* **35**, 237.

16 Eng M., Butler J. & Bonica J.J. (1975) Respiratory function in pregnant obese women. *American Journal of Obstetrics and Gynecology* **123**, 241.

17 Thomson K.J. & Cohen M.E. (1938) Studies on the circulation in pregnancy. II. Vital capacity observations in normal pregnant women. *Surgery, Gynecology and Obstetrics* **66**, 591.

18 Gupta A., Johnson A., Johansson A., Berg G. & Lenmarken C. (1993) Maternal respiratory function following normal vaginal delivery. *International Journal of Obstetric Anaesthesia* **2**, 129.

19 Lehmann V. & Fabel H. (1973) Lungenfunktionsuntersuchungen an Schwangeren, Teil II: Ventilation, Atemmechanik und Diffisionkapazität. *Zeitschrift für Geburtshilfe und Perinatologie* **177**, 397.

20 Pernoll M.L., Metcalfe J., Kovach P.A., Wachter R. & Dunham M.J. (1975) Ventilation during rest and exercise in pregnancy and postpartum. *Respiration Physiology* **25**, 295.

21 Spätling L., Fallenstein F., Huch A., Huch R. & Rooth G. (1992) The variability of cardiopulmonary adaptation to pregnancy at rest and during excercise. *British Journal of Obstetrics and Gynaecology* **99**, 10.

22 Klaften E. & Palugyay J. (1926) Zur Physiologie der Atmung in der Schwangershaft. *Archiv für Gynakologie* **129**, 414.

23 Klaften E. & Palugyay J. (1927) Vergleichende Untersuchungen über Lage und Ausdehnung von Herz und Lunge in der Schwangershaft und im Wochenbett. *Archiv für Gynäkologie* **131**, 347.

24 Möbius W.V. (1961) Abbruch und Schwangerschaft. *Münchener medizinische Wochenschrift* **103**, 1389.

25 McGinty A.P. (1938) The comparative effect of pregnancy and phrenic nerve interruption on the diaphragm and their relation to pulmonary tuberculosis. *American Journal of Obstetrics and Gynecology* **35**, 237.

26 Omatsu Y. (1957) Basal metabolism in pregnancy. *Kobe Journal of the Medical Sciences* **27**, 21.

27 Hughson W.G., Friedman P.J., Feigin D.S., Resnik R. & Moser K.M. (1982) Postpartum pleural effusion: a common radiologic finding. *Annals of Internal Medicine* **97**, 856.

126

28 Wallis M.G., McHugo J.M., Carruthers D.A. & Selwyn Crawford J. (1989) The prevalence of pleural effusions in pre-eclampsia: an ultrasound study. *British Journal of Obstetrics and Gynaecology* **96**, 431.

29 Udeshi U.L., McHugo J.M. & Selwyn Crawford J. (1988) Postpartum pleural effusion. *British Journal of Obstetrics and Gynaecology* **95**, 894.

30 Ihrman K. (1960) A clinical and physiological study of pregnancy in a material from Northern Sweden. VII. The heart volume during and after pregnancy. *Acta Societatis medicorum Upsaliensis* **65**, 326.

31 Krumholz R.A., Echt C.R. & Ross J.C. (1964) Pulmonary diffusing capacity, capillary blood volume, lung volumes and mechanics of ventilation in early and late pregnancy. *Journal of Laboratory and Clinical Medicine* **63**, 648.

32 Cameron S.J., Bain H.H. & Grant I.W.B. (1970) Ventilatory function in pregnancy. *Scottish Medical Journal* **15**, 243.

33 Milne J.A., Mills R.J., Howie A.D. & Pack A.I. (1977) Large airways function during normal pregnancy. *British Journal of Obstetrics and Gynaecology* **84**, 448.

34 Schaeffer G. & Silverman F. (1961) Pregnancy complicated by asthma. *American Journal of Obstetrics and Gynecology* **82**, 182.

35 Juniper E.F., Daniel E.E., Roberts R.S., Kline P.A., Hargreave F.E. & Newhouse M.T. (1989) Improvement in airway responsiveness and asthma severity during pregnancy. *American Review of Respiratory Diseases* **140**, 924.

36 Gordon M., Niswander K.R., Berendes H. & Kantor A.G. (1970) Fetal morbidity following potential anoxigenic obstetric conditions. VII. Bronchial asthma. *American Journal of Obstetrics and Gynecology* **106**, 421.

37 Hiddlestone H.J.H. (1964) Bronchial asthma and pregnancy. *New Zealand Medical Journal* **63**, 521.

38 Gee J.B.L., Packer B.S., Millen J.E. & Robin E.D. (1967) Pulmonary mechanics during pregnancy. *Journal of Clinical Investigation* **46**, 945.

39 Beynon H.L.C., Garbett N.D. & Barnes P.J. (1988) Severe premenstrual exacerbations of asthma: effect of intramuscular progesterone. *Lancet* **2**, 370.

40 Kriesman H., Van de Weil W. & Mitchell C.A. (1975) Respiratory function during prostaglandin-induced labor. *American Review of Respiratory Diseases* **111**, 564.

41 Bevan D.R., Holdcroft A., Loh L., MacGregor W.G., O'Sullivan J.C. & Sykes M.K. (1974) Closing volume and pregnancy. *British Medical Journal* **i**, 13.

42 Farebrother M.J.B. & McHardy G.J.R. (1974) Closing volume and pregnancy. *British Medical Journal* **i**, 454.

43 Littler W.A., Redman C.W.G., Bonnar J., Beilin L.J. & Lee G. de J. (1973) Reduced pulmonary arterial compliance in hypertensive pregnancy. *Lancet* **i**, 1274.

44 Garrard C.G., Littler W.A.W. & Redman C.W.L. (1978) Closing volume during normal pregnancy. *Thorax* **33**, 488.

45 Templeton A. & Kelman G.R. (1976) Maternal blood gases (Pa_{O_2}–Pa_{O_2}) physiological shunt and V_D/V_T in normal pregnancy. *British Journal of Anaesthesia* **48**, 1001.

46 Maclennan F.M. (1986) Maternal mortality from Mendelson's syndrome: an explanation. *Lancet* **1**, 587.

47 Ang C.K., Tan T.H., Walters W.A.W. & Wood C. (1969) Postural influence on maternal capillary oxygen and carbon dioxide tension. *British Medical Journal* **ii**, 201.

48 Bedell G.N. & Adams R.S. (1962) Pulmonary diffusing capacity during rest and exercise: a study of normal persons and persons with atrial septal defect, pregnancy and pulmonary disease. *Journal of Clinical Investigation* **41**, 1908.

49 Milne J.A., Mills R.J., Coutts J.R.T., MacNaughton M.C., Moran F. & Pack A.I. (1977) The effect of human pregnancy on the pulmonary transfer factor for carbon monoxide as measured by the single breath method. *Clinical Science and Molecular Medicine* **53**, 271.

50 Pecora L.J., Putnam L.R. & Baum G.L. (1963) Effects of intravenous estrogens on pulmonary diffusing capacity. *American Journal of the Medical Sciences* **246**, 48.

51 Awe R.J., Nicotra M.B., Newson T.D. & Viles R. (1979) Arterial oxygenation and alveolar–arterial gradients in term pregnancy. *Obstetrics and Gynecology* **53**, 182.

52 Emerson K., Saxena B.N. & Poindexter E.L. (1972) Caloric cost of normal pregnancy. *Obstetrics and Gynecology* **40**, 786.

53 Pernoll M.L., Metcalfe J., Schlenker T.L., Welch J.E. & Matsumoto J.A. (1975) Oxygen consumption at rest and during exercise in pregnancy. *Respiration Physiology* **25**, 285.

54 Döring G.K. & Loeschche H.H. (1947) Atmung und Säure–Basengleichgewieht in der Schwangerschaft. *Pflügers Archiv für die gesamte Physiologie des Menschen und der Tiere* **249**, 437.

55 Bouterline-Young H. & Bouterline-Young E. (1956) Alveolar carbon dioxide levels in pregnant parturient and lactating subjects. *Journal of Obstetrics and Gynaecology of the British Empire* **63**, 509.

56 Lyons H.A. & Antonio R. (1959) The sensitivity of the respiratory centre in pregnancy and after the administration of progesterone. *Transactions of the Association of American Physicians* **72**, 173.

57 Lucius H., Gahlenbeck H., Kleine H.O., Fabel H. & Bartles H. (1970) Respiratory functions, buffer system, and electrolyte concentrations of blood during human pregnancy. *Respiration Physiology* **9**, 311.

58 Kelman G.R. & Templeton A. (1975) Maternal blood gases during human pregnancy. *Journal of Physiology* **244**, 66P.

59 Hellegers A., Metcalfe J., Huckabee W., Meschia G., Prystowsky H. & Barron D. (1959) The alveolar P_{CO} & P_{O_2} in pregnant and non-pregnant women at altitude. *Journal of Clinical Investigation* **38**, 1010.

60 Sobrevilla L.A., Cassinelli M.T., Carcelen A. & Malaga J.W. (1971) Human fetal and maternal oxygen tension and acid-base status during delivery at high altitude. *American Journal of Obstetrics and Gynecology* **111**, 1111.

61 Cross K.W., Hooper J.M.D. & Oppe T.E. (1953) The effect of carbon dioxide on the respiration of the full-term and premature infant. *Journal of Physiology* **119**, 11P.

62 Goodland R.L. & Pommerenke W.T. (1952) Cyclic fluctuations of the alveolar carbon dioxide tension during the normal menstrual cycle. *Fertility and Sterility* **3**, 394.

63 Machida H. (1981) Influence of progesterone on arterial acid base balance in women. *Journal of Applied Physiology* **51**, 1433.

64 Döring G.K., Loescheke H.H. & Ochwadt B. (1950) Weitere Untersuchungen über die Wirkung der Sexualhormone auf die Atmung. *Pflügers Archiv für die gesamte Physiologie der Menschen und der Tiere* **252**, 216.

65 Goodland R.L., Reynolds J.G., McCoord A.B. & Pommerenke W.T. (1953) Respiratory and electrolyte effects induced by estrogen and progesterone. *Fertility and Sterility* **4**, 300.

66 Tyler J.M. (1960) The effect of progesterone on the respiration of patients with emphysema and hypercapnia. *Journal of Clinical Investigation* **39**, 34.

67 Tatsumi K., Hannhart B. & Moore L.G. (1994) Influences of sex steroids on ventilation and ventilatory control. In *Regulation of Breathing*. Ed. J.A. Dempsey & A.I. Pack, p. 829. Lung Biology in Health & Disease Series, **79**, Marcel Dekker, New York.

68 Lurie A.O. & Weis J.B. (1967) Progesterone in cerebrospinal fluid during human pregnancy. *Nature, London* **2**, 1178.

69 Paciorek J. & Spencer N. (1980) An association between plasma progesterone and erythrocyte carbonic anhydrase 1 concentration in women. *Clinical Science* **58**, 161.

70 England S.J. & Fahri L.E. (1976) Fluctuations in alveolar CO_2 and in base excess during the menstrual cycle. *Respiration Physiology* **26**, 157.

71 Wilbrand U., Porath Ch., Matthaes P. & Jaster R. (1959) Der Einfluss der Ovarialsteroide auf die Funktion des Atemzentrums. *Archiv für Gynäkologie* **191**, 507.

72 Prowse C.M. & Gaensler E.A. (1965) Respiratory and acid base changes during pregnancy. *Anaesthesiology* **26**, 381.

73 Kambam J.R., Mandte R.E., Brown W.R. & Smith B.E. (1983) Effect of pregnancy on oxygen dissociation. *Anesthesiology* **59**, A395.

74 Moore L.G., Brodeur P., Clunbe O., D'Brot J., Hofmeister S. & Monge C. (1986) Maternal hypoxic ventilatory response, ventilation and infant birth weight at 4300 m. *Journal of Applied Physiology* **60**, 1401.

75 Moore L.G., Jahniggen D., Round S.S., Reeves J.T. & Grover R.F. (1982) Maternal hyperventilation helps preserve arterial oxygenation during high-altitude pregnancy *Journal of Applied Physiology* **52**, 690–4.

76 Huch R., Baumann H., Fallenstein F., Schneider K.T.M., Holener F. & Huch A. (1986) Physiologic changes in pregnant women and their fetuses during jet travel. *American Journal of Obstetrics and Gynecology* **154**, 996.

77 Leader L.R. & Baillie P. (1988) The changes in fetal habituation patterns due to a decrease in inspired maternal oxygen. *British Journal of Obstetrics and Gynaecology* **95**, 664.

78 Templeton A. (1977) Intrauterine growth retardation associated with hypoxia due to bronchiectasis. *British Journal of Obstetrics and Gynaecology* **84**, 389.

79 Howie A.D. & Milne J.A. (1978) Pregnancy in patients with bronchiectasis. *British Journal of Obstetrics and Gynaecology* **85**, 197.

80 Seeds A.E., Battaglia F.C. & Hellegers A.E. (1964) Effects of pregnancy on the pH, P_{CO_2} and bicarbonate concentrations of peripheral venous blood. *American Journal of Obstetrics and Gynecology* **88**, 1086.

81 Bader R.A., Bader M.E. & Rose D.J. (1959) The oxygen cost of breathing in dyspnoeic subjects as studied in normal pregnant women. *Clinical Science* **18**, 223.

82 Campbell E.J.M., Westlake E.K. & Cherniack R.M. (1959) The oxygen consumption and efficiency of the respiratory muscles of young male subjects. *Clinical Science* **18**, 55.

83 Huch R. & Erkkola R. (1990) Pregnancy and exercise—exercise and pregnancy: a short review. *British Journal of Obstetrics and Gynaecology* **97**, 208.

84 Lotgering F.K., Gilbert R.D. & Longo L. (1984) The interactions of exercise and pregnancy: a review. *American Journal of Obstetrics and Gynecology* **149**, 560.

85 Widlund G. (1945) The cardio-pulmonal function during pregnancy. *Acta Obstetricia et Gynecologica Scandinavica* **25** (Suppl. 1).

86 Seitchik J. (1967) Body composition and energy expenditure during rest and work in pregnancy. *American Journal of Obstetrics and Gynecology* **97**, 701.

87 Artal R., Wiswell R., Romen Y. & Dorey F. (1986) Pulmonary responses to exercise in pregnancy. *American Journal of Obstetrics and Gynecology* **154**, 378.

88 Edwards M.J., Metcalfe J., Dunham M.J. & Paul M.S. (1981) Accelerated respiratory response to moderate exercise in late pregnancy. *Respiration Physiology* **45**, 229.

89 Sørensen K.E. & Børlum K. (1986) Fetal heart function in response to short-term maternal exercise. *British Journal of Obstetrics and Gynaecology* **93**, 310.

90 Clapp J.F. (1985) Fetal heart rate response to running in midpregnancy and late pregnancy. *American Journal of Obstetrics and Gynecology* **153**, 251.

91 Artal R., Rutherford S., Romen Y., Kammula R.K., Dorey F.J. & Wiswell R.A. (1986) Fetal heart rate responses to maternal exercise. *American Journal of Obstetrics and Gynecology* **155**, 729.

92 Alward H.C. (1930) Observations on vital capacity during the last month of pregnancy and puerperium. *American Journal of Obstetrics and Gynecology* **20**, 373.

93 Esteban-Altirriba J. (1960) A comparative study of oxygen saturation of the peripheral arterial blood during pregnancy, labour and the post partum period. *Gynecologica* **150**, 33.

94 Sangoul F., Fox G.S. & Houle G.L. (1975) Effect of regional analgesia on maternal oxygen consumption during the first stage of labor. *American Journal of Obstetrics and Gynecology* **121**, 1080.

128

95 Conn D.A., Moffat A.C., McCallum G.D.R. & Thorburn J. (1993) Changes in pulmonary function tests during spinal anaesthesia for caesarean section. *International Journal of Obstetric Anesthesia* **2**, 12.

96 Milne J.A., Howie A.D. & Pack A.I. (1978) Dyspnoea during normal pregnancy. *British Journal of Obstetrics and Gynaecology* **85**, 260.

97 Campbell E.J.M. & Howell J.B.L. (1963) The sensation of breathlessness. *British Medical Bulletin* **19**, 36.

98 Gilbert R., Epifano L. & Auchincloss J.H. (1962) Dyspnoea of pregnancy: a syndrome of altered respiratory control. *Journal of the American Medical Association* **182**, 1073.

99 Gilbert R. & Auchincloss J.H. (1966) Dyspnoea of pregnancy, clinical and physiological observations. *American Journal of the Medical Sciences* **252**, 270.

100 Adams L., Lane R., Shea S.A., Cockcroft A. & Guz A. (1985) Breathlessness during different forms of ventilatory stimulation: a study of mechanisms in normal subjects and respiratory patients. *Clinical Science* **69**, 663.

The Immune System

I.T. MANYONDA

Basic immunology

The role of the immune system is to protect an individual from pathogenic microorganisms and their toxins, as well as to eliminate cells that have undergone malignant transformation. Therefore, a fundamental requirement of the immune system is that it can distinguish normal healthy cells ('self') from 'non-self' (infected or malignant cells, and toxins). The purpose of this chapter is to allow the reader to achieve a better understanding of the importance of the immune system, how it integrates with and relates to other bodily systems and, in particular, what immunological questions are posed by pregnancy. However, a detailed exposé of basic immunology is beyond the scope of this chapter and a suggested further reading list is given. The section on basic immunology has been divided into three, viz.: cells involved in immune reactions, molecules involved in immune reactions, and effector immune functions.

Cells involved in immune reactions

Lymphocytes and phagocytes, which originate from bone marrow stem cells, are the predominant cells of the immune system, and they interact with each other and other cells of the body to generate the immune response. Various leucocyte populations can be identified via their morphology and the molecules expressed on the cell surface, which are recognizable with monoclonal antibodies. Such molecules are termed *markers*, and a system of nomenclature has been devised for all the major molecules. This is called the cluster of differentiation (CD) system. While CD molecules allow the identification of leucocyte subpopulations, it has become clear that they subserve specific functions e.g. the molecule CD3, found on all mature T cells, is associated with the antigen receptor and acts in transducing activation signals to the cell. Some CD molecules may appear transiently during lymphocyte development (e.g. the CD1 molecule on cortical thymocytes), or following cellular activation (e.g. the interleukin-2 receptor CD25), while others are stable and expressed on particular cell lineages. The key markers of leucocyte subpopulations are listed in Table 5.1.

B lymphocytes are characterized by their expression of surface immunoglobulin (antibody) which acts as a receptor for antigen. They recognize native antigens in solution or on the surface of other cells. B cells, activated by contact with their specific antigen and triggered by cytokines released from T cells, divide and differentiate into antibody-secreting plasma cells. The secreted antibody is of identical antigen specificity to that on the original B cell, although it may become refined during the development of an immune response, resulting

Table 5.1. Key markers of lymphocyte populations.

Marker function	Immunoglobulin antigen receptor	TcR/CD3 T-cell activator	CD4 MHC class II binding	CD8 MHC class II binding	CD8 MHC class I binding	CD5
B cells	+	−	−	−	−	+/−*
T_H cells†	−	+	+	+	−	+
T_C cells†	−	+	+	−	+	+

T_H: helper T cells; T_C: cytotoxic T cells; TcR: T-cell receptor; MHC: major histocompatibility complex.
* A minor subpopulation of B cells is CD+.
† The great majority of helper T cells are CD4+ and the majority of suppressors and cytotoxics, CD8+; exceptions have been found.

in an increasing affinity for the antigen. Antibodies are classified into different biochemical classes (see below). Virgin B cells initially express IgM with or without IgD on their surface. During B-cell differentiation, individual cells may switch to the production of IgG, IgA or IgE while retaining the antigen specificity.

T lymphocytes mature in the thymus and three major events occur during thymic differentiation:
1 the development of a repertoire of T-cell receptors (TcR), and a preferential selection of cells carrying TcRs that may interact effectively with the individual's major histocompatibility complex (MHC) molecules in antigen presentation;
2 the selective removal of cells that recognize the individual's own molecules (i.e. self antigens);
3 the differentiation of different T-cell subpopulations.

T-cell precursors entering the thymus lack specific T-cell markers. They acquire CD2 at an early stage of development and this is retained in mature T cells. Immature thymocytes express both CD4 and CD8, but one of these markers is lost as the cells mature. Thus, T cells leaving the thymus express either CD4 or CD8. A considerable selective pressure is exerted at this stage, and the large majority of thymocytes die without completing differentiation into mature T cells. T-cell subpopulations have been identified by functional studies or by using markers. At least two major sets are described: helper T cells (T_H), predominantly CD4+; cytotoxic T cells (T_C), mostly CD8+. T cells recognize anti-

gens (as peptide fragments) on the surface of other cells, in association with molecules encoded by the MHC (see below). The process by which cells express molecules recognizable by T cells in termed antigen presentation, and the cells are antigen-presenting cells (APCs). Many cell types are capable of presenting antigens in a recognizable form to both B and T lymphocytes, and are thus collectively described as APCs (Table 5.2). CD8+ T cells recognize antigen in association with MHC class I molecules and CD4+ cells recognize antigen in association with MHC class II molecules. T-cell activation causes the cells to divide and secrete various cytokines that modulate immune responses. In addition, cytotoxic T cells secrete molecules called perforins, which polymerize to form holes in the membranes of target cells.

Mononuclear phagocytes are widely distributed throughout the body. They are diverse, including not only blood monocytes, but also microglia of the brain and the Kupffer cells of the liver. Blood monocytes can migrate into the tissues where they develop into macrophages. The latter express receptors for immunoglobulin and complement components, and may be activated by cytokines released from T cells. Their surface molecules facilitate binding to antigens and subsequent phagocytosis. Internalized material (e.g. viruses) is broken down within phagolysosomes (cytoplasmic vesicles), and converted into peptides, which can be recycled to the surface to be presented to T cells by MHC molecules. Macrophages are relatively long lived. Some return from the periphery to secondary lymphoid tissues, thereby transport-

Table 5.2. Characteristics of antigen-presenting cells.

Cell type	Location	MHC Class II	Antigen presentation
Langerhans cell	Skin	+	Weak
Veiled cell	Afferent lymph	+	
Interdigitating dendritic cell	Lymph node, T-cell areas	+	Strong immunostimulation of resting T cells
Non-lymphoid dendritic cell	Connective tissues of most organs	+	? T cells
Follicular dendritic cell	Lymph node follicles	−	B cells
Mononuclear phagocytes and macrophages	Many tissues	$0 \to ++$	B cells and primed T cells
Marginal zone macrophages	Marginal zone of spleen and lymph nodes	−/+	T-independent antigens to B cells
B cells	Lymphoid tissue	$+ \to ++$	To primed T cells

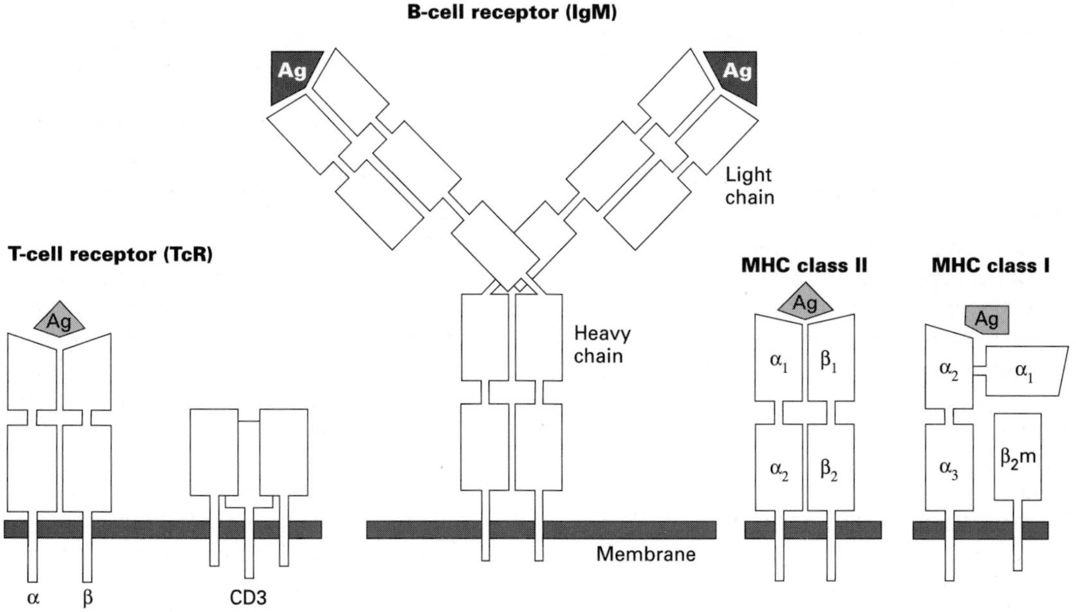

Fig. 5.1. Molecules that bind antigens. Note the domain structure and the similarities among the molecules belonging to the immunoglobulin supergene family.

ing antigen from the periphery into the spleen and lymph nodes. An essential function of these cells is the internal destruction of pathogens and antigens.

Molecules involved in immune reactions

Three groups of molecules are intimately involved in antigen-binding, namely antibodies, TcRs and MHC molecules (Fig. 5.1). Antibodies recognize antigen alone, while TcRs recognize antigen plus MHC, and both are highly specific in their binding. MHC molecules bind peptides which they present to T cells. Other molecules involved in immune responses include complement and cytokines.

132

Antibodies

Antibodies (or immunoglobulins) have a basic structure consisting of four polypeptide chains (Fig. 5.2). There are two identical heavy chains and two identical light chains that are linked by disulphide bonds and non-covalent interactions. Each of these chains is formed of a number of globular domains connected by less tightly folded regions of polypeptide chains. Light chains have two domains and heavy chains four or five, depending on the class of antibody. Each four polypeptide unit has two antigen combining sites, formed by the N-terminal domains of a light chain and heavy chain. Analysis of the amino acid sequences of these N-terminal domains shows them to be very variable between antibodies, the greatest variability being clustered at the extreme ends of the domains where antigen binds. These domains are thus called variable or V domains, while the segments of polypeptide that show the greatest variability (three per V domain) are called hypervariable regions. These hypervariable regions are not contiguous in the polypeptide chain, but are brought into proximity at the antigen-binding site by the overall folding of the polypeptide chain within the domain. The antigen-binding site is sometimes called the antibody paratope, in accordance with the naming of an antigenic determinant as an epitope. With six different hypervariable regions

of different amino acid sequence at the paratope (three from the heavy chain, three from the light), the molecular surfaces of different antibodies are highly variable in shape, charge and amino acid residues: this gives them their antigen specificity.

The remaining domains are less variable between antibodies and are called constant or C domains, but even here there is some variability. Light chains may be one of two different types, namely kappa (κ) or lambda (λ), that are generated from two different gene loci. The heavy chain gene locus of man can generate nine different types of heavy chains that vary in their three domains (in addition to the huge amounts of variation seen in the V domains) and there is a gene for each of these chains. This allows for the formation of antibody isotypes, termed μ, δ, $\gamma 1$, $\gamma 2$, $\gamma 3$, $\gamma 4$, $\alpha 1$, $\alpha 2$, and ϵ. The heavy chain isotype present in an antibody determines the class and subclass of that antibody. Any one of these isotypes can be produced in a membrane bound form to act as a B-cell antigen receptor, or in a secreted form to become part of the effector arm of the immune response. Antibodies can be divided into five classes, or nine subclasses, corresponding to the nine isotypes (Table 5.3). The immunoglobulin G (IgG) class has four isotypes (IgG1, IgG2, IgG3 and IgG4), and IgA class has two subclasses (IgA1 and IgA2), and IgD, IgM and IgE classes are not usually subdivided. While all antibodies can bind antigen, each anti-

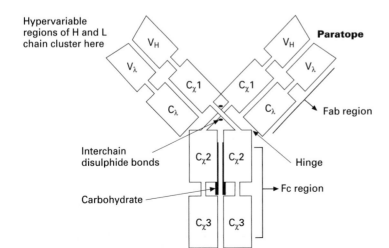

Hypervariable regions of H and L chain cluster here

V_H

V_λ

Paratope

$C_\chi 1$

C_λ

Fab region

Interchain disulphide bonds

$C_\chi 2$

Hinge

Fc region

Carbohydrate

$C_\chi 3$

Fig. 5.2. Structure of immunoglobulin. The structural details of an IgG molecule are illustrated with the names of the domains and different areas of the molecule noted. Interchain disulphide bonds are marked. In this example the light chains are λ.

Table 5.3. Antibody characteristics and functions.

Class	H_2L_2 subunits	H-chain domains	Isotypes	C1q binding	Placental transfer	Cellular binding	Serum concentration in adult (mg/ml)
IgG	1	4	IgG1	++	+	Neutrophils, MOs	9
			IgG2	+	(+)	Neutrophils, MOs weak	3
			IgG3	+++	+	Neutrophils, MOs	1
			IgG4	–	+	Neutrophils, MOs weak	0.5
IgA	1 or 2	4	IgA1	–	–	Neutrophils	3
						Neutrophils	0.5
IgM	5	5	IgM	+++	–		1.5
IgD	1	4	IgD	–	–		0.03
IgE	1	5	IgE	–	–	Mast cells, basophils, MOs weak	0.00005

MOs: mononuclear cells; H_2L_2 = heavy and light chains.

body class, and indeed subclass, has a different set of functions. These functions relate to the capacity of the constant regions of antibody to interact with different tissues expressing Fc receptors, or with C1q of the complement system. Antibodies are therefore bifunctional molecules in which the V domains are responsible for antigen binding, while the C domains allow interaction with various effector systems.

The T-cell receptor

The T-cell receptor (TcR) is an integral membrane protein consisting of a pair of polypeptide chains linked by a disulphide bond. Four genetic loci (α, β, γ, δ) encode for these polypeptide chains, and a T cell may have either an $\alpha\beta$ pair (TcR2) or a $\gamma\delta$ pair (TcR1). Most mature peripheral T cells have TcR2, while TcR1 receptors are seen on a population of thymic T cells and on some T cells located in the peripheral lymphoid tissues such as those in the gut. The functional significance of there being two different types of TcRs is not known. The polypeptide chains each have two extracellular domains, of which the N-terminal domains are variable (V) and form the MHC-antigen recognition site. Each TcR is associated with a number of other polypeptide chains in the cell membrane, and these associated polypeptides (denoted γ, δ, ϵ) appear to be involved in transducing the activation signal to the cell via calcium, and are referred to as the CD3 complex. The CD3 chains are monomorphic and distinct from the chains that form the TcR.

The major histocompatibility complex

The MHC is the human leucocyte antigen (HLA) locus on chromosome 6, and its products are termed MHC antigens or molecules (synonymous with HLA). The MHC can be divided into three distinct regions encoding three classes of molecules (Fig. 5.3). The A, B and C loci (class I genes) encode class I molecules; the DP, DQ and DR loci (class II genes) encode class II molecules; and the class III genes encode a variety of other molecules with diverse functions. The class I loci each encode the α-chain of a single class I molecule. Class II molecules have two polypeptide chains, and there are one or more genes for each pair of chains in each class II locus.

The MHC class I and II molecules share a common molecular ancestry with the domains of immunoglobulin and TcR, and are thus members of the immunoglobulin supergene family of molecules. They are cell surface glycoproteins, each of which has four external domains (Fig. 5.4). Class I molecules have one polypeptide chain (a) encoded within the MHC. Each chain folds into three extracellular domains which are linked non-covalently to the molecule β_2-microglobulin, the latter making the fourth domain of the class I molecule. MHC

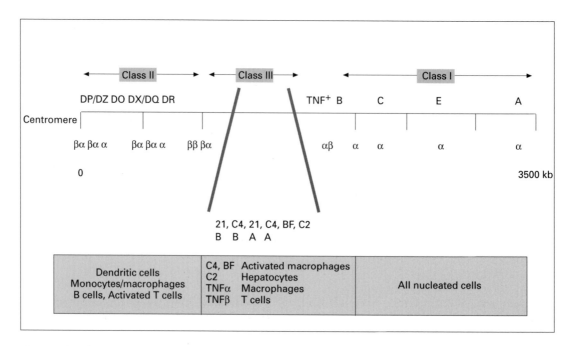

Fig. 5.3. Major histocompatibility complex. Class I genes encode the α/β heterodimer. The β-chain (β₂-microglobulin) is on a different chromosome. The α- and β-chain genes for class II occur in pairs. Class III genes encode four components of the complement system but genes encoding 21-hydroxylase A and B are located in the same region. Tumour necrosis factor (TNF+): α- and β-genes. BF: factor B.

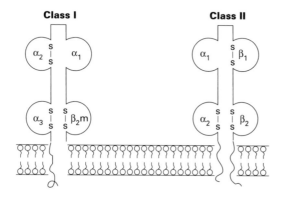

Fig. 5.4. Schematic representation of class I and class II molecules of the MHC. Note the globular domain structure.

class II molecules each consist of two polypeptides (α and β), both encoded in the MHC. They are non-covalently associated and both traverse the membrane. MHC molecules are highly polymorphic (i.e. there is a great deal of genetic varia-

tion between individuals). For example, there are at least 50 structural variants of the HLA B molecule, and at least 25 HLA DR variants. Each of these variants may occur with any combination of the others, thus allowing for a vast number of potential different MHC haplotypes.

MHC molecules are involved in presenting antigen to T cells. Different MHC molecules present different antigens more effectively than others. Consequently, it is advantageous to carry a wide range of MHC molecules that can present the numerous antigens that may be encountered. Analysis of the polypeptide structure of MHC molecules shows that the variability is concentrated in regions in the two domains that are furthest from the membrane; that is the α1 and α2 domains of class I molecules and the N-terminal domains of the α and β chains of the class II molecules.

Following crystallographic analysis of class I molecules, the structure of MHC molecules has recently begun to be elucidated. HLA-A2 molecules have the two domains nearest the membranes folded in a broadly similar way to the immunoglobulin domains, but the more variable distal domains form a peptide binding site, consisting of a base of β-pleated sheet surrounded and enclosed by two loops of an α-helix, one on each side of the binding sites. These loops contain the regions of greatest sequence variability between different class I variants. It is thought that the residues facing into the binding site will determine how the molecule binds to peptides, while residues pointing outwards will control interactions of the MHC antigen complex with the TcR. There is a considerable amount of structural similarity between the class I and II molecules, particularly with respect to the regions surrounding the binding site, and there is increasing evidence to suggest functional similarity between the two classes of molecule.

Complement

Complement is a system of more than 30 interacting proteins and their receptors. There are two pathways by which complement can be activated: the classical pathway involves antibody–antigen complexes, and the alternative

pathway involves the presence of activator surfaces. Activators in the alternative pathway include certain microbial cell walls, carbohydrates and viruses. Complement activation is a complex process, but can be conveniently summarized as depicted in Fig. 5.5. Activation can lead to the covalent attachment of a fragment of the third component of the system (i.e. C3b) to the initiating agent. Mononuclear phagocytes and neutrophils express receptors (mainly CR1 and CR3) for this fragment; thus, complement deposition on particles or antigen–antibody complexes opsonizes them for phagocytosis. The binding of C3b to receptors on phagocytes increases their level of activation, thereby priming them to eliminate the material they have phagocytosed.

The deposition of C3b on membranes can lead to the activation of the complement lytic pathway. This involves the assembly of a membrane attack complex (MAC) that contains components which range from C5 through to C9 and traverse the membranes of the target cell. If MACs become assembled on eukaryotic cells (e.g. on an erythrocyte), they cause osmotic damage to the cells and can lead to their lysis. Other complement components are involved in the development of the inflammatory reaction,

Fig. 5.5. Complement pathways. Complement pathways may be activated by antigen–antibody complexes via the classic pathway or via the alternative pathway. Both routes generate a C3 convertase, which splits C3 into C3a and C3b. C3b deposited on an activator surface in association with a C3 convertase can initiate the lytic pathway to deposit membrane attack complexes (MAC) onto the target membrane.

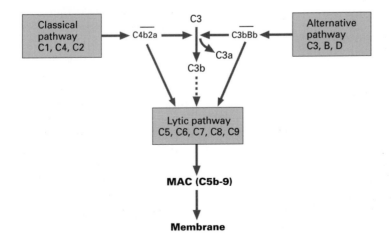

when they act as anaphylatoxins, inducing smooth muscle contraction and mast cell degranulation, and being chemotactic for neutrophils and macrophages. This is thought to be important in the control of the initial influx of phagocytes into sites of acute inflammation.

Cytokines

Cytokines are soluble proteins released by one cell that act on receptors on other cells to affect their functions. Thus, many of the interactions between cells cooperating or participating in an immune response are controlled by cytokines. Cytokine activity is not confined to classical immune responses, and as more and more cytokines are discovered, it becomes increasingly apparent that their actions are wide, complex and intertwined with a wide range of other biological interactions within an organ-

ism. Several cytokines may have the same effect, or they may act synergistically, the action of one potentiating the actions of another, e.g. interferon-γ (IFN-γ) induces MHC class II on many cells and this effect is enhanced by tumour necrosis factor-α (TNFα), while TNFα itself has no class II-inducing ability; interleukin-1 (IL-1), released by macrophages and a number of other cells, enhances the level of IL-2 receptors on the T cell, while IL-2 maintains the T cells in cell cycle. Table 5.4 lists the known functions of the more important cytokines.

Effector functions in the immune response

The theory of clonal selection

The fundamental challenge for the immune system is to be able to protect the body against an almost infinite range of pathogens, some of

Table 5.4. Major cytokines and their functions.

Cytokine	Sources	Targets	Principal effects
IL-1	Macrophages, LGLs, B cells	Lymphocytes	Activation and IL-2 receptor induction
		Macrophages	Activation
		Endothelium	Increased leucocyte adhesion
		Tissue cells	Numerous effects in inflammatory reactions
IL-2	T cells	T cells	T-cell division and differentiation; absolute requirement
		Active B cells	Promotes B-cell division
IL-4 and IL-5	T cells	B cells	Required for B-cell division and differentiation
IL-6	Lymphocytes	B cells	B-cell differentiation
	Macrophages	Hepatocytes	Acute phase protein synthesis
	Fibroblasts		
IFN-γ	T cells	Leucocytes	Macrophage activation
		Endothelium	Increased leucocyte adhesion
		Tissue cells	MHC induction
TNFα	Macrophages	Phagocytes	Activation
TNFβ	T cells	K and NK cells	Activation
		Endothelium	Promotes leucocyte adhesion
		Target cells	Increased susceptibility to cytotoxic cells
IL-3	T cells	Stem cells	Control stem cells division and differentiation pathways
M-CSF	Mononuclear cells	Stem cells	Control stem cells division and differentiation pathways
G-CSF	Endothelium		
GM-CSF	T cells	Stem cells	Control stem cells division and differentiation pathways
	Mononuclear cells		
	Endothelium		
	Fibroblasts		

IL: interleukin; LGLs: large granular lymphocytes; IFN: interferon; TNF: tumour necrosis factor; CSF: colony-stimulating factor; M: macrophage; G: granulocyte; GM: granulocyte-macrophage.

which have the capacity to mutate to evade immune recognition and therefore immune responses. It is now generally accepted that this capacity is based on clonal activation. The basis of an immune response is the stimulation and activation of clones of lymphocytes capable of recognizing the initiating antigen. Although there is only a modest number of genes for immunoglobulin and TcRs, a complex process of genetic recombination generates an enormous diversity of receptors (see suggested further reading). Since this occurs during lymphocyte ontogeny, antigen is not required to generate the repertoire of receptors. Each lymphocyte expresses a receptor of only one specificity, and the entire repertoire is only present when one considers the total population of lymphocytes within the body. It is therefore evident that the

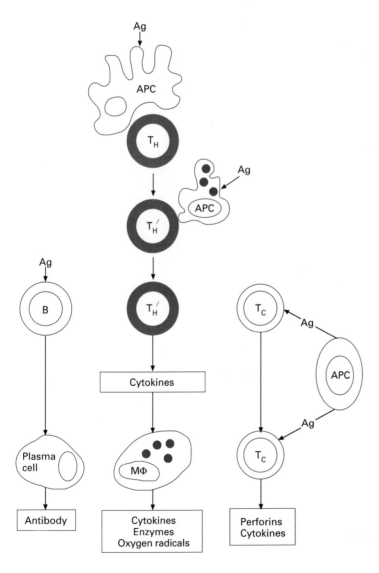

Fig. 5.6. Overview of the immune response. Antigen (Ag) taken up by antigen-presenting cells (APC) stimulates helper T cells (T_H) so that when they encounter the antigen again, they proliferate and release cytokines. These are involved in the differentiation of B cells (B) into antibody-producing plasma cells, the activation of macrophages (MΦ), and the proliferation and activation of cytotoxic T cells (T_C), which recognize antigen on antigen-presenting target cells and can kill them by the action of perforins and cytokines.

system generates receptors for a vast number of antigens, of which the great majority may never be encountered in a lifetime. One consequence of this diversity is that the proportion of lymphocytes expressing receptors for a particular antigen is relatively small. Thus, to mount an effective immune response, one of the first steps is the expansion of clones of antigen reactive cells. In effect, antigen selects and activates those lymphocytes that recognize it. This is called the theory of clonal selection.

Cellular interactions in immune reactions

Figure 5.6 depicts an overview of events occurring during an immune response. The interactions of B cells and macrophages with T cells are particularly important in the development of the immune response. The critical events include: antigen uptake and processing by antigen-presenting cells; antigen presentation to and recognition by antigen-specific B and/or T cells; cooperation between T and B cells (Fig. 5.7), with release of cytokines that subserve a variety of functions including induction of B-

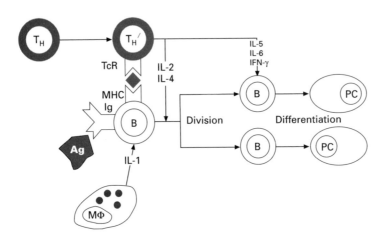

Fig. 5.7. T cell–B cell cooperation. Activated T cells (T_H') can recognize processed antigen (Ag) on B cells (B) associated with MHC class II molecules. IL-2 released by macrophages (MΦ), in association with IL-4 and IL-2 from the T cells, promotes B-cell division and additional cytokines then promote differentiation into plasma cells (PC).

Fig. 5.8. Actions of cytotoxic T cells (T_C). T_C cytotoxic T cells recognize targets primarily by MHC class I-mediated interactions. They can then damage the target cell by the release of perforins, which polymerize to form polyperforin channels, or via other molecules released by the cytotoxic cell, including some cytokines. TcR: T-cell receptor.

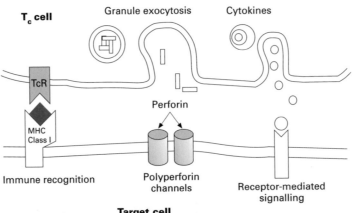

cell differentiation and macrophage activation; and the development of cytotoxic activity (Fig. 5.8). Antibodies produced by plasma cells may neutralize pathogens by direct binding (e.g. blocking viral receptors), but more often they link antigen to cells of the immune system, or activate the complement system. Many of the effects of antibody occur via binding to Fc receptors, which bind to sites in the constant domains of the antibody.

The immunology of pregnancy

From the preceding section it is clear that a fundamental requirement of the immune system is that it can distinguish normal healthy cells ('*self*') from '*non-self*' (infected, malignant or allogeneic cells, and toxins). Nearly 50 years ago, working on the biology of transplantation, Medawar and his colleagues discovered the laws of transplantation immunology. Put simply, these laws state that it is impossible to transplant grafts between genetically dissimilar individuals, and that graft rejection is an immunological phenomenon. It was found that MHC antigens elicited the strongest rejection responses (hence HLA antigens were initially termed '*transplantation antigens*'). It was apparent to Medawar that viviparous pregnancy challenged the laws of transplantation immunology. Medawar [1] paraphrased the paradox thus:

> The immunological problem of
> pregnancy may be formulated thus: how
> does the pregnant mother contrive to
> nourish within itself, for many weeks or
> months, the foetus that is an
> antigenically foreign body? Is pregnancy
> accompanied by any physiological
> changes which may in some degree
> prevent the foetus, qua tissue
> homograph, from immunising the
> mother against itself?

This intriguing situation gave rise to concepts such as the immunological paradox of pregnancy, the fetus being regarded as Nature's perfect allograft. Many scientists thought that the unravelling of Nature's secrets would result in great strides being made in various fields, including transplantation and tumour immunology, not to mention human reproduc-

tion and advances in basic science. Medawar himself, always the philosopher scientist, offered three possible hypotheses: namely, that there may be an anatomical separation of fetus from mother, or that the fetus may be antigenically immature, or that the mother may be immunologically indolent.

That certain parts of the body are not accessed by or lack elements of the immune response, and are therefore immunologically privileged is now well established [2,3]. Thus Billingham [4] suggested that, like the anterior chamber of the eye and certain parts of the brain, the uterus too might be immunologically privileged. Over the past two decades the concept of blocking antibodies captured the imagination of many and resulted in a series of therapeutic measures for women with recurrent abortion.

It is as well to discard those hypotheses that have been categorically shown to be unsustainable. It is now clear that the fetus is antigenically mature from an early stage, and that immunocompetence begins to develop in the first trimester of pregnancy [5]. The uterus is not immunologically privileged: it has an extensive lymphatic and vascular network, especially prominent during pregnancy. Furthermore, elegant experiments using mammalian systems have shown that allografts placed in the uterus are rejected in much the same way as when placed in other sites [6] and that pre-existing systemic allograft immunity can be expressed within the decidua [7]. As regards the remaining hypotheses, a great deal of conflicting data and controversy prevails.

Important issues that must be addressed in trying to understand the apparent immunological paradox of pregnancy include:

1   immunity to sperm and seminal fluid;
2   how the pre-implantation embryo evades the maternal immune system;
3   implantation and placentation: the nature of the maternofetal immunological interface;
4   maternal immunocompetence during pregnancy;
5   maternal immune responses to fetal antigens;
6   whether recurrent miscarriage represents failure of ill-defined immunoregulatory mecha-

140 nisms that normally sustain successful pregnancy. Current ideas on these and other issues are reviewed below.

Sperm and seminal plasma

Antigenicity of spermatozoa

A multiplicity of antigens can be demonstrated on sperm by fluorescent labelling using antibody produced in mice or rabbits. They tend to localize to and be specific for particular areas of the spermatozoon, as shown in Fig. 5.9. Some antigens may only be revealed after capacitation. Whether MHC antigens are or are not expressed on sperm is still not definitively determined [8].

The significance in human reproduction of sperm antigens is not entirely clear. Although some infertile men and women can be shown to possess antibodies against all of these regions, antibodies against surface antigens of the acrosome and main tail piece seem to be of the greatest pathological relevance because they cause immobilization and/or agglutination of sperm [9].

Tolerance to self sperm antigens

Tolerance to self antigens occurs as a result of suppression and/or elimination of potentially self-reactive T cells in the thymus during fetal life. Since spermatogenesis does not commence until long after this self-recognition process is over, spermatozoa should be particularly susceptible to the development of autoimmunity. This can arise and be a cause of male infertility, but among the mechanisms which prevent it from occurring more often are:

1 Physical contact between immunocompetent cells and developing spermatozoa is prevented by the tight junctions between Sertoli cells lining the seminiferous tubules.
2 These same tight junctions prevent the passage of circulating antibody into the tubules.
3 Autoreactivity against the highly immunogenic epididymal sperm may be prevented by suppressor T cells in the epididymal epithelium [10].
4 Once sperm leave the epididymus, they

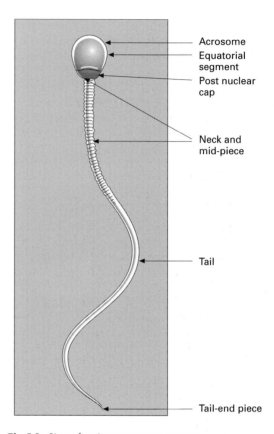

Fig. 5.9. Sites of antigens on spermatozoon.

become coated with seminal plasma components including lactoferrin [9]. This coating reduces their immunogenicity [10], and this is probably relevant both while the sperm are in the seminal vesicles and also once they are deposited in the female vagina.

Tolerance to sperm antigens in the female genital tract

Repeated coitus throughout reproductive life results in the female genital tract being repeatedly exposed to spermatozoa. The former can mount immune responses, while spermatozoa are immunogenic. Clearly the prevention of an antisperm immune response is important for successful reproduction. There is now some evidence to suggest that seminal plasma has a powerful effect on most cells of the immune system and tends to impair the activity of both antibody and complement [10]. Even low concentrations of seminal plasma *in vitro* can inhibit the generation of cytotoxic T cells, the cytotoxic effect of natural killer (NK) cells [11], the phagocytic activity of macrophages and neutrophils, and the generation and activity of antibodies. These studies all have the disadvantage of being *in vitro* and a biological significance for such effects cannot be assumed. Several of the immunosuppressive components of seminal plasma have been characterized. Among these are zinc-containing compounds, the polyamines spermine and spermidine, prostaglandins, transglutaminases and a protein closely related to pregnancy associated protein-A.

The pre-implantation embryo

As the zygote traverses the fallopian tubes and enters the uterus, its protection depends primarily on:

1 Paternal antigens are not expressed at the two-cell stage, but become apparent on the surface from the six- to eight-cell stage.

2 Although the expression of these antigens increases with cellular division, major histocompatability antigens are thought not to be present at this stage in human pregnancy [8].

3 Hormone-dependent non-specific suppressor cells can be found in secretory-phase human endometrium [12]. Supernatants from cultured explants of endometrium, which include these cells, have immunosuppressive effects [13]. Significant immunological problems are, therefore, not posed by the conceptus before implantation.

Immunology of implantation and placentation

The immunological enigma at the heart of viviparity becomes acute during and after implantation. The immunological relationship of mother and fetus is illustrated in Fig. 5.10. In essence, the immunological problem exists because of the intimate juxtaposition of maternal and fetally derived tissue, which is at least partially foreign (semi-allogeneic) to the mother. The following issues must now be considered to try to understand the nature of the mater-nofetal immunological relationship: (i) the anatomy of the maternofetal interface; (ii) control of trophoblast growth; (iii) antigen expression by trophoblast; (iv) the endometrium and decidua.

Anatomy of the maternofetal interface

A detailed description of the embryological development and the anatomical relationships of the interface is beyond the scope of this chapter; here are described those aspects that are relevant to immunological interactions. There is no vascular continuity between the fetal and maternal compartments. The fetus does not come into direct contact with maternal blood, but interacts via the placenta. The process of implantation and subsequent trophoblastic invasion culminates in an intimate interaction between trophoblast and decidua. Figure 5.11 depicts the possible inter-relations between the various trophoblastic subpopulations. The syncytiotrophoblast, the non-mitotic outer layer of the chorionic villi, is bathed in maternal blood, as it also lines the intervillous spaces. Beneath the syncytiotrophoblast is the cytotrophoblast, whose cells are metabolically more active. Some cytotrophoblast cells push through the syncytiotrophoblast to make the cytotrophoblast columns which help anchor the villi to the maternal tissue, while other cytotrophoblast cells break away to form the cytotrophoblast shell, some of these cells subsequently migrating into the myometrium where they are called the interstitial cytotrophoblast cells. Other cytotrophoblast cells invade the spiral arterioles of the uterus and line the vessels as endovascular trophoblast. The cytotrophoblast and syncytiotrophoblast comprise the villous trophoblast. The non-villous trophoblast comprises the rest of the trophoblast tissue, from which the chorion laeve and chorionic plate, the marginal zone and the basal plate of the placenta form. The trophoblast thus represents a continuous frontier over a considerable surface area, up to $15\,m^2$ at 20 weeks' gestation in human pregnancy. It has therefore long been the prime candidate for the role of an immunologically protective or insulating barrier [14].

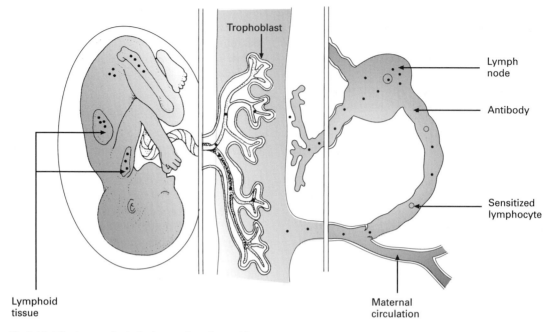

Fig. 5.10. The immunological relation of mother and fetus.

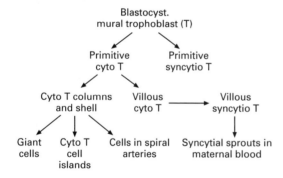

Fig. 5.11. Possible interrelations between the various trophoblastic subpopulations. T: trophoblast.

Control of trophoblast growth

Very little is known currently about the mechanisms which control trophoblast growth and the development of its multiple functions. Ilgren [15] has reviewed cellular and genetic aspects of proliferation and differentiation of trophoblast growth, mostly in the mouse. The next decade will undoubtedly see significant advances in the understanding of the fundamental processess

involved in growth and differentiation in general. Knowledge of trophoblast growth and its control will also increase, not least because the human placenta is so readily available for study.

There is experimental evidence to suggest that, in the mouse, decidual cells secrete substances which promote growth and development of trophoblast and other placental cells [16,17]. Recent reports have provided at least a first glimpse at some very promising areas for future research. The first of these is in relation to proto-oncogenes, which are normal genes involved in cellular growth, proliferation and differentiation. Much of what is currently known about proto-oncogenes has been learnt from studying the rapidly transforming retroviruses. They carry specific genes (oncogenes) which are responsible for the viruses' oncogenic potential and have been designated as, for example, *ras*, *myc*, *erb*, *fis* and *sis*. The puzzle came when specific viral oncogenes (*v-onc*) were used as probes in normal tissues, including that of man, because the oncogenes were found to share some DNA amino acid sequences with those in normal cells. Why should this be so, since such a high degree of conservation of genetic material capable of inducing cancer would be such a disadvantage to the organism? Surely there must be some more fundamental and advantageous reason for the presence of these cellular oncogenes (*c-onc*). This has led to the current thinking that, before viral conversion, the original genes (or proto-oncogenes) function in normal cellular proliferation or differentiation. Circumstantial evidence for this comes from the observation that, of the 20 known proto-oncogenes, at least three have been shown to be related to known growth factors or growth factor receptors [18]. For example, the *c-sis* gene is associated with platelet derived growth factor, and the *c-erb* gene with epidermal growth factor receptor. The *myc* gene is also closely involved in cell proliferation. It is now thought that rapidly transforming retroviruses convert a normal growth gene into one which may be pathogenic, either by altering the gene structure to produce an abnormal gene product, or by amplification, thus increasing to abnormal levels the production of normal products.

The second exciting area is our burgeoning knowledge of the biological importance of growth factors (to which lymphokines and other cytokines belong) and their specific receptors on cells. Proto-oncogenes and growth factors seem to be functionally associated. Questions about their expression on trophoblast are obviously of great interest and some answers are beginning to be produced. The proto-oncogenes *c-myc* and *c-sis* have been found to be co-expressed on extravillous cytotrophoblast [19]. There is evidence that *myc* protein expression and epidermal growth factor (EGF) receptors are associated with trophoblast proliferation and differentiation [20]. EGF receptors are known to be present in large numbers in the human placenta [21] and more detailed studies [22] have localized their expression to the microvillous membrane of syncytiotrophoblast throughout human pregnancy, its basolateral membrane (but only at term) and villous cytotrophoblast cells in the first trimester. As these cells proliferate and migrate towards the maternal tissues, there is a dramatic increase in EGF receptor expression. This is in contradistinction to insulin

receptor expression, which is only to be found on syncytiotrophoblast.

There may be links between tissue differentiation, EGF receptor expression and function on the following basis: syncytiotrophoblast is a non-proliferative and terminally differentiated tissue which expresses EGF receptor; it arises from villous cytotrophoblast which also expresses EGF receptor; as villous cytotrophoblast differentiation alters within the proliferating cell columns, so the expression of EGF receptor decreases; EGF can stimulate the release of human chorionic gonadotrophin and human placental lactogen from syncytiotrophoblast in culture [23]; and villous trophoblast produces most, if not all, of the placental proteins and hormones [24]. Extravillous trophoblast is, in that sense, functionally inert. In the light of the association between proto-oncogenes and growth factors on the one hand, and with retroviruses on the other, it is relevant to note that normal human placentae (like those of other primates) contain retroviral particles [25]. In addition, antisera to human syncytiotrophoblast membranes can cross-react with simian retrovirus-producing cell lines [26]. The significance of these observations remains unclear, but they clearly warrant further exploration.

Another observation which may well be of fundamental importance to the development of the fetus as well as the trophoblast is that development of the mouse embryo depends on distinctive contributions from both parental genomes [27]. Specifically, embryonic development is controlled by the preferential expression of maternal or paternal genes in the embryo, whereas trophoblast development depends on the preferential expression of paternal rather than maternal genes. The mechanism for this is probably differential methylation of genes between embryo and trophoblast. The insertion of a methyl group into the amino acid sequence of a gene causes translation to stop at that point. This is consistent with the clinical observation in human trophoblastic tumours that complete hydatidiform moles are usually genetically androgenetic [28]. The next few years are likely to afford further and clearer insights into the molecular and genetic basis of growth, differentiation and development.

Antigen expression by trophoblast

MHC antigen expression by trophoblast

The biology and role of MHC antigens has already been discussed in the basic immunology section. Since in the human haemochorial placenta trophoblast comes into direct contact with the maternal immune system, MHC antigen expression by trophoblast has been a central focus of investigation. Perhaps the earliest studies were those of Simmons and Russell, who studied murine systems, and transplanted trophoblast tissue alone or embryos without trophoblast into allogeneic hosts and found that trophoblast survived while embryos did not [29]. Trophoblasts survived even in presensitized hosts, and Simmons and Russell concluded that trophoblast did not express histocompatibility antigens. More than a decade later, when reagents that allowed identification of human MHC antigens became available, Faulk and Temple published the first report showing that components of the MHC were selectively absent from villous trophoblast. Antibodies to β_2-microglobulin and to HLA-A2 stained the cells within the chorionic villi but did not stain the surface layers of the trophoblast [30]. These findings were corroborated by Goodfellow et al. [31], and later by Galbraith et al. [32], while other workers demonstrated that there were no class II antigens on trophoblast, although they were present on stromal cells [33].

Thus the concept of an MHC antigen-free trophoblast, able to evade allorecognition, was beginning to emerge, supported by data from functional studies which showed that human syncytiotrophoblast did not stimulate DNA synthesis by allogeneic lymphocytes [34]. However, this view suffered a setback when it was reported that extravillous trophoblast stained strongly with anti-HLA class I antibodies such as W6/32, yet surprisingly failed to stain with antibodies with specificities for paternal antigens [35–37]. It was then realized that W6/32 and similar antibodies had specificities for the non-polymorphic parts of the HLA molecule, while those antibodies that failed to stain were directed at the polymorphic parts of the molecule. There was therefore a possibility that the

HLA molecules expressed on trophoblast were in some way unique. Ellis et al. [38] carried out detailed biochemical studies of this molecule on choriocarcinoma cells and identified a non-polymorphic HLA-like glycoprotein, designated HLA-G, with a heavy chain of 40 kD associated with β_2-microglobulin. They confirmed by gene sequencing and mapping that the same molecular structure was present on placental cytotrophoblast cells [39]. While HLA-G has close homologies with classical HLA class I genes, and the gene products associate with β_2-microglobulin, they are truncated, and show very little, if any, polymorphisms [39]. Thus the current view is that most, if not all, of the HLA molecules expressed on trophoblast are HLA-G.

The regulation of HLA-G expression appears to occur at various levels. The HLA-G gene is transcribed in normal villous and extravillous trophoblast, but not in syncytiotrophoblast [40]. Villous trophoblast can translate the transcribed message into expressed protein [41]. HLA-G mRNA is expressed in first trimester cytotrophoblast and in term chorionic membrane cytotrophoblast, but is seen in low amounts, if at all, in syncytiotrophoblast from both first and third trimester placenta. Unlike most other cell types, cytotrophoblast cannot be induced to up-regulate expression of HLA by cytokines such as IFN-γ or virus infection [40,42,43].

HLA-G: evolutionary vestige, or shield against natural killer cells?

What is the function of this molecule? It would be all too easy to regard it as an evolutionary vestige, a useless molecule which was not subjected to the forces of evolutionary selection because it posed no threat to the continuity of the species. Yet it is odd that regulatory mechanisms seem to have evolved for its expression. Why, for instance, does it only occur predominantly on trophoblast, and why only in certain subsets of trophoblast? If it were simply redundant, it might be expressed on a wider range of tissues along with classical MHC antigens. It has been proposed that HLA-G may play a role in the resistance to lysis by natural killer (NK) cells. The hypothesis is that while lack of classical MHC antigens confers resistance to lysis by allospecific T cells, total lack of MHC antigens would render trophoblast susceptible to lysis by NK cells, which are thought to lyse cells on the basis of recognition of altered self antigens or absence of self. A monomorphic antigen, such as HLA-G, would be recognized as self. This hypothesis will best be explored with transgenic mice expressing predetermined levels of HLA-G. However, there are immediate problems with this hypothesis: how does syncytiotrophoblast, which is devoid of all MHC antigens, escape cytotoxic damage by NK cells? Moreover, not all extravillous trophoblast within decidua express HLA-G, and they should therefore be susceptible to lysis. Nevertheless, this is a potentially exciting area of enquiry, not least because many questions on the nature and role of HLA-G, including whether it can present antigen, may be answered. Already there is intensive research activity to try and answer these questions and more. HLA-transgenic mice, HLA-G transfected cells and the use of protein targeting techniques will now be the obvious tools in the unravelling of the role of HLA-G.

Non-MHC antigen expression by trophoblast

The trophoblast clearly expresses a wide range of antigens, but it is evident that only those antigenic systems that exhibit polymorphism would be of interest to the question of fetal survival, since they would allow the possibility of allogeneic differences between mother and fetus. Such systems include the erythrocyte antigenic systems (e.g. ABO, P, Rh, K) and placental alkaline phosphatase.

Erythrocyte antigenic systems

Human trophoblast does not express the A and B blood group antigens, but Rh (D) is expressed. The paradoxical observation is that this Rh antigen does not appear to sensitize Rh-negative women, any such sensitization occurring only when placental disruption occurs, such as at parturition. The function of Rh (D) on trophoblast is not known, nor the reason for its failure to sensitize. It has been surmised that lack of MHC class II at the maternofetal interface results in

failure to present antigen (Rh-D) to helper T cells, and thus failure of antibody production.

Perhaps the bottom line where erythrocyte antigens are concerned is that although immune responses can be mounted, only in extreme circumstances do they result in fetal compromise (e.g. haemolytic disease of the newborn), but they are not thought to be involved in the fundamental question of fetal survival.

Placental alkaline phosphatase

Although placental alkaline phosphatase has been well characterized, and its polymorphic nature documented, its function is not known. It is found on syncytiotrophoblast but not on other trophoblast cells, and is seen only after the first trimester, thus suggesting that it may not be important in immunoregulation at the maternofetal interface.

Antigens shared by tumours and trophoblast

Certain tumour cells express antigens on the cell surface that are found on trophoblast and embryonic cells [44–46]. From an oncology point of view, these antigens have been of particular importance as they have in some cases acted as tumour markers and allowed monitoring of disease progression and/or response to treatment. When expressed on trophoblast, the maternal immune system might be expected to respond to them in the same way as the immune system responds to tumour cells. However, therein lies the problem. The malignant tumours that produce oncofetal antigens generally escape surveillance by the immune system and it is possible that the mechanisms employed by the tumour are similar to those that allow the fetus to escape maternal immunosurveillance. Thus the mother does not mount a significant response to these antigens.

Complement regulatory proteins on trophoblast

Within such a complex system as the complement system, which acts in a cascade fashion, there is an inherent danger of damage to normal bystander cells, tissues or organs resulting from the fortuitous deposition of activated complement components. Therefore there is a requirement for stringent control mechanisms. The importance of such control systems is reflected in the fact that there are at least as many proteins involved in essential regulatory function as there are components of the pathways themselves. At the cell surface, at least three membrane-bound proteins — decay-accelerating factor (CD55), membrane co-factor protein (MCP, CD46) and CD59 — have been characterized, and their site of action defined.

Perhaps what is likely to turn out to be a very exciting discovery of recent years in reproductive biology is that trophoblast expresses all three proteins in large amounts [47–50]. Furthermore, they are all expressed where trophoblast surfaces are in contact with maternal blood and tissues, and this expression occurs as early as at 6 weeks' gestation. It seems wholly reasonable to assume that the role of these proteins is to protect trophoblast from maternal complement-mediated damage. In addition, it seems that at least part of what used to be regarded as the trophoblast–lymphocyte cross-reactivity (TLX) antigen system is in fact MCP, and this puts paid to the original hypotheses involving cognate recognition of TLX [51], since a maternal antifetal antibody response to trophoblast MCP could interfere with what is likely to be a most crucial function of this protein on trophoblast, namely protecting trophoblast against damage by maternal complement [52]. The potential involvement of these complement regulatory proteins in pregnancy disorders remains a matter for speculation, but research in this area is as yet in its infancy.

Lack of maternal responsiveness to polymorphic non-MHC antigens to trophoblast

By lacking classical MHC antigens, trophoblast cannot elicit allogeneic responses. In addition, assuming that the phenomenon of MHC restriction applies equally to trophoblast, the absence of classical MHC class I antigens would prevent the co-recognition of any other of the wide-ranging trophoblast cell surface antigens. Thus, none of the trophoblast surface antigens would pose a threat to the survival of trophoblast,

while being able to subserve whatever function they are supposed to. The fact that expression of HLA in villous trophoblast cannot be up-regulated by IFN-γ might be an additional fail-safe mechanism to prevent maternofetal allorecognition. Complement regulatory proteins protect trophoblast against fortuitous damage by complement.

The endometrium and decidua

Cell types in the decidua

Decidualization is the response of the uterine endometrium to the implanting embryo, but as yet the nature or precise source of the stimulus is unknown. The site of implantation where the placenta subsequently forms is called the decidua basalis, while the rest of the decidua is designated decidua parietalis. The decidua contains conventional immunological cell types (lymphocytes, macrophages) and non-conventional immunological cell types, most notably the uterine large granular lymphocytes (U-LGLs). Clearly, immunological responses within the decidua are likely to be crucial, as this is the definitive maternofetal interface.

MHC class II+ and CD14+ macrophages, capable of a range of immunological function including antigen presentation, phagocytic activity and secretion of prostaglandins, occur in abundance in the decidua. Conventional T cells are also found, although the proportions of CD4 to CD8 cells appear to be an inverse of the proportions in peripheral blood [53] in that there appear to be relatively more CD8 than CD4 cells. The significance of this is open to conjecture.

U-LGLs have attracted a great deal of interest in recent years. They are CD2+, but unlike conventional T cells, they are CD3−. This absence of CD3 implies the absence of the TcR, suggesting that these cells are not specifically antigen reactive or alloreactive, although they might be activated by another system. They resemble NK cells, but while staining for some NK markers (CD56+, CD57+, HNK-1+), they do not stain for others (CD16−). Functionally, the U-LGLs exhibit NK activity against conventional NK targets, such as the cell line K562 [53,54]. The role of U-LGLs in pregnancy is unknown. Mitotic activity in these cells increases from the proliferative phase through to the late secretory phase of the menstrual cycle [55], and their numbers increase if pregnancy occurs, but decrease if it does not, suggesting a hormonal involvement in the control of their numbers and activity [56].

Conventional NK cells are also found in decidua, but their activity is less than that in peripheral blood. It is known that in the peripheral blood they decrease in number and activity during pregnancy. Their function in the decidua is unknown, although it has been postulated that they may down-regulate maternal antifetal reactions. Of particular interest has been the report that expression of the HLA-G α-chain protein in HLA-A, -B, and -C null cells reduced their susceptibility to NK and Tγδ cell-mediated lysis [57]. There is an evolving idea that HLA-G may function on trophoblast as a recognition molecule to prevent lysis by NK cells.

Suppressor activity in the decidua

The concept of suppressor activity in immunological responses remains a controversial issue. This is largely because although the activity itself is demonstrable, the cells responsible for this effect have not been clearly identified. This suppressive effect can apparently be associated with small non-T non-B granulocytic lymphocytes, the appearance of which is mediated by a soluble factor which blocks lymphocyte responses [58]. Suppressor cells have been observed in two murine models of pregnancy where resorption of embryos occurs: these are when *Mus caroli* embryos transferred to *musculus* uteri and in CBA/J × DBA/2 embryos in a CBA/J uterus. In both cases there appears to be a deficiency of the small non-T non-B granulated suppressor cells [58]. It is claimed that the soluble factor, released by these cells in murine decidua, is related to transforming growth factor-β (TGF-β) [59]. A further factor proposed as a mediator of immunosuppressive activity in murine decidua during pregnancy is prostaglandin PGE$_2$. It has been proposed that NK cells present in decidua become progressively inactivated and by the 12th day of gesta-

tion they are devoid of any killer function against trophoblast cells [60]. These workers claimed that this inactivation comes from local PGE$_2$ production by decidual cells and decidual macrophages and is almost completely reversible when prostaglandin synthesis is inhibited in the presence of indomethacin [60].

Cytokine interactions in the maternofetal relationship

MRL-lpr/lpr homozgous mice have excessive T-cell proliferation along with large placentas that show abnormally high levels of phagocytosis, and the placental phenomena can be reduced to normal by treatment of the pregnant female with anti-T cell antibodies [61]. In normal mice, this treatment reduces placental size and, in some strain combinations, causes fetal resorption. T cells mediate many of their responses via the elaboration of cytokines. Thus, local cytokine production may influence survival and growth of the fetoplacental unit. There is now ample evidence that granolocyte-macrophage colony-stimulating factor (GM-CSF), interleukin-3 (IL-3) and colony-stimulating factor-1 (CSF-1) can promote the growth and/or differentiation of mouse and human trophoblast [62,63], and enhance fetal survival when injected into mice prone to fetal resorption. In contrast, other cytokines, such as IL-2, TNF and interferon-γ (IFN-γ), appear to have deleterious effects. In addition to cells of the immune system, non-immune components of the reproductive tract, including the uterine epithelium and trophoblast, can also elaborate cytokines [64–66]. Thus, the concept has emerged that there are beneficial cytokines which can enhance fetal growth and survival, and deleterious cytokines which can compromise pregnancy, and that such cytokines can be elaborated with or without the involvement of the immune system. Studies into the role of cytokines in pregnancy are in their infancy, but it is becoming increasing clear that many answers will be yielded by these studies.

Maternal immunocompetence during pregnancy

It has been supposed that a change in maternal

148 immunocompetence, presumably a decrease, may be a crucial factor in allowing survival of the fetal semiallograft. However, as outlined below, the extent of such immunomodulation is limited, and could not of its own account for survival of the fetus.

Effect of pregnancy on lymphoid organs

Experiments on laboratory animals have demonstrated clearly that pregnancy affects lymphoid organs. Physiological changes which have been observed in lymphoid organs during both allogeneic and syngeneic murine pregnancy include thymus involution, splenomegaly and changes in humoral and cellular immunity. The thymus is the site of maturation of T lymphocytes and recent intense research activity has given a great deal of insight into the way in which self-reactive T cells are eliminated during ontogeny. Involution of the thymus during pregnancy has been observed in several species, including man, mouse and rat. The mechanism or nature and indeed the significance of this involution remains somewhat unclear. The involution is thought to be due to an exodus of small lymphocytes from the thymic cortex in response to steroid hormones. This involution is a non-specific effect of pregnancy, occurring in both allogeneic and syngeneic pregnancy, and the cellularity of the thymus is thought to return to normal after the period of lactation. Enlargement of the spleen has been reported in human pregnancy. In murine studies, splenomegaly has been clearly documented: it reaches its maximal size at midgestation, returning to normal about 20 days postpartum. In this model, the rate of erythropoiesis in the spleen changes during pregnancy and it would seem that antigens, oestrogen and progesterone as well as erythropoietin affect this rate.

Oestrogen appears to stimulate the production of large and medium erythrocytes in the spleen. The enlargement of the spleen is accompanied by an increase in the numbers of immunoglobulin-producing cells. Teleologically, this increase makes sense, since the increase in circulating maternal immunoglobulin will make extra immunoglobulins available for passive transfer to the fetus. Lymph node changes have been studied in humans and there is histological evidence of a diminution in the germinal centres at term in the para-aortic lymph nodes which drain the uterus. Similar changes have been found in murine studies. The stimulus that produces the increase in the immunoglobulin secretion in para-aortic lymph nodes is not known, but may be of fetal origin, since removal of the fetus without removing the placenta abrogates the observed increase [67].

Maternal response to infection in pregnancy

Perhaps influenced by the general assumption that there must be some form of immunodepression in the mother to allow for the survival of the fetal semiallograft, it has long been assumed that pregnancy increases women's susceptibility to infections. Indeed, there are data suggesting an increase in the clinical severity of certain infections when they are newly acquired in pregnancy [68]. Other infections, such as leprosy, tend to be more severe in late pregnancy, and the incidence of listeriosis is generally increased [69]. Latent viral infections may be reactivated in pregnancy [70]. However, the vast majority of women experience healthy, infection-free pregnancies, and the consensus of opinion is therefore that the maternal immune responses to infection during pregnancy are adequate.

Humoral and cell-mediated responses to conventional antigens

Responses to both novel and recall conventional antigens have been studied in pregnant women. There is general acceptance that both humoral [71] and cellular [72] responses are not significantly different from those in non-pregnant women.

T- and B-cell subpopulations in pregnancy

Since the numbers and relative ratios of circulating immune cells are likely to reflect overall immunocompetence, the effects of pregnancy on these parameters have been widely studied. Some studies have found significant changes

[73–75] while others have not [76–79]. However, the general consensus of opinion is that if indeed there are changes in T- and B-cell numbers and ratios in pregnancy, these changes are not biologically relevant to any putative immunodeficiency of pregnancy [80].

Studies of lymphocyte function have also generated conflicting data, some groups reporting depression of responses to mitogens [81], while other groups failed to corroborate these findings [82]. More importantly, whether these in-vitro findings can be extrapolated to the situation *in vivo* is doubtful.

Natural killer cells in pregnancy

Natural killer cells are capable of killing some tumour cells spontaneously without prior sensitization. They do not seem to have immunological memory and can lyse cells that are syngeneic, allogeneic or xenogeneic to the NK cell donor [83]. During human pregnancy, NK activity decreases from 16 weeks until term [84], returning to control levels after delivery. Studies have shown that in addition to a decrease in NK cell numbers during pregnancy, the cells which remain have less lytic activity. However, as yet the role of this change in number and activity of peripheral NK cells in the success or otherwise of pregnancy is not known. In addition, the factors that directly cause this change have yet to be elucidated. It is thought that NK cells may be suppressed *in vivo* by prostaglandins released by macrophages, and this may be especially true for the U-LGL in the decidua. Of particular interest in this regard has been the observation that the administration of indomethacin *in vitro* blocks NK activity and *in vivo* produces abortion in more than 70% of susceptible mouse strains [85].

Candidate immunosuppressor factors in pregnancy

Pregnancy is accompanied by profound changes in the hormonal milieu including steroid hormones, trophonblast-derived molecules such as chorionic gonadotrophin, and α-fetoprotein (AFP). It is evident that some hormones, especially the steroids, modulate the immune response in pregnancy—the classic observations of Hench [86] on the amelioration of rheumatoid arthritis in pregnancy subsequently led to the use of steroids in the treatment of this condition and to Hench being awarded the Nobel Prize. The mechanism of action of cortisone remains an enigma, and although among animals rodents are particularly susceptible to the immunosuppressive effects of steroids, humans appear to be more resistant [87]. Despite their widespread use in the suppression of autoimmune disease, there is no evidence to suggest that the elevated levels of steroids seen in pregnancy significantly suppress the mother's overall immune response [88].

Of the sex steroids, progesterone has been shown to depress the mixed lymphocyte reaction (MLR) in humans [89], but only at high concentrations equivalent to those reached in the latter stages of pregnancy, so that it is difficult to extrapolate the in-vitro findings to the situation *in vivo*. αFP, a major pregnancy hormone, has been shown to inhibit both the MLR and mitogen responses in mice [90], and in man [91], but in both situations the degree of immunosuppression did not correlate with the concentration of αFP, and the influence of contaminants could not be excluded. While early work suggested that human chorionic gonadotrophin might be a powerful immunosuppressant, subsequent work suggested that the suppressive effects were again due to contaminants [92]. A whole range of other pregnancy-associated proteins have been studied, but the data have remained inconclusive and often contradictory between different centres [93]. Thus, many of the candidate immunosuppressor factors in pregnancy do indeed possess immunosuppressive properties *in vitro*, but whether these are relevant to the survival of the fetal semiallograft is doubtful.

Concluding remarks on maternal immunocompetence in pregnancy

There is ample evidence for some degree of diminution in the maternal immune response in pregnancy, and hormones, steroids and other factors produced in abundance in pregnancy may account for this observation. However, in general, women remain sufficiently immunocompetent during pregnancy to remain healthy, and the degree of immunodepression observed could not account for failure to eradicate as powerful a stimulus as an allograft. While fetal survival could largely be based on an effective physical barrier which, on the one hand, does not express classical HLA antigens while, on the other, expressing large amounts of complement regulatory proteins, yet it is clear that throughout evolution extensive 'fail-safe' mechanisms have evolved in parallel with the evolution of complex biological systems. Reproduction is central to the continuation of the species, and it is therefore not suprising that elaborate mechanisms have evolved to prevent deleterious maternal immunological responses against the fetus. Thus, all the other immune downregulatory phenomena observed within the mother, which by themselves could not explain the survival of the fetal semiallograft, could be viewed as acting synergistically with the central mechanism of an immunologically inert trophoblast, to ensure the continuation of the species. In this way, the immune system allows the propagation of the species without leaving the body open to attack by exogenous pathogens.

Maternal immune responses to fetal antigens

There is now ample evidence that the mother makes both humoral and cellular immune responses to fetal antigens. In this section the mechanisms for sensitizing the mother, the nature and the significance of the immune responses will be reviewed.

Maternal sensitization to fetal antigens

There is irrefutable evidence that at least some, if not all, pregnant women make demonstrable responses to fetal antigens, especially paternally derived MHC antigens. It is interesting to speculate how the mother comes into contact with these antigens. The molecular basis of allorecognition of foreign MHC antigens is thought to be cross-reactivity by antigen-specific, self-MHC-restricted, T cells [94,95]. Allorecognition is thus structurally heterogeneous and influenced by the disparity between the MHC antigens of the responder and stimulator. In disparate responder/stimulator combinations the allo-response may be directed against residues on the MHC molecule itself, while in closely related combinations alloreactive T cells might recognize epitopes of endogenous peptides that are displayed by stimulator but not be responder MHC molecules, seen in a self-restricted manner. This theory would explain both the vigour of alloresponses and the widely reported unusually high precursor frequency of alloreactive T cells [96,97].

It was stated earlier that there is no vascular continuity between the maternal and fetal compartments, and that fetally derived tissue (trophoblast) in direct contact with the maternal immune system is either devoid of MHC antigens, or expresses the monomorphic HLA-G. It has been argued that MHC-bearing fetal cells routinely enter the maternal circulation, and indeed a great deal of research effort has been expended on developing prenatal diagnostic techniques based on isolating these fetal cells from the peripheral blood of pregnant women. However, the passage of fetal cells into the maternal circulation is likely to be a sporadic event due to maternofetal haemorrhage, rather than a facilitated process. This would explain why only a proportion of women develop antibodies to paternal HLA, and why the incidence of these antibodies appears to increase with increasing gestation [98] and parity.

Alloantibody responses

The presence of alloantibodies in pregnancy sera was described independently by two groups [99,100]. The technique used by both groups demonstrated leuco-agglutinating antibodies, but subsequent use of complement-dependent techniques showed the presence of leucocytotoxic antibodies (LCAs). It is now well established that LCAs are directed to paternal, rather than third party, antigens [101], that the incidence of LCAs increases with increasing parity [102], that the frequency of LCA occurrence dips in the last trimester [103], that the LCAs may be IgG as well as IgM [104], and that the placenta acts as a sink for antiallotypic antibodies, and that these antibodies can be eluted from this placental sink [105]. Even among multiparas, some women never make these antibodies, and all studies to date show that no more than 50% of multiparas have these antibodies [98]. The reason for the lack of response is unknown, but it may be that techniques of detection are not sufficiently sensitive, or the LCAs may be made but may be blocked by anti-idiotypes (see below), or these women may be true non-responders, a phenomenon seen in some mice [106]. The role of anti-HLA antibodies in nature is not known. However, they do not seem to be essential for the success of pregnancy [107].

Mixed lymphocyte reaction-blocking antibodies

It has been suggested that mixed lymphocyte reaction (MLR) inhibition might be a more sensitive assay than LCA activity for detecting antipaternal antibodies [108], for in studies of MLR-blocking activity there were fewer sera with LCA activity than were MLR-inhibiting sera [109]. MLR inhibition tends to be specific, and directed at paternal rather than maternal stimulators [110], although inhibition of third-party stimulators may also occur.

The significance of MLR inhibition remains unclear. It could be speculated that since the response is directed at paternal HLA antigens, their role *in vivo* is to mask paternally derived fetal HLA antigens and thereby prevent recognition by maternal alloreactive T cells. However, the fact that MLR inhibition or LCAs are not universal phenomena would tend to militate against their having such a fundamental role.

Anti-idiotypic antibodies

The theory of idiotype and anti-idiotype networks lends itself well to hypotheses in pregnancy, but experiments in this field are difficult to conduct and few laboratories have explored this area. Theoretical considerations are nevertheless fascinating. The evidence from both in-vivo and in-vitro observations above shows that the mother can mount anti-HLA responses to paternally derived fetal antigens. However, such responses are potentially harmful, so the mother may well need to mount another response to block the first one. In idiotype terminology, the

first response produces (anti-HLA) antibody-1, the idiotype, and the second produces (anti-anti-HLA antibody) the anti-idiotype. Some investigators have proposed that this explains the absence of LCAs or MLR-blocking activity in the sera of some multiparas — that they are in fact present but are masked by anti-idiotypic antibodies [111]. This hypothesis is not limited to antibody-antibody responses, but can also be extended to T-cell responses. If the TcR on maternal T-cell clones is regarded as the idiotype, the mother might produce antibodies to this TcR, the anti-idiotype, and experimental evidence has been reported to support this view [112]. In this study, antipaternal alloreactive T cell clones were established. IgG from the mother's pregnancy reacted with these clones, but not with T-cell clones to other unrelated HLA. An MLR between these clones (responders) and paternal cells could be blocked by maternal serum, but not when the responders were control T-cell clones. Interestingly, high concentrations of the fragment, antigen-binding$_2$ (Fab$_2$) of her IgG, bound to a paternal-specific T-cell clone, blocked its cytolytic activity and stimulated the clone to proliferate. Experiments generating similar data had earlier been reported by Suciu-Foca et al. [113].

Thus, in summary, both antibody and cellular responses to paternally derived fetal antigens may be common, but may be masked by anti-anti-paternal (anti-idiotypic) responses.

Antibodies to trophoblast and placental antigens

Antibodies, shown by adsorption studies not to be directed at the HLA system, but binding to trophoblast, have been reported [114]. Some of the antibody occurs in the form of immune complexes, and a degree of specificity has been reported [115], suggesting that perhaps there may be an as yet undefined polymorphic system, distinct from MHC, within trophoblast. However, the explanation may be really quite simple: trophoblast possesses Fc receptors for IgG, and therefore binding of immunoglobulins to trophoblast does not necessarily mean that the Fab fragments are binding to epitopes on trophoblast antigens. The nature, incidence, specificity and possible significance of antitrophoblast antibodies remains to be unravelled.

Antibodies to erythrocyte antigens

Erythrocytes display a wide range of polymorphic antigenic systems to which the maternal immune system can mount a response. However, although such responses, especially responses involving the Rhesus antigens, can compromise the fetus, they are not generally regarded as playing a crucial role in the fundamental question of the immunological paradox. They will therefore not be discussed any further here: suffice it to acknowledge their occurrence.

T-cell responses

Since T cells are thought to be the major effector cells in allograft rejection, they have been an obvious target of investigation with respect to their behaviour in pregnancy. Studies of alloreactive responses are made particularly difficult by a pre-existing high precursor frequency of alloreactive cells, even in the absence of prior exposure to alloantigen [96,97].

In-vivo cell-mediated immune responses

There are obvious ethical constraints to studying cell-mediated immune (CMI) responses to allografts in pregnant women. Most of the available data are therefore based on animal work. The essential experiments have sought to establish whether pre-pregnancy sensitization of a mother to paternal and fetal alloantigens would affect subsequent pregnancies, using sensitization techniques that are known to accelerate subsequent graft rejection. Such sensitization did not affect subsequent pregnancies [4]. These findings parallel the observation in humans that the formation of LCAs (evidence of allosensitization) does not appear to affect subsequent pregnancies.

In-vitro cell-mediated immune responses

In humans, as in other animal models, CMI responses to paternal or fetal antigens have been studied indirectly *in vitro* by means of MLR and cytotoxic T lymphocytes (CTL) assays. Some studies have reported that the antipaternal MLR increased as pregnancy advanced [116], but other studies could find neither an anamnesic MLR in parous women nor significant CTL responses to paternal MHC-bearing cells [117,118]. In more recent studies using the sensitive and quantitative technique of limiting dilution analysis, Manyonda *et al.* [119] demonstrated that presence of wide ranges of antipaternal cytotoxic T cells in the peripheral blood of both primiparal and multiparal, but that the frequencies of these cells did not alter throughout pregnancy.

Thus, the consensus of opinion is that pregnancy is not accompanied by increased T-cell reactivity to fetal antigens, and that when this does occur, it does not prejudice pregnancy outcome.

Graft versus host disease in nature

Due to lack of vascular continuity between the maternal and fetal compartments, in normal pregnancy, no exchange of cellular material occur. However, the trophoblast is a minimal barrier and might be expected to be breached from time to time. Fetal cells entering the maternal circulation might expect to be destroyed, and the worst they could do is elicit formation of antipaternal cytotoxic antibody. The effect of immunocompetent maternal cells entering the fetal compartment would, however, create the possibility of the development of graft versus host disease (GvHD), since the fetus may express paternally derived HLA and its own immune system may be too immature to destroy the maternal cells. It is now clear that what was at one time regarded as a purely theoretical hazard of pregnancy [4] does indeed occur in nature. The first case report [120] described XX/XY lymphoid chimaerism in an infant with an immunodeficiency syndrome, and this was interpreted as a case of GvHD with secondary immunologic failure. Other cases followed [121].

It is well recognized that ABO compatibility between mother and fetus exacerbates Rhesus isoimmunization, since any fetal red cells entering the maternal circulation tend to persist longer. An analogous situation might be expected in maternofetal GvHD: the T cells from a mother homozygous at one or more HLA loci would be able to react against paternally derived HLA antigens on the fetus but the fetus would not react against the maternal T cells because the homozygous HLA gene products will be seen as self. Reports do indeed exist of increased HLA-DR compatibility between mother and child in severe combined immunodeficiency (SCID) and other neonatal haematopoietic diseases [122], and this suggests that instances of SCID where there is no clear autosomal recessive inheritance might represent the outcome of GvHD [123].

Immunology has long been criticized for being largely theoretical and contributing little to practical aspects of clinical practice. For example, some would contend that the major advances in transplantation have not come from immunology, but from improved immunosuppressive therapy and surgical skill [124]. However, there are interesting, if anecdotal, examples of immunologic engineering in the literature: to eliminate maternal cells (graft 1) causing GvHD in a child with SCID, a bone marrow graft (graft 2) from an HLA-identical sibling was given to the SCID child. There was a temporary exacerbation of the GvHD, but the graft-versus-graft situation created resulted in the formation of CTLs which were able to eliminate the maternal T cells (graft 1) [125].

Recurrent spontaneous miscarriage

The corollary of the assumption that immunoregulatory responses may be important for the success of pregnancy is that some defect in this response is the cause of at least some of the cases of otherwise unexplained recurrent spontaneous miscarriage (RSM). The known causes of recurrent miscarriage include chromosomal/genetic disorders in the parents or conceptus, anatomical disorders of the female reproductive tract, endocrinological abnormalities (e.g. polycystic ovaries), infections of the reproductive tract, psychological disorders, and immunological problems such as certain types of autoimmune disease. Texts [126] and reviews [127] have been written on these and a detailed

exposé is beyond the scope of this chapter. Suffice it to state that known causes account for some 60% of recurrent miscarriage [128]. From the point of view of this chapter, the interesting group is the 40% in which there is no apparent cause, for it is within this group that immunological factors are thought to play a role.

RSM as an immunological phenomenon

Whether an intact immune system is crucial for successful pregnancy is pertinent to the issue of the possible role of the immune system in RSM. Doubly homozygous scid/beige mice, which lack all B-cell and T-cell function, and most NK activity, can reproduce successfully in the absence of infection [129]. Mice homozygous for defective β_2-microglobulin genes, and hence incapable of classical MHC class I cell surface expression, can nevertheless develop normally *in utero* [130], suggesting that allorecognition is not important in pregnancy. In humans, it has long been recognized that women with congenital or adult-onset agammaglobulinaemia can have successful pregnancies. Thus it would seem that an intact maternal immune system is not essential for successful reproduction. However, it is well established that fertility and pregnancy success are better when the parents are genetically dissimilar—the concept of hybrid vigour. Furthermore, it is clear that there are circumstances in which the immune system can be detrimental, and others in which it can be beneficial. The obvious examples of harmful effects are seen in certain types of autoimmune disease such as systemic lupus erythematosus, where early pregnancy loss is common, and those pregnancies that proceed to viability often develop complications. A further instructive example are the women with the rare *p* phenotype in the erythrocyte antigenic system: they make anti-PP_1P^k antibodies which cross the placenta and may be responsible for the more than 50% early pregnancy loss [131,132].

The idea that the immune system may be beneficial to pregnancy is central to the immunotrophism hypothesis, the basic concept being that the fetus is immunogenic and evokes a response from the mother that is necessary for successful implantation and growth [133]. It is

154 hypothesized that T-cell activity within the placenta elaborates cytokines, such as GM-CSF, which promote placental and fetal growth [134]. Thus it would seem that optimal pregnancy success depends on the presence of beneficial immunotrophic forces and the absence of deleterious ones. Many investigators are therefore persuaded that immunologic defects are involved in RSM, and this view is supported by evidence from murine studies [135]. It has been observed that CBA females mated with DBA/2 males resorb 30% of the embryos *in vivo*. The fetal resorption rate is 10% if DBA/2 females are mated with CBA males. More intriguingly, the resorption rate in CBA females mated with DBA/2 males can be reduced to 5–6% if the CBA females are immunized with cells from BALB/c mice, while immunization with cells from DBA/2 is not effective. The major histocompatibility complex (H-2) types of the different mouse strains give some interesting clues. CBA mice are H-2^k, and DBA/2 are H-2^d. However, BALB/c mice also carry H-2^d. Thus genes of the MHC may be important, but since DBA/2 cells are not effective but those from BALB/c are, this suggests that background genes associated with the H-2 locus may also be important. The mechanisms involved in both the resorption itself and its prevention remain enigmatic, but some clues are beginning to emerge [134]. Overall, it appears that in certain strain combinations, environmental pathogens activate NK cells which damage trophoblast and possibly other tissues in the placenta, leading to resorption. Immunization may prevent resorption by up-regulating immunotrophism, the final effects being mediated by cytokines such as GM-CSF.

HLA sharing and RSM

There have been numerous investigations into the incidence of HLA sharing between partners in RSM couples compared to couples with successful pregnancies. Earlier studies tended to show an increased incidence of HLA sharing in RSM couples [136–141]. However, other studies failed to find increased HLA sharing [142–147]. Perhaps it is appropriate at this stage to enquire as to the possible significance of HLA in reproduction. Teleologically, increased HLA sharing might be seen as undesirable, as it implies inbreeding, with the risk of expression of lethal or handicapping genes seen with homozygosity. Certainly, some lethal genes have been shown to be linked to the MHC [148,149].

In nature itself, outbred populations, and the resultant genetic diversity, tend to yield more vigorous offspring, while inbred animals tend to have small litters and less robust progeny. Thus RSM might be seen as a method of selecting against the production of homozygous individuals. Why, then, the discrepancy in the above studies? Small sample sizes, inadequate controls, poor definition of groups studied may all be contributory. Studies of closed populations, notably the Hutterites (a religious, highly inbred population which encourages large families) have not resolved the problem. There have been at least four important studies within this group. The first study suggested that increased HLA sharing at the A and B loci was associated with a small decrease in fertility [150]. A subsequent study reported that if couples shared HLA-DR, there was a 27% incidence of miscarriage, compared to 12% in those not sharing and 9% in those who shared at the A or B loci [151]. The third study reported that HLA sharing was associated with smaller families and longer intervals between the second and sixth births [152]. The fourth study found that sharing of HLA-B, not HLA-DR, was associated with increased fetal loss [153]. However, the major problem with data from studies of the Hutterite community is that the influence of non-HLA genes cannot be associated. This is an inbred population in which the incidence of homozygosity is high, yet family sizes are large, and RSM cannot be readily demonstrated.

The issue of primary or secondary aborters is not clearer when examined in relation to HLA. Some investigators make a distinction between primary and secondary aborters, and believe that increased HLA sharing is more important in primary RSM. However, the Hutterite studies involved mainly secondary aborters, and while one study found increased HLA sharing in both primary and secondary aborters [154], another study did not find increased HLA sharing in either primary or secondary aborting couples [146]. In conclusion, the general consensus of opinion appears to favour the notion that there is no evidence of increased HLA sharing in RSM couples.

Suppressor phenomena and RSM

The possible role of suppressor influences in normal pregnancy has already been discussed. Many investigators have been interested in establishing whether these suppressor influences differ in RSM, thereby possibly offering a clue as to the aetiology of RSM. Perhaps the landmark study was that of Rocklin et al. [155] which reported the absence of a blocking factor in the serum of RSM women. Probably this study, more than any other, led to immunological interventions for RSM. Apparently corroborative studies from other groups reported the existence of a serum factor capable of blocking MLR [111] and cytotoxic T-cell responses [156] in the serum of women with successful pregnancies but absent in recurrent aborters. While some reported that leucocyte immunization greatly increased the capacity of RSM sera to block the relevant MLR [140], others [157] found no correlation between the presence or absence of MLR-blocking antibodies and pregnancy outcome. Other investigators have studied the role of cytotoxic and non-cytotoxic anti-paternal (anti-HLA) antibodies. Power et al. [158] found non-cytotoxic antibodies which bound to paternal B cells in 11/11 multiparas, 11/16 primiparas and 1/10 RSM women. However, the lower incidence of anti-paternal HLA antibodies in women who suffer RSM compared to multiparas is more likely to be due to a shorter time of exposure to paternal antigens in RSM women [107]. The consensus of opinion is moving away from the idea of blocking factors.

Rationale for immunotherapy in the treatment of RSM

Since about 1980, women with RSM have been immunized with paternal leucocytes, pooled third-party leucocytes or trophoblast membrane preparations in attempts to prevent further miscarriages. Many reproductive biologists believed, and indeed many still do believe, that the fetus represented Nature's perfect allograft.

Thus, reports of the beneficial effects of pre-transplant blood transfusion in renal transplantation dating back to the pioneering work of Paul Terasaki's group [159] encouraged investigators to believe that similar strategies might be adopted in RSM. It did not seem to matter that the mechanism of the blood transfusion effect was ill-understood. Reports of the absence of a serum-blocking factor in women with RSM, and increased HLA sharing in couples with RSM, resulted in the emergence of the following hypothesis: a high degree of HLA antigen-sharing between couples results in maternal hyporesponsiveness to paternal antigens and thus failure to mount a protective immune response such as production of a blocking antibody. As the placenta was purported to have TLX antigens shared by paternal cells, the belief thus arose that immunization with paternal cells would induce the production of the much needed blocking factor. Belief in these ideas was further strengthened by data from studies using the murine model of RSM, which suggested that immunization of female mice with cells bearing paternal MHC haplotypes significantly reduced resorption rates. Indeed, the preliminary reports of immunotherapy were very encouraging [160,161].

Outcome of treatment with immunotherapy in RSM

Success with immunotherapy is variably reported [160,162,163]. To date, there has only ever been one double-blind, controlled study of immunotherapy that has reported a beneficial effect [164]. This study has been heavily criticized, and subsequent studies have failed to corroborate the findings [165,166]. In a recent meta-analysis of four randomized controlled trials of leucocyte immunotherapy or trophoblast membrane infusion, it was concluded that the prevailing evidence suggests that this treatment should be abandoned unless its efficacy can be established through other randomized controlled trials [167].

Other than success or otherwise in carrying a pregnancy, an additional issue that should be examined regarding immunotherapy is the effect on immune responses of immunizing other-

156 wise healthy immunocompetent women with live allogeneic lymphocytes. Initial immunological investigations of the consequences of alloimmunization were confined to assessing clinical responses [168] and the determination of blocking antibody activity [169,140]. More recent studies by Manyonda *et al.* [170], employing the quantitative technique of limiting dilution analysis, have shown that women with RSM have large numbers of antipaternal specific cytotoxic T cells, and that immunization resulted in increased allosensitization. They concluded that such a response was incompatible with a beneficial effect of immunotherapy.

Reconciling some confounding observations

Thus, discussions argue against a significant role for allo-MHC responses in the success of pregnancy, but there are a number of confounding observations that require explanation. How might the reports of beneficial effects of immunotherapy for recurrent miscarriage be explained? What about the elegant murine studies showing that spontaneous resorption can be reversed by allo-MHC manipulations? Although there is little, if any, evidence for the efficacy of immunotherapy, many centres across the world continue to offer this treatment to women, and it is therefore useful and interesting to speculate how it might achieve a beneficial effect. The theories of blocking antibodies, or hyporesponsiveness of the maternal immune system to fetal antigens, have failed to stand up to scrutiny. Wegmann's theories of 'immunotrophism' are, however, interesting and plausible, and largely involve the existence of cytokine-based 'cross-talk' between the immune and reproductive systems [134]. In essence, Wegmann believes that the basis for the apparent interaction between the immune and reproductive systems is their sharing of certain lymphohaematopoietic cytokines and their receptors. The former appears capable of enhancing or inhibiting the development of the fetoplacental unit. In experimental animals undergoing fetal resorption, immunization with allogeneic lymphocytes and, in some cases, MHC class I molecules [171] leads to enhanced fetoplacental survival and growth. MRL-lpr/lpr

homozygous mice have excessive T-cell proliferation along with large placentas that show abnormally high levels of phagocytosis, and the placental phenomena can be reduced to normal by treatment of the pregnant female with anti-T cell antibodies [61]. In normal mice this treatment reduces placental size and, in some strain combinations, causes fetal resorption.

Most of the above observations involve T cells, which are known to mediate many of their responses via the elaboration of cytokines. Thus, local cytokine production may influence survival and growth of the fetoplacental unit. There is now ample evidence that GM-CSF, IL-3 and CSF-1 can promote the growth and/or differentiation of mouse and human trophoblast [62,63], and enhance fetal survival when injected into mice prone to fetal resorption. In contrast, other cytokines, such as IL-2, TNF and IFN-γ, appear to have deleterious effects. In addition to cells of the immune system, non-immune components of the reproductive tract, including the uterine epithelium and trophoblast, can also elaborate cytokines [64–66]. Thus, the concept has emerged that there are beneficial cytokines which can enhance fetal growth and survival, and deleterious cytokines which can compromise pregnancy, and that such cytokines can be elaborated with or without the involvement of the immune system.

So how might leucocyte immunization be beneficial? Well, MHC antigens are a powerful stimulus, and leucocyte transfusion may cause modulation of the cytokine balance at the maternofetal interface in a manner that results in the preponderance of cytokines that promote development of the fetoplacental unit. This could be true for both the human as well as the murine model, thus explaining how immunotherapy might work, and the observations with the CBA × DBA/2 murine models. It would also explain why, as well as allo-MHC manipulations, a variety of other unrelated treatments achieve similar results in the murine model. Clearly, the difficulty with producing consistent results would lie in not being able to determine the timing and dose of the allo-MHC challenge that would stimulate a beneficial cytokine balance. Even if the above speculation could be shown to be true, it could not justify the continued use of immunotherapy in a blind fashion, because it is a treatment which is potentially harmful, not only because of allosensitization and subsequent problems with tissue cross-matching should this ever be required, or transmission of viruses such as HIV, but also because such blind immunization may result in the production of cytokines that are detrimental to the development of the fetoplacental unit.

Suggested further reading in basic immunology

1 *Essential Immunology*, 9th edn, I.M. Roitt, Blackwell Science, Oxford, 1997.
2 *Advanced Immunology*, 3rd edn, D. Male, A. Cooke, M. Owen, J. Trowsedale and B. Champion, Mosby of Times Mirror International Publishers, 1996.

References

1 Medawar P.B. (1953) Some immunological and endocrinological problems raised by the evolution of viviparity in vertebrates. *Symposium of the Society for Experimental Biology* **11**, 320.

2 Billingham R.E. (1971) Silvers WK. *Immunobiology of Tissue Transplantation*. Prentice-Hall, Englewood Cliffs.

3 Niederkom J.Y. (1990) Immune privilege and immune regulation in the eye. *Advances in Immunology* **48**, 191.

4 Billingham R.E. (1964) Transplantation immunity and the materno-fetal relation. *New England Journal of Medicine* **270**, 720.

5 Lawton A.R. & Cooper M.B. (1989) Ontogeny of Immunity. In *Immunologic Disorders in Infants and Children*. Ed. E.R. Stiehm, p. 1. W.B. Saunders Co., Philadelphia.

6 Beer A.E. & Billingham R.E. (1974) Host responses to intra-uterine tissue, cellular and fetal allografts. *Journal of Reproduction and Fertility* **21**, 49.

7 Dodd M., Andrew T.A. & Coles J.S. (1980) Functional behaviour of skin allografts transplanted to rabbit deciduomata. *Journal of Anatomy* **130**, 381.

8 Heyner S. (1986) Embryonal, gametic and oncofetal antigens. In *Reproductive Immunology*. Eds D.A. Clark & B.A. Croy, p. 289. Elsevier, Amsterdam.

9 Hekman A. & Rumke P. (1969) The antigens of human seminal plasma. *Fertility and Sterility* **20**, 312.

10 James K. & Hargreave T.B. (1984) Immunosuppression by seminal plasma and its possible significance. *Immunology Today* **5**, 357.

11 Vallely P.J., Sharrard R.M. & Rees R.C. (1988) The identification of factors in seminal plasma responsible for suppression of natural killer cell activity. *Immunology* **63**, 451.

12 Daya S., Clarke D.A., Devlin C. & Jarrell J. (1985) Preliminary characteristics of two types of suppressor cells in the human uterus. *Fertility and Sterility* **44**, 778.

13 Wang H.-S., Kanzani H., Yoshida M., Sato S., Tokushige M. & Mori T. (1987) Suppression of lymphocyte reactivity *in vitro* by supernatants of explants of human endometrium. *American Journal of Obstetrics and Gynecology* **157**, 956.

14 Head J.R., Drake B.L. & Zuckerman F.A. (1987) MHC antigens on trophoblast and their regulation: implications in the maternal–fetal relationship. *American Journal of Reproduction and Immunology* **15**, 12.

15 Ilgren E.B. (1983) Review article, control of trophoblastic growth. *Placenta* **4**, 307.

16 Chaouat G., Kolb J.P., Chaffaux S., Riviere M., Lankar D., Anthanassaki I., Green D. & Wegmann T.G. (1987) In *Immunoregulation and Fetal Survival*. Eds T.J. Gill & T.G. Wegmann, p. 239. Oxford University Press, Oxford.

17 Jones W.R. (1980) Immunological factors in male and female infertility. In *Immunological Aspects of Reproduction*. Ed. J.P. Hearn, p. 105. MTP, New York.

18 Slamon D.J. (1987) Proto-oncogenes and human cancers. *New England Journal of Medicine* **317**, 955.

19 Goustin A.S., Betsholtz C., Pfeiffer-Ohlsson S., Persson H., Rydnert J., Bywater M., Holmgren G., Heldin C.H., Westermark B. & Ohlsson R. (1985) Coexpression of the sis and myc proto-oncogenes in developing human placenta suggest autocrine control of trophoblast growth. *Cell* **41**, 301.

20 Marua T. & Mochizuki M. (1987) Immunohistochemical localisation of epidermal growth factor receptor and myc-oncogene product in human placenta: implication for trophoblast proliferation and differentiation. *American Journal of Obstetrics and Gynecology* **156**, 721.

21 Carson S.A., Chase R., Ulep E., Scommegna A. & Benveniste R. (1983) Ontogenesis and characteristics of epidermal growth factor receptors in human placenta. *American Journal of Obstetrics and Gynecology* **147**, 932.

22 Tavare J.M. & Holmes C.H. (1988) Differential expression of the receptors for epidermal growth factor and insulin in the developing human placenta. *Cellular Signalling* **1**, 54.

23 Lai W.H. & Guyda A.J. (1984) Characterisation and regulation of epidermal factor receptors in human placental cell cultures. *Journal of Clinical Endocrilogy and Metabolism* **58**, 344.

24 Loke Y.W., Burland K. & Butterworth B. (1986) Antigen bearing trophoblast in human placental implantation site. In *Reproductive Immunology*. Eds D.A. Clark & B.A. Groy, p. 53. Elsevier, Amsterdam.

25 Kalter S.S., Helmke R.J., Heberling R.L., Panigel M., Fowler A.K., Strickland J.E. & Hellman A. (1973) C-type particles in normal human placenta. *Journal of the National Cancer Institute* **50**, 1081.

26 Thiry L., Loke Y.W., Whyte A., Hard R.C., Sprecher-Goldberger S. & Beukens P. (1981) Heterologous antiserum to human syncytio-trophoblast membrane is cytotoxic to retrovirus producing cells and some

158

cancer cell lines. *American Journal of Reproduction and Immunology* **1**, 240.

27 Surani M.A.H., Barton S.C. & Norris M.L. (1984) Development of reconsituted mouse eggs suggests imprinting of the genome during gametogenesis. *Nature* **308**, 548.

28 Kaufman M.H. (1988) Hydatidiform mole: genetics and practical implications. *Hospital Update* **14**, 1415.

29 Simmons R.L. & Russell P.S. (1962) Antigenicity of mouse trophoblast. *Annals of the New York Academy of Science* **99**, 717.

30 Faulk W.P. & Temple A. (1976) Distribution of b2-microglobulin and HLA in chorionic villi of human placentae. *Nature* **262**, 799.

31 Goodfellow P.N., Barnstable C.J., Bodmer W.F., Snary D. & Crumpton M.J. (1976) Expression of HLA system antigens on placenta. *Transplantation* **22**, 595.

32 Galbraith R.M., Kanto R.S.S., Ferrara G.B., Ades E.W., Galbraith G.M.P. (1981) Differential anatomical expression of transplantation antigens within the normal human placental chorionic villus. *American Journal of Reproduction and Immunology* **1**, 331.

33 Sutton L., Mason D.Y. & Redman C.W.G. (1983) HLA-DR positive cells in the human placenta. *Immunology* **49**, 103.

34 Paul S. & Jailkhani B.L. (1982) Failure of placental syncitiotrophoblast to provoke allogeneic recognition by lymphocytes in-vitro. *Indian Journal of Experimental Biology* **20**, 248.

35 Sunderland C.A., Naiem M., Mason D.Y., Redman C.W.G., Stirrat E.M. (1981) The expression of major histocompatibility antigens by human chorionic villi. *Journal of Reproductive Immunology* **3**, 323.

36 Redman C.W.G., McMichael A.J., Stirrat G.M., Sunderland C.A., Ting A. (1984) Class I MHC antigens on human extravillous trophoblast. *Immunology* **52**, 457.

37 Bulmer J.N. & Johnson P.M. (1985) Antigen expression by trophoblast populations in the human placenta and their possible immunobiological significance. *Placenta* **6**, 127.

38 Ellis S.A., Sargent I.L., Redman C.W.G., McMichael A.J. (1986) Evidence for a novel HLA antigen found on human extra-villous trophoblast and a choriocarcinoma cell line. *Immunology* **59**, 595.

39 Ellis S.A., Palmer M.S. & McMichael A.J. (1990) Human trophoblast and the choriocarcinoma cell line BeWo express a truncated HLA class I molecule. *Journal of Immunology* **144**, 731.

40 Hunt J.S., Yelavarthi K.K., Yangi Y. (1991) Class I major histocompatibility genes in trophoblast cells: studies on expression, regulation and function. In *Cellular and Molecular Biology of the Materno-Fetal Relationship*. Eds G. Chaouat & J. Mowbray, p. 51. INSERM/J. Libbey Eurotext, London.

41 Kovats S., Main E.K., Librach C., Stubblebine M., Fisher S.J., DeMars R. (1990) A class I antigen, HLA-G, expressed in human trophoblasts. *Science* **248**, 220.

42 Head J.R., Drake B.L. & Zuckerman F.A. (1987) MHC antigens on trophoblast and their regulation: impli-

cations in the materno-fetal relationship. *American Journal of Reproduction and Immunology* **15**, 12.

43 Hunt J.S., Andrews G.K. & Wood G.W. (1987) Normal trophoblasts resist induction of class I HLA. *Journal of Immunology* **138**, 2481.

44 Faulk W.P. & Hunt J.S. (1989) Human placentae: view from an immunological bias. *American Journal of Reproduction and Immunology* **21**, 108.

45 Hamilton T.A., Wada H.G. & Sussman H.H. (1980) Expression of human placental cell surface antigens on peripheral blood lymphocytes and lymphoblastoid cell lines. *Scandinavian Journal of Immunology* **11**, 195.

46 Loke Y.W., Whyte A. & Davis S.P. (1980) Differential expression of trophoblast-specific membrane antigens by normal and abnormal human placenta and by neoplasms of trophoblastic and non-trophoblastic origin. *International Journal of Cancer* **25**, 359.

47 Holmes C.H., Simpson K.L., Wainwright S.D., Tate C.G., Houlihan J.M., Sawyer C.H., Rogers I.P. (1990) Preferential expression of the complement regulatory protein decay accelerating factor at the feto-maternal interface during human pregnancy. *Journal of Immunology* **144**, 3099.

48 Purcell D.F.J., McKenzie I.F.C., Lublin D.M., Johnson P.M., Atkinson J.P., Oglesby T.J., Deacon N.J. (1990) The human cell surface glycoproteins HuLy-m5, membrane cofactor protein (MCP) of the complement system and trophoblast-leukocyte common (TLX) antigen are CD46. *Immunology* **70**, 155.

49 Meri S., Waldmann H. & Lachmann P.J. (1991) Distribution of protectin (CD59), a complement membrane attack inhibitor, in normal human tissues. *Laboratory Investigations* **65**, 532.

50 Holmes C.H., Simpson K.L., Okada H., Okada N., Wainwright S.D., Purcell D.F., Houlihan J.M. (1992) Complement regulatory proteins at the feto-maternal interface during human placental development: distribution of CD59 by comparison with membrane cofactor protein (CD46) and decay accelerating factor (CD55). *European Journal of Immunology* **22**, 1579.

51 Faulk W.P., Temple A., Lovins R.E., Smith N. (1978) Antigens of human trophoblasts: a working hypothesis for their role in normal and abnormal pregnancies. *Proceedings of the National Academy of Science USA* **75**, 1947.

52 Holmes C.H., Simpson K.L., Okada H., Okada N., Wainwright S.D., Purcell D.F., Houlihan J.M. (1992) Complement regulatory proteins at the feto-maternal interface during human placental development: distribution of CD59 by comparison with membrane cofactor protein (CD46) and decay accelerating factor (CD55). *European Journal of Immunology* **22**, 1579.

53 Bulmer J.N., Longfellow M. & Ritson A. (1991) Leukocytes and resident blood cells in endometrium. *Annals of the New York Academy of Science* **221**, 57.

54 Ferry B.L., Starkey P.M., Sargent I.L., Redman C.W.G. (1990) Cell populations in the human early pregnancy decidua: natural killer activity and response to interleukin-2 CD56-positive large granular lymphocytes. *Immunology* **70**, 446.

55 Pace D., Morrison L. & Bulmer J.N. (1989) Prolifera-

tive activity in endometrial stromal granulocytes throughout menstrual cycle and early pregnancy. *Journal of Clinical Pathology* **42**, 35.

56 King A. & Loke Y.W. (1990) Uterine large granular lymphocytes: a possible role in embryonic implantation? *American Journal of Obstetrics and Gynecology* **162**, 308.

57 Kovats S., Librach C., Fisch P., Hunt J.S. (1991) Expression and possible function of the HLA-G alpha chain in human cytotrophoblasts. In *Cellular and Molecular Biology of the Materno-Fetal Relationship*. Eds G. Chaouat & J. Mowbray, p. 21. INSERM/J. Libbey Eurotext, London.

58 Clark D.A., Slapsys A.R., Chaput A., Lacroix J. (1986) Immunoregulatory molecules of trophoblast and decidual suppressor cell origin at the materno-fetal interface. *American Journal of Reproduction and Immunology*, **10**, 100.

59 Croy B.A. & Kassouf S.A. (1989) Evaluation of the murine metrial gland for immunological function. *Journal of Reproduction and Immunology* **15**, 51.

60 Lala P.K., Parhar R.S., Kearns M., Annam J. (1986) Immunologic aspects of the decidual response. In *Reproductive Immunology*. Eds D.A. Clark & B.A. Croy p. 190. Elsevier, Amsterdam.

61 Chaouat G., Menu E., Bonneton C. & Kinsky R. (1989) Immunological manipulations in animal pregnancy and models of pregnancy failure. *Current Opinion in Immunology* **1**, 1153.

62 Athanassakis I., Bleackley R.C., Paetkau V., Guilbert L., Barr P.J., Wegmann T.G. (1987) The immunostimulatory effect of T cells and T cell lymphokines on murine fetally derived placental cells. *Journal of Immunology* **138**, 37.

63 Armstrong D.T. & Chaouat G. (1989) Effects of lymphokines and immune complexes on murine placental cell growth in vitro. *Biology of Reproduction* **40**, 466.

64 Pollard J.W., Bartocci A., Arceci R., Orlofsky A., Ladner M.B., Stanley E.R. (1987) Apparent role of the macrophage growth factor, CSF-1, in placental development. *Nature* **330**, 484.

65 Branch D.R., Turc J.M., & Guilbert L.J. (1987) Identification of an erythropoietin-sensitive cell line. *Blood* **69**, 1782.

66 Robertson S.A., Mayrhofer G. & Seamark R.F. Uterine epithelial cells synthesize granulocyte-macrophage colony-stimulating factor and IL-6 in pregnant and non-pregnant mice. *Biology of Reproduction* **46**, 1069.

67 Carter J. & Dressor D.W. (1983) Pregnancy induces an increase in the number of immunoglobulin secreting cells. *Immunology* **49**, 481.

68 Weinberg E.D. (1984) Pregnancy: associated depression of cell-mediated immunity. *Review of Infectious Diseases* **6**, 814.

69 Falkoff R. (1987) Maternal immunologic changes during pregnancy: a critical appraisal. *Clinical Review of Allergy* **5**, 287.

70 Stagno S., Reynolds D.W., Huang E.-S., *et al.* (1977) Congenital cytomegalovirus infection: occurrence in an immune population. *New England Journal of Medicine*, **296**, 1254.

71 Murray D.L., Imagawa D.T., Okada D.M., *et al.*

(1979) Antibody response to monovalent A/New Jersey/8/76 influenza vaccine in pregnant women. *Journal of Clinical Microbiology* **10**, 184.

72 Jones W.R., Hawes C.S. & Kemp A.S. (1983) Studies on cell-mediated immunity in human pregnancy. In *Immunology of Reproduction*. Eds T.G. Wegmann & T.J. Gill III, p. 363. Oxford University Press, New York.

73 Strelkauskas A.J., Wilson B.S., Dray S., *et al.* (1975) Inversion of human T and B cell levels in early pregnancy. *Nature* **258**, 331.

74 Degenne D., Canepa S., Lecomte C., Renoux M., Bardos P. (1988) Serial study of T-lymphocyte subsets in women during very early pregnancy. *Clinical Immunology and Immunopathology* **48**, 181.

75 Tallon D.F., Corcoran D.J.D., O'Dwyer E.M., Greally J.E. Circulating lymphocyte subpopulations in pregnancy: a longitudinal study. *Journal Immunology* **132**, 1784.

76 Moore M.P., Carter N.P. & Redman C.W. (1983) Lymphocyte subsets in normal and pre-eclamptic pregnancies. *British Journal of Obstetrics and Gynaecology* **90**, 32.

77 Bardeguez A.D., McNerney R., Frieri M., Verma U.L., Tejani N. (1991) Cellular immunity in preeclampsia: alterations in T-lymphoycte subpopulations during early pregnancy. *Obstetrics and Gynaecology* **77**, 859.

78 Coulam C., Silverfield J., Kazmar R., Fathman C.G. (1983) T lymphocyte subsets during pregnancy and the menstrual cycle. *American Journal of Reproduction and Immunology* **4**, 88.

79 Lucivero G., Selvaggi A., Dell'osso S., Antonaci S., Lannone A., Bettocchi S., Bonomo L. (1983) Monoclear cell subpopulations during normal pregnancy. I. Analysis of cell surface markers using conventional techniques and monoclonal antibodies. *American Journal of Reproduction and Immunology* **4**, 142.

80 Feinberg B.B. & Gonik B. (1991) General precepts of the immunology of pregnancy. *Clinics in Obstetrics and Gynaecology* **34**, 3.

81 Nelson J.H., Lu T., Hall J.E., Krown S., Nelson J.M., Fax C.W. (1973) The effect of trophoblast on immune state of women. *American Journal of Obstetrics and Gynecology* **117**, 689.

82 Covelli H.D. & Wilson R.T. (1978) Immunologic and medical considerations in tuberculin-sensitized pregnant patients. *American Journal of Obstetrics and Gynecology* **132**, 256.

83 Burns G.F., Cleen B.L., Mackay I.R., Tanner T.W. (1985) Supernatural killer cells. *Immunology Today* **6**, 310.

84 Toder V., Nebel L. & Gleicher N. (1984) Studies of natural killer cell activity in pregnancy. I. Analysis at the single cell level. *Journal of Clinics in Laboratory Immunology* **14**, 123.

85 Lala P.K., Parhar R.S., Kearns M., McKenna J.N. (1986) Immunologic aspects of the decidual response. In *Reproductive Immunology*. Eds D.A. Clark & B.A. Croy, p. 190. Elsevier, Amsterdam.

86 Hench P.S. (1952) The reversibility of certain rheumatic and non-rheumatic conditions by the use of cortisone or of the pituitary adrenocorticotrophic hormone. *Annals of Internal Medicine* **36**, 1.

160

87 Claman H.N. (1972) Corticosteroids and lymphoid cells. *New England Journal of Medicine* **287**, 388.

88 Klopper A. (1989) Pregnancy proteins and hormones in the immune response to pregnancy. In *Immunology of Pregnancy and its Disorders*. Ed. C.M.M. Stern, p. 91. Kluwer Academic Publishers, Dordrecht.

89 Clemons L.E., Siiteri P.K. & Stites D.P. (1979) Mechanisms of immunosuppression of progesterone on maternal lymphocyte activation during pregnancy. *Journal of Immunology* **122**, 1978.

90 Murgita R.A. & Tomasi T.B. (1975) Suppression of immune response by alpha-fetoprotein. *Journal of Experimental Medicine* **141**, 440.

91 Wajner M., Pailha S.S. & Wagstaff T.I. (1986) Inhibition of mitogen and allogeneic stimulated lymphocyte growth by human amniotic fluid: lack of correlation between a-fetoprotein level and in vitro immunosuppression. *European Journal of Obstetrics, Gynecology and Reproductive Biology* **21**, 225.

92 Menu E. & Chaouat G. (1990) Immunoregulatory factors secreted by human or murine placenta or gestational tumors. In *The Immunology of the Fetus*. Ed. G. Chaouat, p. 153. CRC Press, Boca Raton, Fla.

93 Klopper A. (1989) Pregnancy proteins and hormones in the immune response to pregnancy. In *Immunology of Pregnancy and its Disorders*. Ed. C.M.M. Stern, p. 91. Kluwer Academic Publishers, Dordrecht.

94 Gomard E., Henin Y., Sterkers G., Masset M., Fauchet R., Levy J.P. (1986) An influenza A virus-specific and HLA-DRw8-restricted T cell clone cross-reacting with a transcomplementation product of the HLA-DR2 and DR4 haplotypes. *Journal of Immunology*, **136**, 3961.

95 Lechler R.I., Lombardi G., Batchelor J.R., Reinsmoen N. & Bach F.H. (1990) The molecular basis of alloreactivity. *Immunology Today* **11**, 83.

96 Skinner M.A. & Marbrook J. (1976) An estimation of the frequency of precursor cells which generate cytotoxic lymphocytes. *Journal of Experimental Medicine* **143**, 1562.

97 Lindahl K.F. & Wilson D.B. (1977) Histocompatibility antigen-activated cytotoxic T lymphocytes. I. Estimation of the absolute frequency of killer cells generated in vitro. *Journal of Experimental Medicine* **145**, 500.

98 Regan L., Braude P.R. & Hill D.P. (1991) A prospective study of the incidence, time of appearance and significance of anti-paternal lymphocytotoxic antibodies in human pregnancy. *Human Reproduction* **6**, 294.

99 Payne R. & Rolfs M.R. (1956) Fetomaternal leukocyte incompatibility. *Journal of Clinical Investigation* **37**, 1756.

100 van Rood J.J., Eernisse J.G. & van Leeuwen A. (1958) Leucocyte antibodies in sera from pregnant women. *Nature* **181**, 1735.

101 Tongio M.M., Berrebi A. & Mayer S. (1972) A study of lymphocytotoxic antibodies in multiparous women having had at least four pregnancies. *Tissue Antigens* **2**, 378.

102 Doughty R.W. & Gelsthorpe K. (1976) Some parame-

ters of lymphocyte antibody activity through pregnancy and further eluates of placental material. *Tissue Antigens* **8**, 43.

103 Vives J., Gelabert A. & Castillo R. (1976) HLA antibodies and period of gestation: decline in frequency of positive sera during last trimester. *Tissue Antigens* **7**, 209.

104 Koening U.D. & Muller N. (1983) Occurrence and characterization of different types of cytotoxic antibodies in pregnant women in relation to parity and gestational age. *American Journal of Obstetrics and Gynecology* **147**, 671.

105 Doughty R.W. & Gelsthorpe K. (1972) An initial investigation of lymphocyte antibody activity through pregnancy and in eluates prepared from placental material. *Tissue Antigens* **4**, 291.

106 Bell S.C. & Billington W.D. (1983) Anti-fetal alloantibody in the pregnant female. *Immunology Review* **75**, 5.

107 Regan L. & Braude P.R. (1987) Is paternal cytotoxic antibody a valid marker in the management of recurrent abortion? *Lancet* **ii**, 1280.

108 Neppert J., Mueller-Eckhardt G., Neumeyer H., *et al.* (1989) Pregnancy-maintaining antibodies: workshop report (Giessen, 1988). *Journal of Reproductive Immunology* **15**, 159.

109 Jonker M., van Leeuwen A., van Rood I.J. (1977) Inhibition of the mixed leukocyte reaction by alloantisera in man. II. Incidence and characteristics of MLC-inhibitory antisera from multiparous women. *Tissue Antigens* **9**, 246.

110 Hanaoka J.-I. & Takeuchi S. (1986) Individual specificity of blocking antibodies in molar and normal term placenta-bound IgG. *American Journal of Reproduction and Immunology* **3**, 119.

111 Singal D.P., Butler L., Liao S.-K., Lui K. (1984) The fetus as an allograft: evidence for anti-idiotypic antibodies induced by pregnancy. *American Journal of Reproduction and Immunology* **6**, 145.

112 Bonagura V.R., Ma A., McDowell J., Lewison A., King D.W., Suciu-Foca N. (1987) Anti-clonotypic autoantibodies in pregnancy. *Cell Immunology* **108**, 356.

113 Suciu-Foca N., Reed E., Rohowsky C., Kung P., King D.W. Anti-idiotypic antibodies to anti-HLA receptors induced by pregnancy. *Proceedings of the National Academy of Science USA* **80**, 830.

114 Torry D.S., Faulk W.P. & McIntyre J.A. (1989) Regulation of immunity to extraembryonic antigens in human pregnancy. *American Journal of Reproduction and Immunology* **21**, 76.

115 Goto S., Takakuwa K., Kanazawa K., Takeuchi S. (1989) MLR-blocking antibodies are directed against alloantigens expressed on syncytiotrophoblasts. *American Journal of Reproductive Immunology* **21**, 50.

116 Birkeland S.A. & Kristoffersen K. (1980) The fetus as an allograft: a longitudinal study of normal human pregnancies studied with mixed lymphocyte cultures between mother-father and mother-child. *Scandinavian Journal of Immunology* **11**, 311.

117 Sargent I.L., Wilkins T. & Redman C.W.G. (1988) Maternal immune responses to the fetus in early pregnancy and recurrent miscarriage. *Lancet* **ii**, 1099.

118 Sargent I.L. & Redman C.W.G. (1989) Maternal immune responses to the fetus in human pregnancy. In *Immunology of Pregnancy and its Disorders.* Ed. C.M.M. Stern, p. 115. Kluwer Academic Publishers, Dordrecht.

119 Manyonda I.T., Pereira R.S., Pearce J.M. & Sharrock C.E.M. (1993) Limiting dilution analysis of the allo-MHC anti-paternal cytotoxic T cell response. I. Normal primigravid and multiparous pregnancies. *Clinical and Experimental Immunology* **93**, 126.

120 Kadowaki J., Thompson R.L., Zuelzer W.W. (1965) XX/XY lymphoid chimaerism in congenital immunological deficiency syndrome with thymic alymphoplasia. *Lancet* **ii**, 1152.

121 Grogan T.M., Broghton D.D. & Doyle W.F. (1975) Graft-versus-host reaction (GVHR): a case report suggesting GVHR occurred as a result of maternofetal cell transfer. *Archives of Pathology* **99**, 330.

122 Hansen I.A., Good R.A. & DuPont B. (1977) HLA-D compatibility between parent and child: increased occurrence in severe combined immunodeficiency and other hematopoietic diseases. *Transplantation* **23**, 366.

123 Pollack M.S., Kirkpatrick D., Kapoor N., Dupont B., O'Reilly, R.J. Identification by HLA-typing of intrauterine-derived maternal T cell in four patients with severe combined immunodeficiency. *New England Journal of Medicine* **307**, 662.

124 Calne R.Y. (1989) The role of immunology in the development of clinical transplantation. *Immunology Letters* **21**, 81.

125 le Deist F., Raffoux C., Griscelli C., Fischer A. (1987) Graft vs graft reaction resulting in the elimination of maternal cells in a SCID patient with maternofetal GVHD after HLA identical bone marrow transplantation. *Journal of Immunology* **138**, 423.

126 Beard R.W. & Sharp F. (1988) *Early Pregnancy Loss: Mechanisms and Treatment*, p. 351. Royal College of Obstetricians and Gynaecologists, London.

127 Stirrat G.M. (1990) Recurrent miscarriage. I. Definition and epidemiology. *Lancet* **336**, 673.

128 Beer A.E. (1986) New horizons in the diagnosis, evaluation and therapy of recurrent spontaneous abortion. *Clinics in Obstetrics and Gynecology* **13**, 115.

129 Croy B.A., Chapeau C., Reed C. (1990) Is there an essential requirement for bone marrow-derived cells at the feto-maternal interface during successful pregnancy? A study of pregnancies in immunodeficient mice. In *Molecular and Cellular Immunology of the Feto-maternal Interface*. Eds T.G. Wegmann, T.J. Gill & N.E. Brown, p. 44. Oxford University Press, New York.

130 Zijlstra M., Bix M., Simister N.E., Loring J.M., Raulet D.H. & Jaenisch R. (1990) β2-microglobulin deficient mice lack CD4-8+ cytolytic T cells. *Nature* **344**, 742.

131 Cantin G. & Lyonnais J. (1983) Anti-PP1Pk and early abortions. *Transfusion* **23**, 350.

132 Shirey R.S., Ness P.M. & Kickler T.S., Rock T.S., Rock J.A., Callan N.A., Schlaff, W.D. *et al.* (1987) The association of anti-P and early abortion. *Transfusion* **27**, 189.

133 Scott J.R., Rote N.S. & Branch D.W. (1987) Immuno-logic aspects of recurrent abortion and fetal death. *Obstetrics and Gynaecology* **70**, 645.

134 Wegmann T.G. (1990) Placental immunotrophism: the idea and evidence. In *The Immunology of the Fetus*. Ed. G. Chaouat, p. 180. CRC Press, Boca Raton, Fla.

135 Clark D.A. & Chaout G. (1989) What do we know about spontaneous abortion mechanisms? *American Journal of Reproductive Immunology and Microbiology* **19**, 28.

136 Gerencer M., Kastelan A. & Drazancic A., Kerhin-Brkljacic V., Madjaric M. (1978) The HLA antigens in women with recurrent abortional pregnancies of unknown etiology. *Tissue Antigens* **12**, 223.

137 McIntyre J.A., Faulk W.P., Verhulst S.J., Colliver J.A. (1983) Human trophoblast lymphocyte cross-reactive (TLX) antigens define a new alloantigen system. *Science* **222**, 1135.

138 Thomas M.L., Harger J.H., Wagener D.K., Rabin B.S., Gill III T.J. (1985) HLA sharing and spontaneous abortion in humans. *American Journal of Obstetrics and Gynecology* **151**, 1053.

139 Unander A.M., Lindholm A. & Olding L.B. (1985) Blood transfusions generate/increase previously absent/weak blocking antibody in women with habitual abortion. *Fertility and Sterility* **44**, 766.

140 Takakuwa K., Kanazawa K. & Takeuchi S. (1986) Production of blocking antibodies by vaccination with husband's lymphocytes in unexplained recurrent aborters: the role in successful pregnancy. *American Journal of Reproduction, Immunology and Microbiology* **10**, 1.

141 Beer A.E., Quebbeman J.F., Ayers J.W.T., Haines R.F. (1981) Major histocompatibility complex antigens, maternal and paternal immune responses and chronic habitual abortions in humans. *American Journal of Obstetrics and Gynecology* **141**, 987.

142 Lauritsen J.G., Kristensen T. & Grunnet N. (1976) Depressed mixed lymphocyte culture reactivity in mothers with recurrent spontaneous abortion. *American Journal of Obstetrics and Gynecology* **125**, 35.

143 Oksenberg J.R., Pesitz E., Amar A., Schenker J., Segal S., Nelken D., Brautbar C. (1983) Mixed lymphocyte reactivity non-responsiveness in couples with multiple spontaneous abortions. *Fertility and Sterility* **39**, 525.

144 Caudle M.R., Rote N.S., Scott J.R., DeWitt C., Barney M.F. (1983) Histocompatibility in couples with recurrent spontaneous abortion and normal fertility. *Fertility and Sterility* **39**, 793.

145 Sargent I.L., Wilkins T. & Redman C.W.G. (1988) Maternal immune responses to the fetus in early pregnancy and recurrent miscarriage. *Lancet* **ii**, 1099.

146 Cauchi M.N., Tait B., Wilshire M.I., Koh S.H., Mraz G., Kloss M, Pepperell R. (1988) Histocompatibility antigens and habitual abortion. *American Journal of Reproductive Immunology and Microbiology* **18**, 28.

147 Houwert-de Jong M.H., Termijtelen A., Eskes T.K.A.B., Braberg G. (1989) The natural course of habitual abortion. *European Journal of Obstetrics, Gynaecology and Reproductive Biology* **33**, 221.

148 Gill III T.J. (1983) Immunogenetics of spontaneous abortions in humans. *Transplantation* **35**, 1.

162

149 Awdeh Z.L., Raum D., Yunis E.J., Alper C.A. (1983) Extended HLA/complement allelic haplotypes: evidence for a T/t-like complex in man. *Proceedings of the National Academy of Science USA* **80**, 259.

150 Ober C.L., Martin A.O., Simpson J.L., Hauck W.W., Amos D.B., Kostyu D.D., Fotino M. *et al.* (1983) Shared HLA antigens and reproductive performance among Hutterites. *American Journal of Human Genetics* **35**, 994.

151 Ober C.L., Hauck W.W., Kostyu D.D., O'Brien E., Elias S., Simpson J.L., Martin A.O. (1985) Adverse effects of human leukocyte DR sharing on fertility: a cohort study in a human isolate. *Fertility and Sterility* **44**, 227.

152 Ober C., Elias S., O'Brien E., Kostyu D.D., Hauck W.W., Bombard A. (1988) HLA sharing and fertility in Hutterite couples: evidence for prenatal selection against compatible fetuses. *American Journal of Reproductive Immunology and Microbiology* **18**, 111.

153 Ober C., Elias S., Kostyu D.D., Hauck W.W. (1992) Decreased fecundability in Hutterite couples sharing HLA-DR. *American Journal of Human Genetics* **50**, 6.

154 Ho H.-N., Gill III T.J., Hsieh R.-P., Yang Y.S., Lee T.Y. (1990) Sharing of human leukocyte antigens (HLA) in primary and secondary recurrent spontaneous abortions. *American Journal of Obstetrics and Gynecology* **163**, 178.

155 Rocklin R.E., Kitzmiller J.L., Carpenter C.B., Garovoy M.R., David J.R. (1976) Maternal–fetal relation: absence of an immunologic blocking factor from the serum of women with chronic abortions. *New England Journal of Medicine* **295**, 1209.

156 Fizet D. & Bousquet J. (1983) Absence of a factor blocking cellular cytotoxicity reactions in the serum of women with recurrent abortions. *British Journal of Obstetrics and Gynaecology* **90**, 453.

157 Sargent I.L., Wilkins T. & Redman C.W.G. (1988) Maternal immune responses to the fetus in early pregnancy and recurrent miscarriage. *Lancet* **ii**, 1099.

158 Power D.A., Catto G.R.D., Mason R.J. (1983) The fetus as allograft: evidence for protective antibodies to HLA-linked paternal antigens. *Lancet* **ii**, 701.

159 Opelz G., Sengar D.P.S., Mickey M.R. & Terasaki P.I. (1973) Effect of blood transfusions on subsequent kidney transplants. *Transplantation Proceedings* **5**, 1973.

160 Taylor C. & Faulk W.P. (1981) Prevention of recurrent abortion with leukocyte transfusion. *Lancet* **ii**, 68.

161 Beer A.E., Semprini A.E., Xiaoyn Z., Quebbeman J.F. (1985) Pregnancy outcome in human couples with recurrent spontaneous abortion: HLA antigen profiles, HLA antigen sharing, female serum MLR blocking factors and paternal leukocyte immunization. *Experimental and Clinical Immunogenetics* **2**, 137.

162 Unander A.M. & Lindholm A. (1984) Transfusions of leukocyte rich erythrocyte concentrates: a successful treatment in selected cases of habitual abortion. *American Journal of Obstetrics and Gynaecology* **154**, 516.

163 Reznikoff-Etievant M.F., Durieux I., Huchet J., Salmon C. & Netter A. (1988) Human MHC antigens and paternal leucocyte injections in recurrent spontaneous abortion. In *Early Pregnancy Loss: Mechanisms and Treatment*. Eds F. Sharp & R.W. Beard, p. 375. Royal College of Obstetricians and Gynaecologists, London.

164 Mowbray J.F., Gibbings C., Liddel H., Reginald P.W., Underwood J.L., Beard R.W. (1985) Controlled trial of treatment of recurrent spontaneous abortion by immunisation with paternal cells. *Lancet* **i**, 941.

165 Cauchi M.N., Lim C., Young D.E., Kloss M., Pepperell R.J. (1991) Treatment of recurrent aborters by immunization with paternal cells: controlled trial. *American Journal of Reproductive Immunology* **25**, 16.

166 Ho H.-N., Gill III T.J., Hsieh H.-J., Jiang J.J., Lee T.Y., Hsieh C.Y. (1991) Immunotherapy for recurrent spontaneous abortions in a Chinese population. *American Journal of Reproductive Immunology* **25**, 10.

167 Fraser E.J., Grimes D.A. & Schulz K.F. (1993) Immunization as therapy for recurrent spontaneous abortion: a review and meta-analysis. 82:854–859. *Obstetrics and Gynaecology* **82**, 854.

168 Hofmeyr G.J., Joffe M.I., Bezwoda W.R. & van Iddekinge B. (1987) Immunologic investigation of recurrent pregnancy loss and consequences of immunizating with husbands' leukocytes. *Fertility and Sterility* **48**, 681.

169 Unander A.M. & Lindholm A. (1986) Transfusions of leukocyte-rich erythrocyte concentrates: a successful treatment in selected cases of habitual abortion. *American Journal of Obstetrics and Gynecology*, **154**, 516.

170 Manyonda I.T., Pereira R.S., Pearce J.M. & Sharrock C.E.M. (1993) Limiting dilution analysis of the allo-MHC anti-paternal cytotoxic T cell response. II. Recurrent spontaneous abortion and the effect of immunotherapy. *Clinical and Experimental Immunology* **93**, 132.

171 Chaouat G., Kolb J.P., Kiger N., Stanislawki M., Wegman T.G. (1985) Immunologic consequences of vaccination angainst abortion in mice. *Journal of Immunology* **134**, 1594.

PART 2

Nutrition and Metabolism

Nutrition

MARY CAMPBELL-BROWN & F.E. HYTTEN

Nutritional needs

Assessment of dietary or nutritional needs is based on two types of information.

Physiological requirements

Physiological requirements are based on knowledge of the relations between food intake and health, or of metabolic data derived from healthy people. An intake below the physiological requirement is likely to result in impairment of health and efficiency.

It is convenient to distinguish physiological requirements specific to pregnancy from total physiological requirements. The specific requirements are those which are imposed by the growth and development of the product of conception together with associated changes in maternal structure and metabolism; for example, expansion of blood volume and enlargement of the reproductive organs. Total physiological requirements during pregnancy are not necessarily the sum of ordinary non-pregnant requirements and those specific to pregnancy. For example, there is now evidence that the additional energy required during pregnancy can be compensated, in whole or in part, by economies in maternal metabolism and by reduced physical activity [1].

Social requirements

In the absence of physiological information, it is possible to construct a schedule of requirements that is compatible with health by measuring the habitual food intakes of healthy persons. Requirements so assessed may be considerably higher than physiological requirements, and an intake below the standard will not necessarily lead to impaired health. Suppose, for example, that healthy women are found to take an average of 60 mg of vitamin C daily. Such an intake, being compatible with health, is perfectly acceptable as a nutritional standard, and has the practical advantage that it conforms to the current food habits of the population from which it was derived. But we know, from experimental information and observations on other populations, that much lower intakes of vitamin C will prevent signs of deficiency.

It may be difficult to differentiate clearly between physiological and social requirements, and the requirements recommended by official bodies, especially in the past, have tended to reflect both in some measure. Even when average physiological needs can be precisely assessed, it is customary to add to them an arbitrary safety allowance, and perhaps also to adjust them in order to conform with ordinary dietary practices in the population concerned.

Recommendations by official bodies are not intended for application to individuals, but are guides to the needs of populations and groups. Individuals undoubtedly vary widely in their requirements, and it would be wrong to conclude, without clinical evidence, that because the diet of an individual woman falls somewhat short of the standard, it is therefore necessarily inadequate. But a population or group whose average diet falls much below a physiological standard may be expected to show signs of impairment in some individuals.

The specific requirements of pregnancy

The specific nutritional costs of pregnancy can be divided into capital gains, the value of tissue laid down by the mother and the product of conception, and running costs, the cost of the extra metabolism of pregnancy.

The organic components of added maternal tissue and the uterine contents are simply and conveniently grouped as protein (N × 6.25) and fat. Table 6.1, adapted from the work of Hytten and Leitch [2] on the components of weight gain in pregnancy for Scottish women, shows the mean daily increments of protein and fat for the four quarters of pregnancy, and the total increments for pregnancy.

Table 6.2 and Fig. 6.1 show the net energy equivalents of those increments as their heats of combustion, and the net energy cost of maintaining the fetus and added maternal tissues, computed from their oxygen consumption as set out in Table 6.3. In the last line of Table 6.2, the total net energy is converted to metabolizable energy, in terms of which the energy of food is usually expressed. The efficiency of conversion is not known; 10% has been allowed as a reasonable approximation.

Extension of this work by others [1], to allow comparison between centres in five countries, determined the total energy cost of pregnancy by measuring the increase in basal metabolic rate (BMR) which gives the energy equivalent of the increased oxygen consumption and then adding the energy cost of the estimated 'capital gains'. The outcome can be seen in Table 6.4 with the differences between the countries in their total energy costs of pregnancy. Those for the two European countries (Scotland, 281 MJ, and the Netherlands, 286 MJ), although lower, are similar to the value determined for the earlier group of Scottish women, 323 MJ (shown in Table 6.2), whereas the total for women in the circumstances of a subsistence farming economy in the Gambia, 78 MJ, indicates a pro-

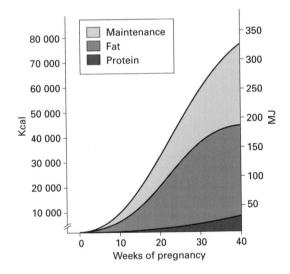

Fig. 6.1. The cumulative energy cost of pregnancy and its components.

Table 6.1. Mean daily increments of protein and fat in the fetus and maternal body.

	Weeks of pregnancy				
	0–10	10–20	20–30	30–40	Cumulative total
Protein, g	0.64	1.84	4.76	6.1	925.0
Fat, g	5.85	24.80	21.85	3.3	3825.0

For the first 10-week period, total increment is divided by 56 since pregnancy is dated from the last menstrual period.

Table 6.2. Cumulative energy cost (equivalent kcal/day) of pregnancy computed from the energy equivalents of protein **167** and fat increments and the energy cost of maintaining the fetus and added maternal tissues. The total is derived from oxygen consumption figures (see Table 6.3) and assumes an RQ of 0.90. *Source*: Hytten and Leitch [2].

	Weeks of pregnancy				Cumulative total kcal (MJ)*
	0–10	10–20	20–30	30–40	
Protein	3.6	10.3	26.7	34.2	5 186 (22)
Fat	55.6	235.6	207.6	31.3	36 329 (152)
Oxygen consumption	44.8	99.0	148.2	227.2	35 717 (144)
Total net energy	104.0	334.9	382.5	292.7	77 234 (323)
Metabolizable energy (total net energy + 10%)	114.0	379.0	421.0	322.0	84 957 (355)

For the first 10-week period, total increment is divided by 56 since pregnancy is dated from the last menstrual period.
* Taken as 5.6 kcal/g (0.023 MJ) for protein and 9.5 kcal/g (0.040 MJ) for fat.

Table 6.3. The extra components of oxygen consumption in pregnancy. *Source*: Hytten and Leitch [2].

Source of extra energy output	Increment at given week of pregnancy				Estimated cost, ml O₂/min	Increment of O₂ consumption ml/min at given week of pregnancy			
	10	20	30	40		10	20	30	40
Cardiac output, l/min	1.0	1.5	1.5	1.5	About 20 at 4.5l/min*	4.5*	6.8*	6.8*	6.8*
Respiration, l/min	0.75	1.50	2.25	3.00	1.0/l ventilation	0.8	1.5	2.3	3.0
Uterine Muscle, g	140	320	600	970	3.7/kg	0.5	1.2	2.2	3.6
Placenta, g									
Wet	20	170	430	650	3.3 per 100 g	0	0.5	2.2	3.7
Dry	2	17	65	110	dry weight				
Fetus, g	5	300	1500	3400	3.65/kg	0	1.1	5.5	12.4
Breast, g	45	180	360	410	3.3/kg	0.1	0.6	1.2	1.4
Kidneys, (mmol Na reabsorbed)	7†	7†	7†	7†	1.0/mmol	7†	7†	7†	7†
					Total ml/min	12.9	18.7	27.2	37.9

* Increase pro rata.
† Kiil *et al.* [17].

Table 6.4. Energy cost (in MJ) of pregnancy in different centres. *Source*: Durnin [1].

	Scotland	Netherlands	Gambia	Thailand*	Philippines*
Fetus	34.00	34.40	29.90	29.90	28.90
Placenta	3.05	3.10	2.34	2.51	2.51
Expanded maternal tissue	12.10	12.30	10.40	10.40	10.10
Maternal fat*	106.00	92.00	27.60	64.40	59.80
Increase in BMR	126.00	144.00	7.90	100.00†	79.00†
Total	281.15	285.80	78.14	207.21	180.31

* Estimated from 10 weeks.
† Estimated from 13 weeks.

found adaptation to adverse circumstances. Thailand with 207 MJ and the Philippines with 188 MJ lie between these two extremes. When standardized for maternal body weight, the total energy costs in four of the five centres were about 250 MJ, with the small differences between them explained by variation in the amount of fat stored. The exception was the Gambia where additional economies in the running costs of pregnancy were found to have been possible.

Protein

The quality of a protein depends on its amino acid composition. In practice, the value of a protein or protein mixture in the diet depends not only on its amino acid composition, but also on the proportion absorbed from the intestine described as the digestibility and the conditions under which it is eaten. Utilization for the construction of new tissue will be diminished if, for example, the energy supplied by the diet is so low that protein must be used as fuel or if the protein supply is uneconomically large. Many devices and conventions have been adopted in order to express the usefulness of dietary protein mixtures in practice, but this is not the place to describe the complexities of the procedures. The interested reader may be referred to the report of an FAO/WHO/UNU Expert Group [3]. The point of reference is a protein which can be utilized completely, such as that of whole egg or of milk. The value of other proteins is then expressed as a proportion of the reference protein by calculation from tables which give comparative values for its amino acid content, and digestibility. In an ordinary British diet, the protein it contains has a value of about 70%, whereas in many developing countries, the value of their dietary protein is between 60–70% of the reference protein; where the protein of the staple is notably poor, as with diets where cassava predominates, it may be as low as 50–60%.

The increments of protein shown in Table 6.1 are proteins that have been fully assimilated. The amounts therefore correspond to a dietary protein with a value of 100%. It is seen that the mean daily increment of stored protein during the final weeks of pregnancy averages about 6 g. Where only 70% is assimilated, as in Britain, that corresponds to an additional daily requirement of about 8.5 g dietary protein. In countries where the value of the protein is lower, the daily addition would be proportionately increased, unless it can be assumed that, with smaller mothers and babies, the increments of new tissue during pregnancy are smaller than those reported.

This calculation, that the average British woman will need an additional 8.5 g of dietary protein daily to remain in balance during late pregnancy, assumes that there is no alteration in the metabolism of protein. That assumption has been questioned by Naismith [4], who showed in the pregnant rat that there are enzyme changes in the liver which reduce its capacity to form urea, thus sparing protein for anabolic purposes. In women, the characteristically low blood urea level, which hitherto has been attributed to changed renal function, is consistent with this possibility. If they can be shown to share this adaptation with the rat, then protein requirements for pregnancy may be substantially less than the calculated 8.5 g per day. More recently it has been suggested from an ^{15}N stable isotope study of protein turnover and retention in Jamaican women [5] that the weight of protein deposited during pregnancy may be more than the amounts shown in Table 6.1. But the difficulties in measuring and the dangers of extrapolating the small changes in nitrogen retention during pregnancy, in studies which, because of their complexity, cover short periods of time and with the subjects away from their normal diet and environment, has meant that many uncertainties remain as to what extent economies made in nitrogen metabolism can contribute to the amount of protein required to support a pregnancy and whether the size of this requirement may be greater than that calculated by Hytten and Leitch [2,5,6].

Fat and energy

Under ordinary conditions, protein is required for structural purposes only, and not for activity. Carbohydrate as fuel is required by the maternal brain, which uses glucose, and by the fetus, since it burns carbohydrate almost exclusively. Apart from that, only an extremely small amount of carbohydrate is required, as structural material in the brain, cartilage and connective tissue. Apart from requirements for fat as fuel for muscular work, there is a need for long chain unsaturated fatty acids which are essential, both as components of cellular and subcellular membranes and as precursors of biologically active metabolites which include the prostaglandins, prostacyclins, thromboxanes and leukotrienes [7]. Fats also act as a vehicle for the carriage and the efficient absorption of fat-soluble vitamins and some other substances. As the need for fats other than as a fuel makes up only a small proportion of the total fat intake, the requirements for both carbohydrate and fat as fuel are included in the calculated energy allowance.

Disregarding carbohydrate, increased stores of which during pregnancy are trivial, the additional requirement for energy specific to pregnancy comes from two demands: the protein and fat accumulated by the fetus and the mother, and the addition to metabolism which the new tissues incur. The energy represented by the new tissue can be expressed as its heat of combustion, and the added cost of metabolism as oxygen consumption. Table 6.1 summarizes the daily amounts of protein and lipid added during normal pregnancy, and the first two lines of Table 6.2 give their heats of combustion. The third line of Table 6.3 gives estimates of increased energy expenditure due to the extra work of the maternal heart, respiratory and renal effort and in maintaining the new tissues. No allowance has been made for the possible cost of maintaining the higher body temperature characteristic of pregnancy, but it may not be negligible although there is evidence that postprandial thermogenesis, a further source of energy expenditure, is reduced in well-fed women in late pregnancy [8].

Bisdee and James [9] showed that a rise in sleeping metabolic rate of some 80 kcal/24 hours was linked to the rise in progesterone in the luteal phase of the menstrual cycle, though not directly to the rise in basal body temperature. During the third quarter of pregnancy, the extra energy requirement attributable to laying down new tissues (chiefly maternal fat) is at a maximum, about 240 kcal (1 MJ) daily on average, and the additional oxygen consumption is estimated to average about 150 kcal (0.6 MJ) daily, giving a total of about 390 kcal (1.6 MJ) daily. During the final quarter of pregnancy, fetal tissue is increasing rapidly but the rate of maternal fat storage is considerably reduced. The energy represented by daily increments of new tissue is only about 65 kcal (0.3 MJ), on average. The total average addition to energy requirements imposed during the final weeks of pregnancy is thus about 300 kcal (1.3 MJ) daily.

It used to be thought that the energy needs specific to pregnancy would be greatest during the final weeks, the period when the fetus grows most rapidly. Table 6.2 and Fig. 6.1 make it clear that this is not the situation. Specific energy requirements are greatest during the two middle quarters of pregnancy, when relatively large amounts of maternal fat are being laid down to form an energy bank. During the final quarter, such fat storage practically stops, and most of the energy required for the formation of new tissue is that due to the growth of the fetus, which is accompanied by a considerable rise in oxygen consumption. The overall effect is to spread the additions to total energy needs over about three-quarters of pregnancy, and there is no increase in demand in the final weeks.

The estimated additional cost of pregnancy during its final quarter, 300 kcal (1.3 MJ) daily on average, is thus only about one-quarter of the ordinary expenditure on activity envisaged for the non-pregnant woman, proposed as being $0.56 \times BMR$ by FAO/WHO/UNU [3]. The energy costs of pregnancy could therefore be met without additional supplies from the diet, by reducing activity. Although the energy cost of activity increases in late pregnancy, some reduction in the amount of activity seems to be usual and appears to be a physiological characteristic rather than a conscious change of behaviour or due to taking advice to rest. This is what appears to have occurred in the women of the Gambia who were part of the Five Country Study (Table 6.4); they reduced their energy expenditure during the second and third trimesters at least in part by reducing the rate at which they carried out their heavier work such as bending and digging and by reducing their leisure activity [10].

Calcium

The specific increment of calcium requirements is about 30 g, almost all in the fetal skeleton, with most of it being deposited during the third trimester [11]. That amount is only 2.5% of the calcium in the maternal skeleton and can be provided from that reservoir if necessary. The exception may be with teenage pregnancies, where the mother is herself still growing, so that supplements may be advisable.

Iron

Of all the nutrients, iron is the most subject to controversy and it is surprising that even the basic physiological estimates are far from agreed.

The iron requirement specific to pregnancy is that which is lost to the mother at parturition, i.e. iron in the fetus and placenta and in any maternal blood lost. Estimates of the iron content of the term fetus have ranged from 200 to 600 mg [12–14] and the content of the placenta from under 30 mg [15] to as much as 170 mg [16]. The estimate by the joint FAO/WHO Expert Group [17] of 315 mg for the fetus plus placenta seems as good as any. Both the FAO/WHO Expert Group and Pritchard and Scott [18] give the average iron content of blood lost at parturition as 250 mg, corresponding to 500 ml or more of blood. That seems excessive, but, added to the iron content of the fetus, comes to something less than 600 mg of iron lost to the mother as a result of pregnancy; it corresponds to roughly 4 mg iron daily during the second half of pregnancy.

Whether iron required for the expansion of maternal red cell mass should be added to the estimate seems to be a question of philosophy rather than of science, in the present state of knowledge. An estimate of the physiological increase of red cell mass (Chapter 3) corresponds to an increase of 290 mg iron. The Joint FAO/WHO Expert Group suggests 500 mg, apparently based on the expansion of red cell mass, which is possible when therapeutic doses

of iron are given [19]. Whatever the figure, the iron involved is presumably available to the mother when pregnancy is over, apart from that lost by haemorrhage at parturition, which has already been allowed for. There seems to be no evidence that a maximum red cell response is necessary for healthy pregnancy nor, conversely, that a moderate fall in haemoglobin concentration is harmful. At all events, the iron needed for the extra red cells is to some extent compensated by iron saved during the cessation of menstruation, some 120 mg per pregnancy [20].

Other minerals and trace elements

The specific increments of the major elements such as sodium and potassium can be readily calculated and were assessed by Hytten et al. as 947 and 320 mmol (about 22 and 12 g). The magnesium content of the healthy full-term fetus was measured by Widdowson and Dickerson [21] as approximately 1 g, most of which is acquired in the last 2 months of pregnancy. This, together with the small amount needed for the growth in maternal tissues, is about 5% of the 20 g in the body of an adult woman and can be met without difficulty from the maternal diet.

With recent advances in technology, the increment in some essential trace elements has been calculated [22]. Swanson and King [23] estimated this to be 100 mg for zinc, and Schroeder et al. [24], assuming a 5 kg gain in lean tissue, estimated the increment for selenium as 1.25 mg. The copper contained in a full-term fetus is 14 mg, with approximately half of it stored in the liver at a concentration eight times that in the maternal liver and thought to provide reserve to provide for the early months of life [14]. Manganese, molybdenum, chromium and cobalt are also confirmed as being essential trace elements and of these the fetal liver concentration is available for manganese, chromium and cobalt and has been found to be similar to maternal levels, again suggesting a need for a fetal reserve [14].

Vitamins

Much has been written about requirements in pregnancy, chiefly to show that it is easier to induce deficiency in the pregnant than in the non-pregnant woman, the difference being attributed to the demands of the fetus. Until recently there has been little or no information about specific requirements but with evidence that there is teratogenic risk from excessive intakes of vitamin A there is now interest in this area of research [25]. The possible effect of the increased losses of vitamins in the urine remains uninvestigated. The indiscriminate use in clinical practice of the fat-soluble vitamins is now being called into question and women planning a pregnancy are now advised to avoid other than recommended doses of vitamin A [26]. Of the B vitamins, it is probably safe to assume that, during pregnancy as in the non-pregnant state, requirements of thiamin, riboflavin and pyridoxine are related to energy intake. With the now unimpeachable evidence that the use of folic acid supplementation before conception and during the first trimester will prevent most neural tube defects [27], attention is being paid as to how this can best be given. The size of the supplement is more than can be achieved through dietary change so at present the advice is for all women planning a pregnancy to take 0.4 mg folic acid daily as a tablet.

Vitamin C and vitamin E both have among other essential roles anti-oxidant activity in common with several other nutrient-derived compounds. These include the trace elements zinc, copper, selenium and manganese which are essential components of antioxidant enzymes and the carotenoids which can also be precursors of vitamin A [28]. Through their antioxidant capacity, tissues are protected from damage by the highly reactive free radicals produced during oxidative metabolism which, if not adequately controlled, are involved in a variety of disease processes. Among these there is now sufficient evidence to include the pathophysiological processes of pre-ecalampsia [29,30].

Recommended dietary allowances during pregnancy

During recent decades, numerous official bodies and individual authorities have published schedules which specify the amounts of energy and of nutrients that ought to be provided to maintain populations in health. As explained in the introduction to this chapter, such schedules may be based on estimated physiological needs, or the observed dietary habits of healthy people, or on a mixture of evidence. As new information accumulated, the schedules were revised, and the emphasis on physiology became more explicit. An interesting fact is that the recommended allowances of energy and of nutrients have usually become smaller as knowledge has improved. With respect to pregnancy, most of the early schedules appeared to assume that additional requirements over and above those of the non-pregnant woman were imposed only during the final half or final third of pregnancy.

Tables 6.5, 6.6 and 6.7 summarize recommended allowances for non-pregnant and pregnant women proposed by agencies of the United Nations and by official bodies in the UK and the US. The recommendations of official bodies in developing countries have tended to follow those of the United Nations agencies, and need not be described here.

The UK's Department of Health [31], with the exception of energy, defined its allowances, defined the reference nutrient intake (RNI), as:

> an amount of nutrient that is enough, or more than enough, for about 97% of people in a group. If average intake of a group is at RNI, then the risk of deficiency in the group is small. The RNI is a notional 2 standard deviations above the Estimated Average Requirement (EAR) in a group of individuals. It does not cover any additional needs arising from diseases, such as infections, disorders of the gastrointestinal tract or metabolic abnormalities.

There is no evidence to suggest that intakes in excess of the recommendations confer any benefit; indeed for energy and certain nutrients, intakes in excess may be harmful, and, where there is evidence for this, official bodies have included upper limits to the safe intakes shown in Table 6.7. With some evidence of health risk from excessive intake of protein over the longer term, the UK's Department of Health recommends that intakes for adults should not be more than twice the RNI [32]. 'The recom-

Table 6.5. Daily recommended allowances for non-pregnant women doing light work and the increment recommended to support a pregnancy. *Sources*: WHO [3,35,36], US National Research Council [32] and UK Department of Health [31].

	WHO, NR		US, RDA		UK, RNI	
	Non-pregnant	Pregnancy increment	Non-pregnant	Pregnancy increment	Non-pregnant	Pregnancy increment
Weight, kg	55.0 [3]	12.5 [3]	58.0–63.0	12.5	60.0	12.5
Energy,						
kcal	1990.0* [3]	200.0* [3]	2200.0†	300.0†	1940.0*	200.0*
MJ	8.30* [3]	0.84* [3]	9.2†	1.26† in trimesters 2 and 3	8.10*	0.84* in trimester 3
Protein, g	45.0 [3]	6.0 [3]	46.0–50.0	10.0	45.0	6.0
Thiamin, mg	0.9 [35]	0.1‡ [35]	1.0	0.4	0.8	0.1 for trimester 3
Riboflavin, mg	1.3 [35]	0.2‡ [35]	1.2	0.3	1.1	0.3
Niacin, mgEq	14.5 [35]	2.3‡ [35]	15.0	2.0	13.0	None
Vitamin B_6, mg	–	–	1.6	0.6	1.2	None
Vitamin B_{12}, µg	1.0 [36]	0.4 [36]	2.0	0.2	1.5	None
Folate, µg	170 [36]	200–300 [36]	180	220	200	100
Vitamin C, mg	30 [35]	20 [35]	60	10	40	10
Vitamin A, µg						
retinol equivalent	500 [36]	100 [36]	800	None	600	100
Vitamin D, µg	2.5 [35]	10 in later half [35]	5	5	0 if exposed to sun	10

NR: nutritional requirements; RDA: recommended daily allowance; RNI: reference nutrient intakes.
* Estimated Average Requirement (EAR).
† Average Energy Allowance (AER).
‡ Second half of pregnancy.

mended intake of energy . . . is equated with the estimated average requirement, and therefore does not refer to individuals but only to groups'. That is to say, the allowance for energy has not been increased so as to cover individuals with requirements above the population average; it is assumed that individuals, with needs below the average will balance those with extra needs.

In a similar vein, the US National Research Council's recommended allowances [32], excepting calories, 'are defined to afford a margin sufficiently above average physiological requirements to cover variations among practically all individuals in the general population. The allowances provide a buffer against common stresses . . . but they are not necessarily adequate to meet the additional requirements of persons depleted by disease, traumatic stress, or prior dietary inadequacies.'

Inevitably, such recommendations are tentative and are bound to be revised as knowledge improves, but the following points should not be forgotten. The US National Research Council's recommendations for any one nutrient 'presuppose that requirements for energy and other

Table 6.6. Daily recommended allowances for minerals and trace elements for non-pregnant women and the increment recommended to support a pregnancy. *Sources*: WHO [34–37], US National Research Council [32] and UK Department of Health [31].

Mineral	WHO, NR		USA, RDA		UK, RNI	
	Non-pregnant	Pregnancy increment	Non-pregnant	Pregnancy increment	Non-pregnant	Pregnancy increment
Calcium, mg (mmol)	400–500 [34]	700 [34]	800	400	700 (17.5)	None
Magnesium, mg (mmol)	200–300 [35]	None [35]	280	20	270 (10.9)	None
Iron, mg (μmol)	14 [36]	None [36]	15	15	14.8 (260)	None
Zinc, mg (μmol)	6.5 [37]	0.8–6.8 [37]	12	3	7.0 (110)	None
Copper, mg (μmol)	1.15 [37]	None [37]	1.5–3.0	None	1.2 (19)	None
Selenium, μg (μmol)	30 [37]	9 [37]	55	10	60 (0.8)	None
Iodine, μg (μmol)	120–150 [37]	25 [37]	150	25	140 (1.1)	None

Table 6.7. Daily safe intakes of those nutrients where there is insufficient information to recommend intakes. *Sources*: WHO [35], US National Research Council [32] and UK Department of Health [31].

Nutrient	Pantothenic acid, (mg)	Biotin, μg	Vitamin E, mg	Vitamin K, μg	Manganese, mg (μmol)	Molybdenum, μg	Chromium, μg (μmol)
WHO	—	—	—	—	—	2/kg	—
US	4–7	30–100*	8*; pregnancy increment, 2*	1/kg*	2–5	75–250	50–200
UK	3–7	10–200	>3	1/kg	1.4 (26)	50–400	25 (0.5)

* RDA [32].

nutrients are met'. Official recommendations are intended as guides to the planning and assessment of diets and food supplies on a large scale; *they do not provide yardsticks against which to assess the diets of individual women.*

Since their initiation during the 1930s, all requirement schedules have had as their principal aim the maintenance of health. At one time it seemed as if targets for attainment in the supply of essential nutrients and desirable foods could not be fixed too high, as if it were axiomatic that we cannot have too much of a good thing. This is bad physiology. An excess of some nutrients is harmful, and an excess of energy intake over expenditure notoriously leads to obesity. Furthermore, it is bad psychology: the very high recommended allowances

174 originally proposed, especially in the US, scarcely helped to bolster the morale of less well fed and physically smaller people, and caused some overdiagnosis of malnutrition where little existed. The current trend towards a more realistic appraisal of requirements in terms of physiological needs is therefore timely and helpful. It is perfectly legitimate, of course, to add a safety factor to a physiological average, provided that it is specified and is known to be harmless. And it would do no harm to adopt a still higher social target, provided the basis of the formulation is explicit, and there is known to be no danger in excess. Acceptability and palatability remain desirable in dietetic matters.

A practical implication is that the routine administration of protein, mineral or vitamin supplements to the diets of women who are basically healthy and adequately fed should never be necessary unless there is a clear and specific clinical indication.

Whatever the role of malnutrition in causing morbidity and mortality associated with pregnancy, millions of women in the developing countries and in the poorer sections of more affluent countries have reproduced so successfully on diets far below those recommended that a population explosion has resulted. This is not a reason for brushing aside the importance of improving nutrition wherever possible; but it is a reason for maintaining a sense of perspective, and for remembering that nutritional policies have social as well as clinical implications.

Diets taken by pregnant women

Many surveys of dietary intake in pregnancy from many parts of the world have been and continue to be published. All that need be said here is that the techniques of dietary survey are extremely difficult, that very few have used truly quantitative techniques, and that they are, of necessity, like nutrient balance studies applicable to a small and often unrepresentative part of the population [33].

In general, the evidence is that pregnant women consume diets whose energy value is considerably less than the calculated specific increment for pregnancy given in Table 6.2. The deficit is about 200 kcal (0.84 MJ) per day, but some recent studies suggest that many women may eat little if any more than before pregnancy [38,39]. The difference is made up from savings in energy expenditure.

A considerable amount has also been written about qualitative peculiarities of diets eaten by pregnant women, in particular those enforced by food taboos [2,40]. The effects of food habits and taboos have been poorly studied and may be important where, for example, vegetarians and vegans immigrate to a country with varieties of food to which they are unaccustomed. There is evidence from Asians coming to the UK in the 1960s and 70s that their diet had adjusted to locally available foods and seemed to be adequate in all except vitamin D. Here, lack of sunshine may have been more important than nutrient intake, and in vitamin B_{12} among those who were strict vegetarians [41,42]. Nevertheless, this low intake of vitamin B_{12} appears sufficient to protect them from any nutritional deficiency, probably through the capacity for reabsorption from the enterohepatic circulation which can rise to close to 100% [43].

The effect of inadequate diet

This chapter has so far dealt with the nutrient needs of pregnancy based on reasonably well grown, healthy women with an adequate food supply and living in normally comfortable conditions; such women are able not only to provide for the growth of the fetus, but also to accumulate reserves which would, if need be, protect it against at least short periods of deprivation.

When measured food intakes are compared with estimated needs the agreement is, on the whole, reassuring, and is confirmed by the rarity of reported deficiency disease among pregnant women. Iron deficiency appears to be a notable exception and is discussed in Chapter 3. Evidence that inadequate diet in pregnancy has adverse effects on childbearing is largely epidemiological: the fact that the poorer and presumably less well fed sections of the population have greater perinatal morbidity and mortality, and smaller babies than the more affluent and presumably better-fed classes. But although it is usually assumed in this context that differences of socioeconomic circumstances are predominantly differences of nutrition, they are much more complex: women who eat a poor diet in adult life have generally eaten a poor diet as children and are poorly grown; moreover, they often smoke more and have living standards which fall short of those of more affluent women in many respects.

The direct evidence of a cause-and-effect relation that could be provided by a feeding experiment is also unsatisfactory; those that have been reported have generally been poorly designed and the results have been neither consistent nor statistically convincing. Rush [44] concluded that:

> attempts at nutritional supplementation, while well-intentioned, have not always had the desired effect. First, it is clear that high-density protein supplements are consistently associated with depression, rather than increase in mean birth weight. Second, only small increments in mean birthweight (on average, about 50 g) have been found in association with programmes of aggressive nutritional counselling and/or supplementation with preparations of lower protein density.

Rush's conclusions are supported by Kramer in a meta-analysis which included more recent supplementation trials [45] and gave maternal weight gain with the mean increase being 21 g per week. In a randomized trial, one of those included in these two overview studies, Campbell-Brown [46], found an increase of less than 40 g in birthweight when a group of Aberdeen primigravidae, judged to be of poor nutritional status, were given a supplement averaging 189 kcal per day. It is possible that women in underdeveloped countries who have low birthweight babies do not benefit as much as expected from dietary supplementation because lack of food is not the basic problem. These women usually work hard under hot conditions, a situation which will tend to cause a reduction in uteroplacental blood flow and provide an additional reason for their small babies [47].

The opposite situation, where basically healthy, well-nourished women are subjected to severe dietary deprivation, occurred during the famine in northwest Holland from September 1944 to May 1945. During this period an unusually severe winter and a blockade of food supplies caused daily energy intake to fall below 1000 kcal (4.2 MJ). The most obvious effect of severe undernutrition on reproduction is infecundity; the famine was followed 9 months later by a massive fall in the birth rate [48], but large numbers of women were pregnant during all or part of the famine. When the last trimester or last two trimesters of pregnancy coincided with the famine, the birthweight of the babies was reduced on average by some 350 g [49]. Linear growth was little affected, which raises the possibility that these babies were not particularly stunted, merely thin, and the 350 g deficit which distinguished them from the babies whose mothers escaped the famine may have been largely the luxury of a subcutaneous fat store. Furthermore, these babies appeared to have suffered no permanent effect on their subsequent growth and intellectual development [49,50].

There is now however disquieting evidence of more subtle damage from exposure *in utero* to this famine, with long-term consequences for the individual. When the male children entered military service at age 18, those exposed during the last trimester of pregnancy and the first few months of life were found to have lower rates of obesity when compared with the young men not exposed to the famine, and those whose exposure was during the first half of pregnancy with no deficit in birth weight, had higher obesity rates; the inference being that nutritional deprivation had affected the factors which in later life control obesity [51]. When the female fetuses reached childbearing age, those who were exposed during the first half of pregnancy without any deficit in their own birthweight had babies of considerably reduced birthweight, by contrast those who were exposed during the second half of pregnancy with their own birthweight conspicuously reduced had babies of normal birthweight [52]. These longer term outcomes give support to Barker's hypothesis that the nourishment the fetus receives from its mother influences its health in later life [53].

Further evidence that rate of growth *in utero*, which reflects at least in part maternal nutrition, is associated with risk of adult disease has now been found in several studies which examined in adulthood birth cohorts where there are records of fetal and sometimes infant growth with or without information on maternal nutrition. These associations include coronary artery disease, diabetes and chronic bronchitis and risk factors for these diseases: carbohydrate tolerance, blood pressure, lipid metabolism, haemostasis and lung function, all giving further support to Barker's hypothesis, and, moreover, where there is information on the maternal diet the quality as well as the quantity appears to be important [54].

At the time of birth, the fetus appears remarkably unaffected by maternal dietary inadequacy during pregnancy. The reasons may lie in the profound metabolic readjustments which characterize pregnancy and are made by the mother to provide for the fetus under a wide range of circumstances. Where these fail, the fetus may make adaptive changes in order to survive and these are reflected in an increased risk of disease in later life.

Metabolic adjustments

Metabolism during pregnancy was for long interpreted, implicitly or explicitly, as the superimposition of a parasite (the product of conception) upon normal non-pregnant metabolism. Maternal changes were accordingly regarded as reactions to stress or to depletion of reserves by the fetus. That concept is no longer tenable, for several reasons.

In the first place, many of the metabolic adjustments of pregnancy are well established, often fully, during the early weeks and months of pregnancy when the product of conception is still too small to make significant demands on maternal reserves. Such changes cannot be explained by stress; they seem, rather, to be anticipatory, preparing the way for much greater fetal demands that will have to be met at a later stage. The increase of maternal depot fat during midpregnancy is a striking example.

Secondly, the metabolic adjustments are too widespread, complex and fundamental. It is now well recognized that the changes in the composition of blood which characterize pregnancy cannot be explained by apparent haemodilution and that some metabolic changes appear to involve a radical resetting of hypothalamic control centres. For example, body temperature rises and the P_{CO_2} falls, with considerable effects on the protein-binding of thyroxine and perhaps on other aspects of metabolism. The entire maternal metabolism is working from a different base, the mother is almost another species.

Thirdly, the concept of competition between the product of conception and the maternal organism is not as simple as may appear at first sight. Under ordinary conditions pregnancy is a period in which overall nutritional balances are positive, that is anabolic even under the most adverse circumstances [1]. It is difficult, without carcass analysis, to separate the maternal and the fetal components of the nutritional balance sheet, but the estimates already given indicate that, in general, the physiological state is one in which both mother and fetus are gaining. Competition for nutrients, if it occurs, is probably limited to the final weeks of pregnancy, when the product of conception is large and increasing rapidly and when the maternal food intake may be limited by lack of appetite or by shortage of supplies. Even then, evidence of maternal depletion is by no means unequivocal or easy to interpret. The situation may well be otherwise if the pregnant woman is young enough to be still growing herself. Harrison [55] has provided evidence that maternal growth during pregnancy in very young teenage Nigerians, and the birthweight of their babies, was enhanced by nutritional supplements.

There are other, more subtle nutritional influences on pregnancy, through placental size, for example, which is positively correlated with birthweight. The growth of the placenta is increased in early pregnancy and at birth where there is a low maternal haemoglobin in basically well-fed British women and also at birth in pregnancies at high altitude, but it is reduced at birth where there is severe iron deficiency with anaemia in Indian women. The physiological influences determining the placental size are clearly different in the three circumstances, that underlying the British pregnancies may be a response to the growth potential of the pregnancy, that at high altitude to a relative anoxia, and that in India to a poor nutritional environment [53,56,57].

In practice, the situation is complicated by the fact that many of the physiological changes which characterize pregnancy simulate pathology in the non-pregnant state. Pathology is a deviation from the normal, and under ordinary conditions the normal is defined by reference to Claude Bernard's concept of an unchanging *milieu intérieur*. But during healthy pregnancy, the *milieu intérieur* undergoes substantial change, and new reference standards of normality are essential. Even then, the fact remains that in pregnancy the normal tends to merge gradually into the abnormal with no sharp boundary. This means that it is sometimes impossible to discuss the physiological without reference to pathology; for example, in discussing carbohydrate metabolism it is necessary to review the relation of pregnancy to diabetes mellitus.

Knowledge and understanding of metabolic adjustments during pregnancy is still so incomplete that it is not possible to do more than indicate trends from the few areas that have been studied. Information on the renal excretion of nutrients is in Chapter 10. Carbohydrate metabolism and calcium metabolism merit chapters to themselves (Chapters 7 and 8, respectively).

Overall energy balance

One of the more important protective devices for the fetus is a major modification of the mother's energy balance which leads to the storage of some 3.5 kg of depot fat. Energy storage in body fat occurs in other species where high energy costs are anticipated: in birds before migration and in mammals before hibernation, but storage on this scale in man is quite unknown in healthy adult life apart from pregnancy. It obviously makes biological sense; the average woman will enter the last trimester of pregnancy with a considerable buffer against possible food shortage amounting to more than 30000 kcal (126 MJ). Figure 6.1 shows that fat accumulation dominates the overall specific energy cost of pregnancy; it is greatest at

a time when maintenance costs of extra metabolism are relatively slight and stops in late pregnancy when maintenance costs are high, so that it has a smoothing effect on costs. Moreover, Fig. 6.1 shows clearly that the energy costs of maintenance could be completely subsidized during late pregnancy by the stored fat.

Evidence suggests that the stimulus to accumulate this large extra fat store is not simply through the appetite-satiety centres driving the mother to eat more, but by a more fundamental change in the control of energy balance, probably caused by progesterone. In female rats the hypothalamic centre controlling total body fat is reset by progesterone so that the new level of body fat store is achieved either by eating more or by expending less energy, or both [58]. The pregnant woman usually does both, increasing her daily food intake up to 200 kcal (0.84 MJ) and reducing energy output in several ways: she is relatively listless, spends more time at rest and performs tasks with more economy of effort. There is a general relaxation of voluntary muscle, and a reduction in free thyroid hormone (Chapter 13), possibly allowing all maternal tissue to metabolize at a slightly reduced tempo. Whether there are other, more subtle ways in which the woman can economize remains to be investigated. Some basic metabolic processes may be reduced which could explain the reduction in resting metabolic rate in early to mid-pregnancy shown by Lawrence *et al.* [10] and by Durnin [1], and Illingworth *et al.* [8] found that the thermogenic response to a meal was reduced in midpregnancy.

It has to be said that most of the evidence given here is derived from studies of well-nourished Western women for whom the anticipatory storage of fat as a buffer is least likely to be appropriate. But from a more recent study (Table 6.4), it would seem that in different parts of the world and in their different circumstances women are able to make adaptations to their energy economy which reflect the adequacy of the food available to meet their energy needs. This does not seem to be a genetic trait, rather a response to immediate circumstances; the Gambian women, for example, were able to store more fat and increase their basal energy

178 expenditure when their subsistence diet was supplemented.

Nutrient metabolism

Apart from glucose (Chapter 7), there are relatively few data about the metabolism of individual nutrients in pregnancy. Knowledge is still at an early stage, and is almost entirely restricted to a description of changing plasma levels.

Nutrients in blood

Protein

There is little disagreement about the general pattern of plasma protein changes in pregnancy but considerable dispute about absolute values. What follows is, firstly, from the review of the literature up to 1970 by Hytten and Leitch [2], during which time almost all the studies were made using simple paper electrophoresis and, secondly, from the more recent study by Studd [59] using gel immunoelectrophoresis which is capable of separating many more protein fractions.

Total protein The total protein content of serum falls within the first trimester and reaches a plateau at midpregnancy which is about 1 g per 100 ml below non-pregnant levels. In round figures the fall is from about 7 to 6 g per 100 ml (70–60 g/l).

Albumin Albumin concentration falls, usually quite abruptly in early pregnancy and then more slowly until late pregnancy. The overall fall is about 1 g per 100 ml, typically from about 3.5 to 2.5 g per 100 ml (35–25 g/l). It is this fall which is largely responsible for the fall in total protein concentration.

Albumin plays an important role both because of its influence on colloid osmotic pressure and as a non-specific carrier protein for several hormones, drugs, free fatty acids, unconjugated bilirubin and various ions. The relation between albumin concentration and colloid osmotic pressure is shown in Fig. 6.2, from the study of Robertson [60]. Colloid osmotic pressure must be clearly distinguished from total

osmolality. In somewhat oversimplified terms, it is a measure of the effect in attracting water to large molecules such as protein which cannot diffuse across semipermeable membranes such as cell walls. The pressure is measured as the hydrostatic pressure which has to be applied to the colloid-containing solution to prevent water moving across a semipermeable membrane; the technique requires relatively elaborate equipment. A fall in colloid osmotic pressure will therefore allow water to move from the plasma into the cells or out of vessels and it undoubtedly plays a part in the increased fragility of red cells which have become somewhat more distended by water [61], in oedema of the lower limbs, and possibly also in the glomerular filtration rate (see Chapter 10).

In terms of carrier capacity of drugs, for example, the fall in concentration of albumin probably makes little overall difference. The total circulating albumin will fall by about 10 g, from around 90 to 80 g in the first half of pregnancy, but then rises again as the plasma volume expands, to reach levels in late pregnancy at least as great as in the non-pregnant state (Fig. 6.3).

The reason for the fall in albumin concentration is unknown. Tovey [62] suggested, without evidence, that the fall might be due to increased breakdown in the kidney, but Hønger [63] could find no evidence of changed rates of either catabolism or synthesis of albumin, although his conclusion that total intravascular albumin was unchanged was a fortuitous observation based on his choice of late pregnancy to compare with

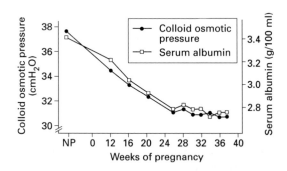

Fig. 6.2. The relation between albumin concentration and serum colloid osmotic pressure. NP: non-pregnant.

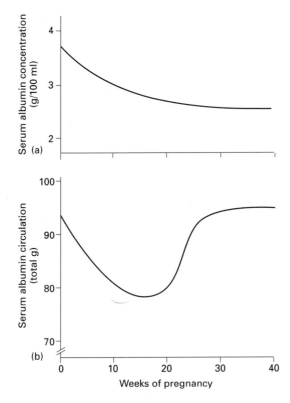

Fig. 6.3. Serum albumin in pregnancy. (a) The concentration. (b) The total in circulation.

the non-pregnant state. A woman of average size is synthesizing and catabolizing about 10 g of albumin each day. A drop of 10 g in, say, the first 100 days of pregnancy represents a decreased synthesis or increased breakdown of only about 1%, too small to be estimated by current methods. Alternatively, the 10 g of intravascular protein could be transferred to the extravascular compartment where at least half the albumin normally resides, without any change of metabolism at all.

The globulins In total, the globulins show a rise of about 10% in concentration during pregnancy from about 0.2 to 0.3 g per 100 ml (2–3 g/l) in the non-pregnant state [59], but there are large individual variations and the patterns of change are complex.

Of particular interest is caeruloplasmin, an α_2-globulin, which binds copper in a non-

exchangeable form and contains most of the copper present in plasma. It increases in concentration early in pregnancy rising to twice the pre-pregnancy level by term and accounting for the rise in copper concentration when that of most non-lipid nutrients falls (Figs 6.4 and 6.5) [64,65]. Other well-defined physiological functions of the globulins are referred to elsewhere: for example, the immunoglobulins (Chapter 5), transferrin (Chapter 3), thyroxine-binding globulin (Chapter 13) and the specific pregnancy proteins (Chapter 16); the remainder are listed by Studd [59].

Lipids

Pregnancy is characterized by a considerable rise in most plasma lipids to the extent that the picture is frequently referred to as a hyperlipidaemia. An extensive study of changing lipid metabolism in pregnancy has been published by Fahraeus [66].

Total lipids The total lipids are a heterogeneous collection of compounds which have in common only their solubility in solvents such as chloroform, alcohols and ethers. The main components are triglycerides, cholesterol, phospholipids and non-esterified (free) fatty acids. Other lipids of physiological importance are present in smaller amounts; they include the steroid hormones and the fat soluble vitamins. During pregnancy, the total lipid concentration rises from about 600 to 1000 mg per 100 ml maternal serum.

Triglycerides (neutral fat) Triglycerides rise progressively throughout pregnancy in keeping with the rise in total lipids [66–68] but their distribution in lipoproteins is altered [68].

Cholesterol There is general agreement that a linear increase in the serum cholesterol level takes place from early pregnancy until the last few weeks, when it appears to stop. A consistent finding which cannot yet be explained is the fall in concentration which occurs in the first trimester before the more obvious rise begins [66,67,69–72] (Fig. 6.4). The similarity of the curves in all the published studies is the more

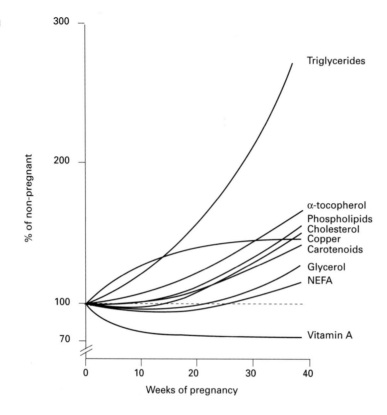

Fig. 6.4. A schematic representation of the relative changes in the concentrations of lipid moieties and of the trace element copper in the plasma in pregnancy. 100% = the normal non-pregnant level. NEFA: non-esterified fatty acids.

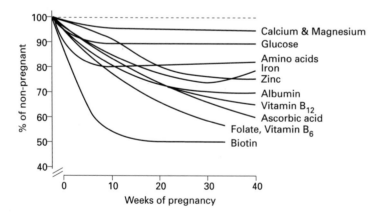

Fig. 6.5. A schematic representation of the relative changes in the concentrations of water-soluble nutrients in the plasma during pregnancy. 100% = the normal non-pregnant level.

surprising in that they were not made under standardized conditions either in respect of fasting or of time of day. The regulation of cholesterol concentration during pregnancy is not well understood. Potter and Nestel [73] could find no change in cholesterol metabolism and no increase in the rate of cholesterol synthesis, although there was a rise in bile acid output bal-anced by a fall in neutral steroid excretion which resembled that reported in other hyperlipaemic states. Nor does diet appear to exert any influ-ence; among pregnant Indian women, vegetari-ans showed the same rise as meat eaters [74]. While a diet low in saturated fats and high in polyunsaturated fats has been shown to have no effect [70], such a diet invariably reduced serum cholesterol in the same women before pregnancy. Moreover, the injection of glucose or insulin or both, which normally has the effect of lowering serum cholesterol, raises it instead [75].

Roth *et al.* [76] have shown that serum cholesterol binding reserve, 'the serum's capacity to solubilize additional cholesterol', rises even more in pregnancy than does cholesterol.

Phospholipids The concentration of total phospholipids rises during pregnancy in a fashion similar to that of cholesterol, from about 250 to 350–400 mg per 100 ml of serum [71,76–79] although the first trimester fall was apparent only in the data of de Alvarez *et al.* [70] and Sattar *et al.* [67].

That overall rise conceals a considerable variation in the behaviour of individual phospholipid fractions; thus the cephalins rise to almost three times, the lecithins and sphingomyelins to less than twice their normal level, while the lysolecithins fall [77]. Samsioe *et al.* [80] showed a change in the fatty acid composition of the phospholipids with a rise in palmitic and oleic acids and a fall in the essential fatty acids linoleic and arachidonic acids; they suggest without any satisfactory evidence that the changes may be an effect of diet. Others have confirmed the steady fall in essential fatty acids and found in addition after delivery a relatively slow return of more than 6 months to pre-pregnancy levels [81]. Whether these changes found in a cross-sectional study are of functional importance is still not clear but there remains the possibility that they reflect a maternal adaptation to pregnancy similar to that found for other essential nutrients, although the authors suggested it may indicate that time is required after pregnancy to replete the maternal pool.

Non-esterified (free) fatty acids A measurement of non-esterified fatty acids (NEFA) in plasma is valid only for the circumstances at the time of sampling. There is no physiological situation analogous to the basal or fasting state for plasma glucose where homeostatic forces ensure an almost constant level. NEFA are extremely labile — rising continuously during fasting and highly sensitive to numerous other influences including exertion [82,83], emotional stress [84], the temperament of the subject, whether or not she smokes, and even the effect of an indwelling needle [85]. For these reasons, and because the details of sampling are seldom mentioned in the literature, the interpretation of published data is difficult. Nevertheless, studies have been almost unanimous in showing that NEFA levels in late pregnancy are considerably above those in early pregnancy or in the non-pregnant women [85–93].

Beyond that simple fact unanimity ceases. Mean levels in late pregnancy cover a range from under 500 μM (0.5 mmol/l) [93] to 1255 μM (1.3 mmol/l) [86]. The lower levels reported reflect a move to more specific analytical methods; two papers [85,93] which showed late pregnancy levels below 600 μM (0.6 mmol/l) used gas chromatography, while most of the earlier studies used non-specific methods which are likely to have included other lipid fractions. Very high values, in excess of 1000 μM (1.0 mmol/l), have been found during labour [86,88,94]—a possible effect of oxytocin which has been shown to cause a marked increase in serum NEFA postpartum [95].

The effect appears to be sex dependent; in men, oxytocin induces a fall in NEFA. Earlier studies have reported that the pattern of NEFA changes in pregnancy: the proportion of unsaturated acids falls while that of saturated acids rises; and there is an increase in the proportion of palmitic and stearic acids and a decrease in oleic, linoleic and arachidonic acids [96,97]. More recent papers show no change in the proportions [85,93].

The pattern of change in NEFA levels generally described — a fall in early pregnancy, followed by rising levels in late pregnancy (Fig. 6.4) — makes physiological sense. The low, even below normal, levels in midpregnancy are consistent with the storage of neutral fat in adipose tissue which occurs at that time. The rising levels in late pregnancy are consistent with a parallel rise in glycerol [85] which reflects the cessation of storage and the beginning of lipolysis which typifies the last trimester. Such a pattern accords closely with that shown for the rat by Knopp *et al.* [98]; their explanation was that in the first half of pregnancy there is twice the usual conversion of glucose to storage triglyceride and a diminished release of NEFA, while in the second half of pregnancy, as insulin effectiveness deteriorates, the formation of fatty acids from glucose falls and matenal fat stores are increasingly mobilized. But more recently the suggestion of 'insulin resistance' has been discounted [99]; adipose tissue retains its sensitivity to the antilipolytic effects of insulin in late pregnancy and some other lipolytic factor must be at work. Human placental lactogen (hPL) has been suggested since it appears to be effective *in vitro* with rat adipose tissue, but the same effect could not be shown for human adipose tissue [100].

Further, it does not seem that the level of NEFA influences hPL secretion. High levels of NEFA depress, and low levels stimulate human growth hormone (hGH) secretion, suggesting a negative feedback between this metabolic fuel and hGH secretion, but the same effect cannot be shown for hPL [101].

Lipoproteins Because they are insoluble in water, most of the lipids in the blood are transported as protein–lipid complexes: the lipoproteins. These have at their centre a non-polar core of triglyceride and cholesteryl esters with a surface layer of phospholipids, cholesterol and proteins. They are classified by their densities, with chylomicrons (CM) being the least dense, then very low density lipoprotein (VLDL), intermediate density lipoprotein (IDL), low density lipoprotein (LDL) through to high density lipoprotein (HDL). There are at least seven different proteins, the apolipoproteins, which determine the type of complex, the way in which the lipids are metabolized and, because they can bind with receptors, the tissue in which this occurs. In general, apolipoproteins A are in the HDL fraction, the apolipoprotein B in the IDL and LDL fraction and in VLDL and CM, apolipoproteins C and B. During pregnancy with VLDL and IDL there are increases in triglyceride, cholesterol and phospholipid, but in LDL and HDL triglyceride increases much more than either cholesterol or phospholipid [67,68,79]. The proportional increases in all three lipids of the VLDL and IDL fractions are consistent with the increased VLDL production in pregnancy.

The increase in HDL triglyceride without reducing HDL cholesterol distinguishes pregnancy from any of the five conventional types of hyperlipoproteinaemia.

Amino acids

There have been relatively few systematic studies of the changing levels of amino acids in the maternal plasma. In making comparisons with levels in umbilical cord blood, most studies have looked only at blood at term or at delivery [102–105], or compared that in women in early and late pregnancy with that in non-pregnant women [106]. Two studies have compared amino acid levels in women at different stages of pregnancy with those in non-pregnant women [107,108] and only one [109] was a wholly serial study. Although there is general agreement about the changing pattern of amino acids, there are considerable differences in the reported figures and every investigator has noted large differences both in level and in pattern between subjects. There is little point in attempting a synthesis of these results and Table 6.8 lists only the data of Hytten and Cheyne [107].

It is obvious that most amino acids fall in concentration with particularly pronounced drops in ornithine, glycine, taurine and proline, but nothing useful can be said at this stage about the relation of patterns of change to types of amino acids or their biological role. A particularly closely observed subject reported by Cox and Calame [109] has shown that there is a fall in amino acid concentration throughout the menstrual cycle from just after the menses with an abrupt rise about the time of menstruation unless pregnancy intervenes, in which case the fall continues. They describe three patterns of cyclic change with, firstly, the main glucogenic amino acids and methionine falling continuously and to the greatest extent; secondly, those largely involved in the urea cycle falling less; and (only after a delay) a third group of mostly ketogenic branched chain or non-glucogenic amino acids starting with a delayed fall and rising again before the other groups. The exceptions to the continued fall in pregnancy were glutamic acid and alanine, which rose to

Table 6.8. Plasma amino acid concentrations in pregnancy and postpartum from 10 normal subjects (mean ± SD). Units are mmol/l. Data from Hytten and Cheyne [107].

	Under 20 weeks	20–29 weeks	30 weeks and over	8 weeks postpartum
Alanine	295 ± 56	338 ± 69	341 ± 89	382 ± 128
Arginine	80 ± 24	68 ± 31	59 ± 23	75 ± 33
Asparagine	28 ± 9	28 ± 13	27 ± 13	32 ± 23
Cystine	22 ± 9	37 ± 24	24 ± 11	33 ± 21
Glutamic acid	145 ± 56	148 ± 79	167 ± 64	162 ± 71
Glycine	161 ± 37	154 ± 37	132 ± 44	246 ± 105
Histidine	92 ± 22	92 ± 11	93 ± 17	92 ± 34
Isoleucine	58 ± 19	50 ± 15	49 ± 11	56 ± 23
Leucine	100 ± 27	99 ± 20	85 ± 18	105 ± 46
Lysine	163 ± 41	170 ± 31	152 ± 26	212 ± 99
Methionine	12 ± 8	13 ± 7	12 ± 5	18 ± 15
Ornithine	46 ± 10	53 ± 13	46 ± 15	93 ± 43
Phenylalanine	54 ± 18	56 ± 13	50 ± 9	61 ± 24
Proline	150 ± 58	151 ± 62	167 ± 51	251 ± 88
Serine	135 ± 50	143 ± 62	118 ± 44	169 ± 73
Taurine	80 ± 34	75 ± 26	62 ± 15	104 ± 69
Threonine	295 ± 46	378 ± 75	354 ± 106	400 ± 118
Tyrosine	47 ± 18	42 ± 6	45 ± 6	68 ± 31
Valine	186 ± 45	178 ± 41	156 ± 33	204 ± 93

early cycle levels by 10 weeks and continued to rise thereafter. It would be imprudent to speculate on such a straw in the wind but glutamic acid shows other evidence of eccentric behaviour and deserves special study: for example, red cell levels of amino acids rise in pregnancy to give relatively high erythrocyte to plasma ratios and no doubt reflect increased tissue uptake by the mother, a phenomenon not shared by the fetus. But glutamic acid stands out as not showing the enhanced tissue uptake of the other amino acids [110].

Another phenomenon which cannot yet be interpreted is the difference between pregnant and non-pregnant women in their response to starvation. Felig and his colleagues [111] have examined the plasma amino acid changes in 23 women between 16 and 22 weeks of pregnancy (awaiting termination) and 11 healthy controls who were starved for 84–90 hours except for water. In both groups there was a two- or threefold rise in valine, leucine, isoleucine and α-aminobutyric acid; alanine levels fell but less in the pregnant women; and glycine levels fell in the non-pregnant women to 50% of the postabsorptive level, although they rose by 25% in the pregnant women.

Fat-soluble vitamins

There is a general tendency for the plasma concentrations of the fat-soluble vitamins, like the other lipid components of the blood, to rise during pregnancy (Fig. 6.4) and for the water-soluble vitamins to fall like most other nutrients (Fig. 6.5). Data for the fat-soluble group are limited and blood levels are variable and influenced by diet.

Vitamin A This is a generic term for a number of compounds showing vitamin A activity, retinol (vitamin A) and its esters, and carotenoids (carotene) with pro-vitamin A activity. In pregnancy, levels of vitamin A itself have been shown to be somewhat below non-pregnant levels whereas carotenoids are considerably raised [112–114].

It is perhaps worth noting in relation to Fig.

184 6.4 that the early pregnancy fall in the plasma concentration of carotenoids, while not in itself particularly remarkable compared to the more conspicuous rise which is the main feature of the pattern, is curiously similar to the dip which has been noted in cholesterol, phospholipids, fatty acids and glycerol. This point deserves further study.

Tocopherol (vitamin E) Vitamin E concentration almost doubles during pregnancy to a maximum at term some 60% above non-pregnant levels [115,116]. The place of supplements of vitamin E is still uncertain but again until there is firm evidence of benefit, the same guidelines as for any intervention during pregnancy should apply before any wholesale supplementation is offered.

Vitamin D The complex question of vitamin D is discussed in Chapter 8.

Vitamin K There appears to be no published data on vitamin K. Recently there has been concern that therapeutic doses of vitamin K may have adverse effects on the newborn, there is now general agreement that the benefits well outweigh any known risks [117].

Water-soluble vitamins

There are few data about the behaviour of the water-soluble vitamins in pregnancy, and most of what has been written has been concerned with demonstrating deficiency rather than with examining physiological changes.

Thiamine (vitamin B_1) Lockhart *et al.* [118] estimated by means of the thiamine excretion test that the thiamine needs of pregnant women were three times those of non-pregnant women, and a more recent paper [119] suggested that when 'vitamin B_1 status' was estimated by the erythrocyte–transketolase activation test, some 25–30% of pregnant women in Tübingen were thiamine depleted. Subsequent work has not supported their conclusion from this evidence that dietary deficiency is widespread and this is reflected in the recommendation of the official

bodies on dietary intakes as they recommend a small increment, if any, for pregnancy.

Riboflavin Similar studies [120,121] of riboflavin status using the erythrocyte–glutathione reductase activation test showed between 20 and 40% of healthy pregnant women to be depleted. Some studies [119,120] were promoted by a commercial organization which makes vitamin supplements; the needs for thiamine and riboflavin are raised only in proportion to energy intake and widespread deficiency seems unlikely. It is more probable that these changes are further examples of metabolic adaptations characteristic of pregnancy.

Nicotinic acid (niacin) Nicotinic acid is available from a wide variety of foods and is also able to be manufactured in the body from tryptophan. There is some evidence [122] that pregnant women can convert tryptophan into nicotinic acid more efficiently.

Biotin Blood levels of biotin are approximately half the non-pregnant level throughout pregnancy [123].

Vitamin B_6 Contractor and Shane [124] measured the levels of five vitamin B_6 compounds in a small number of women at an unstated stage of pregnancy. For pyridoxal 5-phosphate, the co-enzyme form of the vitamin, and an interchangeable form, pyridoxamine, the levels were about half the normal non-pregnant level, but for the other three interchangeable forms — pyridoxamine 5-phosphate, pyridoxal and 4-pyridoxic acid—the levels did not differ from the non-pregnant.

Vitamin B_{12} Plasma levels of vitamin B_{12} also fall continuously from about 300 pg per ml in early pregnancy to about 240 pg per ml at term [125]. Similar levels were found by Low-Beer *et al.* [126], who also demonstrated an important genetic difference: British black people of West Indian origin, although having an apparently smaller dietary intake of vitamin B_{12} than white Europeans, have plasma levels which are twice as high. The vitamin B_{12}-binding capacity was also greatly increased in the West Indians, presumably because of genetic differences in binding protein.

Vitamin B_{12} levels have also been shown to be lower at all stages of pregnancy in cigarette smokers [127]. That may be an effect of the cyanide in tobacco smoke since cyanide is detoxified by a mechanism which depletes vitamin B_{12} stores.

Folate The most studied vitamin in blood, folate, also falls in concentration during pregnancy. The study by Hansen [128] is typical in showing a fall from about 6 ng/ml plasma in early pregnancy to about 3 ng/ml in late pregnancy, with considerable individual variation. Whole blood levels, which include the much higher concentration in red cells, fall less, from 58 ng/ml to about 50 ng/ml of whole blood, a reduction which is probably due to the fall in packed cell volume. The folate content of the red cells themselves appears to change little [129].

Because of the increased, though small, incidence of megaloblastic anaemia in pregnancy which responds to treatment with folic acid, the interpretation of the reduced levels is subject to the same controversy which surrounds haemoglobin concentration. Almost all recent reviews of the subject start from the assumption that pregnancy is a state of folic acid deficiency and that the majority of low serum levels which are not associated with megaloblastic erythropoiesis represent preclinical deficiency. It was on this basis that folic acid supplements were offered to women and it is now accepted that given periconceptually in amounts well in excess of that available from a normal diet it can prevent neural tube defects. An alternative explanation in keeping with present understanding of nutrient metabolism in pregnancy has been been put forward by Scott *et al.* [130]: neural tube defects which are known to have a genetic component may result from a metabolic block in folate metabolism in susceptible individuals and this can be overcome by supplementatation with supraphysiological doses of folate.

Ascorbic acid (vitamin C) Plasma ascorbic acid levels fall progressively during pregnancy even in women on a high vitamin C diet [131–133] and while there is evidence for a moderate increase in intake during pregnancy there is little to support the supraphysiological doses proposed in the past.

Trace elements

There are now seven elements present in trace amounts in the body recognized as essential nutrients: zinc, copper, selenium, manganese, molybdenum, chromium and cobalt [24]. The cobalt is almost all contained in the vitamin B_{12}, of which it is an essential component. Eight others which may be essential are: fluorine, arsenic, boron, bromine, lithium, nickel, silicon and vanadium. It continues to be difficult to determine their part in metabolism or to carry out balance studies because they are present in the body in trace amounts that lie at the limits of the capacity of present-day technology to measure them with any accuracy. In addition, most are present in large amounts in the environment leading to problems with contamination. As with the vitamins, most research has examined the possibility of dietary deficiency, but with zinc, copper and selenium, the three present in in the greatest amounts, frank deficiency has only been shown in unusual circumstances which include inborn errors of metabolism, parenteral nutrition, unusual diets, malabsorption or, as with selenium, depleted content of the soil in particular geographic areas of China [134–136]. There remains concern that deficiency or excess of the trace elements may affect either the pregnancy itself or be teratogenic to the fetus and there is some support for these effects, mostly from animal studies by veterinarians involved in animal husbandry. The changes in the concentrations in the maternal plasma are shown for copper in Fig. 6.4 where there is a rise associated with the copper-containing globulin caeruloplasmin, and for zinc in Fig. 6.5, showing a fall similar to that of albumin, the main zinc transport protein in plasma [65].

Homeostasis

The composition of blood and tissue fluids reflects two kinds of physiological need: the need to have a certain total quantity of a substance available in the circulation, and the need to have a substance at a particular concentration; both can be subject to homeostatic control.

Thus it is the total quantity of fibrinogen available to the circulation which is important to haemostasis, and for haemoglobin the total is adjusted to the demand for oxygen carriage with some precision. For other substances, the efficient function of the body depends on a precisely controlled concentration: ionized calcium and hydrogen ion are examples.

In pregnancy, both types of control are affected. For example, Ca^{2+} and H^+ are preserved at the usual non-pregnant concentrations, but osmolality and P_{CO_2}, whose levels are subject to equally careful control, are maintained during pregnancy at much lower levels. As examples of changes in total quantity, there is a greatly increased amount of fibrinogen held ready in the circulation, enough considerably to raise the concentration in the expanded volume of plasma; and there is also a considerable rise (20%) in the total circulating haemoglobin which is more than enough to cater for the 15% increase in the need for oxygen carriage, but not enough to maintain the concentration in the blood at the pre-pregnancy level.

How the levels of most nutrients are controlled is unclear. If there is a homeostatic mechanism controlling nutrients in blood, it is not known whether the total amount or the concentration is important. In pregnancy, most nutrients that have been measured — with the exception of the lipid components (Fig. 6.4) — occur at a lower concentration than in the non-pregnant subject but the changes in level and the patterns of change are variable (Fig. 6.5).

The almost universal reduction in the blood levels of nutrients suggests a common mechanism or perhaps a common purpose. No mechanism is known; dietary deficiency or failure of absorption is certainly not responsible, at least for most of the low levels described, although many can be artificially raised by large dietary supplements. Nor is it likely that the kidney plays more than a marginal role: all women show a reduced fasting blood sugar but not all have increased glycosuria. There is little relation between amino acid excretion and blood levels. For example, histidine which is lost in greatest amounts has unchanged blood levels in pregnancy.

It is perhaps worth stressing the general implausibility of dietary deficiency as a cause of reduced nutrient levels in normal pregnancy. First, it is hardly rational to claim that a phenomenon affecting all healthy, well-nourished women having normal pregnancies and healthy babies is due to dietary inadequacy. Secondly, the reduced concentrations often occur in the presence of greatly increased total circulating quantities.

The changes in blood concentrations are so widespread and varied in detail that we are left with the impression that levels of many different nutrients are reduced by a resetting of many different homeostatic mechanisms, which suggests a common purpose. It may be that a general lowering of nutrient levels in the blood produces a balance which favours transfer to the fetus rather than to the maternal tissues. The placenta is clearly able to take up nutrients with considerable efficiency from maternal blood and store within its cells particularly high concentrations of the nutrients we are discussing; it is perhaps better able to do so at the low levels in blood in pregnancy than are the maternal tissues. That is to say, the nutritional symbiosis between a mother and her fetus seem to involve a deliberate change of nutrient levels in the maternal blood to shift the balance of advantage to the fetus.

Peripheral thyroid activity is reduced, so saving on the turnover of a number of metabolites in maternal tissues. Muscle generally is relaxed, saving the cost of maintaining high tone. The evidence, in fact, is that there is a general quiescence of metabolism in maternal tissues.

It is reasonable to assume that, in health, the body maintains in its fluid environment the amounts and concentrations of the substances it needs for maximum efficiency of function; that is the purpose of homeostasis. If that is so, then the greatly altered amounts and concentrations which are characteristic of pregnancy cannot reasonably be assumed to be equally advantageous to the mother's metabolism. The most plausible explanation is that they represent changes which allow maximum efficiency of fetal growth and metabolism.

The fetus, using hormones as manipulators, over-rides and resets the mother's homeostatic mechanisms in its own interests and the mother must therefore alter her entire physiological and biochemical environment in order to provide conditions which are best suited to the fetus for whom she is hostess. That is the price of viviparity.

References

1 Durnin D.V.G.A. (1987) Energy requirements of pregnancy: an integration of the longitudinal data from the five country study. *Lancet* **2**, 1131.

2 Hytten F.E. & Leitch I. (1971) *The Physiology of Human Pregnancy*, 2nd edn. Blackwell Scientific Publications, Oxford.

3 FAO/WHO/UNU (1985) *Energy and Protein Requirements*. Report of a joint FAO/WHO/UNU expert consultation. WHO Technical Report Series; No. 724. WHO, Geneva.

4 Naismith D.J. (1977) Protein metabolism in pregnancy. In *Scientific Foundations of Obstetrics and Gynaecology*. Eds E.E. Philipp, J. Barnes & M. Newton, p. 503. Heinemann, London.

5 de Benoist B., Jackson A.A., Hall J.S. & Persaud C. (1985) Whole body protein turnover in Jamaican women during normal pregnancy. *Human Nutrition, Clinical Nutrition* **39**, 167.

6 Fitch W.L. & King J.C. (1987) Protein turnover and 3 methyl histidine in non-pregnant, pregnant and gestational diabetic women. *Human Nutrition, clinical Nutrition* **41C**, 327.

7 Olsen S.F., Sorensen J.D., Secher N.J. (1992) Randomised controlled trial of effect of fish-oil supplementation on pregnancy duration. *Lancet* **339**, 1003.

8 Illingworth P.J., Jung R.T., Howie P.W. & Isles T.E. (1987) Reduction in postprandial energy expenditure during pregnancy. *British Medical Journal* **294**, 1573.

9 Bisdee J.T. & James W.P.T. (1984) Menstrual cycle hormonal changes and energy expenditure. *Proceedings of the Nutrition Society* **43**, 143A.

10 Lawrence M., Lawrence F., Coward W.A., Cole T.J. & Whitehead R.G. (1987) The energy requirements of pregnancy in The Gambia. *Lancet* **ii**, 1072.

11 Pitkin R.M. (1985) Calcium metabolism in pregnancy and the perinatal period: a review. *American Journal of Obstetrics and Gynecology* **151**, 99.

12 Garry R.C. & Stiven D. (1935–36) Review of recent work on dietary requirements in pregnancy and lactation with attempt to assess human requirements. *Nutrition Abstracts and Reviews* **5**, 855.

13 Fullerton H.W. (1937) The iron deficiency anaemia of late pregnancy. *Archives of Disease in Childhood* **12**, 91.

14 Widdowson E.M. & Spray C.M. (1951) Chemical development in utero. *Archives of Disease in Childhood* **26**, 205.

15 Mischel W. (1957–58) Die anorganischen Bestandteile der Placenta. 6. Der Gesamt und Gewebseisengehalt der reifen und unreifen, normalen und pathologischen menschlichen Placenta. *Archiv für Gynäkologie* **190**, 638.

16 McCoy B.A., Bleiler R.E. & Ohlson M.A. (1961) Iron content of intact placentas and cords. *American Journal of Clinical Nutrition* **9**, 613.

17 FAO/WHO (1970) *Requirements of Ascorbic Acid, Vitamin D, Vitamin B_{12} Folate and Iron*. Report of a joint FAO/WHO Expert Group. WHO Technical Report Series No. 452, Geneva; also FAO Nutrition Meetings Report Series No. 47, Rome.

18 Pritchard J.A. & Scott D.E. (1970) Iron demands during pregnancy. In *Iron Deficiency*. Eds L. Hallberg, H.-G. Hawerth & A. Vannotti. Academic Press, London.

19 Kiil F., Aukland K. & Refsum H.E. (1961) Renal sodium transport and oxygen consumption. *American Journal of Physiology* **201**, 511.

20 Hytten F.E., Cheyne G.A. & Klopper A.I. (1964) Iron loss at menstruation. *Journal of Obstetrics and Gynaecology of the British Commonwealth* **71**, 255.

21 Widdowson E.M. & Dickerson J.W.T. (1964) Chemical composition of the body. In *Mineral Metabolism*, Vol. II, *The Elements*, Part A. Eds C.L. Comar & F. Bronner. Academic Press, New York.

22 Hallberg L., Sandstrom B. & Aggett P.J. (1993) Iron zinc and other trace elements. In *Human Nutrition and Dietetics*. Eds J.S. Garrow & W.P.T. James, p. 196. Churchill Livingstone, Edinburgh.

23 Swanson C.A. & King J.C. (1987) Zinc and pregnancy outcome. *American Journal of Clinical Nutrition* **46**, 763.

24 Schroeder H.A., Frost D.V. & Balassa J.J. (1970) Essential trace metals in man: selenium. *Journal of Chronic Disease* **23**, 227.

25 Rosa F.W., Wilk A.L. & Kelsay F.O. (1986) Teratogen update: vitamin A cogeners. *Teratology* **33**, 355.

26 American College of Obstetrics and Gynecology (1993) Vitamin A supplementation during pregnancy. ACOG opinion: committee on obstetrics: maternal and fetal medicines. *International Journal of Gynaecology and Obstetrics* **40**, 175.

27 Wald N.J. (1994) Folic acid and neural tube defects: the current evidence and implications for prevention. In *Neural Tube Defects*, p. 192 (Ciba Foundation symposium 181). Chichester, Wiley.

28 Jackson M.J. (1994) Can dietary micronutrients influence tissue oxidant capacity? *Proceedings of the Nutrition Society* **53**, 53.

29 Chen G., Wilson R., Cumming G., Walker J.J., Smith W.E. & McKillop J.H. (1994) Intracellular and extracellular antioxidant buffering levels in erythrocytes from pregnancy-induced hypertension. *Journal of Human Hypertension* **8**, 37.

30 Uotila J.T., Tuimala R.J., Aarnio T.M., Pyykkö K.A. & Ahotupa M.O. (1993) Findings on lipid peroxidation and antioxidant function in hypertensive complications of pregnancy. *British Journal of Obstetrics and Gynaecology* **100**, 270.

31 Department of Health (1991) *Dietary Reference Values for Food Energy and Nutrients for the United*

188

Kingdom. Committee on Medical Aspects of Food Policy. Report on Health and Social Subjects, 41. HMSO, London.

32 National Research Council, Food and Nutrition Board, Commission on Life Sciences (1989) *Recommended Dietary Allowances,* 10th edn. National Academy Press, Washington, D.C.

33 Livingstone M.B.E., Prentice A.M., Strain J.J., Coward W.A., Black A.E., Barker M.E., McKenna P.G. et al. (1990) Accuracy of weighed dietary records in studies of diet and health. *British Medical Journal* **300**, 708.

34 WHO (1961) *FAO/WHO Expert Group on Calcium Requirements.* WHO Technical Report Series No. 230 (Rome).

35 WHO (1974) *Handbook on Human Nutritional Requirements.* Monograph Series No. 61. WHO, Geneva.

36 WHO (1988) *Requirements of Vitamin A, Iron, Folate and Vitamin B_{12}.* Report of a Joint FAO/WHO Expert Consultation. FAO Food and Nutrition Series No. 23.

37 WHO Expert Committee on Trace Elements in Human Nutrition (1996) *Trace Elements in Human Nutrition.* WHO Technical Report Series No. 532.

38 Anderson A.S. & Lean M.E.J. (1986) Dietary intake in pregnancy: a comparison between 49 Cambridgeshire women and current recommended intake. *Human Nutrition, Applied Nutriton* **40A**, 40.

39 Durnin, J.V.G.A., McKillop F.M., Grant S. & Fitzgerald G. (1985) Is nutritional status endangered by virtually no extra intake doing pregnancy? *Lancet* **2**, 823.

40 Ploss H.H., Bartels M. & Ploss P. (1935) *Woman,* vol. II, p. 448. Heinemann, London.

41 Abraham R., Brown M.C., North W.R. & McFadyen I.R. (1987) Diets of Asian pregnant women in Harrow: iron and vitamins. *Human Nutrition, Applied Nutrition* **41**, 164.

42 Chanarin I., Malkowska V., O'Hea A.-M., Rinsler M.G. & Price A.B. (1985) Megaloblastic anaemia in a vegetarian Hindu community. *Lancet* **ii**, 1168.

43 Herbert V. (1994) Staging vitamin B_{12} (cobalamin) status in vegetarians. *American Journal of Clinical Nutrition* **59** (Suppl.), 1213S.

44 Rush D. (1989) Effects of changes in protein and calorie intake during pregnancy on the growth of the human fetus. In *Effective Care in Pregnancy and Childbirth.* Eds I. Chalmers, M. Enkin & M.J.N.C. Kierse, vol. 1, p. 255. Oxford University Press, Oxford.

45 Kramer M.S. (1993) Effects of energy and protein intakes on pregnancy outcome: an overview of the research evidence from controlled clinical trials. *American Journal of Clinical Nutrition* **58**, 627.

46 Campbell-Brown M. (1983) Protein energy supplements in primigravidae women at risk of low birthweight. In *Nutrition in Pregnancy.* Eds D.M. Campbell & M.D.G. Gillmer. R.C.O.G., London.

47 Hytten F.E. (1984) The effect of work on placental function and fetal growth. In *Pregnant Woman at Work.* Ed. G. Chamberlain. Macmillan, London.

48 Stein Z. & Susser M. (1975) Fertility, fecundity, famine: food rations in the Dutch famine 1944/5

have a causal relation to fertility and probably to fecundity. *Human Biology* **47**, 131.

49 Stein Z. & Susser M. (1975) The Dutch famine 1944–45, and the reproductive process. I. Effects on six indices at birth. *Pediatric Research* **9**, 70.

50 Stein Z., Susser M., Saenger G. & Marolla F. (1975) *Famine and Human Development: the Dutch hunger winter of 1944–1945.* Oxford University Press, New York.

51 Ravelli G.-P., Stein Z.A. & Susser M.W. (1976) Obesity in young men after famine exposure in utero and early infancy. *New England Journal of Medicine* **295**, 349.

52 Lumey L.H. (1992) Decreased birthweights in infants after maternal *in utero* exposure to the Dutch Famine of 1944–1945. *Paediatric and Perinatal Epidemiology* **6**, 240.

53 Barker D.J.P. (1994) *Mothers, Babies and Disease in Later Life.* BMJ Publishing Group, London.

54 Campbell D.M., Hall M.H., Barker D.J.P., Cross J., Sheill A.W. & Godfrey K.M. (1996) Diet in pregnancy and the offspring's blood pressure 40 years later. *British Journal of Obstetrics and Gynaecology* **103**, 273.

55 Harrison K.A. (1985) Childbearing, health and social priorities. *British Journal of Obstetrics and Gynaecology* **92** (Suppl. 5), 40.

56 Singla P.N., Chand S., Khanna S. & Agarwal K.N. (1978) Effect of maternal anaemia on the placenta and the newborn infant. *Acta Paediatrica Scandinavia* **67**, 645.

57 Howe D.T., Wheeler T. & Osmond C. (1995) The influence of maternal haemoglobin and ferritin on mid-pregnancy placental volume. *British Journal of Obstetrics and Gynaecology* **102**, 213.

58 Hervey G.R. (1969) Regulation of energy balance. *Nature* **222**, 629.

59 Studd J. (1975) The plasma proteins in pregnancy. *Clinics in Obstetrics and Gynaecology* **2**, 285.

60 Robertson E.G. (1970) The natural history and physiology of oedema occurring during pregnancy. MD thesis, University of Newcastle upon Tyne.

61 Robertson E.G. (1968) Increased erythrocyte fragility in association with osmotic changes in pregnancy serum. *Journal of Reproduction and Fertility* **16**, 323.

62 Tovey J.E. (1959) The significance of electrophoretic serum protein changes in pregnancy. *Journal of Obstetrics and Gynaecology of the British Empire* **66**, 981.

63 Hønger P.E. (1968) Albumin metabolism in normal pregnancy. *Scandinavian Journal of Clinical and Laboratory Investigation* **21**, 3.

64 O'Leary J.A., Novalis G.S. & Vosburgh G.J. (1966) Maternal serum copper concentrations in normal and abnormal gestations. *Obsterics and Gynaecology* **28**, 112.

65 Campbell-Brown M., Ward R.J., Haines A.P., North W.R., Abraham R., Turnlund J.R. & King J.C. (1985) Zinc and copper in Asian pregnancies: is there evidence for a nutritional deficiency? *British Journal of Obstetrics and Gynaecology* **92**, 875.

66 Fahraeus I., Larsson-Cohn U. & Wallentin L. (1985) Plasma lipoproteins including high density lipopro-

tein subfractions during normal pregnancy. *Obstetrics and Gynaecology* **66**, 1468.

67 Sattar N., Greer I.A., Louden J., Lindsay G., McConnell M., Shepherd J. & Packard C.J. (1997) Lipoprotein subfraction changes in normal pregnancy: threshold effect of plasma triglyceride on appearance of small, dense low density lipoprotein. *Journal of Clinical Endocrinology and Metabolism* **82**, 2483.

68 Warth M.R., Arky R.A. & Knopp R.H. (1975) Lipid metabolism in pregnancy. III. Altered lipid composition in intermediate, very low, low and high-density lipoprotein fractions. *Journal of Clinical Endocrinology and Metabolism* **41**, 649.

69 Mazurkiewicz J.C., Watts G.F., Warburton F.G., Slavin B.M., Lowy C. & Koukkou E. (1994) Serum lipids, lipoproteins and apolipoproteins in pregnant non-diabetic patients. *Journal of Clinical Pathology* **47**, 728.

70 de Alvarez R.R., Gaiser D.F., Simkins D.M., Smith E.K. & Bratvold G.E. (1959) Serial studies of serum lipids in normal human pregnancy. *American Journal of Obstetrics and Gynecology* **77**, 743.

71 Green J.G. (1966) Serum cholesterol changes in pregnancy. *American Journal of Obstetrics and Gynecology* **95**, 387.

72 Von Studnitz W. (1955) Studies on serum lipids and lipoproteins in pregnancy. *Scandinavian Journal of Clinical and Laboratory Investigation* **7**, 329.

73 Potter J. & Nestel A.J. (1978) Cholesterol balance during pregnancy. *Clinica Chimica Acta* **87**, 57.

74 Mullick S., Bagga O.P. & Du Mullick V. (1964) Serum lipid studies in pregnancy. *American Journal of Obstetrics and Gynecology* **89**, 766.

75 Dannenburg W.N. & Burt R.L. (1965) The effect of insulin and glucose on plasma lipids during pregnancy and the puerperium. *American Journal of Obstetrics and Gynecology* **92**, 195.

76 Roth M.S., Donato D.M., Lansman H.H., Robertson E.G., Hsia S.L. & Lemaire W.J. (1978) Effect of steroids on serum lipids and serum cholesterol binding reserve. *American Journal of Obstetrics and Gynecology* **132**, 151.

77 Svanborg A. & Vikrot O. (1965) Plasma lipid fractions, including individual phospholipids at various stages of pregnancy. *Acta Medica Scandinavica* **178**, 615.

78 Oliver M.F. & Boyd G.S. (1955) Plasma lipid and serum lipoprotein patterns during pregnancy and puerperium. *Clinical Science* **14**, 15.

79 Becker H., Berle P., Wallé A. & Volgt K.D. (1971) Influence of late gestation and early puerperium on lipid and carbohydrate metabolism in normal females. *Acta Endocrinologica* **67**, 570.

80 Samsioe G., Johnson P. & Gustafson A. (1975) Studies in normal pregnancy. I. Serum lipids and fatty acid composition of serum phospholipids. *Acta Obstetricia et Gynecologica Scandinavica* **54**, 265.

81 Hornstra G., Al M.D.M., v-Houwelingen A.C. & Foreman-von Drongelen M.M.H.P. (1995) Essential fatty acids in pregnancy and early human development. *European Journal of Obstetrics and Gynaecology* **61**, 57.

82 Greaves M.W., McDonald-Gibson W.H. & McDonald-Gibson R.G. (1972) The effect of venous occlusion, starvation and exercise on prostaglandin activity in whole human blood. *Life Science* **11**, 919.

83 Carlson L.A., Ekelund L.-G. & Orö L. (1963) Studies on blood lipids during exercise. IV. Arterial concentration of plasma free fatty acids and glycerol during and after prolonged exercise in normal men. *Journal of Laboratory and Clinical Medicine* **61**, 724.

84 Bogdonoff M.D., Estes E.H. & Trout D. (1959) Acute effect of psychological stimuli upon plasma non-esterified fatty acid levels. *Proceedings of the Society for Experimental Biology and Medicine* **100**, 503.

85 McDonald-Gibson R.G., Young M. & Hytten F.E. (1975) Changes in plasma non-esterified fatty acids and serum glycerol in pregnancy. *British Journal of Obstetrics and Gynaecology* **82**, 460.

86 Burt R.L. (1960) Plasma non-esterified fatty acids in normal pregnancy and the puerperium. *Obstetrics and Gynecology* **15**, 460.

87 Bleicher S.J., O'Sullivan J.B. & Freinkel N. (1964) Carbohydrate metabolism in pregnancy. 5. The interrelations of glucose, insulin and free fatty acids in late pregnancy and post partum. *New England Journal of Medicine* **271**, 866.

88 Nelson G.H. (1965) Serum non-esterified fatty acid levels in human pregnancy as determined by various titration procedures. *American Journal of Obstetrics and Gynecology* **92**, 202.

89 Picard C., Ooms H.A., Balasse E. & Conard V. (1968) Effect of normal pregnancy on glucose assimilation, insulin and non-esterified fatty acid levels. *Diabetologica* **4**, 16.

90 Fioretti P., Genazzani A.R., Aubert M.L., Gragnoli G. & Pupillo A. (1970) Correlations between human chorionic somatomammotrophin (lactogen), immuno-reactive insulin, glucose and lipid fractions in plasma of pregnant women. *Journal of Obstetrics and Gynaecology of the British Commonwealth* **77**, 745.

91 Fairweather D.V.I. (1971) Changes in levels of serum non-esterified fatty acid and blood glucose in pregnancy. *Journal of Obstetrics and Gynaecology of the British Commonwealth* **78**, 707.

92 Potnis A.V. & Purandare B.N. (1972) Serum nonesterified (free) fatty acids in pregnancy. *Journal of Obstetrics and Gynaecology of India* **22**, 120.

93 Hagenfeldt L. & Hagenfeldt K. (1976) Individual free fatty acids in amniotic fluid and in plasma of pregnant women. *British Journal of Obstetrics and Gynaecology* **83**, 383.

94 Laron Z., Manrheimer S., Nitzan M. & Goldmann J. (1967) Growth hormone, glucose and free fatty acid levels in mother and infant in normal diabetic and toxaemic pregnancy. *Archives of Disease in Childhood* **42**, 24.

95 Burt R.L., Leake N.H. & Dannenburg W.N. (1963) Effect of synthetic oxytocin on plasma non-esterified fatty acids, triglycerides and blood glucose. *Obstetrics and Gynecology* **21**, 708.

96 Hasen A.E., Wiese H.F., Adam D.J.D., Boelsche A.N., Haggard M.E., Davis H., Newsom W.T. *et al.* (1964) Influence of diet on blood serum lipids in pregnant

190

women and newborn infants. *American Journal of Clinical Nutrition* **15**, 11.

97 Bottiglioni F., Flamigni C., Caramazza G. & Tirelli R. (1966) Richerche gas-chromatografiche negli acidi grassi liberi del plasma nello stato puerperale. *Bolletino della Società italiana di biologia sperimentale* **42**, 893.

98 Knopp R.H., Saudek C.D., Arky R.A. & O'Sullivan J.B. (1973) Two phases of adipose tissue metabolism in pregnancy: maternal adaptations for fetal growth. *Endocrinology* **92**, 984.

99 Coltart T.N. & Williams C. (1976) Effect of insulin on adipose tissue lipolysis in human pregnancy. *British Journal of Obstetrics and Gynaecology* **83**, 241.

100 Elliott J.A. (1975) The effect of pregnancy on the control of lipolysis in fat cells isolated from human adipose tissue. *European Journal of Clinical Investigation* **5**, 159.

101 Gaspard U.J., Luyckx A.S., George A.N. & Lefebvre P.J. (1977) Relationship between plasma free fatty acid levels and human placental lactogen secretion in late pregnancy. *Journal of Clinical Endocrinology and Metabolism* **45**, 246.

102 Lindblad B.S. & Baldesten A. (1967) The normal venous plasma free amino acid levels of non-pregnant women and of mother and child during delivery. *Acta Paediatrica Scandinavica* **56**, 37.

103 Cockburn F., Blagden A., Michie E.A. & Forfar J.O. (1971) The influence of pre-eclampsia and diabetes mellitus on plasma free amino acids in maternal umbilical vein and infant blood. *Journal of Obstetrics and Gynaecology of the British Commonwealth* **78**, 215.

104 Dallaire L., Potier M., Melancon S.B. & Patrick J. (1974) Fetomaternal amino acid metabolism. *British Journal of Obstetrics and Gynaecology* **81**, 761.

105 Velazquez A., Rosado A., Bernal A., Bernal A., Noriega L. & Arevaldo N. (1976) Amino acid pools in the fetomaternal system. *Biology of the Neonate* **29**, 28.

106 Young M. & Prenton M.A. (1969) Maternal and fetal plasma amino acid concentrations during gestation and in retarded fetal growth. *Journal of Obstetrics and Gynaecology of the British Commonwealth* **76**, 333.

107 Hytten F.E. & Cheyne G.A. (1972) The aminoaciduria of pregnancy. *Journal of Obstetrics and Gynaecology of the British Commonwealth* **79**, 424.

108 Schoengold D.M., Defiore R.H. & Parlett R.C. (1978) Free amino acids in plasma throughout pregnancy. *American Journal of Obstetrics and Gynecology* **131**, 490.

109 Cox B.D. & Calame D.P. (1978) Changes in plasma amino acid levels during the human menstrual cycle and in early pregnancy: a preliminary report. *Hormone and Metabolic Research* **10**, 428.

110 Björnesjö K.B. (1968) The distribution of amino acids between erythrocytes and plasma in fetal and maternal blood. *Clinica Chimica Acta* **20**, 11.

111 Felig P., Kim Y.J., Lynch V. & Hendler R. (1972) Amino acid metabolism during starvation in human pregnancy. *Journal of Clinical Investigation* **51**, 1195.

112 Darby W.J., McGanity W.J., Martin M.P., Bridgforth E., Denson P.M., Kaser M.M., Ogle P.J. *et al.* (1953) The Vanderbilt cooperative study of maternal and infant nutrition. IV. Dietary laboratory and physical findings in 2129 delivered pregnancies. *Journal of Nutrition* **51**, 565.

113 Pulliam P.R., Dannenburg W.N., Burt R.L. & Leake N.H. (1962) Carotene and vitamin A in pregnancy and the early puerperium. *Proceedings of the Society for Experimental Biology and Medicine* **109**, 913.

114 Lund C.J. & Kimble M.S. (1943) Vitamin A during pregnancy, labor and the puerperium. *American Journal of Obstetrics and Gynecology* **46**, 486.

115 Ferguson M.E., Bridgforth E., Quaife M.L., Martin M.P., Cannon R.O., McGanity W.J., Newbill J. *et al.* (1955) The Vanderbilt cooperative study of maternal and infant nutrition. VII. Tocopherol in relation to pregnancy. *Journal of Nutrition* **55**, 305.

116 Vobecky J.S., Vobecky J. & Munan L. (1973) Alpha-tocophérol sérique pendant la grossesse et l'état du nouveau-né. *Proceedings of the Canadian Federation of Biological Societies* **16**, 268.

117 Zipursky A. (1996) Vitamin K at birth. *British Medical Journal* **313**, 179.

118 Lockhart H.S., Kirkwood S. & Harris R.S. (1943) The effect of pregnancy and the puerperium on the thiamine status of women. *American Journal of Obstetrics and Gynecology* **46**, 358.

119 Heller S., Salkeld R.M. & Körner W.F. (1974) Vitamin B_1 status in pregnancy. *American Journal of Clinical Nutrition* **27**, 1221.

120 Heller S., Salkeld R.M. & Körner W.F. (1974) Riboflavin status in pregnancy. *American Journal of Clinical Nutrition* **27**, 1225.

121 Vir S.C., Love A.H.G. & Thompson W. (1981) Riboflavin status in pregnancy. *American Journal of Clinical Nutrition* **34**, 2699.

122 Wertz A.W., Lojkin M.E., Bouchard B.S. & Derby M.B. (1958) Tryptophan-niacin relationships in pregnancy. *Journal of Nutrition* **69**, 339.

123 Bhagavan N.H. (1969) Biotin content of blood during gestation. *International Journal of Vitamin Research* **39**, 235.

124 Contractor S.F. & Shane B. (1970) Blood and urine levels of vitamin B6 in the mother and fetus before and after loading of the mother with vitamin B6. *American Journal of Obstetrics and Gynecology* **107**, 635.

125 Ball E.W. & Giles C. (1964) Folic acid and vitamin B_{12} levels in pregnancy and their relation to megaloblastic anaemia. *Journal of Clinical Pathology* **17**, 165.

126 Low-Beer T.S., McCarthy C.F., Austad W.I., Brzechwa-Ajdukiewicz A. & Read A.E. (1968) Serum vitamin B_{12} levels and vitamin B_{12} binding capacity in pregnant and non-pregnant Europeans and West Indians. *British Medical Journal* **iv**, 160.

127 McGarry J.M. & Andrews J. (1972) Smoking in pregnancy and vitamin B_{12} metabolism. *British Medical Journal* **ii**, 74.

128 Hansen H.A. (1967) On the diagnosis of folic acid deficiency. *Acta Obstetrica et Gynaecologica Scandinavica* **46** (Suppl. 7), 13.

129 Landon M.J. (1975) Folate metabolism in pregnancy. *Clinics in Obstetrics and Gynaecology* **2**, 413.

130 Scott J., Kirke P., Molloy A., Daly L. & Weir D. (1994)

The role of folate in the prevention of neural tube defects. *Proceedings of the Nutrition Society* **53**, 631.

131 Khalil A. & Waly G. (1949) Vitamin C in the nutrition of infants, pregnant and lactating women. *Journal of the Egyptian Medical Association* **32**, 158.

132 McGanity W.J., Bridgforth E.B. & Derby W.J. (1958) The Vanderbilt cooperative study of maternal and infant nutrition. XII. Effect of reproductive cycle on nutritional status and requirements. *Journal of the American Medical Association* **168**, 2138.

133 Mason M. & Rivers J.M. (1971) Plasma ascorbic acid levels in pregnancy. *American Journal of Obstetrics and Gynecology* **109**, 960.

134 Mills C.F. (1991) The significance of copper deficiency in human health and disease. In *Trace Elements in Man and Animals* vol. 7. Ed. B. Momcilovic, p. 1. IMI, Zagreb.

135 Yang G., Ge K., Chen J. & Chen X. (1988) Selenium-related endemic diseases and the daily selenium requirement of humans. *World Review of Nutrition and Dietetics* **3**, 98.

136 Prasad A.S. (1996) Zinc deficiency in women. *Journal of the American College of Nutrition* **15**, 113.

Carbohydrate Metabolism

J.P. O'HARE

The physiology of carbohydrate metabolism in pregnancy involves the study of the availability of glucose for the fetus from the maternal plasma.

Maternal glucose homeostasis

Glucose is the major substrate for the human fetus throughout pregnancy. Maternal glucose levels determine fetal levels which are 15–20% lower [1]. The blood glucose level in the mother is regulated by maternal insulin. The amount of insulin will depend on the secretion rate from the β-cells of the pancreas together with the insulin clearance rate. The blood glucose level in the mother will depend not only on the prevailing insulin level but the activity of that insulin in delivering glucose to the insulin sensitive tissues of the mother (muscle, fat and liver).

Insulin is involved not only in glucose regulation but also in the regulation of amino acids and fats. Figure 7.1 shows the effects of insulin on the metabolic and anabolic pathways. Increased amounts of insulin or enhanced insulin action lower plasma glucose by moving it into cells and inhibiting its release from stores, but also will reduce amino acids and free fatty acids. On the other hand, reduced insulin or a loss of its action and effectiveness will lead to increased plasma concentrations of glucose and amino acids. Furthermore, enhanced lipolysis because of the reduction of glucose within cells will increase free fatty acid oxidation and the production of ketones if there is extreme deficiency of insulin or its action.

In pregnancy the changes in carbohydrate metabolism are achieved through increased production of insulin combined with increased resistance to its action. The concept of hormonal resistance is the reduced ability of that hormone to exert its effects on its target organ or tissue [2]. In decreased sensitivity an increase in hormone concentration is required to produce a normal biological response. In decreased responsiveness the hormone concentration is unchanged, but the maximal possible biological response is reduced. Both decreased sensitivity and responsiveness appear to contribute to insulin resistance in pregnancy (Fig. 7.2) where, despite increases in maternal insulin production, blood glucose rises in the second half of pregnancy. These concepts are discussed in more detail below.

192

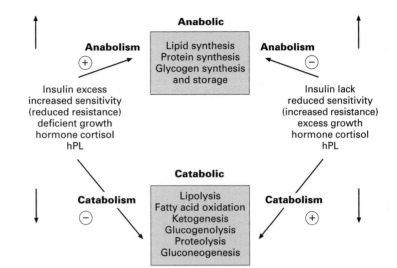

Fig. 7.1. The effects of insulin on maternal metabolic pathways.

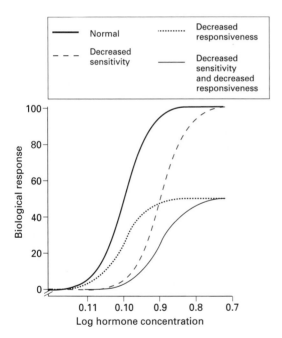

Fig. 7.2. Types of insulin resistance as defined by theoretical dose–response curves. Effects of decreases in insulin sensitivity, insulin responsiveness or both. From Kahn [2], with permission.

Maternal glucose homeostasis in the fasting state

During normal pregnancy the fasting blood glucose levels decrease. Lind's [3] longitudual studies (Fig. 7.3) show a fall in the level of plasma glucose with advancing pregnancy. The fasting glucose concentrations reached their nadir at about 12 weeks and represent a fall of about 0.5–1 mmol/l on the pre-pregnancy blood glucose. This fall in blood glucose is associated with a rise in plasma insulin levels but this occurs in the third trimester, not measurably in the first (Fig. 7.4a). The fasting insulin levels increase from 5 µU/l to 8 µU/l (Fig. 7.4b). Other workers [4,5] have also reported decreases of about 0.8 mmol/l in glucose levels of pregnant women after an overnight fast. Kühl [6] has demonstrated that during pregnancy the insulin to glucagon ratio increases significantly when compared with that in the non-pregnant state. These data suggest that the increased levels of insulin are not just part of an overall increase in the levels of hormones or secondary to a rise in counter-regulatory hormones such as glucagon.

Response to glucose load

After carbohydrate ingestion there is, as a result of insulin release and action on sensitive tissues, a suppression of endogenous glucose production (from liver and muscle) and an acceleration of glucose utilization. In the non-pregnant normal woman the plasma glucose load levels reach their peak at 30 minutes after the ingestion of the glucose load and have returned to the base-

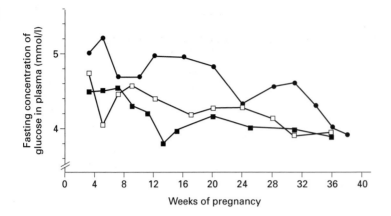

Fig. 7.3. Decrease in fasting plasma glucose concentration throughout pregnancy in three healthy women in whom the non-pregnancy value was the mean of 12 weekly determinations prior to conception in each individual.

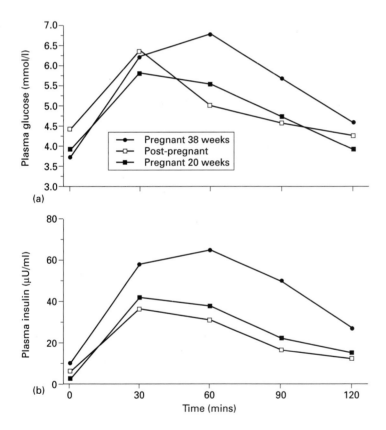

Fig. 7.4. Longitudinal study of (a) plasma glucose and (b) insulin responses to 50 g load in 19 healthy primigravidae at 20 and 38 weeks' gestation, and 10–12 weeks postpartum. Redrawn from data from Lind [3].

line fasting concentration at approximately 60 minutes [3,7]. The same women tested during the third trimester showed higher peak glucoses that were slower to reach their peak and decline. The peaks occurred 60 minutes after the glucose load and fasting levels were only achieved after about 2 hours [5,7].

The data for glucose in the study by Lind are presented in graphical form together with insulin responses in Fig. 7.4a. Insulin levels reach their peak at 1 hour (Fig. 7.4b) after the glucose load (50 g) when glucose values are also peaking. Insulin levels then decline slowly and are still not back to baseline by the 2-hour point.

Thus, for any given glucose challenge the pregnant woman will produce extra insulin but the blood glucose levels remain elevated despite this insulin. This insulin resistance through a loss of insulin sensitivity can be seen from the study of Lind et al. [3] in 19 healthy women (Table 7.1). Early in pregnancy the fasting plasma glucose level falls and the peak level and the 2-hour levels are lower than in the non-pregnant (postnatal) state. Glucose homeostasis in the first trimester is improved as is sensitivity to insulin (Table 7.1). In contrast, after 20 weeks during the second half of pregnancy there are higher peak values, a delayed time to reach the peak and a higher 2-hour value than in the non-pregnant postpartum state. This deterioration in postload glucose homeostasis is accompanied by increased levels of plasma insulin, thereby indicating insulin resistance, a change specific to the second half of pregnancy, and represents a loss of insulin sensitivity in humans. This insulin resistance during the second half of pregnancy is not seen in African women eating a non-Westernized diet [8,9] which raises the question as to whether reducing glucose loads with a less refined carbohydrate and fibre-enriched diet (the principle of a diabetic diet) in healthy pregnant Western women might reduce postprandial hyperglycaemia and hyperinsulinaemia.

While the glucose tolerance test (variously with a load at different times and places of 50, 75 or 100 g) is the standard method used to challenge the system, it is unphysiological as most food is taken in mixed form with a diet of carbohydrate protein and fat in ordinary meals. Gillmer et al. [10] studied mixed meal feeding and showed a postprandial response similar to glucose load with a return to lower fasting levels. In this study in normal pregnant women it was interesting to note the normal fasting blood glucoses seen at 4.5 mmol/l in early pregnancy and 4.8 even in the third trimester. In a much larger epidemiological study of normal pregnancy in the Wessex area in the UK, Hatem et al. [11] reported similar fasting values for glucose with the 97.5 centiles for pregnant women being 4.88 mmol/l in the second trimester and 4.8 in the third trimester. In this study, the 2-hour value after the 75 g glucose load of the glucose tolerance test (GTT) had a 97.5 centile of 7.5 during the second trimester (weeks 14–20) and 9.6 during the third (weeks 28–37).

The obese mother comes to pregnancy with a pre-existing state of insulin resistance and this resistance increases under the influence of the pregnancy hormones, particularly cortisol and human placental lactogen. As a group, obese pregnant women require much higher peripheral insulin levels to overcome the resistance and maintain glucose levels and stop them from rising. If this fails, the pregnant woman will

Table 7.1. Mean glucose and insulin concentration during the course of oral glucose tolerance tests in 19 healthy women, throughout pregnancy and 10–12 weeks after delivery.

| Sampling time (minutes) | Glucose (mmol/l) | | | | | Insulin (µU/ml) | | | | |
| | During pregnancy (weeks) | | | | 10–12 weeks after delivery | During pregnancy (weeks) | | | | 10–12 weeks after delivery |
	10	20	30	38		10	20	30	38	
0	4.2	4.9	4.1	3.8	4.4	4.2	4.2	7.6	7.8	5.8
15	5.8	5.3	5.6	5.0	6.1	28.3	27.6	37.1	37.7	27.7
30	6.2	5.9	6.6	6.3	6.4	41.4	40.4	55.9	57.6	38.8
45	6.2	6.0	6.8	6.8	6.1	42.6	45.3	67.1	63.0	42.0
60	5.6	5.5	6.2	6.8	5.1	34.8	38.7	61.4	66.4	32.7
75	5.2	5.2	5.6	6.2	4.7	31.4	34.3	52.8	56.8	23.2
90	5.0	4.7	5.4	5.7	4.6	32.0	23.4	40.6	51.6	19.5
120	4.8	3.9	4.4	4.5	4.3	16.9	15.8	22.7	28.2	13.4

develop a chronically elevated blood glucose and be classified as having impaired glucose tolerance of pregnancy or gestational diabetes.

The metabolic response to feeding in pregnancy is associated with hyperinsulinaemia, hyperglycaemia and hypertriglyceridaemia accompanied by a decrease in circulating glucagon. Freinkel *et al.* [12] coined the phrase 'facilitated anabolism' for these pregnancy changes where the increased resistance is overcome by increased insulin production. The ability to increase insulin production can fail in some mothers, particularly those with insulin deficiency or enhanced insulin resistance or antagonism. In these mothers, if the deficiency is extreme there is an enhanced catabolic process with lipolysis, ketogenesis, glycogenolysis, proteolysis and gluconeogenesis (Fig. 7.1). These mothers exhibit maternal hyperglycaemia which results in fetal hyperglycaemia and, consequent to this, fetal hyperinsulinaemia. These are the pathophysiological changes thought to contribute to fetal macrosomia and neonatal complications in gestational and insulin-dependent diabetic women.

Insulin resistance in pregnancy

Early studies showed that for a given dose of insulin (0.02 units/kg body weight) there was a reduced blood glucose lowering effect in the third trimester (36 weeks) compared to post pregnancy (0.9. v. 1.8 mmol/l) [13]. Euglycaemic insulin clamp studies have been carried out using both high and low rates of insulin infusion which are countered to maintain fasting blood glucoses at a clamped level by a variable infusion of glucose [14]. The amount of glucose needed to maintain the plasma glucose clamped for a given load of insulin will thus give an idea of the sensitivity of the tissue to insulin action. In pregnancy in the third trimester it can be seen from Table 7.2 that insulin resistance is a feature and less glucose needs to be infused than in the non-pregnant state (about 25–35% less) [14]. Ryan *et al.* have also shown in this study that women with gestational diabetes have further reduced glucose infusion rates (increased resistance) of 50–75% [15]. Catalano [16] has found using clamp techniques that about 50% of women with gestational diabetes who are normal on glucose tolerance testing postpartum will show insulin resistance (Fig. 7.5). This is most marked in the obese mothers and with increasing maternal age [15].

Insulin resistance occurs in most women as a normal physiological change as pregnancy progresses. Those women who exhibit a more marked insulin resistance as defined by a more rapid and prolonged glucose response to challenge and are above defined pragmatic criteria have been labelled as having impaired glucose tolerance of pregnancy or gestational diabetes. These criteria are specified in Table 7.2. Clearly an understanding of the mechanism of insulin resistance in normal pregnancy is central to progress in understanding the clinical problem of gestational diabetes.

It is conventional when considering hormone action to analyse the action at the prereceptor, receptor and postreceptor levels. Any factor which reduces free insulin concentration would

Table 7.2. Euglycaemic clamp studies of normal non-diabetic non-pregnant and pregnant women. An increased glucose infusion rate for a fixed blood glucose and constant insulin infusion represents increased insulin sensitivity. At high insulin doses sensitivity is considered to be maximal and different infusion rates represent altered responsivity (from Ryan *et al.* [14]; see also Fig. 7.2).

	Glucose infusion rate—clamped at 4.2 mmol/l (mg/m²/min)	
	Non-pregnant	Pregnant
Low dose insulin (40 mU/m²/min)	11.8 ± 0.6	7.9 ± 1.3
High dose insulin (240 mU/m²/min)	20.7 ± 0.6	15 ± 1.7

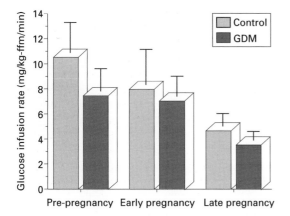

Fig. 7.5. Longitudinal changes in glucose infusion rate required to maintain euglycemia (90 mg/d) during insulin infusion (mean ± SD). $P = 0.0001$: changes over time from pre-pregnancy through late pregnancy. $P_g = 0.03$: differences between groups. From Catalano [16].

lation cascade. The following sections address these various points.

197

Reduced insulin concentration

The ability of the mother to secrete more insulin to meet the increased demands of the second and third trimesters of pregnancy has been clearly shown in the early classic papers of Lind [3,7]. Table 7.3 represents the data of experiments in which glucose was infused in normal mothers over 80 minutes. Blood glucose was held close to 11 mmol/l and the studies were performed at 16, 26, 36 weeks and in the postpartum period as a control. Fasting levels of insulin doubled from the postnatal to the 26th week and almost trebled at 36 weeks' gestation. There was a magnified insulin secretion as pregnancy advanced following the glucose load. Insulin secretion has now been shown to consist of a biphasic response with an early first phase response that reaches its peak within 5–10 minutes of carbohydrate ingestion and is followed by a slower secretion rate (Fig. 7.6). A defect in the first phase of insulin response can lead to an overall impairment of insulin action even when the overall total (through an increased slower second phase response) is increased.

cause a loss of action at the prereceptor level. At the receptor level, reductions in binding affinity or the number of receptors would lead to insulin resistance with a reduced biological response for a given concentration of free hormone. Postreceptor effects found within the cells of insulin-sensitive tissue include mechanisms such as defects in the transfer of glucose from the receptor to the site of utilization or defects in the enzymes involved in the metabolism of glucose, particularly those involved in the phosphory-

In a study designed to analyse the phase of insulin response using a hyperinsulinaemic euglycaemic clamp, six women were studied preconception and then in early (12–14 weeks) and late (34–36 weeks) pregnancy. Catalano and col-

Table 7.3. Plasma glucose (mmol/l) and insulin (µU/ml) concentrations during glucose infusions at various stages of pregnancy (from Lind [7]).

Weeks of gestation		Infusion time (minutes)			
		0	40	60	80
10–12 post natal	Glucose	4.9	12.7	12.3	12.7
	Insulin	5.7	35.1	48.9	66.4
16	Glucose	4.2	9.9	9.7	9.7
	Insulin	6.6	79.5	87.5	89.5
26	Glucose	4.3	10.8	10.7	10.8
	Insulin	12.7	93.0	94.2	115.6
36	Glucose	4.6	11.0	11.7	11.8
	Insulin	16.0	130.2	163.2	198.6

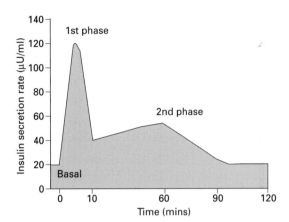

Fig. 7.6. Biphasic insulin response to a constant glucose stimulus. The peak of the first phase in the human is between 3 and 5 minutes and lasts 10 minutes. The second phase begins at 2 minutes but is not evident until after 10 minutes and continues to increase slowly for at least 60 minutes until the stimulus stops.

leagues [17] reported a significant 3.0- to 3.5-fold increase throughout gestation in both first and second phase insulin release in response to the intravenous glucose tolerance test (Fig. 7.7). Similar studies have reported that there is the reduced insulin sensitivity of pregnancy, but that the normal insulin secretion rate and the qualitative nature of the response and phases remain intact [13,18].

Reduced receptor affinity

An altered affinity or reduced number of insulin receptors produced during the second half of pregnancy might explain the insulin resistance that is apparent, particularly if this occurred in muscle cells, adipocytes or hepatocytes.

Reduced insulin binding in isolated adipocytes from healthy pregnant women has been reported [19]. Furthermore, in this study, obese women had binding that was further reduced, as did women with non-insulin dependent diabetes. Evidence is mounting that hyperinsulinaemia produced by the resistance to insulin action itself is a potent cause of down-regulation of both the number of insulin receptor sites and the affinity of the receptor binding. In addition, this area is further complicated by the fact that maximum biological effects of insulin are

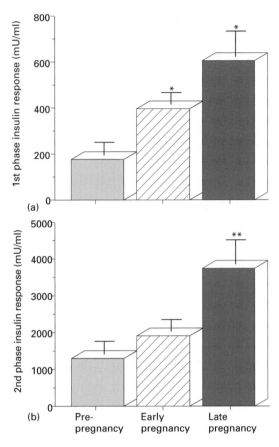

Fig. 7.7. (a) Changes in first-phase insulin response during the intravenous glucose tolerance test (mean ± SD); *$P = 0.025$. (b) Changes in second-phase insulin response during the intravenous glucose tolerance test (mean ± SD); **$P = 0.0001$. Reproduced from Catalano [17].

achieved with only 2–5% occupancy of available binding sites making this a rather crude mechanism for regulation.

Post-receptor insulin action

Recently the techniques of molecular biology have increased knowledge in this area. A study of adipocytes in pregnancy concluded that basal and stimulated lipolysis are enhanced in late pregnancy as a result of insulin resistance [15]. The glucose transporters, especially GLUT 1, 2 and GLUT 4, and their function in human pregnancy in adipocyte muscle and liver cells represent an exciting area for future research in insulin resistance [20]. These proteins are known to be regulated directly by insulin and are each the product of single genes. Under basal conditions, about 95% of GLUT 4 is located in an intracellular pool but with insulin stimulation, 40–50% of this pool moves to the cell surface, giving rise to a 20- to 30-fold increase in cell-surface GLUT 4 levels and thereby accounting for a large increase in glucose transport into cells.

Potential sites for insulin resistance such as occurs in pregnancy could be:

1 impaired receptor binding or impaired activation of receptor associated tyrosine kinase [21];

2 a defective signal from insulin to mobilize glucose transporters to cell surface;

3 defective translocation of GLUT 4 to the cell surface;

4 a reduction in the intracellular pool of GLUT 4 [20].

In adipocytes from women with gestational diabetes, a combination of defects in GLUT 4 has been observed [22]. Garvey *et al.* [22] noticed reduced GLUT 4 expression in half the subjects examined and a novel mistargeting of the transporter in the rest of the cohort. Figure 7.8 illustrates these possible sites within an insulin-sensitive cell.

The role of hormones antagonistic to insulin in pregnancy

Normal pregnant women are thus insulin resistant and can be shown to be one-fifth as sensitive to insulin as in their non-pregnant state [23]. The hormonal changes in pregnancy with an increase in hormones that could antagonize insulin action at the postreceptor level in muscle and liver cells could clearly play a role as mediators of this effect. There are increases in cortisol, progesterone, human placental lactogen (human chorionic somatomammotrophin), prolactin and oestradiol. The diabetogenic potential of these hormones can be summarized on a scale of 5 and is illustrated in Fig. 7.9.

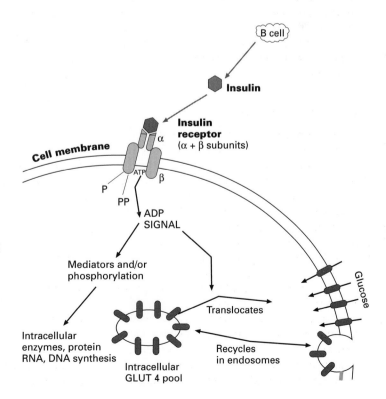

Fig. 7.8. Insulin-stimulated glucose transport in adipocytes. Under basal conditions, 95% of GLUT 4 is located intracellularly in a pool of vesicles but with insulin stimulation, 40–50% of this pool translocates rapidly (within minutes) giving rise to a 20- to 30-fold increase in the cell surface GLUT 4 levels and a large increase in glucose transport. As insulin levels fall GLUT 4 is resequestered back into the intracellular pool.

Cortisol

Free cortisol and bound cortisol both increase during human pregnancy. Glucocorticosteroids can inhibit peripheral glucose uptake in muscles and increase liver gluconeogenesis, thus contributing to antagonism to insulin effects and producing insulin resistance. Levels of cortisol increase with duration of pregnancy and are maximal by the third trimester but no direct correlation between free cortisol levels and insulin resistance as measured by changes in insulin in response to glucose challenge can be demonstrated [24].

Progesterone

Progesterone is produced by the placenta in pregnancy and it has a direct effect on glucose metabolism [21]. In normal fasting women, progesterone infusions increase insulin concentrations but glucose remains unchanged. Levels of 17-OH progesterone do not peak until about the 32nd week of gestation. As glucose levels remain unchanged despite stimulating insulin release, it is likely that progesterone could be involved in mediating the insulin resistance of pregnancy.

Oestrogens and prolactin

Oestrogens have weak insulin antagonistic properties and their effect is largely derived from stimulating the liver to produce more cortisol-binding globulin, with a consequent enhanced maternal adrenal cortisol production to maintain free cortisol levels. This is likely to be the mechanism of insulin resistance of exogenous steroids seen in the combined oral contraceptive which can provoke a deterioration of glucose homeostasis in some normal women [25].

Prolactin has a role in early pregnancy and may be involved in enhancing cell-to-cell communication among the β-cells of the pancreatic islets [26]. While at this stage it may be involved in stimulating both maternal and fetal β-cell hypertrophy, it does not appear to increase in parallel with the rising insulin resistance during pregnancy or assume a further role in the second half of pregnancy.

Glucagon

In pregnancy, most observers report enhanced suppression of glucagon [27]. Despite its physiological role of a counter-regulatory hormone to insulin it is, therefore, unlikely to be important as a mediator of insulin antagonism during pregnancy.

Catecholamines

Plasma levels of catecholamines (noradrenaline and adrenaline) are the same in pregnancy as in the non-pregnant state [28]. There is no evidence that sensitivity to the metabolic effects of these hormones increases in pregnancy so it is unlikely that these hormones through their actions to release glucogon or inhibit insulin secretion play a role in the insulin resistance of pregnancy.

Growth hormone

The levels of growth hormone decrease during pregnancy with a blunted response to provocative stimuli [29]. This suppression is probably mediated by human placental lactogen. Antagonism by growth hormone of insulin is therefore

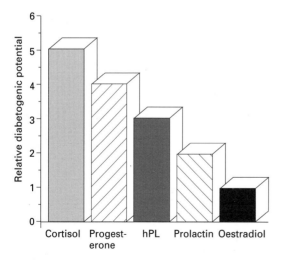

Fig. 7.9. The relative diabetogenic potential of the pregnancy-related hormones. From Mulford *et al.* [23].

an unlikely explanation of the insulin resistance of pregnancy.

Leptin

The size of fat stores in the body reflects changes in energy balance. Leptin is a protein of MW ~16000. The *ob* gene which codes for leptin is only expressed in the white adipose tissue outside pregnancy, its expression is stimulated by insulin and glucocorticoids and suppressed by activation of the β-adrenoceptors of the sympathetic nervous system. The leptin receptor is present in the hypothalamus, where it may react with the neuropeptide Y system, and is also in peripheral tissues. It is thought that leptin acts as a signal to the brain about the extent of the fat stores (see Tritos and Mantzoros [30]). Human placental syncytiotrophoblast and amniotic cells have also been shown to synthesize leptin [31] which may explain the markedly raised circulating leptin concentrations observed in human pregnancy. Maternal leptin concentrations correlate strongly with term body mass index and plasma insulin concentration but not with birthweight.

Neonatal leptin concentrations are raised by comparison with non-pregnant values, but are usually lower than maternal: maternal and fetal concentrations are not correlated with each other. Umbilical venous plasma leptin concentrations are directly correlated with each other and placental weight, but not with plasma insulin concentration [32]. It seems likely that leptin has a role in intrauterine and neonatal development and that the placenta provides a source of leptin for the fetus.

Human placental lactogen

Human placental lactogen (hPL) is a protein hormone produced by the placenta with immunological epitopes and biological properties similar to growth hormone [29]. It has growth hormone-like effects both in the mother and the fetus. In the fetus it has effects on tibial epiphyseal growth, body weight gain and effects on fetal fat and carbohydrate metabolism [33]. In the mother, insulin-like growth factor (IGF1) concentrations increase markedly in the third trimester to concentrations frequently seen in acromegaly and this is, at least in part, due to placental lactogen [33]. hPL has effects on maternal carbohydrate and protein metabolism similar to growth hormone. There is inhibition of peripheral glucose uptake and stimulation of insulin release [33,34]. hPL acts as an antagonist of insulin action by enhancing insulin resistance in the mother and increasing lipolysis and proteolysis, with the net effect of promoting the transfer of glucose and amino acids to the fetus. The changes in circulating hPL levels which are detected in maternal plasma by about 6 weeks and then increase linearly until a peak at the 30th week coincide temporally with the insulin resistance in successive periods of pregnancy [34] and with its rapid disappearance when the placenta is removed in the puerperium. This hormone is clearly a major mediator of the insulin resistance of the mother in pregnancy and has important metabolic effects (Fig. 7.10).

It may play a role in the pathophysiology of disturbance in fetal metabolism in mothers with diabetes mellitus or impaired tolerance. Reductions in levels of hPL have been reported in diabetic pregnancies. Recently [34], the physiological role of apoA1, the apoprotein constituent of high density lipoprotein, in the regulation of the synthesis and release of hPL has been described raising the possibility that reduction of hPL and this apoprotein in diabetes mellitus, particularly when poorly controlled, may contribute to the pathogenesis of intrauterine growth retardation or macrosomia in these pregnancies.

The puerperium

That placental hormones are the mediators of the insulin resistance of pregnancy is supported by the rapid return to normal carbohydrate metabolism once the placenta is separated [35,36].

Fasting plasma insulin and insulin response curves had returned to non-pregnant values within 48 hours of delivery in Lind and Harris's study [36], but the glucose values did not return to normal until the 6th week postpartum. By convention, following a pregnancy in which impaired glucose tolerance or gestational dia-

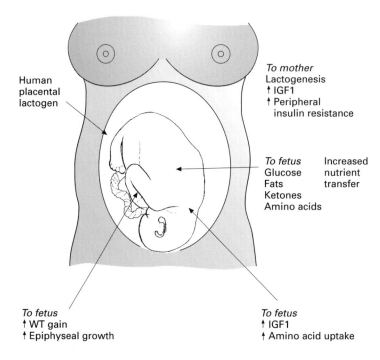

Human placental lactogen

To mother
Lactogenesis
↑ IGF1
↑ Peripheral insulin resistance

To fetus   Increased
Glucose   nutrient
Fats   transfer
Ketones
Amino acids

To fetus
↑ WT gain
↑ Epiphyseal growth

To fetus
↑ IGF1
↑ Amino acid uptake

Fig. 7.10. Important metabolic effects of placental lactogen to ensure optimal supply of nutrients to the fetus and utilization of the nutrients by fetal tissues.

betes is found, the testing of the mother post-pregnancy with an oral glucose tolerance test is carried out about 6 weeks postpartum. Gestational diabetes is defined as having occurred in those returning to normal values and impaired glucose tolerance and pre-existing diabetes or those developing diabetes can then be diagnosed using the conventional World Health Organization (WHO) criteria (Table 7.4).

Clinical implications

Definitions of diabetes mellitus

Diabetes mellitus has been defined as a chronically elevated blood glucose. The cut-off points for the diagnosis are based on the likelihood of that person developing the complications of diabetes, either microvascular or large vessel disease and have been agreed internationally. The WHO Expert Committee (Table 7.4) set the blood glucose values based on a 75g GTT as either a fasting of greater than 7.8 mmol/l or a 2-hour postload of greater than 11.1 mmol/l [37]. This organization has recognized that within the remaining population there is a

group whose glucose tolerance is not entirely normal, and who can be identified as having impaired glucose tolerance. This group will often progress to frank diabetes over time and share some of the risks of large vessel disease [39]. They have recommended the 2-hour postload values to determine this group and suggest that it delineates those women with values 2 hours postload between 7.8 and 11.1 mmol/l on venous plasma and slightly higher (between 8.9 and 12.2 mmol/l) for capillary plasma. Normality is defined as those less than 7.8 mmol/l following challenge. Assessment of the fasting sample has recent guidance from the WHO and the American Diabetes Association (ADA) who now consider impaired glucose tolerance if fasting levels lie between 6.1 and 7.8 and normal defined as less than 6.1 mmol/l. This definition of a fasting value recently changed and remains an area of some controversy [40]. All definitions need to take account of the fact that capillary plasma glucose values are higher than venous plasma and this introduces another area of potential for misunderstanding in interpreting the literature.

Table 7.4. International criteria for the diagnosis of diabetes in pregnancy.
a 75 g glucose load after overnight fast (glucose measurements in mmol/l) WHO Expert Committee [37].

	Fasting		2 hours post load	
	Venous plasma	Capillary plasma	Venous plasma	Capillary plasma
Normal	<6.1	<6.1	<7.8	<8.9
Impaired glucose tolerance	<7.8	<7.8	7.8–11.1	8.9–12.2
Diabetes	>7.8	>7.8	>11.1	>12.2

b Gestational diabetes diagnosed if two or more of the following values are met or exceeded; 100 g glucose load after overnight fast (glucose measurements in mmol/l) National Diabetes Data Group [38].

		Time post load		
	Fasting	1 hour	2 hour	3 hour
Gestational diabetes (venous plasma)	5.8	10.6	9.2	8.1

Diabetes in pregnancy

During pregnancy, women with diabetes can be classified as having established (those having diabetes before the pregnancy), developing (diabetes presenting in pregnancy and persisting afterwards), or gestational diabetes (diabetes presenting in pregnancy). Taking into account the normal reduction in glucose tolerance during pregnancy, there is a further group where glucose intolerance is excessive, but not frankly diabetic, who have been labelled impaired glucose tolerance in pregnancy. Women with established diabetes will be those mothers diagnosed as having diabetes before pregnancy. This group in Europe and North America will be largely insulin-dependent diabetics, but in certain young women and particularly in certain races (for example, Indian, Chinese, Japanese and Afro-Caribbean), there may be non-insulin dependent diabetes which has presented at an early age. This is particularly seen with the advancing age of the mother, a situation becoming more prevalent in Europe and North America, where women are increasingly becoming pregnant above the age of 30 [41].

Strict blood glucose control aiming to render blood glucose levels within the range to achieve premeal values below 5 mmol/l and postprandial values below 7 mmol/l has been shown to reduce the mortality and morbidity for the infants of diabetic mothers. Perinatal mortality for these infants has declined dramatically, from 197 per 1000 live births in 1967 [42] to 20 per 1000 in 1984 [43] in the US, with similar figures in Europe. This improvement towards the normal rate can be seen in Fig. 7.11. It needs to be considered in the light of the overall reduction in the fetal death rate which, through changes in maternal health and obstetrical practice, have resulted in a 70% decline in the rate of fetal death among pregnant women of all ages since the 1960s [44].

Macrosomia, defined as a baby larger than 4.5 kg, is an obvious but rather crude index of the effects of maternal hyperglycaemia in the infant. It can occur in mothers with normal glucose tolerance especially in the obese, those with excessive weight gain in pregnancy, multiparous women, and older mothers. It makes no allowance for maternal build, race, gestation length, or the gender of the baby and is associated with protracted labour, shoulder dystocia, perinatal asphyxia, and skeletal and nerve injuries at birth. In the macrosomic infant of the diabetic mother, the increase in the size of viscera through an increase in cell number and size can lead to organ dysfunction such as a

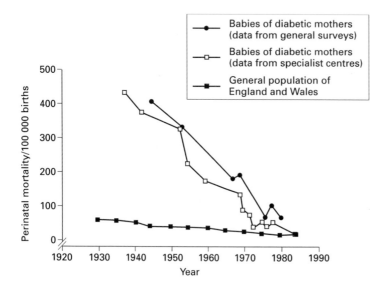

Fig. 7.11. The improvement in diabetic perinatal mortality (adapted from Lowy [40]).

hypertrophic cardiomyopathy with septal hypertrophy causing both ventricular outflow obstruction and heart failure (hydrops fetalis) [45].

Poor control of diabetes periconceptually in established diabetes increases the rate of major and minor congenital malformations and fetal wastage through miscarriage. The combined risk of congenital abnormalities and first-trimester spontaneous abortion in poorly controlled diabetes in early pregnancy can approach 65% [46]. The incidence of major congenital malformations among infants of diabetic mothers is 6% whereas that in a normal population is 2% [47]. This incidence reduces in diabetic women who plan pregnancy and are well controlled but remains above the normal rate, suggesting that other factors apart from glycaemic control are involved.

Pederson proposed in 1954 that maternal hyperglycaemia produces fetal hyperglycaemia and fetal hyperinsulinaemia and that the fetal hyperinsulinaemia stimulates fetal growth [42–44]. It is now recognized [46] that increased amino acids passing to the fetus have a synergistic effect with high glucose concentrations to promote fetal hyperinsulinaemia and macrosomia. The pathophysiology of these changes is represented in Fig. 7.12. Strict blood glucose control in the mothers during weeks 20–30 of gestation can reduce macrosomia, whereas good

glycaemic control in the third trimester may not have as large an effect [45]. Poor intrauterine growth can occur in 20% of diabetic pregnancies, particularly associated with mothers with hypertension or documented microvascular disease. The infants of poorly controlled diabetic mothers, particularly those macrosomic or dysmature, have increased rates of respiratory distress syndrome due to underdevelopment of the lung and a lack of alveolar surfactant; they have hypoglycaemia, sometimes severe, following birth, and hypocalcaemia, hypomagnesaemia, jaundice, and polycythaemia.

Screening for abnormal glucose tolerance

The success of the treatment of mothers with established diabetes with strict metabolic control achieving normoglycaemia during pregnancy has led to the concept particularly prevalent in the US that strict normalization of blood glucose in mothers who have any degree of glucose intolerance in pregnancy should be achieved and that mothers should be screened to achieve this. There can be little doubt that this approach discussed in more detail below will be valuable for the minority of mothers labelled in pregnancy as having glucose intolerance or gestational diabetes, who are in fact developing diabetes, or those who have previously unrecog-

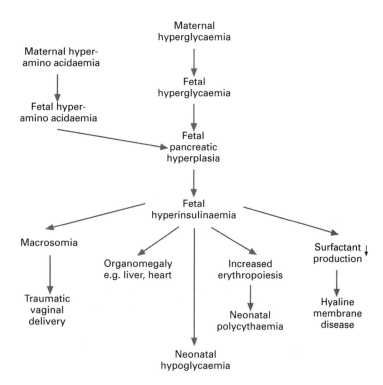

Fig. 7.12. Pederson's hypothesis on macrosomia [45].

nized diabetes. In this group of women, the pregnancy with its additional physiological stress to glucose tolerance produces hyperglycaemia. This group of women developing diabetes will include some type I insulin-dependent diabetics, since it has been shown that pregnancy can unmask this.

In countries that are multiethnic, young women may present during pregnancy who are early presentations of non-insulin dependent diabetes. During the pregnancy these women will be labelled gestational diabetics or as having impaired glucose tolerance of pregnancy, and it will be only with the postnatal check or blood glucoses taken after delivery that the fact that they have remained diabetic or glucose intolerant becomes apparent and this diagnosis can be made. It is likely that the babies of this small group would have the same risk if left untreated as the infants of other diabetic mothers and strict glycaemic control to reduce fasting values below 5 mmol/l and postprandial below 7 mmol/l are required for this group to reduce neonatal morbidity and mortality.

Gestational diabetes and impaired glucose tolerance in pregnancy

Gestational diabetes is defined as the development of abnormal glucose tolerance during pregnancy in a woman who was normal before and whose glucose tolerance returns to normal after pregnancy. As we have previously described, the tendency to postprandial hyperglycaemia is a physiological adaptation of normal pregnancy and there appears to be a spectrum of glucose tolerance influenced towards intolerance during the second half of pregnancy. Risk factors for the pregnant population include the age of the mother, ethnicity, family history of diabetes, and obesity. The definition of where on the upper end of this spectrum glucose tolerance can be considered abnormal and to constitute pathology is a matter of considerable debate. Despite many international conferences and attempts at agreement, there is no standard test based on an agreed fixed glucose load or, indeed, any consensus on interpretation. What has emerged is a division between the European and

North American approach and both will be described.

The WHO suggested that the 75 g oral GTT should be used and that investigators apply the diagnostic criteria as for impaired glucose tolerance outside pregnancy to diagnose gestational diabetes. This would imply that those with a 2-hour postglucose load of greater than 7.8 mmol/l would be abnormal [37]. The WHO Expert Committee's criteria are probably too low for the 2-hour postprandial state in pregnancy and too high for the fasting state (6.1–7.8 mmol/l) and identify two to three times more women as having gestational diabetes mellitus than the US and UK methods used in clinical practice that are validated in pregnancy [47,48]. Proponents of this definition argue that lesser degrees of glucose intolerance have been shown to be associated with adverse pregnancy outcome than the original O'Sullivan and Mahan criteria [49] modified in the US by the National Diabetes Advisory Board [38]. More recently, the Third International Workshop conference on gestational diabetes mellitus recommended that a 75 g glucose challenge be adopted and 'the highest priority should be given to efforts to develop international consensus on methods and definitions' [51]. This has not yet resulted in any agreed methodology or interpretation of results.

The American approach is to favour the 100 g load and there has been agreement to accept the original criteria based on studies by O'Sullivan and Mahan [49] and endorsed by the National Diabetes Data Group [38]. O'Sullivan and Mahan's original study is seminal as it was the first attempt to relate the abnormality of glucose tolerance during pregnancy to fetal outcome and the prediction of subsequent diabetes in the mothers during later life. The predictive value was based not only on a 100 g GTT but on two values being abnormal in a 3-hour test (Table 7.5).

In Europe, a study group of the European Association for the Study of Diabetes (EASD) recommended using the 75 g oral load with a 1-hour and 2-hour cut-off and that carbohydrate intolerance (labelled 'impaired glucose tolerance of pregnancy') be assigned to women showing a 2-hour venous plasma or capillary whole blood of

Table 7.5. Upper limits of normality (**a**) in O'Sullivan's work following 100 g oral glucose tolerance test in 752 women [49]; (**b**) in Abell and Beischer's following a 50 g in 200 women at 32–34 weeks [52] (**c**) a multicentre EASD study group using 75 g in 513 women after 28 weeks [51]; (**d**) UK study (within **c**) excluding first degree relatives of diabetics in 168 women at 28–37 weeks [11].

Glucose (mmol/l)	Time (hours)			
	0	1	2	3
a 100 g	5.0	9.2	8.1	6.9
b 50 g (32–34 weeks)	5.2	9.2	7.1	5.9
c 95 centile, 75 g (28–40 weeks)	5.2	10.5	9.0	8.0
d 97.5 centile, 75 g (28–37 weeks)	4.8	11.0	9.6	

9 mmol/l or more when it is combined with a 1-hour value of greater than 10.5 mmol/l [51]. They recommended that the term 'gestational diabetes' should be reserved for those in whom blood glucose levels are diagnostic of diabetes, using the existing agreed international criteria outside pregnancy (fasting greater than 7.8 or 2-hour greater than 11.1 mmol/l). This group, led by Lind, point out that 10% of pregnant women will exceed a value of 8 mmol/l at 2 hours but it is unlikely that 10% of the European population have abnormal carbohydrate metabolism. By insisting on a 1-hour value of 10.5 mmol/l as necessary to define an abnormal response, 15 women out of 500 were identified instead of the 79 who would have been identified if a 2-hour concentration of 9.0 mmol/l alone was chosen.

A further study from the UK [11] stresses the importance of gestational age in assessing glucose tolerance and defines the 97.5 centile after a 75 g oral glucose load as 7.5 mmol/l for the second trimester (weeks 14–20), but 9.6 mmol/l for the third trimester (weeks 28–36). In this physiological study, the second trimester postload values are close to the WHO suggestion of 7.8 mmol/l and the third trimester results are close to the EASD and American groups' 2-hour values of 9.0 mmol/l. The 1-hour value in the study for the second trimester was 8.8 and for the third trimester was 11.0 mmol/l. The fasting value was not different for the second and third trimester and the 97.5 centile during these trimesters was 4.9 and 4.8 respectively.

Much of the apparent disagreement on the definition of abnormal glucose tolerance in pregnancy may be related to differences in the timing during pregnancy when screening occurs. Impaired glucose tolerance in pregnancy could be defined during the second trimester as fasting above 5, 1 hour above 9, and 2 hours above 7.8 mmol/l, and in the third trimester fasting above 5, 1 hour above 10.5, and 2 hours above 9 mmol/l. Gestational diabetes might be reserved for those with 2-hour values greater than 11.1 or fasting values greater than 5.8. These criteria, which are the author's own practice, try to synthesize the many different values adopted by different bodies and to approximate the 97.5 centiles for normal pregnant populations. Clearly a consensus and international agreement is needed to establish a baseline for further research and evidence based clinical practice.

Implications for the infant

It has been claimed that the pregnancy-related morbidity and perinatal mortality in gestational diabetes defined on O'Sullivan and Mahan's criteria are less than those for established diabetic women but that if these women are left untreated they are significantly higher than for non-diabetic women [47,48,52]. Maternal obesity is a co-existing risk factor in this increase in perinatal morbidity associated with fetal macrosomia [53]. Figure 7.13 shows a macrosomic infant with a mother who had impaired glucose tolerance during pregnancy which was relatively mild.

Maternal obesity does not contribute to the other aspects of morbidity seen in the diabetic mothers' offspring so that neonatal hypoglycaemia, polycythaemia, jaundice and hypocalcaemia are all related to the degree of maternal hyperglycaemia. There remains a small increase of unexplained late stillbirths in gestational diabetes and impaired glucose tolerance in pregnancy. Reports from the Second International Workshop Conference [54] suggest that gesta-

tional diabetes can show macrosomia, hypoglycaemia, polycythaemia and jaundice in up to 25% of infants of mothers with this condition. The wide fluctuations in perinatal mortality reported at this workshop (0–28.5%) presumably reflect the differences in both obstetric and perinatal care, ethnic risk, and social factors such as the nutrition of the mothers across the world. In the most recent large series from Canada of pregnancy diabetes that could be adequately treated with diet, between 1961 and 1974 or between 1978 and 1993, it was found not to be a significant risk factor for fetal death [41].

Macrosomia is the most common condition cited in the reports of perinatal mortality in

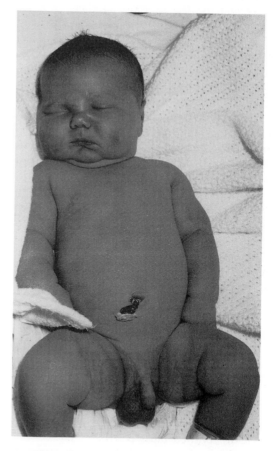

Fig. 7.13. Macrosomic infant of mother with impaired glucose tolerance during pregnancy which was relatively mild.

pregnant women with glucose intolerance or gestational diabetes mellitus [48,54–57]. Despite some reports to the contrary [55], it is generally accepted that there is no increase in congenital malformations in true gestational diabetes because significant maternal hyperglycaemia in this group occurs after organogenesis has taken place [58]. Some reports that suggest an increase probably includes mothers with pre-existing diabetes recognized only in the later stages of pregnancy. O'Sullivan's original work was carried out in Boston, a city centre population of multiethnic origin, in the 1950s, in which there may have been a significant number of women discovered during pregnancy who were not really gestational but were unrecognized early presenters of non-insulin dependent diabetes. This, and the fact of obese mothers as a co-existing variable, may explain the relatively high perinatal mortality. O'Sullivan had reported this as 6% in the 1950s and most recent reports indicate values well below 1%, approximating the normal rate for the background pregnant population.

With the general improvement in perinatal outcomes, all recently published studies [41,57,58] have failed to detect an increase in the perinatal mortality rate among women defined as having gestational diabetes. Most US authorities [57,58] interpret this as implying that now that there is earlier identification of gestational diabetes through screening combined with better obstetric care, there has been success in lowering the risk of perinatal mortality. In a recent large study in the UK [59] Hadden showed no difference in fetal outcome or neonatal morbidity or in the incidence of antenatal complications between the normal or gestational and impaired glucose tolerance group.

Is identification of mothers with impaired glucose tolerance or gestational diabetes worthwhile?

A more sceptical approach has emerged and Jarret [60] has argued that there is little evidence to support an increased perinatal mortality in this group of women, proposing that the increase reported in the early studies [47] arose in the absence of correction for the variables of maternal obesity, race or age. He argues that screening, and indeed the whole concept of gestational diabetes, causes more maternal stress and wastes health care resources than it produces in health benefit for the infants of these mothers.

Indirect support for the view that attempts to prevent macrosomia may produce no significant improvement in the health care of infants of these mothers and may even harm them in the long term has recently been produced by the epidemiological studies of Barker et al. [61]. Previous studies [62,63] claimed that gestational diabetes or impaired glucose tolerance in pregnancy changed the intrauterine milieu to influence the later development of type 2 diabetes and obesity in the infants of these mothers. The argument proposed was that more individuals with impaired glucose tolerance or non-insulin dependent diabetes later in life occur if there is a maternal rather than a paternal history of diabetes. This was interpreted as suggesting that maternal hyperglycaemia in pregnancy may be an important influence as well as the expected parental genetic factors. However, maternally inherited diabetes mellitus may be largely genetic and has been associated with a form of non-insulin dependent diabetes with a mitochondrial abnormality and deafness [64].

Clearly these data also need to be interpreted in the light of the fact that 20% of the offspring of mothers with diabetes will suffer intrauterine growth retardation and not macrosomia. Barker's work is difficult to reconcile with these results, as he examined birthweight and development of non-insulin dependent diabetes and impaired tolerance later in life (by middle age) in a cohort of offspring identified from 1911 to 1930 in Hertfordshire in the UK. His data showed that the larger the baby in terms of birthweight, the lower the risk of developing diabetes or impaired tolerance in later life and the lower the risk of hypertension and coronary heart disease. These studies at a time when screening and treatment of gestational diabetes did not exist must have included those women who on the present criteria would have been defined as having gestational diabetes or impaired glucose tolerance in pregnancy. While it is possible that selection bias may exist in these studies in as much as some of the pregnancies complicated by severe gestational diabetes pregnancies may not have resulted in live births, these studies do suggest that intrauterine growth retardation and small babies rather than macrosomia may be storing up later health problems in the progeny. They raise the possibility that the over-zealous attempts to reduce fetal macrosomia pursued in even minor degrees of glucose intolerance [65] could interfere with what is in fact a normal homeostatic adaptation of the mother to pregnancy. There could be the potential to cause harm if growth retardation is produced and these offspring are left with an increased chance of developing serious diseases in later life.

Implications for the mother of the diagnosis of gestational diabetes

Identifying mothers with impaired glucose tolerance or gestational diabetes during a pregnancy may not improve fetal outcome in modern obstetric practice, but should protect the mother's health in the future. This group of women have been shown to constitute a high risk group for hypertension and pre-eclampsia in pregnancy [65], a risk that appears to increase with intolerance.

Those women in the process of developing diabetes or who were previously unrecognized until the screening during pregnancy should benefit by allowing the introduction of strict metabolic control, often with insulin, prior to any future pregnancy. This group should also benefit if earlier treatment and optimizing glycaemic and lipid control reduces the risk of long-term microvascular and macrovascular complications of diabetes.

True gestational diabetes, those that show normal glucose tolerance postpartum, remain at a greatly increased risk of diabetes in future pregnancies [66] and for the development of diabetes later in life [67,68]. About 5% will develop diabetes requiring insulin within 5 years of the index pregnancy [67,68]. O'Sullivan recorded that as many as 40% of all women classifying as gestational diabetes on his criteria develop either impaired glucose tolerance or non-insulin dependent diabetes within 20 years [69]. An important influence on the percentage that will subsequently develop diabetes later in life will be the ethnicity of the population reported [70,71]. Among Asian women, 50% of those identified as having gestational diabetes develop non-insulin dependent diabetes within 4 years [71]. Other high risk factors are obesity, a family history of diabetes, a high fasting glucose in pregnancy, and those in pregnancy requiring insulin [67]. Obese mothers who show further weight gain following a pregnancy in which there was gestational diabetes have a twofold increased risk of subsequent impaired tolerance or diabetes mellitus, while mothers exhibiting weight loss showed only half this rate [68]. In contrast to these studies, diabetes in later life was observed in only 2% in a Belfast population over a 10-year follow-up [70]. The racial mix and presence of the other risk factors clearly influences these population figures.

Health education for the obese, the need to avoid smoking and encouraging exercise in this group has the potential to prevent or delay the onset of diabetes in later life [72]. Encouraging these women to engage in regular screening for diabetes or impaired glucose tolerance should lead to earlier diagnosis and a reduced chance of damage to the future health of these mothers from undiagnosed diabetes [72].

References

1 Hagay Z.J. & Reece E.A. (1992) Diabetes mellitus in pregnancy. In *Medicine of the Fetus and Mother*. Eds E.A. Reece, J.C. Hobbins, J.M. Mahoney & R.H. Petrie, p. 982. Lippincott, Philadelphia.

2 Kahn C.R. (1978) Insulin resistance, insulin insensitivity and insulin unresponsiveness: a necessary distinction. *Metabolism* **27** (Suppl. 2), 1893.

3 Lind T., Billewicz W.Z. & Brown G. (1973) A serial study of changes in the oral glucose tolerance test during pregnancy. *Journal of Obstetrics and Gynaecology of the British Commonwealth* **80**, 1033.

4 Felig P. & Lynch V. (1970) Starvation in human pregnancy: hypoglycaemia, hypoinsulinaemia and hyperketonaemia. *Science* **170**, 900.

5 Cousins L., Rigg L., Hollingsworth D., Brink G., Auran J. & Yen S. (1980) The 24 hour excursion and diurnal rhythm of glucose insulin and C-peptide in normal pregnancy. *American Journal of Obstetrics and Gynaecology*, **136**, 483.

6 Kühl C. (1977) Serum insulin and plasma glucogon in

210

human pregnancy: on the pathogenesis of gestational diabetes. *Acta Diabetologia* **14**, 1.

7 Lind T. (1975) Changes in carbohydrate metabolism during pregnancy. *Clinical Obstetrics and Gynaecology* **2**, 395.

8 Fraser R.B. (1981) The normal range of the OGTT in the African female: pregnant and non-pregnant. *East African Medical Journal* **58**, 90.

9 Okonofua F.E., Amole F.A., Ayangade S.O. & Ninalaraj T. (1988) Criteria for the oral glucose tolerance test in pregnant and non-pregnant Nigerian women. *International Journal of Obstetrics and Gynaecology* **27**, 85.

10 Gillmer M.D.G., Beard R.W., Broske F.M. & Oakley N.W. (1975) Carbohydrate metabolism in pregnancy: the diurnal profile in normal and diabetic women. *British Medical Journal* **3**, 399.

11 Hatem M., Anthony F., Hogston P., Rowe D.J. & Dennis K.J. (1988) Reference values for 75g oral glucose tolerance test in pregnancy. *British Medical Journal* **296**, 676.

12 Freinkel N., Metzger B. & Nitzan M. (1974) Facilitated anabolism in late pregnancy: some novel maternal compensations for accelerated starvation. *In Diabetes*. Eds W.J. Mallaise & J. Pirart, p. 474. Excerpta Medica, Amsterdam.

13 Lind T., Bell S., Gilmore E., Huisjes H.J. & Schally A.V. (1977) Insulin disappearance rate in pregnant and non-pregnant women and in non-pregnant women given GHRIH. *European Journal of Clinical Investigation* **7**, 47.

14 Ryan E.A., O'Sullivan M.J. & Skyler J.S. (1985) Insulin action during pregnancy: studies with the euglycaemic clamp technique. *Diabetes* **34**, 380.

15 Elliot J.A. (1975) The effect of pregnancy on the control of lipolysis in fat cells isolated from human adipose tissue. *European Journal of Clinical Investigation* **5**, 159.

16 Catalano P.M., Bernstein I.M., Wolfe R.R. Srikanta S., Tyzbir E. & Sims E.A. (1986) Subclinical abnormalities of glucose metabolism in subjects with previous gestational diabetes. *American Journal Obstetrics and Gynaecology* **155**, 1255.

17 Catalano P.M., Tyzbier E.D. & Roman N.M. (1991) Longitudinal changes in insulin release and insulin resistance in non-obese pregnant women. *American Journal of Obstetrics and Gynaecology* **165**, 1667.

18 Buchanan T.A., Metzgen B.E., Freinkel N. & Bergman R.N. (1990) Insulin sensitivity and B-cell responsiveness to glucose during late pregnancy in lean and moderately obese women with normal GTT or mild gestational diabetes. *American Journal of Obstetrics and Gynaecology* **162**, 1008.

19 Pagano G., Cassader M., Massobrio M., Bozzo C., Trossarelli G.F., Menato G. & Lenti G. (1980) Insulin binding to human adipocytes during late pregnancy in healthy obese and diabetic state. *Hormone and Metabolic Research* **12**, 177.

20 Livingstone C., Dominiczak A.F., Campbell I.W. & Gould G.W. (1995) Insulin resistance, hypertension and the insulin responsive glucose transporter, GLUT 4. *Clinical Science* **89**, 109.

21 Kalkhoff R.K., Jacobson M. & Lemper D. (1970) Progesterone, pregnancy and the augmented plasma insulin response. *Journal of Clinical Endocrinology and Metabolism* **31**, 24.

22 Garvey W.T., Maianu L., Zhu J.-H., Golichowski A.M. & Hancock J.A. (1993) Herterogeneity in the number and a novel abnormality in subcellular localisation of GLUT 4 glucose transporters. *Diabetes* **42**, 1773.

23 Mulford M.I., Jovanovic-Peterson L. & Peterson C.M. (1993) Alternative therapies for the managment of gestational diabetes. *Clinic in Perinatology* **20**, 619.

24 Kühl C., Horness P.J. & Anderson O. (1985) Aetiology and pathophysiology of gestational diabetes mellitus. *Diabetes* **34** (Suppl. 2), 66.

25 Wynn V., Adams P.W., Godsland I., Melrose J., Niththyananthan R., Oakley N.W. & Seed M. (1979) Comparison of effects of different combined oral contraceptive formulations on carbohydrate and lipid metabolism. *Lancet* **i**, 1045.

26 Michaels R.L., Sorenson R.L., Parsons J.A. *et al.* (1987) Prolactin enhances cell to cell communication among beta cells in pancreatic islets. *Diabetes* **36**, 1098.

27 Hornnes P.J., Kuhl C. & Lauritsen K.B. (1981) Gastrointestinal insulinotropic hormones in normal and gestational diabetic pregnancy. *Diabetes* **30**, 504.

28 Lederman R.P., McCann D.S. & Work B. (1977) Endogenous plasma epinephrine and norepinephrine in last trimester pregnancy and labor. *American Journal of Obstetrics and Gynecology* **129**, 5.

29 Mintz D.H., Stock R., Finster J.L. & Taylor A.L. (1968) The effect of normal and diabetic pregnancies on growth hormone responses to hypoglycaemia. *Metabolism* **17**, 54.

30 Tritos N.A. & Mantzoros C.S. (1997) Leptin, its role in obesity and beyond. *Diabetologia* **40**, 1371.

31 Masuzaki H., Ogawa Y., Sagawa N. Hosoda K., Matsumoto T., Mise H., Nishimura H. *et al.* (1997) Nonadipose tissue production of leptin: leptin as a novel placenta-derived hormone in humans. *National Medical* **3**, 1029.

32 Hassink S.G., de Lancey E., Sheslow, D.V. Smith-Kirwin S.M., O'Connor D.M., Considine R.V., Openianova I. *et al.* (1997) Placental leptin: An important new growth factor in intrauterine and neonatal development? *Paediatrics* **100**, E1.

33 Gaspard V.J., Sandront H.M. & Luychz A.S. (1975) The control of human placental lactogen (HPL) secretion and its inter-relation with glucose and lipid metabolism in late pregnancy. In *Diabetes in Early Life*. Eds R.H. Camerini-Davalos & H.S. Coles, p. 273, Academic Press, New York.

34 Handwerger S. (1991) Clinical counterpoint: the physiology of placental lactogen in human pregnancy. *Endocrine Reviews* **12**, 329.

35 Spellacy W.N. & Goetz F.C. (1963) Plasma insulin in normal late pregnancy. *New England Journal of Medicine* **268**, 988.

36 Lind T. & Harris V.G. (1976) Changes in the oral glucose tolerance test during the puerperium. *British Journal of Obstetrics and Gynaecology* **83**, 460.

37 WHO Study Group (1997) Report of the expert committee on diagnosis of diabetes mellitus. *Diabetes Care* **20**, 1183.

38 National Diabetes Data Group (1985) *Report of an Expert Committee on Diabetes*. Bethesda, National Institutes of Health.

39 Keen H., Jarrett R.J. & McCartney P. (1982) The ten

year follow up of the Bedford study glucose tolerence and diabetes (1962–72). *Diabetologia* **22**, 73.

40 Pickup J. & Williams G. (Eds) (1991) *Textbook of Diabetes*. Blackwell Scientific Publishers, Oxford.

41 Freets R.C., Schmittriel J., McLean F.H., Usher R. & Goldman M.B. (1995) Increased maternal age and the risk of fetal death. *New England Journal of Medicine* **333**, 953.

42 Pedersen J.F. (1967). *The Pregnant Diabetic and Her Newborn*. Williams and Wilkins, Baltimore. p. 126.

43 Landon M.B. (1991) Diabetes mellitus and other endocrine diseases. In *Obstetrics*. Eds S.G. Gabbe, J.R. Niebyl & J.L. Simpson, p. 112. Churchill Livingstone, New York.

44 Greene M.F. (1993) Prevention and diagnosis of congenital abnormalities in diabetic pregnancies. *Clinics in Perinatology* **20**, 533.

45 Pedersen J.F. (1954) Weight and length at birth of infants of diabetic mothers. *Acta Endocrinologica* **18**, 330.

46 Freinkel N. (1980) Of pregnancy and progeny: Banting Lecture 1980. *Diabetes* **29**, 1023.

47 O'Sullivan J.B., Mohan C.M., Charles D. & Dandrow R.V. (1973) Gestational diabetes and perinatal mortality rate. *American Journal of Obstetrics and Gynaecology* **116**, 901.

48 Pettitt D.J., Knowler W.C., Baird H.R. & Bennet P.H. (1980) Gestational diabetes: infant and maternal complications of pregnancy in relation to third trimester glucose tolerance in the Pima Indians. *Diabetes Care* **3**, 458.

49 O'Sullivan J.B. & Mahan C.B. (1964) Criteria for the oral glucose tolerance test in pregnancy. *Diabetes* **13**, 278.

50 Metzger B.E. & Organising Committee (1991) Summary and recommendations of the 3rd International Workshop, Conference on Gestational Diabetes Mellitus. *Diabetes* **40**, 197.

51 Lind T., Sutherland H.W., Stowers J.M. & Pearson D.W.M. (1989) A prospective multi-centre study to determine the influence of pregnancy upon the 75 g oral glucose tolerance test (OGTT). In *Carbohydrate Metabolism in Pregnancy and the Newborn*. Diabetic Pregnancy Study Group of the EASD, p. 209. Churchill Livingston, New York.

52 Abell D.A. & Beischer N.A. (1975) Evaluation of the three-hour oral glucose tolerance test in detection of significant hyperglycaemia and hypoglycaemia. *Diabetes* **24**, 874.

53 Green J.R., Schumacher L.B. & Pawson I.G. (1991) Influence of maternal body habitus and glucose tolerance on birth. *Obstetrics and Gynecology* **78**, 235.

54 The Organising Committee (1985) Summary and recommendations of the Second International Workshop Conference on Gestational Diabetes Mellitus. *Diabetes* **34**, 123.

55 Oats J.N., Abell D.A., Beischer N.A. & Broomhale G.R. (1980) Maternal glucose tolerance during pregnancy with excessive size infants. *Obstetrics and Gynaecology* **55**, 184.

56 Willman S.P., Leveno K.J. & Guzick D.S. (1986) Glucose threshold for macrosomia in pregnancy complicated by diabetes. *American Journal of Obstetrics and Gynaecology* **154**, 470.

57 Hod M., Merlob P., Friedman S., Schoenfeld A. & Ovadia J. (1991) Gestational diabetes mellitus: a survey of perinatal complications in the 1980s. *Diabetes* **40** (S2), 74.

58 Coustan D.R. (1994) Screening and diagnosis of gestational diabetes. *Seminars in Perinatology* **18**, 407.

59 Roberts R.N., Mohan I.M., Foo R.L.K., Harley J.M.G., Traub A.I. & Hadden D.R. (1993) Fetal outcome in mothers with impaired glucose tolerance in pregnancy. *Diabetic Medicine* **10**, 438.

60 Jarret R.J. (1993) Gestational diabetes: a non-entity? *British Medical Journal* **306**, 37.

61 Barker D.J.P., Hales C.N., Fall C.H.D., Osmond C. & Winter P.D. (1993) Type 2 (non-insulin dependent) diabetes mellitus, hypertension and hyperlipidaemia (syndrome X): relation to foetal growth. *Diabetologia* **36**, 62.

62 Pettit D., Aleck K., Baird H., Carreher M., Bennett B. & Knowler W. (1988) Congenital susceptibility to NIDDM: role of intra-uterine environment. *Diabetes* **37**, 622.

63 Pettit D.J., Bennett P.H., Knowler W.C., Baird H.C. & Aleck K.A. (1985) Gestational diabetes mellitus and impaired glucose tolerance during pregnancy: long term effects on obesity and glucose intolerance in the offspring. *Diabetes* **34** (S2), 119.

64 Alcolado J.C. & Alcolado R. (1991) Importance of maternal history of non-insulin dependent diabetic patients. *British Medical Journal* **302**, 1178.

65 Tallarigo L., Giam Petro O., Penno G. *et al.* (1986) Relation of glucose to complications of pregnancy in non-diabetic women. *New England Journal Medicine* **315**, 989.

66 Philipson E.H. & Super D.M. (1989) Gestational diabetes mellitus: does it recur in subsequent pregnancy? *American Journal of Obstetrics Gynaecology* **160**, 1324.

67 Damm P.D., Molsted-Pedersen L.M.P. & Kuhl C.K. (1989) High incidence of diabetes mellitus and impaired glucose tolerance in women with previous gestational diabetes (abstract). *Diabetologia* **32**, 479a.

68 Dornhurst A., Bailey P.C., Anyaoku V., Elkeles R.S., Johnston D.G. & Beard R.W. (1990) Abnormalities of glucose tolerance following gestational diabetes. *Quarterly Journal of Medicine* **284**, 1219.

69 O'Sullivan J.B. (1984) Subsequent morbidity among gestational diabetic women. In *Carbohydrate Metabolism in Pregnancy and Newborn*. Eds H.W. Sutherland & J.M. Stowers, p. 174. Churchill Livingston, New York.

70 Hadden D.R. (1980) Screening for abnormalities of carbohydrate metabolism in pregnancy 1966–1977: the Belfast experience. *Diabetes Care* **3**, 440.

71 Motala A.A., Omar M.A.R. & Gouws E. (1993) High risk of progression of NIDDM in South African Indians with impaired glucose tolerance. *Diabetes* **42**, 556.

72 Dornhorst A. (1994) Implications of gestational diabetes for the health of the mother. *British Journal of Obstetrics and Gynecology* **101**, 286.

Calcium Metabolism

D.J. HOSKING

Normal pregnancy is associated with substantial changes in maternal mineral metabolism but since calcium is the most important element, both physiologically and quantitatively, it will be the focus of this review. However, the regulation of other elements, particularly magnesium and phosphate, also needs to be considered and this will be done in the context of their inter-relationship with calcium. Zinc, copper and other trace elements are reviewed in Chapter 6.

The driving force behind the changes in maternal calcium homeostasis is the need to provide for the mineralization of the fetal skeleton. However, mineral homeostasis is also important because its derangement may also have a substantial influence on the development of clinical disorders such as pre-eclampsia or maternal osteoporosis.

It is necessary to begin with a review of normal calcium homeostasis so that the changes which occur as pregnancy advances can be seen in context. The unique features of fetal mineral metabolism are then discussed in detail before considering the pathophysiological basis of mineral disorders of pregnancy.

Calcium, magnesium and phosphate homeostasis

The body contains about 1000 g of calcium, all of which is in bone except for 9 g (225 mmol) in the soft tissues and 1 g (25 mmol) in the extracellular fluid (ECF). The ionized calcium (Ca^{2+}) concentration of the ECF (1.0–1.3 mmol) is closely regulated by the co-ordinated actions of the parathyroid hormone–vitamin D endocrine system acting on the kidney, intestine and bone. Although stability of the ECF Ca^{2+} is required for its role in blood coagulation and the maintenance of plasma membranes, it is also important as a source of intracellular calcium which is an essential regulator of a variety of cellular functions. The cytosolic free calcium concentration in resting cells is about 100 nmol but rises 10- to 100-fold with activation [1]. Intracellular calcium concentrations are regulated by a series of channels, pumps and other transport mechanisms which control the movement of Ca^{2+} in and out of cells and determine the partition between the various intracellular compartments [2].

The essential characteristic of the calcium

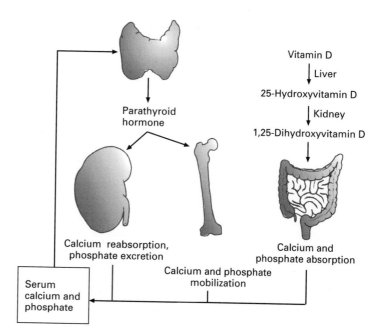

Vitamin D

Liver

25-Hydroxyvitamin D

Kidney

1,25-Dihydroxyvitamin D

Parathyroid
hormone

Calcium reabsorption,
phosphate excretion

Calcium and
phosphate absorption

Calcium and phosphate
mobilization

Serum
calcium and
phosphate

Fig. 8.1. Parathyroid
hormone–vitamin D endocrine
system.

homeostatic system is the ability of the parathyroid cells to sense, and respond to, alterations in ECF Ca^{2+} with an appropriate change in the rate of parathyroid hormone (PTH) secretion [1]. These responses are extremely rapid, occurring over a few seconds, and involve two types of end organ response. There is an immediate effect on calcium transport in kidney and bone to effect short-term buffering of the calcium concentration. There is also a more sustained homeostatic response acting through regulation of the renal production of 1,25-dihydroxyvitamin D $(1,25(OH)_2D)$ which modulates calcium transport in intestine and bone [3]. This system is also integrated in such a way that the ECF Ca^{2+} concentration can be regulated independently of magnesium and phosphate (Fig. 8.1).

Parathyroid hormone–vitamin D endocrine system

Parathyroid cell calcium receptor

It has been recognized for many years that ECF Ca^{2+} acts directly on the parathyroid cell to regulate the secretion of PTH but it is only recently that the molecular basis for this effect has been identified [1]. The cell surface Ca^{2+} receptor which enables the parathyroid cell to detect and respond to ECF Ca^{2+} is a member of the G protein coupled receptor (GPCR) superfamily. These cell surface receptors share a common structure of a single polypeptide chain which has an extracellular amino terminus, seven membrane spanning domains and an intracellular terminus [4] (Fig. 8.2). The human parathyroid cell Ca^{2+} receptor is made up of 1078 amino acids, with high sequence homology (93%) with the bovine calcium receptor. GPCRs respond to a wide variety of agonists and this diversity is reflected in differences in the structure of the receptor–ligand binding domain. Small agonists like calcium bind in a pocket formed by the extracellular loops and this is assumed to cause a conformational change in the receptor which activates the associated G protein [5]. This in turn is coupled to a variety of downstream pathways including adenylate cyclase/cAMP and phospholipase C/phosphoinositol, which mediate the actions of the ligand within the cell [6].

There is no convincing evidence that cyclic adenosine monophosphate (cAMP) plays a

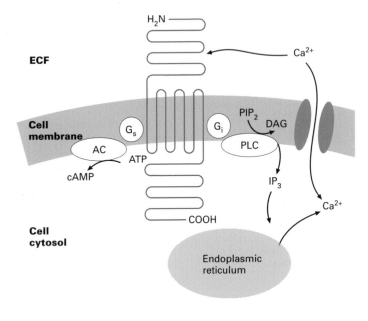

Fig. 8.2. Cell surface calcium receptor. AC: adenylate cyclase; ATP: adenosine triphosphate; cAMP: cyclic adenosine monophosphate; DAG: diacylglycerol; ECF: extracellular fluid; G_s, G_i: stimulatory and inhibitory G proteins; IP_3: inositol triphosphate; PIP_2: phosphatidylinositol bisphosphate; PLC: phospholipase C.

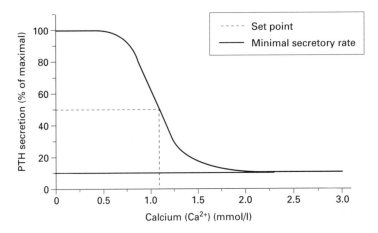

Fig. 8.3. Relationship between parathyroid hormone (PTH) secretion and extracellular fluid Ca^{2+} [1].

significant role in PTH secretion and attention has focused on the phosphoinositol pathway. Activation of the calcium receptor is thought to stimulate phospholipase C which hydrolyses phosphatidylinositol 4,5-bisphosphate to inositol 1,4,5-triphosphate (IP_3) and diacylglycerol (DAG). The increase in IP_3 leads to the mobilization of intracellular calcium, probably from the endoplasmic reticulum while DAG, perhaps controlled by receptor activation itself, may play a key role in regulating PTH secretion [7].

Persistent agonist stimulation of the GPCR leads to phosphorylation of the C-terminus and cytoplasmic loops of the calcium receptor by protein kinase C and as a consequence its sensitivity to activation by ECF Ca^{2+} is decreased. More chronic receptor down-regulation may be modulated at a transcriptional level by cAMP responsive elements in the promotor region of the GPCR gene [8].

There is a steep inverse sigmoidal relationship between PTH secretion and ECF Ca^{2+} (Fig. 8.3) which encompasses a number of important physiological characteristics of the parathyroid cell

[1]. The set point is the Ca^{2+} at which secretion is half maximally inhibited (about 1 mmol) and determines the concentration around which ECF Ca^{2+} is regulated (1.1–1.3 mmol). The steep slope at the set point ensures a large change in PTH secretion for a small change in Ca^{2+} which helps maintain tight control of homeostasis. Secretory rates cover a fourfold range from minimum to maximum and as a result the gland has a large secretory reserve which can respond to a hypocalcaemic stimulus. However, under normal circumstances, relatively low secretory rates are required to maintain ECF Ca^{2+} homeostasis. ECF Mg^{2+} concentrations are principally regulated by the kidney which excretes the excess in hypermagnesaemia and conserves Mg^{2+} when there is a deficit. Despite this close homeostatic function there is no evidence that it is regulated by either PTH or $1,25(OH)_2D$ [9].

Synthesis of parathyroid hormone

The initial product of the parathyroid cell is a 115 amino acid polypeptide (pre-pro-PTH) which is subsequently cleaved, initially to pro-PTH (1–90) and then to PTH (1–84) as the hormone passes through the endoplasmic reticulum to the Golgi apparatus prior to secretion [10].

The PTH gene (on the short arm of chromosome 11) contains three exons separated by two introns; the first contains the 5′ non-coding region while exon II and part of III contain the coding region for pre-pro-PTH. Transcription produces an RNA precursor which undergoes post-transcriptional modification to produce pre-pro-PTH mRNA, which is translated on polyribosomes within the cell matrix. As the growing pre-proPTH emerges from the ribosome, the first two amino terminal methionines are removed. The remaining leader sequence of 23 amino acids facilitates transport through the endoplasmic reticulum to the Golgi apparatus but this is removed, prior to arrival, by a specific protease to produce pro-PTH. In the Golgi, pro-PTH undergoes a final post-translational modification to remove the amino terminal sequence of six amino acids to produce PTH. At this point the hormone is either packaged and stored in vesicles prior to secretion or is enzymatically degraded and secreted as biologically inactive fragments.

The immediate parathyroid response to a fall in ECF Ca^{2+} depends on release of stored hormone because it takes about 30 minutes for newly synthesized PTH to become available for secretion [11]. However, under normal circumstances a substantial proportion (about 50%) of newly synthesized PTH is degraded intracellularly but this process is inhibited when the demands on the gland increase. Although this adaptive response also takes about 40 minutes [12], it is rapid enough, supported by the release of stored and newly synthesized PTH, to allow the cell to respond appropriately without exhaustion.

Cellular actions of parathyroid hormone

PTH regulates the function of target cells through several signal transduction mechanisms initiated by binding of the hormone to specific cell surface receptors. The first to be identified was the adenylate cyclase/cAMP system but PTH may also act through the phosphoinositol pathway in some target cells. A more recent possibility is the non-receptor tyrosine kinase c-src which has been studied in cultured osteoblast-like cells [13]. It is uncertain whether these systems couple to a single or multiple receptor but present evidence favours a single receptor common to all target organs [10].

Binding of PTH to a specific cell surface receptor activates guanyl nucleotide binding proteins (G proteins) in the cell membrane. The G proteins, which may be stimulatory (G_s) or inhibitory (G_i), are made up of three guanyl nucleotide binding polypeptides, α, β and γ, which cycle between an active guanosine triphosphate (GTP) binding form and an inactive guanosine diphosphate (GDP) binding moiety [14]. Activation of the receptor leads to an exchange of GTP for GDP on the α-chain which then dissociates from the β–γ chains (Fig. 8.4). $G_{s\alpha}$ modulates the activity of adenylate cyclase located on the cytoplasmic side of the plasma membrane: the response is terminated by intrinsic hydrolytic activity of the α-chain which converts GTP to GDP [15]. This mechanism is

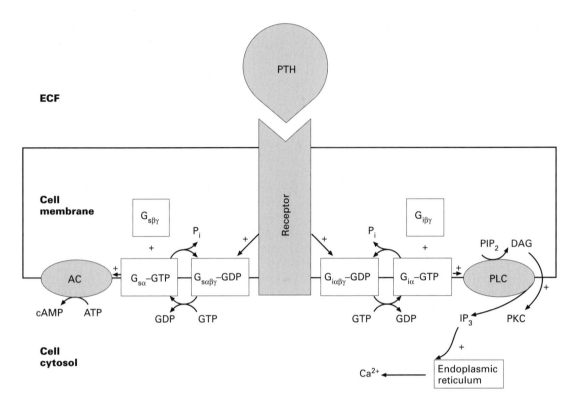

Fig. 8.4. PTH receptor and activation of adenylate cyclase and phospholipase C pathways. GDP: guanosine diphosphate; GTP: guanosine triphosphate; PKC: protein kinase C. See Fig. 8.2 for further abbreviation definitions.

distinct from that which occurs in response to repeated exposure to PTH which leads to a reduction in the number of available cell surface receptors with a consequential decrease in hormone sensitivity (down-regulation). However, it is uncertain whether this is a physiologically important mechanism or one only seen after exposure to pharmacological doses of PTH.

Activation of adenylate cyclase catalyses the production of cAMP which acts through a series of protein kinases made up of two catalytic and two regulatory subunits. Binding of cAMP to the regulatory units induces a conformational change which allows the subunits to dissociate from the complex. These catalyse the phosphorylation of serine and threonine residues on target proteins which subsequently express the effects of PTH on the target cell.

PTH also seems to act through agonist-receptor mediated hydrolysis of plasma membrane phosphoinositol with the production of IP_3

and DAG [16]. IP_3 seems responsible for release of calcium from intracellular stores such as the endoplasmic reticulum. Calcium then binds to calmodulin (molecular weight 16.7 kDa) and the calcium–calmodulin complex, which has no intrinsic enzyme activity, binds to protein kinases. These catalyse the phosphorylation of proteins which mediate the initial cellular response to PTH [17]. DAG, acting within the plane of the plasma membrane, activates protein kinase C which is believed to be involved in the sustained cellular response to PTH.

The current view is that PTH activates both adenylate cyclase and the phosphoinositol pathway through an effect on a single cell surface receptor. It is clear that activation of adenylate cyclase requires the first two amino acid residues (and acts through G_s) while the phosphoinositol pathway is activated by part of the sequence between residues 3 and 34 acting through G_i [18].

Vitamin D

Biochemistry

A major function of PTH is to regulate the renal production of $1,25(OH)_2D$, the major active metabolite of vitamin D. This in turn enhances calcium absorption from the intestine, reabsorption from the kidney, and mobilization from bone.

Vitamin D_3 (cholecalciferol) is either taken in the diet or synthesized by non-enzymic photolysis of 7-dehydrocholesterol in the Malpighian layer of the skin. This forms pre-vitamin D_3 which slowly isomerases to vitamin D_3. Dairy produce, eggs and oily fish are the main dietary sources of D_3 while vitamin D_2 (ergocalciferol) from plant sources is largely obtained from margarine. For practical purposes, vitamins D_3 and D_2 are biologically interchangeable, although there are differences in their rates of metabolism [19]. The daily requirement for vitamin D is in the region of 2.5 μg for an adult and 10 μg during pregnancy or for a child.

Vitamin D, from endogenous synthesis or upper small intestinal absorption, is transported to the liver bound to a specific α-globulin, and to a small extent albumin or lipoproteins, where it is hydroxylated to 25-hydroxyvitamin D (25-OHD) by microsomal and mitochondrial mixed function oxidases. This step requires reduced nicotinamide adenine dinucleotide phosphate (NADPH), molecular oxygen and magnesium, and increases the biological potency by two to five times, relative to parent vitamin D. This step is not tightly product inhibited and high circulating levels of 25-OHD may occur where substrate supply is increased.

Synthesis of 1,25-dihydroxyvitamin D

25-OHD passes to the proximal convoluted tubule (PCT) where it is hydroxylated by a mitochondrial mixed function oxygenase (1α-hydroxylase) to form $1,25(OH)_2D$. This is the rate limiting step in $1,25(OH)_2D$ synthesis and it is regulated predominantly by PTH and intracellular phosphate but also to a lesser degree by calcium, calcitonin, growth hormone, oestrogen, prolactin and $1,25(OH)_2D$ itself [19]. PTH mediates its effects through cAMP but the molecular pathways which form the basis of this action are unknown. Changes in ECF Ca^{2+} also influence $1,25(OH)_2D$ synthesis partly through reciprocal changes in PTH but also by a direct effect on the 1α-hydroxylase [1]. Recent studies have shown that monoclonal antibodies thought to bind to the parathyroid cell calcium receptor also cross-react with PCT cells [20]. This might provide a mechanism whereby a fall in ECF Ca^{2+} results in corresponding changes in intracellular Ca^{2+} which in turn may increase the activity of adenylate cyclase. Such a process might tie in with the effect of PTH stimulating $1,25(OH)_2D$ synthesis through the generation of cAMP.

The 1α-hydroxylase is strongly product inhibited and shows a reciprocal relationship with the renal 24-hydroxylase which converts 25-OHD to $24,25(OH)_2D$ and $1,25(OH)_2D$ to $1,24,25(OH)_3D$. The latter metabolite is considered to be the first step in the catabolic inactivation of $1,25(OH)_2D$. Although the function of $24,25(OH)_2D$ is uncertain, it is a major renal metabolite when circulating concentrations of $1,25(OH)_2D$ are high but has much less calcium-mobilizing effect on target organs than $1,25(OH)_2D$.

Vitamin D receptor

$1,25(OH)_2D$ exerts its biological effect through vitamin D receptors (VDR) which are members of the steroid–thyroid receptor gene superfamily of nuclear transcription factors. The VDR is predominantly located in the nucleus and contains a hormone-binding domain at the carboxy terminus and a DNA-binding region at the amino terminus. The steroid–receptor complex interacts with the promoter regions (vitamin D response elements: VDRE) of a number of genes including those of calcium-binding protein, the plasma membrane calcium pump, and the osteoblast product osteocalcin. This interaction may be either stimulatory or inhibitory. An interesting observation is that PTH suppresses VDR transcription in renal cells but not enterocytes which lack a PTH receptor.

Effect of parathyroid hormone and 1,25-dihydroxyvitamin D on target organs

Intestine

Calcium, magnesium and phosphate are absorbed both proximally in the duodenum and jejunum, where transport is active, and in the distal bowel, where the greater length and surface area make a significant contribution despite a less active transport process. Proximal absorption is an energy dependent and saturable process regulated by $1,25(OH)_2D$ and involves increased luminal permeability, intracellular calcium transport and active extrusion at the basolateral membrane [21]. In the distal intestine, calcium is absorbed by both a $1,25(OH)_2D$ modulated carrier process and by passive paracellular diffusion down a concentration gradient partially dependent on the luminal calcium concentration. Calcium may also be transported by an endocytic-exocytic vesicular flow process which allows calcium to be transported through the enterocyte without disturbance of cytosolic Ca^{2+} concentration [19].

Calcium transport in the enterocyte is facilitated by vitamin D dependent calcium-binding proteins (CaBP-D) which belong to the troponin-C superfamily, of which calmodulin (CaM) is also a member [22]. There are two calcium-binding proteins in the intestine, one of molecular weight 9 kDa (CaBP-D_{9k}) which is the most abundant, and one of 28 kDa (CaBP-D_{28k}). There is no sequence homology between these binding proteins each of which, despite differences in molecular weight, binds two Ca^{2+}/molecule of protein.

The first vitamin D dependent phase of active calcium absorption involves transport across the brush border membrane into the enterocyte (Fig. 8.5). This response is specific to $1,25(OH)_2D$ and is too rapid (seconds–minutes) to be a result of gene transcription and seems to depend on an opening of voltage-gated calcium channels in the enterocyte membrane [19]. This may be linked with an increase in phosphatidylcholine synthesis which may enhance membrane fluidity and increase the accessibility of calcium channels on the surface of the brush border membrane [23].

The second step in active calcium absorption involves transportation of calcium through the cell from apical to basolateral membrane (BLM) and involves both $1,25(OH)_2D$ and calcium-binding protein. $1,25(OH)_2D$ leads to an immediate and rapid transcription of the CaBP-D_{9k} gene followed by post-transcriptional effects which prevent degradation of CaBP-D_{9k} [24]. The subsequent accumulation, over a period of hours, of CaBP-D leads to an accelerated transfer of calcium from the apical brush border to CaBP-

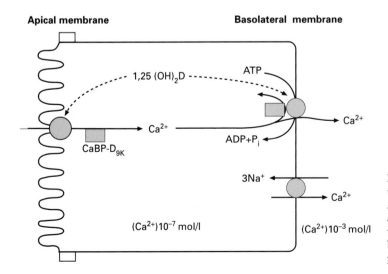

Fig. 8.5. Calcium transport across the enterocyte (see text for details). ADP: adenosine diphosphate; ATP: adenosine triphosphate; CaBP-D: vitamin D-dependent calcium-binding proteins; P_i: inorganic phosphate.

D_{9k} which has a fourfold greater affinity for Ca^{2+}. Since the plasma membrane calcium pump has a 2.5-fold greater affinity for Ca^{2+} than CaBP-D_{9k} there develops a progressively increasing gradient of calcium binding affinity from brush border to BLM which facilitates transcellular calcium transport [19].

The final step involves movement of calcium out into the ECF against a concentration gradient (low in enterocyte cytosol, 10^{-7} mol/l; high in ECF, 10^{-3} mol/l). This depends on the activity of the plasma membrane calcium pump and a Na^+-Ca^{2+} exchanger in the BLM. Expression of the plasma membrane Ca^{2+} pump mRNA and protein is vitamin D dependent. The pump itself is a Ca^{2+}-Mg^{2+}-dependent adenosine triphosphatase (ATPase) which uses adenosine triphosphate (ATP) to pump Ca^{2+} out of the cell into the ECF [25]. The activity of the duodenal pump is partially dependent on calmodulin but CaBP-D_{9k} has also been shown to stimulate this type of ATPase in a dose-dependent manner. It may be that CaBP-D_{9k} provides an alternative activator of the plasma membrane ATPase at cytosolic calcium concentrations which are too low for the calmodulin effect [26].

These cellular mechanisms are integrated with the needs of calcium homeostasis by the PTH–vitamin D endocrine system. Although PTH has no direct effect on the enterocyte, a change in secretion rate due to a deviation of ECF calcium from its set point is translated into a change in renal $1,25(OH)_2D$ production which, in turn, ensures an appropriate absorptive response. Although this process of adaptation is initiated within hours of a challenge to calcium homeostasis, it may take days or weeks to reach a new steady state [27].

About 30–50% of the dietary magnesium is absorbed and this occurs throughout the gastrointestinal tract but is maximal in the small intestine. Both active (saturable) and passive (unsaturable) mechanisms are involved although active transport becomes more important at lower magnesium intakes [9]. Magnesium transport is much less tightly regulated by $1,25(OH)_2D$ than calcium although a number of dietary constituents such as phosphate (but not calcium), fibre, phytate and oxalate may reduce the efficiency of absorption.

Transport of inorganic phosphate (P_i) across the luminal brush border membrane depends on a Na^+-P_i co-transporter. This produces an accumulation of sodium within the enterocyte which provides the driving force for phosphate transport. This step is the site at which $1,25(OH)_2D$ regulates phosphate absorption [28]. The mechanism which leads to transcellular P_i transport and extrusion at the basolateral membrane into the ECF is currently poorly understood.

Kidney

Although the major portion of the filtered load of calcium is reabsorbed by hormone-independent mechanisms in the proximal nephron, it is now clear that the calcium homeostatic function of the kidney resides in the distal convoluted tubule (DCT). The recognition that CaBP-D plays an important role in DCT transcellular transport [19] illustrates that in the kidney, as in bone and intestine, the interrelationship between PTH and $1,25(OH)_2D$ is central to the maintenance of homeostasis. In contrast to bone and intestine, where calcium and phosphate are co-transported, the kidney (under the influence of PTH which enhances the reabsorption of calcium and promotes the excretion of phosphate) is the only target organ where the transport of these two ions moves in opposite directions. A more recent development has been the emergence of evidence that a calcium receptor mechanism, similar to that in the parathyroid cell, may also be involved in the proximal tubular production of $1,25(OH)_2D$ and the distal tubular maintenance of calcium homeostasis [1].

Filtered load of calcium, magnesium and phosphate

In order to reach the urinary space the filtered fluid must cross the capillary endothelium, the glomerular basement membrane and the visceral epithelium of Bowman's capsule. The capillary endothelium is not a significant permeability barrier, except to blood cells. The visceral epithelial cells are not joined to form a single sheet but are separated from the basement membrane by processes (podocytes) through the gaps in which filtration occurs. The main barrier

220 to filtration is the basement membrane and the major determinants are molecular size and charge. Approximately 40% of the total serum calcium is albumin bound and since the latter does not pass through the basement membrane, only the ultrafilterable portion (50% ionized, 10% diffusable salts of citrate and lactate) passes into the urinary space. Magnesium is similarly protein bound and at a plasma concentration of 1 mmol/l about 50% is filtered at the glomerulus. In contrast, the phosphate concentration of the glomerular filtrate is approximately equal to that in serum. This is a consequence of a limited degree of protein binding (13%) and the effects of the Donnan equilibrium where the presence of protein in the glomerular capillaries, but not in the urinary space, induces an electrochemical gradient and an unequal distribution of ions across the basement membrane [29].

Proximal nephron

Calcium and magnesium reabsorption

Calcium and magnesium are predominantly reabsorbed paracellularly through the tight junctions between the PCT cells, driven by the concentration gradient established by sodium and water transport (Fig. 8.6). Both active and passive transport processes are involved [30]. Sodium crosses the luminal brush border of the PCT both through a co-transporter mechanism,

using other solutes such as glucose, phosphate or amino acids and via a counter transporter with H^+. These processes, which account for 30–60% of the PCT Na^+ reabsorption, are enhanced by the favourable concentration gradient due to the activity of a Na^+-K^+ ATPase pump in the basolateral membrane which maintains intracellular Na^+ substantially below (30 mmol/l) that of the tubular lumen (145 mmol/l). This is an expensive, energy-consuming process and is supplemented by passive sodium diffusion linked to chloride reabsorption. In the early PCT Cl^- is relatively poorly reabsorbed relative to other solutes, with the result that its concentration rises in more distal segments. Here the permeability of the tight junctions is relatively greater for Cl^- compared to other solutes leading to preferential reabsorption down a concentration gradient. Water and sodium follow passively down osmotic and electrochemical gradients respectively and this mechanism accounts for about 30% of PCT sodium and water reabsorption. These processes in the PCT and early diluting segment of the loop of Henle provide the driving force for the passive reabsorption of about 80% of the filtered load of calcium. The tight junctions of the PCT are relatively less permeable to Mg^{2+} where only about 30% of the filtered load is reabsorbed, the remainder (except for about 3% of the filtered magnesium load which is excreted) being reabsorbed in the early diluting segment of the loop of Henle [31].

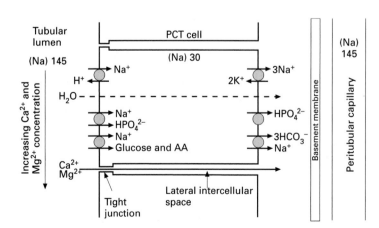

Fig. 8.6. Proximal tubular reabsorption of calcium and magnesium. AA: amino acids; PCT: proximal convoluted tubule.

Phosphate reabsorption

Phosphate transport differs from that of calcium in that active regulation is centred on the PCT where up to 70% of the filtered load is reabsorbed while the remainder of the nephron is relatively impermeable. The major component of the absorptive mechanism is a specific $2Na^+-HPO_4^{2-}$ electroneutral co-transporter in the luminal membrane (Fig. 8.6). The transport capacity of this system is primarily regulated by PTH but changes in plasma phosphate, metabolic acidosis and $1,25(OH)_2D$ may also be involved. The molecular basis for these effects is incompletely understood but the PTH response seems mediated through the activated subunits of the cAMP-dependent protein kinase which phosphorylates specific membrane proteins. Modulation of co-transporter activity may be due to binding to regulatory sites which are separated from those which bind phosphate (allosteric regulation) or there may be reversible covalent modification of the enzyme (activation–inactivation). Chronic or adaptive changes may depend on the synthesis of new transporter protein leading to a sustained increase in activity which outlasts the initiating stimulus [29]. Entry of phosphate at the luminal membrane would lead to increases in cytosolic concentration with damage to a wide range of metabolic processes without some coupling to exit at the basolateral membrane. Such a process has been inferred from animal studies but understanding of the transcellular and basolateral transport of phosphate is incomplete.

Distal nephron

Calcium reabsorption in the cortical portions of the ascending limb, diluting segment and early collecting duct occurs by a sodium independent process against a steep concentration and electrical gradient. It is at this site that $1,25(OH)_2D$ and PTH regulate calcium reabsorption according to the needs of homeostasis. The essential features of active calcium transport across the distal tubular cell are similar to those in the enterocyte. CaBP-D$_{28k}$ binds calcium at the luminal border of the cell and by maintaining a low cytosolic free Ca^{2+} enhances membrane–

Ca^{2+} transport. A specific vitamin D regulated plasma membrane calcium pump localized to the basolateral membrane with a greater affinity for Ca^{2+} relative to CaBP-D$_{28k}$ transports Ca^{2+} out of the cell into the peritubular capillary. Whether these processes are sufficient to maintain transcellular calcium transport or whether some other mechanism is involved is currently unknown.

PTH modulates distal calcium transport through activation of basolateral membrane receptors which couple to adenylate cyclase. The subsequent increase in intracellular cAMP acting through specific receptors, enhances the calcium permeability of the luminal membrane. Calcium transport is also enhanced by $1,25(OH)_2D$ which binds to a specific low-capacity cytosolic receptor. The ligand–receptor complex is then transported to the nucleus where it stimulates the expression of CaBP-D. This process is potentiated by an increase in ECF Ca^{2+} but it is uncertain whether it is due to an action upon a calcium receptor mechanism [1]. $1,25(OH)_2D$ may also have a stimulatory effect on the synthesis of the plasma membrane calcium pump as well as regulating its activity. Active transport of calcium in the distal nephron is therefore dependent on the presence of both PTH and $1,25(OH)_2D$.

Phosphate is almost completely (80–95%) reabsorbed in the proximal tubule and since the distal nephron is relatively impermeable to this ion, that which escapes proximal reabsorption appears in the final urine.

A substantial proportion of the filtered load of magnesium (50–60%) is reabsorbed in the loop of Henle although the mechanism involved is poorly understood. There is evidence to suggest the presence of a calcium receptor in the medullary thick ascending limb which couples to adenylate cyclase [32]. An increase in peritubular Mg^{2+} reduces absorption in this segment [31] and may act through such a divalent cation receptor.

Bone

The skeleton contains a huge store of mineral potentially available for the maintenance of calcium homeostasis. Short-term buffering, over hours or days, depends upon exchange of soluble calcium salts between a labile pool in bone and the ECF. This system, regulated by PTH, calcitonin and 1,25(OH)$_2$D involves the osteocyte–lining cell system. Longer term homeostatic mechanisms depend on a shift in the balance between bone resorption and formation of the remodelling cycle which maintains the mechanical integrity of the skeleton.

Osteocyte–lining cell system

Bone surfaces not undergoing active remodelling are covered by a continuous layer of flattened lining cells which are of the osteoblast lineage. These cells are in communication with osteocytes lying within lacunae and connecting with other similar cells to form a syncytium throughout the bone (Fig. 8.7) [33]. The lining cells separate the bulk ECF (Ca^{2+} = 1.0–1.3 mmol/l) from bone ECF (Ca^{2+} = 0.4 mmol/l) and as a consequence Ca^{2+} tends to diffuse down its concentration gradient into bone. This influx is balanced by an active calcium transport mechanism in the lining cells which is stimulated by PTH and inhibited by calcitonin (CT). The capacity of this system has been estimated at 25–150 mmol/day [34]. A fall in ECF Ca^{2+} will increase PTH secretion which will stimulate the lining cell pump and increase the calcium efflux from bone. Since PTH also stimulates renal calcium reabsorption, the calcium pumped out of bone will be retained within the ECF to restore homeostasis. An increase in ECF Ca^{2+} will both suppress PTH and stimulate CT secretion with inhibition of the lining cell pump and a decrease in calcium efflux from bone, again leading to a restoration of calcium homeostasis. The role of 1,25(OH)$_2$D in this system is uncertain but the presence of CaBP-D in the osteocytes suggests that vitamin D may be involved in transcellular calcium movement which would facilitate calcium supply to the lining cell pump [35].

Bone remodelling

The skeleton is subjected to repeated physical stress leading to microdamage and these areas are continually remodelled to maintain structural and mechanical integrity. An essential feature of this reparative process is that bone mass should be preserved. This is ensured by the initial phase of resorption being exactly balanced by, and coupled to, the subsequent bone formation. Under normal circumstances,

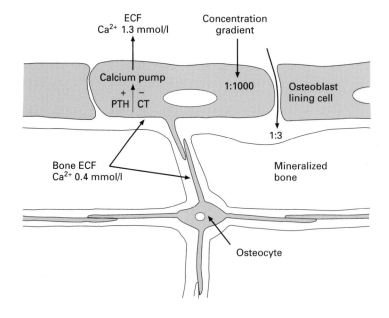

Fig. 8.7. Osteocyte-lining cell system and calcium homeostasis. CT: calcitonin; ECF: extracellular fluid; PTH: parathyroid hormone.

calcium released by reabsorption is deposited elsewhere at sites of formation so that calcium is recycled within the bone micro-environment and does not perturb ECF homeostasis.

The osteocyte–lining cell system has a finite capacity to support calcium homeostasis and when this is exhausted the remodelling cycle is recruited to support the ECF calcium concentration. The essential feature of this response is that by increasing the rate of bone turnover there is a reversible loss of bone (and calcium) because of expansion of the remodelling space [36]. This efflux of calcium over a period of days or weeks supports homeostasis while other long-term mechanisms (for example, gastrointestinal absorption) up-regulate to take over the defence of calcium homeostasis.

Homeostatic function of bone remodelling and its regulation by calcitropic hormones

Remodelling begins by proliferation and differentiation of stem cells of the monocyte–macrophage lineage to form mature osteoclasts. The early phase is regulated by a number of colony-stimulating factors including granulocyte macrophage colony-stimulating factor (GMCSF) while later stages are stimulated by 1,25(OH)$_2$D and other cytokines [37]. Bone resorption is stimulated by PTH, parathyroid hormone-related protein (PTHrP) and 1,25(OH)$_2$D as well as locally acting cytokines such as interleukin-3, interleukin-6, transform-

ing growth factor-β (TGF-β), lymphotoxin and tumour necrosis factor [38]. Receptors for 1,25(OH)$_2$D have not been found on mature osteoclasts and the effect of this hormone on bone resorption may either be through an increase in osteoclast differentiation and maturation, or indirectly through cytokine production by other cells including osteoblasts [39].

Osteoclasts become closely attached to bone around the perimeter of the cell through interaction with integrins (Fig. 8.8). The space so enclosed contains the ruffled border which creates an acid environment through the action of proton pumps leading to removal of the mineral phase of bone by acid hydrolysis. Secretion of proteolytic enzymes, including acid phosphatase and collagenase by the ruffled border, removes the organic matrix [37]. The resorption cavity is then invaded by macrophages whose function is unknown but may be implicated in the initiation of formation.

Bone formation begins by differentiation of mesenchymal stromal cells to form mature osteoblasts which secrete Type I collagen, forming the major portion (>90%) of the bone matrix. The remaining organic component is made up of a variety of non-collagenous proteins such as osteocalcin, osteonectin, osteopontin and bone sialoprotein, which play a subsequent role in mineralization. The major regulators of osteoblast differentiation include PTH, 1,25(OH)$_2$D, growth hormone, thyroid hormones and growth

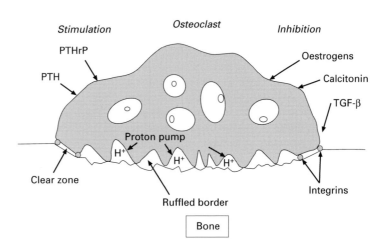

Fig. 8.8. Osteoclastic bone resorption. PTH: parathyroid hormone; PTHrP: parathyroid-hormone related protein; TGF-β: transforming growth factor-β.

224 factors such as transforming growth factor-β (TGF-β) [37].

Mineralization begins by the formation of calcium phosphate and CaBP-D$_{9k}$ containing vesicles within the osteoblast microvilli and cell processes directed towards the mineralization front [35]. These vesicles are pinched off from the cell and migrate extracellularly to the zone of mineralization. Prior to extrusion, growth of the apatite crystals depends on osteoblast mineral transport and the presence of CaBP-D$_{9k}$, which implies a functional role of 1,25(OH)$_2$D in this process. After extrusion, crystal growth depends on the mineral content of the bone ECF [40], which is regulated by PTH and 1,25(OH)$_2$D at the bone surface as well as in intestine and kidney. As mineralization proceeds some of the osteoblasts become incorporated in bone as osteocytes while others remain as lining cells covering the trabecular surface.

Remodelling space and calcium homeostasis

The processes of bone resorption and formation are tightly coupled both in time and space. This seems to depend on latent growth factors, such as TGF-β, deposited in bone being released and activated by resorption and then regulating the subsequent reparative process [41]. However, there is a delay between the end of resorption and the completion of formation leading to a focal deficit of bone which will progressively diminish with time. The size of this remodelling space depends on the rate of activation of new remodelling sites, their lifespan and the depth of resorption [36].

In a steady state, calcium liberated from the remodelling space will be deposited at other sites of formation. However, a change in the size of the remodelling space will lead to a transient imbalance where there will be either an excess or deficit of calcium in bone. This process can be used for the needs of calcium homeostasis since the rate of remodelling, a major determinant of the size of the remodelling space, is under the control of the calciotropic hormones. A reduction in ECF Ca^{2+} stimulates PTH secretion, which increases the rate of remodelling and the size of the remodelling space. During this period of change there will be a net excess of calcium removed by resorption which can be used for the maintenance of homeostasis. As other defence mechanisms (intestine and kidney) are recruited, the stimulus to PTH secretion will diminish, the rate of bone remodelling will fall and, as a consequence, the remodelling space will decrease in size with a net influx of calcium into bone and restoration of bone mass. Since resorption lasts about 1 month and formation about 3 months at each individual site, this process allows time for intestinal absorption to adapt to the need for increased calcium.

Although these inter-relationships between PTH, 1,25(OH)$_2$D and their target organs relate to the normal adult human, so little is known about the corresponding processes in pregnancy and the fetus that they have to be assumed to be similar unless there is evidence to the contrary.

Calcitonin

Synthesis and secretion

Calcitonin (CT) is a 32 amino acid peptide secreted by the parafollicular 'C' cells of the thyroid in response to an increase in ECF Ca^{2+}. The initial translation product is a 17.5 kDa (136 amino acid) peptide with a leader sequence at the amino terminus and a flanking peptide at the carboxy terminus. Both are cleaved at dibasic amino acid residues to produce the 3.5 kDa secreted hormone. The calcitonin gene (short arm of chromosome 11) also expresses an alternative product, calcitonin gene-related peptide (CGRP) in the central nervous system. CGRP is a 37 amino acid peptide which shares homology with CT at the amino terminus and is a widely distributed neuropeptide but its role in calcium homeostasis is uncertain [42].

The C cell is capable of responding directly to a change in ECF Ca^{2+} because of the presence of a cell surface calcium receptor. In common with the parathyroid cell, an increase in ECF Ca^{2+} results in an increase in intracellular Ca^{2+}, but unlike PTH this leads to a stimulation of hormone secretion [1]. The initial rise in C cell intracellular Ca^{2+} is prevented by calcium channel blockers, suggesting that it is due to an influx of calcium rather than the mobilization of endoplasmic reticulum Ca^{2+} seen in the parathyroid cell. It is uncertain whether the calcium receptor couples to adenylate cyclase and the phosphoinositol systems. There is some evidence that a high ECF Ca^{2+} raises cAMP in the C cell [43] and this could enhance CT secretion. The effect on the phosphoinositol system is poorly understood but available data do not support a role for IP_3-mediated mobilization of Ca^{2+} similar to that seen in the parathyroid cell [1].

Effect on target organs

Since CT lowers ECF Ca^{2+} in experimental animals after the removal of the kidneys and the intestine, it is clear that the hormone has an effect on bone. CT inhibits the resorbing activity of osteoclasts through an increase in cAMP production. This is accompanied by morphological changes which include withdrawal of the cells from the bone surface, loss of the ruffled border, and a decrease in liposomal enzyme activity [44]. The magnitude of the hypocalcaemic effect of CT depends on the prevailing rate of bone resorption which under physiological conditions declines with age. Thus, although CT may have an effect on calcium homeostasis in the growing animal, its role in the adult is more difficult to assess.

It is possible that CT may have an effect on the lining cell–osteocyte system because the hormone causes shrinkage of osteocytes within their lacunae. However, CT receptors have not been demonstrated on cells of the osteoblast lineage from which the lining cell osteocytes are derived [42]. CT receptors have been demonstrated in a subclone of an osteogenic sarcoma cell line which shows CT responsiveness [45], and this raises the possibility that some cells of the osteoblast lineage possess CT receptors and could fulfil a homeostatic role.

CT causes a transient increase in calcium excretion considered to be due to a distal renal tubular effect on the basis of the presence of CT sensitive adenylate cyclase in the thick ascending limb of the loop of Henle and the early distal convoluted tubule [46]. CT may also contribute to the regulation of $1,25(OH)_2D$ production in the proximal convoluted tubule by stimulating the 1α-hydroxylase [47].

An interesting hypothesis, based on animal experiments [48], is that CT may be implicated in the homeostatic response to feeding. CT release is stimulated by enteric hormones and, as a consequence, calcium efflux out of bone could be inhibited as calcium is ingested. Before calcium absorption is established, there will be a transient fall in ECF Ca^{2+} which will induce a PTH response. This will stimulate renal tubular calcium reabsorption, with the consequence that when calcium is absorbed it will be retained within the ECF rather than otherwise elevating the ECF Ca^{2+} and being excreted in the urine.

In quantitative terms, the role of CT is difficult to assess because loss of CT secretion in adults does not seem to be attended by any measurable disturbance of calcium homeostasis.

Parathyroid hormone-related protein

Biochemistry

Parathyroid hormone-related protein (PTHrP) was first isolated from a human squamous lung cancer cell line associated with hypercalcaemia but it is now known to be a major calciotropic hormone of the fetus. Its physiological role in the human adult is less certain but it may be involved in cell differentiation, particularly in skin. The commonest clinical expression is through actions on the kidney and bone in the humoral hypercalcaemia of malignancy [47].

The PTHrP gene is located on the short arm of chromosome 12 in a position homologous to the PTH gene on chromosome 11 [49]. It is a single copy gene but alternative splicing at the carboxy terminus results in peptides of 139, 141 and 173 amino acids in length [50]. PTH and PTHrP share considerable sequence homology at the amino terminus where eight of the first 13 amino acids are identical while many of the differences in the 14–34 region represent conservative substitutions: thereafter, the sequences diverge completely [51]. The strong homology at the amino terminus and the evidence that PTH and PTHrP share a common receptor [52] is the basis for their similar effects on bone and kidney. However, the variable regions of both peptides appear to serve distinct biological functions.

Actions on kidney and bone

The qualitative and quantitative similarities between the renal effects of PTH and PTHrP have been demonstrated in a variety of animal and cellular models. In opossum kidney cells, PTH (1–34) and PTHrP (1–34) were found to be equipotent in suppressing sodium-dependent phosphate transport and stimulating cAMP production [53]. This pointed towards an action through a common PTH receptor and this appeared confirmed by inhibition of these responses by a PTH antagonist [54]. In intact rats, PTHrP (1–34) and PTHrP (1–141) stimulated calcium reabsorption, cAMP production and phosphate excretion [55] as well as enhancing 1,25(OH)$_2$D production [56].

PTHrP binds to osteoblasts as shown by studies using radiolabelled PTHrP (1–34) [57]. In osteoblast cell lines (UMR106 rat osteosarcoma cells), it enhances intracellular cAMP production and sodium-dependent phosphate transport [58]. PTHrP (1–34) also increases cytosolic Ca^{2+} due to mobilization of intracellular calcium [59]. Bone resorption is also increased although osteoclasts lack PTH receptors and binding of radiolabelled PTHrP (1–34) could not be demonstrated [57]. Increased resorption is assumed to be indirect either through stimulation of recruitment and differentiation of osteoclasts or through an osteoblast effect due to cell-cell contact or cytokine production [37]. A recent observation that the carboxy terminus peptide PTHrP (107–111) inhibited activity in pure osteoclast cultures [60] emphasizes the uncertainty about the precise regulatory role of PTHrP (and PTH) on bone remodelling.

Mineral homeostasis in pregnancy

Maternal mineral homeostasis

The full-term human fetal skeleton contains 25–30 g of calcium, 1 g of magnesium and 16 g of phosphorus [61], most of which is acquired in the third trimester. This equates with a transplacental flux at term in the region of 6.5 mmol/day of calcium and 4.6 mmol/day of inorganic phosphate which have to be met by adaptation of maternal mineral homeostasis. Changes occur early with a progressive fall in maternal total calcium (and inorganic phosphate and magnesium) and an increase in urinary calcium excretion. The former is due to haemodilution of the protein bound calcium but ionized calcium [62] or albumin-corrected calcium [63] are maintained. The rise in urinary calcium excretion from 2.5–6.25 mmol/day in the non-pregnant woman to 8.75–15 mmol/day in pregnancy [64] is largely due to a physiological increase in glomerular filtration rate [61]. This will place an additional burden on intestinal calcium absorption which will have to compensate for these increased urinary losses.

Serum magnesium falls below the lower limit of the non-pregnant reference range during early pregnancy, probably largely due to dilution of serum albumin. Magnesium remains subnormal until after delivery when levels rapidly increase into the normal range [65]. Although reduced, the serum inorganic phosphate remains within the reference range throughout pregnancy before rising back to the pre-pregnancy level after delivery. CT also increases but the explanation for this change is uncertain because levels are preserved in pregnancy after total thyroidectomy [66], which would suggest some other source of hormone production such as the placenta [67].

Circulating concentrations of the major calciotrophic hormones show significant changes in pregnancy with a doubling of 1,25(OH)$_2$D, a fall in PTH with a rise in CT and PTHrP. Target organ responses include a doubling of calcium absorption and an early, but transient, increase in bone remodelling.

PTH-like bioactivity [68] and its sensitive marker, nephrogenous cAMP [69], are normal or increased in pregnancy, while a fall in intact PTH has been a consistent finding [62,70]. Although a study using a C-terminal assay for PTHrP found no difference between pregnant and non-pregnant women [62], another, using an N-terminal assay, showed a significant increase [63]. This is likely to be the most stringent test since the maternal target organ responses to PTH and PTHrP depend on the amino terminus 1–34 sequence. PTHrP tends to increase in the first trimester and this would account for the early rise in 1,25(OH)$_2$D, which would otherwise be difficult to explain given the fall in PTH. The rise in 1,25(OH)$_2$D, due to an increase in the free hormone as well as in the protein-bound fraction, is also apparent as early as the first trimester and increases two- to threefold by term [64]. 1,25(OH)$_2$D is also synthesized by the placenta [71] and this may contribute to the rise in maternal plasma concentrations. On the other hand, 25 OHD is unchanged during pregnancy.

The early fall in serum calcium, rise in PTHrP and PTH bioactivity, and the increase in 1,25(OH)$_2$D reflect a series of inter-related responses culminating in enhanced intestinal calcium absorption. This increases in early pregnancy, from the 20–25% absorption of the pre-pregnant state to 50% by 24 weeks, thereafter remaining stable until delivery [72]. Despite the increased absorption, the current recommended daily allowance for calcium in pregnancy is 1200 mg (30 mmol), although a maternal calcium deficit is probably unlikely until intakes fall below 600 mg/day [73]. Phosphate and magnesium are so plentiful in most diets that no specific recommendations are needed. They are assumed to follow calcium passively in terms of their intestinal absorption.

There is bone biopsy evidence of an increase in osteoclastic resorption and loss of volume in early pregnancy (8–10 weeks of gestation) which appears to subside by term [74]. This biphasic response is difficult to equate with the steady rise in alkaline phosphatase which begins in early pregnancy and continues until delivery, by which time levels are considerably elevated [65]. This pattern of response would be more consistent with placental alkaline phosphatase production [75], although an early increase due to bone resorption could make a contribution.

These changes reflect a co-ordinated shift in maternal physiology aimed at preserving maternal calcium homeostasis and providing the calcium required for fetal growth [61]. While the very earliest phase of fetal growth may be met by a transient increase in maternal bone resorption, the major source of calcium for growth in later pregnancy is derived from enhanced maternal intestinal calcium absorption.

Fetal mineral metabolism

Since the circulating concentrations of calcium, inorganic phosphate and magnesium are higher in the fetus than in the mother [76], their accumulation against a concentration gradient implies an active placental transport mechanism. The placental transfer of calcium and magnesium is predominantly regulated by PTHrP [77], presumably acting through an appropriate receptor, while the relative contributions of PTH and 1,25(OH)$_2$D are likely to be small. In contrast, PTHrP and PTH do not seem to be involved in phosphorus transport [77] where the underlying mechanisms remain uncertain.

Of necessity, much of the available information relating to human fetal metabolism is based on studies in premature or term infants. Important insights into the changes in early fetal life can only be obtained from animal studies. However, great care must be exercised when extrapolating from animals to humans because of the well-documented species variation under apparently identical experimental conditions.

Placental mineral transfer

Calcium transport across the placental membrane is bidirectional, but animal experiments show considerable species variation in the relative magnitudes of the unidirectional maternal-fetal and feto-maternal components which determine the net flux into the fetus [78]. Calcium transport involves at least three components (Fig. 8.9).

Influx of calcium ion from the maternal circulation across the trophoblast microvillous membrane is aided by a specific membrane carrier and a favourable concentration gradient between maternal serum (10^{-3} mmol/l) and trophoblast cytosol (4.2×10^{-8} mmol/l) [78].

Movement of calcium through the trophoblast cytosol requires some buffering mechanism to avoid large changes in Ca^{2+} concentration which might otherwise disrupt cellular processes. Some sequestration may occur

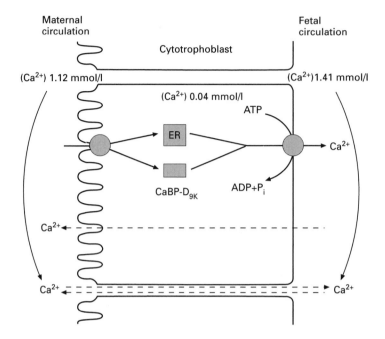

Maternal circulation

Fetal circulation

Cytotrophoblast

(Ca^{2+}) 1.12 mmol/l

(Ca^{2+}) 1.41 mmol/l

(Ca^{2+}) 0.04 mmol/l

ATP

ER

Ca^{2+}

CaBP-D$_{9K}$

ADP+P$_i$

Ca^{2+}

Ca^{2+}

Ca^{2+}

Ca^{2+}

Fig. 8.9. Placental calcium transfer. ADP: adenosine diphosphate; ATP: adenosine triphosphate; CaBP-D: vitamin D-dependent calcium-binding proteins; ER: endoplasmic reticulum; P$_i$: inorganic phosphate.

within intracellular organelles such as the endoplasmic reticulum [79], but calcium-binding proteins (CaBP-D) are also likely to be involved [80]. Such a mechanism is supported by the observation that placental CaBP-D and its mRNA increase during the last trimester of pregnancy, when calcium transport is at its height [81]. While there are tempting analogies between the trophoblast and the enterocyte in terms of the mechanisms of calcium transport, an element of caution is needed. In the human intestine, the precise relationship between active calcium transport, CaBP-D and $1,25(OH)_2D$ are not entirely clear and as yet a direct role for $1,25(OH)_2D$ in placental calcium transport has not been established [77].

Efflux of calcium across the trophoblast basement membrane into the fetal circulation depends on the presence of a high-affinity calcium pump in the basolateral membrane [82]. This has been confirmed by immunohistochemical and fractionation techniques in both human and rat placentas and has the features of a calcium- and magnesium-dependent ATPase pump. It has a calcium sensitivity in the nanomolar range similar to those in erythrocytes and other cells.

Placental magnesium transport seems to share many of the characteristics of calcium [77], but there may be some differences. Maternal serum magnesium concentrations have been shown to influence fetal concentrations, implying either that the magnesium pump is not normally saturated or that there is increased diffusion across the placenta [78]. However, neither maternal hypermagnesaemia nor hypomagnesaemia affect the maternofetal flux of calcium [83].

The mechanism underlying the net maternofetal flux of phosphorus is less certain than those of calcium and magnesium. Transfer seems to be an active process in that it is inhibited by anoxic conditions or metabolic poisons and seems to be sodium dependent [84].

Regulation of placental mineral transfer

Regulation of calcium transport across the placenta was initially considered to be a function of $1,25(OH)_2D$ produced by the fetal kidney but subsequent studies have indicated that PTHrP is the main regulator [85]. Although PTH bioactivity is increased in cord blood compared to maternal serum [68], PTH immunoreactivity is only about one-quarter of the maternal level, which in turn is only half the non-pregnant concentration [62]. This discrepancy between bioactivity and immunoreactivity is due to the presence of PTHrP, the major calciotrophic hormone of the fetus.

PTHrP is secreted both by the placenta [86,87] and the fetal parathyroid glands [85], but since umbilical arterial concentrations exceed venous levels [62], it is likely that the parathyroids are the dominant source. This is supported by the observation that removal of fetal PTHrP by thyroparathyroidectomy results in a rapid loss of the placental calcium gradient. Since under these conditions there is no consistent change in fetal plasma $1,25(OH)_2D$ and the calcium gradient cannot be restored by exogenous $1,25(OH)_2D$, this points to a dominant role for PTHrP [88]. The current view is therefore that a direct role for $1,25(OH)_2D$ in active placental calcium and magnesium transport has not been established.

Parathyroid hormone-related protein polyhormone

The traditional view of peptide hormones is that they only contain a single biologically active region within which resides the specific function of the hormone. This view has had to be modified as it becomes apparent that different peptide sequences of hormones such as PTH and PTHrP embody different functions [51]. This concept is well illustrated by PTHrP which appears to have a multifunctional role in maintaining fetal hypercalcaemia and ensuring adequate skeletal mineralization during the rapid phase of growth.

Studies in sheep [77] suggest that placental calcium and magnesium transfer are dependent on a midmolecular fragment of PTHrP distal to the 1–34 amino terminus. This was based on the observation that bovine PTH (1–84), rat PTH (1–34) and human PTH (1–34) all failed to stimulate placental calcium and magnesium transfer while human PTHrP (1–84, 1–108 and 1–141) are all effective in this system [89]. Subsequent studies showed that a number of midmolecular fragments reproduce this effect but that human PTHrP (67–86 amide) appeared to exert a more rapid effect which was also demonstrable in the

less sensitive intact, rather than thyroparathyroidectomy fetus [90]. This suggests that this peptide may resemble the PTHrP sequence which activates the placental calcium and magnesium pumps. This would also be consistent with the finding that the concentration of PTHrP (1–86) immunoreactivity in fetal pig plasma was inversely correlated to the serum ionized calcium, consistent with an endocrine role in calcium homeostasis [91].

Doses of hPTHrP (1–86) which stimulate calcium transfer were unable to influence placental phosphate transport [92]. However, it is known that PTH produces a cAMP-mediated decrease in inorganic phosphate uptake into human placental microvillous membrane vesicles [93]. This raises the possibility that placental phosphate transport depends on a different peptide sequence to that controlling calcium and magnesium. Recent studies have shown that PTH (1–34) and PTHrP (1–34) both activate placental cAMP production and, by analogy with the previous PTH experiments, could regulate phosphate transport [94]. In the same experiments, PTHrP (67–86 and 107–138) did not activate placental cAMP, suggesting that their action on calcium and magnesium transport must depend on a messenger system other than cAMP. These different functions of PTHrP fit neatly into the concept of the polyhormone but further studies are needed to confirm the current hypotheses.

Non-hormone regulators

Other potential regulators of placental mineral transfer include uterine blood flow and maternal serum mineral concentration. The major component of the fetal accumulation of calcium occurs in the last trimester. At this time the uterine blood flow is around 500 ml/min and since the total fetal calcium could be provided by the clearance of 170 litres of plasma, uterine blood flow is unlikely to be a rate-limiting factor [78]. Chronic reduction in blood flow leading to placental ischaemia may have an indirect effect through impairment of active metabolic processes.

Clinical experience suggests that changes in maternal serum calcium may also influence placental transfer. Maternal hypocalcaemia due to vitamin D deficiency or hypoparathyroidism may be associated with transient fetal hyper-parathyroidism, while the converse situation pertains with maternal hypercalcaemia due to hyperparathyroidism. Whether less extreme variations in serum calcium are of physiological importance is unknown.

Renal function

It is unlikely that fetal hypercalcaemia could be maintained solely by placental calcium transfer without some contribution from the kidneys. The demonstration of specific PTHrP staining in the developing distal renal tubule and collecting duct [95] and the identification of PTHrP messenger RNA transcripts in early second trimester human fetal kidney [96] support a role in fetal calcium homeostasis.

Thyroparathyroidectomy in fetal lambs led to a fall in serum calcium, a rise in fractional calcium excretion (urinary calcium expressed as a fraction of the filtered load: $U_{Ca}V/GFR \times$ total plasma calcium) and a decrease in cAMP excretion [97]. The implication that these changes were a consequence of the loss of PTHrP was supported by amelioration of these changes by infusions of PTH (1–34), PTHrP (1–34) and PTHrP (1–141), each of these peptides being equally potent. Calcium reabsorption increased both when measured as an absolute excretion rate or as a ratio of the fractional excretion rates of calcium and sodium, a measure of distal tubular calcium transport.

Since the 1–34 peptides of PTH and PTHrP have no effect on placental calcium transfer, the rise in serum calcium in these experiments implied the presence of a hormone-mediated efflux of calcium from the skeleton and previous studies had shown that the dose of PTHrP (1–34) used in the renal experiments was able to mobilize bone calcium [98]. Other observed renal effects of PTH and PTHrP in these experiments included an increase in urinary pH and a decrease in free water clearance, all of which are consistent with the known actions of these peptides in the adult.

A surprising occurrence was the diversity of results pertaining to the phosphaturic effect of PTHrP, a recognized property in the human adult [51]. This diversity may be a result of dose differences and uncertainty whether they were physiological or pharmacological. In one study giving a 3 nmol bolus of hPTHrP (1–34) followed by 3 nmol over the next 30 minutes, produced a rise in serum calcium, a fall in serum phosphate and phosphaturia [99]. Urine flow rate also increased and this was attributed to a vasorelaxant effect of PTHrP on the renal arteries [100] but glomerular filtration rate (GFR) was not measured directly. Although these effects were blocked by the PTH antagonist (Tyr[34]) bPTH (7–34)NH$_2$, it is not possible to separate a specific tubular effect of PTHrP from phosphaturia due to an increase in GFR and filtered load. Using smaller doses of PTHrP (1–34 and 1–141) — 1 nmol bolus followed by 1 nmol/hour for 2 hours — phosphaturia was not evident although serum calcium rose [97]. In this latter study GFR was unchanged and there was no evidence of a natriuresis, both of which would exclude changes in filtered phosphate load.

These studies contrast with those on the placenta and underlie the differing functions of peptide sequences within the PTHrP molecule. Amino terminal fragments, which share homology with PTH, are responsible for the renal actions of the hormone while midmolecular sequences regulate placental mineral transfer.

Skeletal contribution of mineral homeostasis

PTHrP immunoreactivity has been demonstrated in both endochondral and intramembranous bone in second trimester human fetuses [86]. Both osteoblast-like cells and chondrocytes stained with PTHrP, consistent with previous evidence for PTHrP receptors on these cells [57]. Material immunologically similar to PTHrP with adenylate cyclase-stimulating activity can also be identified in fetal rat bone matrix. This activity could be blocked by antiserum to PTHrP (1–11) but not by antiserum to PTH (1–34) [101]. Identification of PTHrP by immunohistochemistry identifies targets of action of a hormone but does not confirm synthesis at that site. The expression of PTH mRNA in a tissue is more positive evidence of site-specific secretion and this has been shown for fetal bone [52].

Thyroparathyroidectomy of the lamb fetus with thyroxine replacement leads to the development of rickets, which can be prevented by supplemental calcium and phosphate [102]. However, bone remodelling and development remain impaired, suggesting that PTHrP is essential for these functions. Whether PTHrP found in bone comes from osteoblastic synthesis or from the parathyroid gland is uncertain but neither source is mutually exclusive. PTHrP deposited in bone and released by resorption could act as a local regulator of bone remodelling in the fetus [101].

Lactation

High levels of oestrogen, progesterone and prolactin during pregnancy prime the breast and lactation begins with the sudden fall in oestrogen and progesterone concentrations at delivery. Thereafter, lactation is maintained by a high but declining secetion of prolactin. Suckling provides the stimulus for prolactin secretion and also for that of oxytocin which is needed for milk expulsion. Prolactin is also the driving force for the production of PTHrP mRNA in the breast [103].

The progressive increase in mammary PTHrP as gestation advances suggests that the hormone exerts a functional role. Its presence at the 14th day of gestation in the rat suggests that it may have a role in breast growth and development [104]. In the later stages of pregnancy, and during lactation, PTHrP can be demonstrated in the epithelial cells lining the alveoli and in the milk, where its concentration increases with the duration of lactation. The physiological role of PTHrP in the mammary gland is uncertain but there are several possibilities [52,104].

PTHrP may serve a paracrine/autocrine function regulating the secretion and flow of milk. Stimulation of calcium (and phosphate) transport into milk is an active process since it occurs against a concentration gradient (milk Ca^{2+} > ECF Ca^{2+}). Milk calcium concentration is maintained within a tight range independent of maternal calcium intake. PTHrP seems the major regulator since there is no evidence for a role of PTH, CT or $1,25(OH)_2D$ [52]. Other roles in milk secretion could include increasing

mammary blood flow through an action on vasorelaxation, maintenance of secretory epithelia in the mammary gland or contractility of the myoepithelial cells and milk expression [104].

PTHrP may also serve an endocrine function in the lactating mother through its actions on bone and kidney. Lactation imposes a huge demand on the maternal supply of calcium for milk production. Circulating concentrations of PTHrP are higher during lactation than in control women [105] and this could serve a role in calcium delivery. Such a response could centre around the stimulation of bone resorption and renal conservation of calcium and there is evidence in humans for both of these effects [106].

Much less certain is whether PTHrP serves an endocrine function in the neonate. The high concentrations of PTHrP in milk could have a local effect on the differentiation of gastrointestinal cells in the suckling infant. Although milk is known to contain a variety of growth factors and hormones, it is not certain whether PTHrP is absorbed in a physiologically active form. PTHrP reaches its peak concentration in milk towards the end of lactation [107] at a time when the ability of the neonatal gut to absorb macromolecules is rapidly declining. This temporal discordance may militate against such an endocrine function in the neonate.

Physiopathology

Skeletal disorders

Since mineral homeostasis in pregnancy is directed towards optimization of fetal skeletal growth and preservation of maternal calcium balance, it is to be expected that attention would focus on clinical consequences of failure.

The development of bone pain, fractures and low bone mass (measured by dual energy X-ray absorptiometry, DEXA) towards the end of pregnancy or during lactation is well described [108]. However, there is considerable uncertainty about the pathogenesis of this pregnancy-associated osteoporosis, although there seem two possibilities.

The earliest assumption was that the

osteoporosis reflected a failure of calcium homeostasis during pregnancy in a woman with a previously normal skeleton. It is difficult to understand why the loss of 30 g of calcium to the fetus should cause fractures when the maternal skeleton contains 1000 g of calcium and pregnancy is accompanied by a complex hormonal response to meet the increased need for calcium. In normal pregnancies, total body calcium generally remains unchanged [109]. Another problem with this hypothesis is the lack of a consistent pattern of change in the concentration of the major calciotropic hormones or in the rates of bone remodelling [110–112]. The same heterogeneity of findings is seen during lactation and the condition is well described in the absence of breast feeding [108]. Failure of the calcium homeostatic responses also seems an unlikely cause of the osteoporosis since many of the described cases had adequate dietary calcium intakes [108,112].

The other possibility is that pregnancy is an aggravating factor which unmasks a pre-existing defect in the maternal skeleton. In this context it is interesting that the mothers of women with pregnancy-associated osteoporosis have a higher prevalence of fractures which develop at an earlier age compared to controls [108]. This raises the possibility that genetic influences on peak bone mass may be a major determinant of the presence of osteoporosis. It remains uncertain whether transient changes in bone mass during pregnancy or lactation contribute to additional bone loss or perforation of trabeculae which lead to the development of fractures.

Primary hyperparathyroidism is uncommon in pregnancy, largely because it is a disease of an older age group. Mild hyperparathyroidism in pregnancy may be missed because of the fall in serum albumin, although ionized and protein-corrected calcium will be raised. Calcium crosses the placenta and maternal hypercalcaemia will lead to suppression of the fetal parathyroid glands and the occurrence of neonatal tetany [113]. Other consequences of primary hyperparathyroidism include stillbirth and abortion.

Hypoparathyroidism in pregnancy is even less common but illustrates several facets of the altered calcium homeostasis at this time. Mater-nal requirements for vitamin D (as part of their treatment for hypoparathyroidism) may decline during pregnancy because of transfer of $1,25(OH)_2D$ from the placenta. Conversely, treatment of the hypoparathyroid patient with parent vitamin D leads to supraphysiological levels of 25 OHD in the maternal circulation which will cross the placenta and may have an unpredictable effect on fetal $1,25(OH)_2D$ synthesis [73]. During lactation, maternal renal synthesis of $1,25(OH)_2D$ is enhanced by prolactin with a marked reduction in the requirement for exogenous $1,25(OH)_2D$ [114]. These changes make it important to monitor serum calcium closely during pregnancy so that the treatment of hypoparathyroidism can be adjusted. The short half-life of $1,25(OH)_2D$ (calcitriol) makes it the preparation of choice for treatment during pregnancy and lactation.

Pure dietary calcium deficiency of a magnitude to overcome the calcium homeostatic system is probably rare in pregnancy [73] unless there is evidence of malabsorption or a defect in vitamin D metabolism. Although diminished production of $1,25(OH)_2D$ may be a consequence of chronic renal failure or hypoparathyroidism, the commonest problem is that of marginal vitamin D deficiency exacerbated by the increased demands of pregnancy. Maternal vitamin D stores may be depleted by transfer of 25 OHD to the fetus [115], which may lead to overt maternal deficiency. In populations with marginal vitamin D intakes, maternal serum calcium tends to be lower than in those that are replete while neonatal serum calcium also tends to be lower [116]. Where this is a problem it seems prudent to advise supplementation of the diet with 400 i.u. vitamin D daily.

Since the fetus gains the majority of its calcium in the last trimester, it is to be expected that undermineralization of the skeleton is a well-recognized complication of prematurity. Cross-sectional studies measuring the bone mineral content (BMC) (mg/cm) of premature infants and varying lengths of gestation suggest a mineralization rate in the later stages of pregnancy of about 4.5 mg/cm/100 g weight gain [117]. This study also showed that BMC was strongly correlated with body weight. Replenishing the mineral deficit in preterm infants may present some problems relating to the type of calcium supplement. Calcium absorption from cows' milk is very variable but is low in preterm infants and may take 60 days to reach 50% [118]. Breast milk may be relatively deficient in inorganic phosphate, with the result that calcium incorporation into bone is incomplete and some is wasted by being excreted in the urine [119]. On the other hand, special care formulas for the preterm infant may be relatively calcium deficient and may lead to marginal hypocalcaemia, hypocalciuria and secondary hyperparathyroidism with spillage of phosphate into the urine.

Hypertension

There is a substantial body of evidence showing a close inverse relationship between the mean calcium intake in a population and the incidence of pre-eclampsia [120]. However, a caveat is in order for these studies, since the early work was done in Central/South American populations who were first-generation city dwellers in very poor areas. For generations they had had a high Ca^{2+} diet because they hand-milled their grain in limestone querns but their intake dropped dramatically in the towns. Thus their whole Ca^{2+} metabolism may be atypical nor was their vitamin D status considered. It is at least possible to argue that the improved antenatal care given to the study women improved outcome. Systematic review of a number of randomized trials of calcium supplementation suggests that it was associated with a substantial reduction in the risk of hypertension and pre-eclampsia during pregnancy [121]. There was also promising evidence of a reduction in the risk of preterm delivery, although it was not possible to identify the protective mechanism responsible. Many of these trials were small and the data are not so compelling that routine calcium supplementation during pregnancy can currently be recommended, however, a randomized controlled study of 4789 nulliparae allocated 2 g elemental calcium or placebo in second trimester onwards showed no difference on pre-eclampsia or outcomes of perinatal death, small for gestational age or preterm deliveries [122].

The other interesting facet of these epidemiological studies is the question for what physiological mechanisms might lie behind these associations. A number of studies have drawn attention to the presence of hypocalciuria in women with pre-eclampsia [64,123] and there is also a suggestion that a urinary calcium excretion below 5 mmol/day before the 20th week of gestation might predict the subsequent development of pre-eclampsia [124]. This contrasts with the hypercalciuria of early normal pregnancy and the lack of hypocalciuria in pregnant women with chronic essential hypertension [122]. Various changes in the calcium homeostatic system have been described in pre-eclampsia, including reductions in ionized calcium and $1,25(OH)_2D$ with elevated levels of PTH [64]. Interestingly, intracellular (Ca^{2+}) is increased in platelets from women with pre-eclampsia and the rise evoked by angiotensin II (A II) is greater [125]. What is currently uncertain is whether these changes are the result of pre-eclampsia or its cause.

Pre-eclampsia is accompanied by a reduction in placental perfusion and this, together with renal damage from hypertension, could lead to reduced synthesis of $1,25(OH)_2D$. Active calcium absorption would fall as a consequence, as would ECF Ca^{2+}, leading to a rise in PTH and the development of hypocalciuria. The essential question is which, if any, of these changes is implicated in the production of hypertension. PTH (or PTHrP) might be a candidate if they increased intracellular calcium in vascular smooth muscle, or other components of the vascular system, which resulted in a pressor effect [63]. In this context the well-recognized effect of magnesium infusions in lowering blood pressure (and PTH) in pre-eclampsia might give clues to potential mechanisms.

Increased levels of ECF Mg^{2+} inhibit PTH secretion through an action on the parathyroid cell calcium receptor [1], although in-vivo studies show a subsequent return to baseline levels [125]. High levels of ECF Mg^{2+} also stimulate CT secretion and inhibit PTH-mediated stimulation of proximal tubular cAMP production [1]. This latter mechanism may be implicated in $1,25(OH)_2D$ production and its inhibition, together with the fall in PTH and a rise in CT, could contribute to the consistent fall in ECF Ca^{2+} which follows Mg^{2+} therapy. An additional contributory factor to the fall in ECF Ca^{2+} might be the development of hypercalciuria because of inhibition of divalent ion reabsorption in the thick ascending limb of the loop of Henle by an increase in peritubular Mg^{2+} concentration [32].

The development of hypertension in pregnancy may be multifactorial and relate more to the complex interplay between divalent cations and the major calciotrophic hormones rather than result from an isolated change in one element of the calcium homeostatic system. The ease of calcium supplementation in pregnancy makes it an ideal candidate for the prevention of pre-eclampsia but its widespread introduction is inhibited by poor results of large-scale clinical trials [122] and uncertainty about the pathophysiology of the condition.

References

1 Brown E.M. (1991) Extracellular Ca^{2+} sensing, regulation of parathyroid cell function and role of Ca^{2+} and other ions as extracellular (first) messengers. *Physiological Reviews* **71**, 371.

2 Borle A.B. (1981) Control, modulation and regulation of cell calcium. *Review of Physiology, Biochemistry and Pharmacology* **90**, 13.

3 Parfitt A.M. (1987) Bone and plasma calcium homeostasis. *Bone* **8** (Suppl. 1), S1.

4 Baldwin J.M. (1994) Structure and function of receptors coupled to G proteins. *Current Opinion in Cell Biology* **6**, 180.

5 Pearce S.H.S. & Trump D. (1995) G protein-coupled receptors in endocrine disease. *Quarterly Journal of Medicine* **88**, 3.

6 Simon M.I., Strathmann M.P. & Gautam N. (1991) Diversity of G proteins in signal transduction. *Science* **252**, 802.

7 Nemeth E.F. (1995) Ca^{2+} Receptor-dependent regulation of cellular functions. *News in Physiological Sciences* **10**, 1.

8 Collins S., Caron M.G. & Lefkowitz R.J. (1992) From ligand binding to gene expression: new insights into the regulation of G protein-coupled receptors. *Trends in Biological Science* **17**, 37.

9 Rude R.K. (1993) Magnesium metabolism and deficiency. *Endocrinology and Metabolism Clinics of North America* **22**, 377.

10 Habener J.F. & Potts J.T. (1990) Fundamental considerations in the physiology, biology and biochemistry of parathyroid hormone. In *Metabolic Bone Disease and Clinically Related Diseases*. Eds L.V. Avioli & S.M. Krane, p. 69. WB Saunders Company, Philadelphia.

11 Habener J.F., Rosenblatt M. & Potts J.T. (1984) Parathyroid hormone: biochemical aspects of biosyn-

thesis, secretion, action and metabolism. *Physiological Reviews* **64**, 985.

12 Cohn D.V. & MacGregor R.R. (1981) The biosynthesis, intracellular processing and secretion of parathormone. *Endocrine Reviews* **2**, 1.

13 Izbicka E., Niewolna M., Yoneda T., Lowe C., Boyce B. & Mundy G. (1994) C-Src expression and activity in MG-63 osteoblastic cells modulated by PTH, but not required for PTH-mediated adenylate cyclase response *Journal of Bone and Mineral Research* **9**, 127.

14 Gilman A.G. (1984) Guanine nucleotide inhibiting regulatory proteins and dual control of adenylate cyclase. *Journal of Clinical Investigation* **73**, 1.

15 Stryer L., & Bourne H.R. (1986) G proteins: a family of signal transducers. *Annual Review of Cell Biology* **2**, 391.

16 Berridge M.J. (1984) Inositol trisphosphate and diacylglycerol as second messengers. *Biomedical Journal* **220**, 345.

17 Rasmussen H. (1986) The calcium messenger system. *New England Journal of Medicine* **314**, 1094, 1164.

18 Litosch I. & Fain J.N. (1986) Mini review: regulation of phosphoinositol breakdown by guanine nucleotides. *Life Sciences* **39**, 187.

19 Johnson J.A. & Kumar R. (1994) Renal and intestinal calcium transport: roles of vitamin D and vitamin D-dependent calcium binding proteins. *Seminars in Nephrology* **14**, 119.

20 Juhlin C.R., Holmdahl R., Johansson H., Rastad J., Akerstrom G. & Klaresog G. (1987) Monoclonal antibodies with exclusive reactivity against parathyroid cells and tubule cells of the kidney. *Proceedings of the National Academy of Science USA* **84**, 2990.

21 Wasserman R.H., Brindak M.E., Buddle M.M., Cia Q., Davis F.C., Fullmer C.S., Gilmour R.F. *et al.* (1990) Recent studies on the biological actions of Vitamin D on intestinal transport and the electrophysiology of peripheral nerve and cardiac muscle. *Progress in Clinical and Biological Research* **332**, 99.

22 Gross M. & Kumar R. (1990) Physiology and biochemistry of vitamin D-dependent calcium binding proteins. *American Journal of Physiology* **259**, F195.

23 McCarthy J.T., Barham S.S. & Kumar R. (1984) 1.25-dihydroxy vitamin D_3 rapidly alters the morphology of the duodenal mucosa of rachitic chicks: evidence for novel effects of 1.25-dihydroxy vitamin D_3. *Journal of Steroid Biochemistry* **21**, 253.

24 Dupret J.M., Brun P., Perret C., Lomri N., Thomasset M. & Cuisinier-Gleizes P. (1987) Transcriptional and post-transcriptional regulation of Vitamin D-dependent calcium-binding protein gene expression in the rat duodenum by 1.25 dihydroxy cholecalciferol. *Journal of Biological Chemistry* **262**, 16553.

25 Carafoli E. (1992) The Ca^{2+} pump of the plasma membrane. *Journal of Biological Chemistry* **267**, 2115.

26 Reisner P.D., Christakos S. & Vanaman T.C. (1992) In vitro enzyme activation with calbindin-D_{28k}, the vitamin D dependent 28 kDa calcium binding protein. *FEBS Letters* **297**, 127.

27 Kanis J.A. & Passmore R. (1989) Calcium supplementation of the diet. I. *British Medical Journal* **298**, 137.

28 Murer H. & Hildmann B. (1981) Transcellular trans-

port of calcium and inorganic phosphate in the small intestinal epithelium. *American Journal of Physiology* **240**, G409.

29 Hruska K.A. & Kurnik B.R. (1990) Regulation of renal phosphate transport. In *Metabolic Bone Diseases and Clinically Related Disorders*. Eds L.V. Avioli & S.M. Krane, p. 222. WB Saunders, Philadelphia.

30 Rose D.B. (1989) *Clinical Physiology of Acid Base and Electrolyte Disorders*. McGraw-Hill, New York.

31 Quamme G.A. & Dirks J.H. (1986) The physiology of renal magnesium handling. *Renal Physiology* **9**, 257.

32 Quamme G.A. (1989) Control of magnesium transport in the thick ascending limb. *American Journal of Physiology* **256**, F197.

33 Parfitt A.M. (1976) The action of parathyroid hormone on bone: relation to bone remodelling and turnover, calcium homeostasis and metabolic bone disease. II. PTH and bone cells: bone turnover and plasma calcium regulation. *Metabolism* **25**, 909.

34 Parfitt A.M. (1989) Plasma calcium control at quiescent bone surfaces: a new approach to the homeostatic function of bone lining cells. *Bone* **10**, 87.

35 Balmain N. (1991) Calbindin-D_{9k}: a vitamin-D dependent, calcium binding protein in mineralised tissues. *Clinical Orthopaedics and Related Research* **265**, 265.

36 Mosekilde L., Eriksen E.F. & Charles P. (1991) Hypercalcaemia of malignancy; pathophysiology, diagnosis and treatment. *Critical Reviews in Oncology/Hematology* **11**, 1.

37 Mundy G.R. (1995) *Bone Remodelling and its Disorders*. Martin Dunitz, London.

38 Raisz L.G. (1988) Local and systemic factors in the pathogenesis of osteoporosis. *New England Journal of Medicine* **318**, 818.

39 Stern P.H. (1990) Vitamin D and bone. *Kidney International* **38** (Suppl. 29), S17.

40 Wuthier R.E. (1982) A review of the primary mechanism of endochondral calcification with special emphasis on the role of cells, mitochondria and matrix vesicles. *Clinical Orthopaedics* **169**, 219.

41 Bonewald L.F. & Mundy G.R. (1990) Role of transforming growth factor beta in bone remodelling. *Clinical Orthopaedics* **250**, 261.

42 Martin T.J. & Moseley J.M. (1990) *Calcitonin in Metabolic Bone Disease and Clinically Related Disorders*. Eds L.V. Avioli & S.M. Krane, p. 131. WB Saunders Company, Philadelphia.

43 Zeytin F.N. & Delellis R. (1987) The neuropeptide-synthesizing rat 44-2C cell line: regulation of peptide synthesis, secretion, 3', 55–cyclic adenosine monophosphate efflux and adenylate cyclase activation. *Endocrinology* **121**, 352.

44 Friedman J. & Raisz L.G. (1967) Thyrocalcitonin: inhibitor of bone resorption in tissue culture. *Science* **150**, 1465.

45 Forrest S.M., Ng K.W., Findlay D.M., Michelangeli V.P., Livesey S.A., Partridge N.C., Zajac J.D. (1985) Characterisation of an osteoblast-like clonal line which responds to both parathyroid hormone and calcitonin. *Calcified Tissue International* **37**, 51.

46 Chabardes D., Gagnan-Brunette M., Imbert-Teboul M., Gontcharevskai O., Montegut M., Clique A. & Morel F. (1980) Adenylate cyclase responsiveness to hormones in various portions of the human nephron. *Journal of Clinical Investigation* **65**, 439.

47 Moseley J.M., Kubota M., Diefenbach-Jagger H., Wettenhall R.E.H., Kemp B.E., Suva L.J., Rodda C.P. et al. (1987) Parathyroid hormone-related protein purified from a human lung cancer cell line. *Proceedings of the National Academy of Science USA* **84**, 5048.

48 Talmage R.V., Cooper C.W. & Toverud S.V. (1983) The physiological significance of calcitonin. In *Bone and Mineral Research Annual 1*. Ed. W.A. Peck, p. 74. Excerpta Medica, Amsterdam.

49 Mangin M., Webb A.C., Dreyer B.E., Posillico J.T., Ikeda K., Weir E.C., Stewart A.F. et al. (1988) Identification of a cDNA encoding a parathyroid hormone-like peptide from a human tumor associated with humoral hypercalcaemia of malignancy. *Proceeedings of the National Academy of Science USA* **85**, 597.

50 Mangin M., Ikeda K., Dreyer B.E., Milstone L. & Broadus A.E. (1988) Two distinct tumor-derived, parathyroid hormone like peptides result from alternative ribonucleic acid splicing. *Molecular Endocrinology* **2**, 1049.

51 Mallette L.E. (1991) The parathyroid polyhormones: new concepts in the spectrum of peptide hormone action. *Endocrine Reviews* **12**, 110.

52 Law F., Ferrari S., Rizzoli R. & Bonjour J.-P. (1993) Parathyroid hormone-related protein and calcium phosphate metabolism. *Pediatric Nephrology* **7**, 827.

53 Pizurki L., Rizzoli R., Moseley J.M., Martin T.J., Caverzasio J. & Bonjuour J.-P. (1988) Effects of synthetic tumoral PTH-related peptide on cAMP production and Na-dependent Pi transport. *American Journal of Physiology* **255**, F957.

54 Pizurki L. Rizzoli R. & Bonjour J.-P. (1990) Inhibition by (D-Trp[12], Tyr[34]) bPTH (7–34 amide) of PTH and PTHrP effects on Pi transport in renal cells. *American Journal of Physiology* **259**, F389.

55 Zhou H., Leaver D.D., Moseley J.M., Kemp B., Ebeling P.R. & Martin T.J. (1989) Actions of parathyroid hormone-related protein on the rat kidney in vivo. *Journal of Endocrinology* **122**, 229.

56 Rizzoli R., Caverzasio J., Chapuy M.C., Martin T.J. & Bonjour J.-P. (1989) Role of bone and kidney in parathyroid hormone-related peptide induced hypercalcaemia in rats. *Journal of Bone and Mineral Research* **4**, 759.

57 Evely R.S., Bonomo A., Schneider H.-G., Moseley J.M., Gallagher J. & Martin T.J. (1991) Structural requirements for the action of parathyroid-hormone-related protein (PTHrP) on bone resorption by isolated osteoclasts. *Journal of Bone and Mineral Research* **6**, 85.

58 Pizurki L., Rizzoli R., Caverzasio J. & Bonjour J.-P. (1991) Stimulation by parathyroid hormone-related protein and transforming growth factor of phosphate transport in osteoblast-like cells. *Journal of Bone and Mineral Research* **6**, 1235.

59 Civitelli R., Martin T.J., Fausto A., Gunsten S.L.,

236

Hruska K.A. & Avioli L.V. (1989) Parathyroid hormone-related peptide transiently increases cytosolic calcium in osteoblast-like cells: comparison with parathyroid hormone. *Endocrinology* **125**, 1204.

60 Fenton A.J., Kemp B.E., Hammonds R.G., Mitchelhill K., Moseley J.M., Martin T.J. & Nicholson G.C. (1991) A potent inhibitor of osteoclastic bone resorption with a highly conserved pentapeptide region of parathyroid hormone-related protein: PTHrP (107–111). *Endocrinology* **129**, 3424.

61 Pitkin R.M., Reynolds W.A., Williams G.A. & Hargis G.K. (1979) Calcium metabolism in normal pregnancy: a longitudinal study. *American Journal of Obstetrics and Gynecology* **133**, 781.

62 Seki K., Wada S., Nagata N. & Nagata I. (1994) Parathyroid hormone-related protein during pregnancy and the perinatal period. *Gynecologic and Obstetric Investigation* **37**, 83.

63 Bertelloni S., Baroncelli G.I., Pelletti A., Battini R. & Saggese G. (1994) Parathyroid hormone-related protein in healthy pregnant women. *Calcified Tissue International* **54**, 195.

64 Seely E.W. & Graves S.W. (1993) Calcium homeostasis in normotensive and hypertensive pregnancy. *Comprehensive Therapy* **19**, 124.

65 Dahlman T., Sjoberg H.E. & Bucht E. (1994) Calcium homeostasis in normal pregnancy and puerperium: a longitudinal study. *Acta Obstetrica et Gynaecologica Scandinavica* **73**, 393.

66 Bucht E., Telenius-Beg M., Lundell G. & Sjoberg H.E. (1986) Immunoextracted calcitonin in milk and plasma from totally thyroidectomized women: evidence of monomeric calcitonin in plasma during pregnancy and lactation. *Acta Endocrinologica (Copenhagen)* **113**, 529.

67 Galan F.G., Balbontin F.C., Cano R.P., Rubio A.J., Anon M.G. & Peralta M.G. (1984) Is there an extrathyroidal source of calcitonin during pregnancy? *Acta Endocrinologica (Copenhagen)* **105**, 266.

68 Allgrove J., Adami S., Manning R.M. & O'Riordan J.L.H. (1985) Cytochemical bioassay of parathyroid hormone in maternal and cord blood. *Archives of Diseases in Childhood* **60**, 110.

69 Gillette M.E., Insogna K.L., Lewis A.M. & Baran D.T. (1982) Influence of pregnancy on immunoreactive parathyroid hormone levels. *Calcified Tissue International* **34**, 9.

70 Davis O.K., Hawkins D.S., Rubin L.P., Posillico J.T., Brown E.M. & Schiff I. (1988) Serum parathyroid hormone (PTH) in pregnant women determined by an immunoradiometric assay for intact PTH. *Journal of Clinical Endocrinology and Metabolism* **67**, 850.

71 Zerwekh J.E. & Breslau N.A. (1986) Human placental production of 1,25 dihydroxy vitamin D_3 biochemical characterisation and production in normal subjects and patients with pseudohypoparathyroidism. *Journal of Clinical Endocrinology and Metabolism* **62**, 192.

72 Heaney R.P. & Skillman T.G. (1971) Calcium metabolism in normal human pregnancy. *Journal of Clinical Endocrinology and Metabolism* **33**, 661.

73 Reeve J. (1991) Calcium metabolism. In *Clinical Physiology in Obstetrics*, 2nd edn. Ed. F.E. Hytten & G. Chamberlain, p. 213. Blackwell Scientific Publications, Oxford.

74 Purdie D.W., Aaron J.E. & Selby P.L. (1988) Bone histology and mineral homeostasis in human pregnancy. *British Journal of Obstetrics and Gynaecology* **95**, 849.

75 Sadowsky E. & Zucherman H. (1965) An alkaline phosphatase specific to normal pregnancy. *Obstetrics and Gynaecology* **26**, 211.

76 Schauberger C.W. & Pitkin R.M. (1979) Maternal-perinatal calcium relationships. *Obstetrics and Gynaecology* **53**, 74.

77 MacIsaac R.J., Heath J.A., Rodda C.P., Moseley J.M., Care A.D., Martin T.J. & Caple I.W. (1991) Role of the fetal parathyroid glands and parathyroid hormone-related protein in the regulation of placental transport of calcium, magnesium and inorganic phosphate. *Reproduction, Fertility and Development* **3**, 447.

78 Husain S.M. & Mughal M.Z. (1992) Mineral transport across the placenta. *Archives of Diseases in Childhood* **67**, 874.

79 Croley T.E. (1973) The intracellular localisation of calcium within the mature human placental barrier. *American Journal of Obstetrics and Gynecology* **77**, 10.

80 Tuan R.S. (1985) Calcium-binding protein of the human placenta, characterisation, immunohistochemical localisation and function involvement in Ca^{2+} transport. *Biochemical Journal* **227**, 317.

81 Delorme A.C., Marche P. & Garel J.M. (1979) Vitamin D-dependent calcium binding protein: changes during gestation, prenatal and postnatal development in rats. *Journal of Development Physiology* **1**, 181.

82 Borke J.L., Caride A., Verma A.K., Kelly L.K., Smith C.H., Penniston J.T. & Kumar R. (1989) Calcium pump epitopes in placental trophoblast basal plasma membranes. *American Journal of Physiology* **257**, C341.

83 Mimouni F. & Tsang R.C. (1991) Perinatal magnesium metabolism: personal data and challenges for the 1990s. *Magnesium Research* **4**, 109.

84 Stulc J. & Stulcova B. (1984) Transport of inorganic phosphate by the fetal barrier of the guinea-pig placenta perfused in situ. *Placenta* **5**, 9.

85 Abbas S.K., Pickard D.W., Illingworth D., Storer J., Purdie D.W., Moniz C., Dixit M. *et al.* (1990) Measurement of parathyroid-related protein in extracts of fetal parathyroid glands and placental membranes. *Journal of Endocrinology* **124**, 319.

86 Moseley J.M., Hayman J.A., Danks J.A., Alcorn D., Grill V., Southby J. & Horton M.A. (1991) Immunohistochemical detection of parathyroid hormone-related protein in human fetal epithelia. *Journal of Clinical Endocrinology and Metabolism* **73**, 478.

87 Bowden S.J., Emly J.F., Hughes S.V., Powell G., Ahmed A., Whittle M.J. Ratcliffe J.G. *et al.* (1994) Parathyroid hormone-related protein in human term placenta and membranes. *Journal of Endocrinology* **142**, 217.

88 Care A.D., Caple I.W. & Pickard D.W. (1985) The roles of the parathyroid and thyroid glands on calcium homeostasis in the ovine fetus. In *The Physiological Development of the Fetus and Newborn.* Eds C.T. Jones & P.W. Nathaniels, p. 135. Academic Press, London.

89 Rodda C.P., Kubota M., Heath J.A., Ebeling P.R., Moseley J.M., Care A.D., Caple I.W. *et al.* (1988) Evidence for a normal parathyroid hormone-related protein in fetal lamb parathyroid glands and sheep placenta: comparison with a similar protein implicated in humoral hypercalcaemia of malignancy. *Journal of Endocrinology* **117**, 261.

90 Care A.D., Abbas S.K., Pickard D.W., Barri M., Drinkhill M., Findlay J.B.C., White I.R. *et al.* (1990) Stimulation of ovine placental transport of calcium and magnesium by mid-molecular fragments of human parathyroid hormone-related protein. *Experimental Physiology* **75**, 605.

91 Abbas S.K., Ratcliffe W.A., Moniz C., Dixit M., Caple I.W., Silvers M., Fowden A. *et al.* (1994) The role of parathyroid hormone-related protein in calcium homeostasis in the fetal pig. *Experimental Physiology* **79**, 527.

92 Barlet J.-P., Davicco M.-J., Rouffet J., Coxam V. & Lefaivre J. (1994) Parathyroid hormone-related peptide does not stimulate phosphate placental transport. *Placenta* **15**, 441.

93 Brunette M.G., Auger D. & Lafond J. (1989) Effect of parathyroid hormone on PO_4 transport through the human placenta microvilli. *Pediatric Research* **25**, 15.

94 Williams J.M.A., Abramovich D.R., Dacke C.G., Mayhew T.M. & Page K.R. (1991) Parathyroid hormone (1–34) peptide activates cyclic adenosine 3′, 5′ monophosphate in the human placenta. *Experimental Physiology* **76**, 297.

95 Moseley J.M., Danks J.A., Grill V., Southby J., Hayman J.A. & Horton M.A. (1989) Immunohistochemical localisation of parathyroid hormone-related protein in fetal tissues. *Journal of Bone and Mineral Research* **4** (Suppl. 1), S134.

96 Burton P.B.J., Moniz C., Zuirke P., Tzannatos C., Pickles A., Dixit M., Triffit J.T. *et al.* (1990) Parathyroid hormone-related peptide in the human fetal urogenital tract. *Molecular and Cellular Endocrinology* **69**, R13.

97 MacIsaac R.J., Horne R.S.C., Caple I.W., Martin T.J. & Wintour E.M. (1993) Effects of thyroparathyroidectomy, parathyroid hormone, and PTHrP on kidneys of ovine fetuses. *American Journal of Physiology* **264**, E37.

98 Caple I.W., Heath J.A., Pham T.T., MacIsaac R.J., Rodda C.P., Farrugia W., Wark J.D. *et al.* (1990) The roles of the parathyroid glands, parathyroid hormone (PTH) parathyroid hormone related protein (PTHrP), and elevated plasma calcium in bone formation in fetal lambs. In *Calcium Regulation and Bone Formation.* Ed. D.V. Cohn, F.H. Glorieux & T.J. Martin, p. 455. Oxford University Press, New York.

99 Davicco M.-J., Coxam V., Lefaivre J. & Barlet J.-P. (1992) Parathyroid hormone-related peptide increases urinary phosphate excretion in fetal lambs. *Experimental Physiology* **77**, 377.

100 Winquist R.J., Baskin E.P. & Vlasuk G.P. (1987) Synthetic tumor-derived human hypercalcaemic factor exhibits parathyroid hormone-like vasorelaxation in renal arteries. *Biochemical and Biophysical Research Communications* **149**, 227.

101 Nijs-Dewolf N., Pepersack T., Corvilain J., Karmali R. & Bergmann P. (1991) Adenylate cyclase stimulating activity immunologically similar to parathyroid hormone-related peptide can be extracted from fetal rat long bones. *Journal of Bone and Mineral Research* **6**, 921.

102 Aaron J.E., Abbas S.K., Colwell A., Eastell R., Oakley B., Russell R.G.G. & Care A.D. (1992) Parathyroid gland hormones in the skeletal development of the ovine foetus: the effect of parathyroidectomy with calcium and phosphate infusion. *Bone and Mineral* **16**, 121.

103 Thiede M.A. (1989) The mRNA encoding a parathyroid hormone-like peptide is produced in mammary tissue in response to elevations in serum prolactin. *Molecular Endocrinology* **3**, 1443.

104 Rakapoulos M., Vargas S.J., Gillespie M.T., Ho P.W.M., Diefenbach-Jagger H., Leaver D.D., Girll V. *et al.* (1992) Production of parathyroid hormone-related protein by the rat mammary gland in pregnancy and lactation. *American Journal of Physiology* **263**, E1077.

105 Grill V., Hillary J., Ho P.M.W., Law F.M.K., MacIsaac P.J., MacIsaac I.A., Moseley J.M. *et al.* (1992) Parathyroid hormone-related protein: a possible endocrine function in lactation. *Clinical Endocrinology* **37**, 405.

106 Kent G.N., Price R.I., Gutteridge D.H., Smith M., Allen J.R., Bhagat C.I., Barnes M.P. *et al.* (1990) Human lactation: forearm trabecular bone loss, increased bone turnover, and renal conservation of calcium and inorganic phosphate with recovery of bone mass following weaning. *Journal of Bone Mineral Research* **55**, 361.

107 Yamamoto M., Fisher J.E., Thiede M.A., Caulfield M.P., Rosenblatt M. & Duong L.T. (1992) Concentration of parathyroid hormone-related protein in rat milk change with duration of lactation and interval from previous suckling but not with milk calcium. *Endocrinology* **130**, 741.

108 Dunne F., Walters B., Marshall T. & Heath D.A. (1993) Pregnancy associated osteoporosis. *Clinical Endocrinology* **39**, 487.

109 Christiansen C., Rodbro P. & Heinild B. (1976) Unchanged total body calcium in normal human pregnancy. *Acta Obstetrica Gynaecologica Scandinavica* **55**, 141.

110 Gruber H.E., Gutteridge D.H. & Baylink D.J. (1984) Osteoporosis associated with pregnancy and lactation: bone biopsy and skeletal features in three patients. *Metabolic Bone Disease and Related Research* **5**, 159.

111 Smith R., Stevenson J.C., Winearls C.G., Woods C.G. & Wordsworth B.P. (1985) Osteoporosis in pregnancy. *Lancet* **i**, 1178.

112 Blanch J., Pacifici R. & Chines A. (1994) Pregnancy-associated osteoporosis: report of two cases with long-term bone density follow up. *British Journal of Rheumatology* **33**, 269.

238

113 Delmonico F.L., Neer R.M., Cosimi A.B., Barnes A.B. & Russell P.S. (1976) Hyperparathyroidism during pregnancy. *American Journal of Surgery* **131**, 328.

114 Cundy T., Haining S.A., Guilland-Cumming D.F., Butler J. & Kanis J.A. (1987) Remission of hypoparathyroidism during lactation: evidence for a physiological role for prolactin in the regulation of vitamin D metabolism. *Clinical Endocrinology* **26**, 667.

115 Teotia M., Teotia S.P.S. & Singh R.K. (1979) Maternal hypovitaminosis and congenital rickets. *Bulletin of the International Pediatric Association* **3**, 39.

116 Turton C.W.G., Stanley P., Stamp T.C.B. & Maxwell J.D. (1977) Altered vitamin D metabolism in pregnancy. *Lancet* **i**, 222.

117 Pohlandt F. & Mathers N. (1989) Bone mineral content of appropriate and light for gestational age preterm and term newborn infants. *Acta Paediatrica Scandinavica* **78**, 835.

118 Day G.M., Chance G.W., Radde I.C., Reilly B.J., Park E. & Sheepers J. (1975) Growth and mineral metabolism in very low birth weight infants. II. Effects of calcium supplementation on growth and divalent cations. *Pediatric Research* **9**, 568.

119 Pohlandt F. (1993) Prevention of postnatal bone demineralisation in very low birth weight infants by individually monitored supplementation with calcium and phosphorus. *Pediatric Research* **35**, 125.

120 Belizan J.M. & Villar J. (1980) The relationship between calcium intake and edema, proteinuria, and hypertension-gestosis: an hypothesis. (1994) *American Journal of Clinical Nutrition* **33**, 2202.

121 Carroli G., Duley L., Belizan J.M. & Villar J. (1994) Calcium supplementation during pregnancy: a systematic review of randomised and controlled trials. *British Journal of Obstetrics and Gynaecology* **101**, 753.

122 Sanchez-Ramos L., Jones D.C. & Cullen M.T. (1991) Urinary calcium as an early marker for preeclampsia. *Obstetrics and Gynecology* **77**, 685.

123 Taufield P.A., Ales K.L., Resnick L.M., Druzin M.L., Gertner J.M. & Laragh J.H. (1987) Hypocalciuria in pre-eclampsia. *New England Journal of Medicine* **316**, 715.

124 Kilby M.D., Broughton Pipkin F. & Symonds E.M. Calcium and platelets in normotensive and hypertensive human pregnancy. *Journal of Hypertension* **10**, 997.

125 Cholst I.N., Steinberg S.F., Tropper P.J., Fox H.E., Segre G.V. & Bilezikian J.P. (1984) The influence of hypermagnesaemia in serum calcium and parathyroid hormone levels in human subjects. *New England Journal of Medicine* **310**, 1221.

Pharmacokinetics

FELICITY REYNOLDS
WITH ADDITIONAL MATERIAL BY
THE EDITORS

Everyone prescribing drug treatment for a female patient needs to consider whether she might be pregnant. This is such an important step that its omission must be regarded as negligent. Pregnancy affects the therapeutic situation, both because it alters drug handling, and because of the risk of harming the embryo by exposing it to a teratogenic substance. Since the thalidomide disaster of the early 1960s, avoidance of all but essential drugs in early pregnancy has been mandatory. Moreover, drugs given in later pregnancy can cause behavioural anomalies [1,2] — thus therapeutic caution should be exercised throughout pregnancy. Despite wide acceptance of these principles, pregnant women may inadvertently be exposed to medication, both prescribed and across the counter. Known or suspected teratogenic substances that may still be inappropriately used in pregnancy include cold cures, oral contraceptives, sex hormones and tetracyclines [3,4].

Nevertheless, the use of drugs during pregnancy is sometimes inescapable: for example, maintenance therapy of chronic medical conditions such as epilepsy, asthma and diabetes, anticoagulation following valve replacement, and drug therapy specific to obstetric problems such as preterm labour and pre-eclampsia. Still other women will benefit from short-term therapy for intercurrent illness or will need anaesthesia. In these circumstances it must be remembered that pregnancy itself may alter the patient's response to drug treatment.

A key factor in understanding drug action in clinical medicine has been the realization that patients respond in a similar way to the same concentration of drug in their blood; most individual variations in response are due to pharmacokinetic processes such as absorption, distribution and elimination, and not to a variable susceptibility of target organs to the drug. The physiological changes that take place throughout pregnancy can modify every aspect of pharmacokinetics. If the differing capacity of the pregnant woman to distribute and metabolize drugs is taken into account in planning treatment, then the management of such conditions as epilepsy can be greatly improved.

Pharmacokinetic measurements

The most commonly reported pharmacokinetic measurements are the plasma half-life ($T_{1/2}$), the distribution volume (V_D) and the clearance (C).

The plasma half-life is the time taken for the plasma concentration to fall by half. In some studies an initial or distribution half-life may be quoted but this is of relevance only to drugs given by single bolus intravenous injection, and it is the elimination or terminal half-life which

Table 9.1. Changes in the pharmacokinetic values of some drugs from the non-pregnant state.

	V_D	Cl	$T_{1/2}$	Reference
Polar compounds $T_{1/2}$ ↓				
Antibiotics: penicillins	↑	↑	↓	13,64,65
cephalosporins	=	↑	↓	68,69
Pancuronium	=	↑	↓	140
Oxazepam	↑	↑	↓	18
Transitional $T_{1/2}$ =				
Phenytoin (late pregnancy)	↑	?↑	?=	12,76–78
Paracetamol	↑	↑	=	141
Sotalol	?↑	↑	=	137
Metoprolol	↑	↑	=	138
Labetalol	=	=	=	87
Propanolol	=	=	=	142
Phenobarbitone	=	=	=	80
Pethidine	=	=	=	60
Lipophilic compounds $T_{1/2}$ ↑				
Thiopentone	↑	↑	↑	9,54
Diazepam	=	↓	↑	133
Bupivacaine			↑	134,136
Caffeine	=	↓	↑	130,131

Data may be equivocal because not all are derived from internally controlled trials, and V_D is not always calculated per kilogram body weight.

is of more general importance. It is measured in hours or sometimes minutes.

The distribution volume is a hypothetical concept and may be defined as that volume that a drug would occupy if the concentration throughout the body were equal to that in plasma. Thus the figure may appear impossibly large if the drug is more concentrated in tissues than in the plasma. It should be measured in litres/kg.

The clearance, which may also be termed the total clearance, is the volume of plasma cleared of drug in unit time. It is usually measured in ml/min, but should perhaps be measured in $ml.kg^{-1}min^{-1}$.

The three are interrelated thus:

$$C = \frac{V_D \times 0.693}{T_{1/2}} \qquad (0.693 = \log_e 2)$$

For a drug that is given chronically, clearance is easily derived:

$$C = \frac{\text{drug absorbed in unit time}}{\text{plasma concentration at steady state}}$$

or, for a single dose: $C = dose/AUC$, where AUC = the area under the plasma concentration

versus time curve. Clearance is an important concept for chronic drug administration because it determines what dose of drug is necessary to maintain a certain plasma concentration, but it cannot indicate how rapidly a drug will disappear when treatment is stopped. For a drug given in a single dose, $T_{1/2}$ may be more important than C.

A high clearance rate is not necessarily associated with a short elimination half-life, for if the distribution volume is large, relatively little of the total amount of drug in the body is to be found in the plasma, and only that which is in the circulation can pass through liver and kidneys in order to be eliminated. In pregnancy, an increase in V_D may be a dominant change, and for some drugs, C may be increased but $T_{1/2}$ prolonged, or one may change without the other (see Table 9.1).

Drug disposition

Drugs that are hydrophilic and poorly lipid soluble, such as antibiotics, do not readily enter cells. They therefore tend to have a smaller V_D than lipid soluble drugs, and are mainly eliminated by renal excretion. The more lipid soluble drugs usually have larger V_D values and are readily reabsorbed in the renal tubule. They must therefore be broken down to more polar (water-soluble) compounds, usually in the liver, prior to elimination. Many drugs are bound to plasma proteins, which influences tissue distribution and may in some cases limit hepatic extraction.

The drugs whose pharmacokinetics are of particular importance are those that are given for more than just an isolated dose, and those whose therapeutic effects are not clear but whose margin of safety is narrow. For example, on the one hand, drug effects on blood pressure and blood sugar are continuously measurable, while on the other, convulsions come and go, and anticonvulsant monitoring is dependent upon drug concentration measurement. Antibiotic treatment requires adequate plasma levels but the effects cannot be immediately detected clinically. Thus, where drug administration cannot be directly titrated against clinical effect, a knowledge of drug kinetics is crucial to management. Pregnant women are, moreover, notoriously variable in their drug handling, and direct monitoring of drug therapy by drug concentration measurement can be vitally important.

The influence of physiological changes in pregnancy

Ingestion

Fear of adverse effects may deter some pregnant women from taking any drugs. An additional factor may be the common symptoms of nausea and heartburn, while vomiting may reject a drug once it is taken. Thus if it is assumed that the dose prescribed is equal to that absorbed, all these factors may lead to an apparent increase in clearance during the first trimester. This may particularly be so for anticonvulsants (Fig. 9.1), whose teratogenic potential may be overrated by women starting pregnancy.

Absorption

The major part of absorption of all drugs occurs in the small intestine and is therefore accelerated by gastric emptying. Gastric motility may be reduced in pregnancy, though functionally the change is slight until late labour. Gastric emptying is always markedly slowed after pethidine has been given [5,6]. Delayed gastric emptying slows the absorption and reduces the peak plasma level of readily absorbed drugs such as

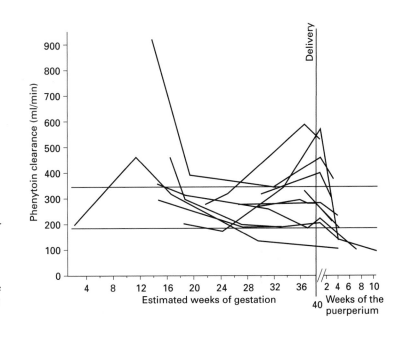

Fig. 9.1. Clearance of unbound phenytoin derived from:

$$\frac{\text{dose } (\mu g/min)}{\text{saliva phenytoin concentration } (\mu g/ml)}$$

during pregnancy and the puerperium in 11 epileptic women. Horizontal lines represent the normal range of phenytoin clearance. High clearance in the first trimester may not be genuine but simply reflect poor compliance or reduced absorption. From Knott et al. [12].

paracetamol, while reduced overall intestinal motility which undoubtedly occurs in pregnancy might in theory actually enhance the bioavailability of slowly absorbed drugs such as digoxin. Most drugs that are given by mouth on a regular basis are, however, well absorbed and little affected by gastrointestinal motility. Reduced absorption of anticonvulsants given by mouth has been reported [7], but antacids, which are frequently taken in pregnancy and labour, can reduce the absorption of phenytoin [8].

Delayed absorption of drugs given by mouth shortly before labour may lead to greatly increased plasma levels postpartum, and can therefore contribute to a fall in drug clearance that may be observed in the puerperium (Fig. 9.1).

Distribution

Part of the weight gain of pregnancy is accounted for by an increase of 6–8 litres in body water, the major part being extracellular fluid. The distribution volume of all drugs therefore increases, and in many cases reports do not take into account the overall increase in body weight. The proportional increase in V_D for polar drugs, which are limited in their distribution to the extracellular space, is probably greater than that of lipophilic drugs, whose V_D is larger and probably more determined by protein and lipid binding (Table 9.1).

Body fat also tends to increase in pregnancy (Chapter 16), and an exception to the above general rule is the highly lipophilic thiopentone, whose V_D actually rises in real terms, and whose clearance increases, though $T_{1/2}$ is prolonged [9].

The distribution volume of a drug is of course increased by the products of conception which are generally included in estimates of total body water. The fetal compartment equilibrates more slowly than maternal tissues, and can probably be neglected when considering maternal requirements for a single dose of drug, particularly that given by intravenous bolus. It must, however, be taken into account in longer term treatment with all but the most polar drugs.

Protein binding

Many drugs are reversibly bound to plasma protein. Of the various protein components that may take part, albumin is the most important, having a large capacity and being the major protein binding acidic drugs (salicylates, non-steroidal anti-inflammatory drugs, warfarin, anticonvulsants) and some essentially neutral compounds such as diazepam. The principal agent for binding many basic drugs (β-blockers, opioid analgesics, local anaesthetics) is, however, α_1-acid glycoprotein, one of the acute phase proteins, which though of smaller capacity shows, in general, relatively high affinity binding.

Albumin concentration falls during pregnancy, partly due to dilution. In addition, there is competition between ligands for albumin, and the rise in free fatty acids that occurs in late pregnancy [10] could also contribute to the observed decrease in binding in late pregnancy of salicylate [11] and phenytoin [12]. Binding to albumin during pregnancy is therefore very variable, and cannot be predicted even given a knowledge of the plasma albumin. For drugs that require accurate monitoring and are highly bound to plasma albumin, the wide variation in free fraction makes plasma concentration measurement an inaccurate predictor of the active free concentration. This applies particularly to phenytoin (Fig. 9.2). Saliva monitoring is, in such circumstances, more informative, as it bears a constant relation to free phenytoin [12].

A reduction in albumin binding can contribute to an increase in V_D and clearance for drugs such as phenytoin which undergo restrictive elimination [13].

In contrast to albumin, there is an increase in the concentration of a number of specific carrier proteins such as transferrin and thyroxine-binding globulin in pregnancy. The plasma concentration of α_1-acid glycoprotein does not change significantly in pregnancy [14] but shows wide inter-individual variation and increases with stress [15]. The large transplancental concentration gradient that exists for α_1-acid glycoprotein has an important effect on the placental transfer of drugs that are highly bound to it.

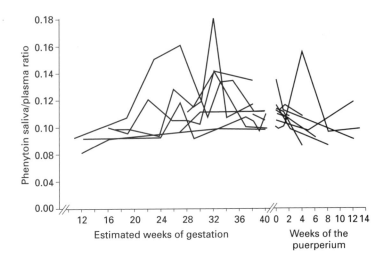

Fig. 9.2. Changes in protein binding of phenytoin in pregnancy and the puerperium in nine epileptic women. Phenytoin saliva to plasma ratios accurately reflect the free (unbound) fraction of phenytoin. From Knott *et al.* [12].

Elimination

Drugs that act within cells must be lipid soluble to gain access to their site of action. Such drugs cannot effectively be excreted by the kidney since they undergo renal tubular reabsorption. Moreover, the large distribution volume of such compounds within the body would make renal elimination extremely slow. They must therefore first undergo conversion to more hydrophilic compounds.

Biotransformation

The maternal liver

The liver is the principal site of conversion, mostly employing the non-specific mixed function oxidases of the microsomal enzymes system. Two phases are commonly involved in the process. Phase I metabolism involves oxidation, reduction or hydrolysis, yielding products whose activity is usually diminished, though not absent. Phase II metabolism involves conjugation, and the products are completely water-soluble and commonly inactive. Drugs possessing phenolic hydroxyl groups can be conjugated directly and therefore their metabolites are largely inactive.

Some drugs that are broken down in the liver have a high extraction ratio, so that more than 70% of the drug in the circulation reaching the liver is cleared by the first pass. The rate of hepatic clearance of such drugs (chlormethaziole, pethidine, lignocaine) is therefore dependent upon liver blood flow. Others are broken down more slowly, at a rate less dependent on blood flow than on liver enzyme activity (phenytoin, theophylline, caffeine). The breakdown of such drugs is accelerated by enzyme induction. It appears that for certain drugs (for example, phenytoin and propranolol) the liver only handles the unbound fraction, therefore a change in protein binding may alter hepatic extraction [16].

Changes in pregnancy Liver size and liver blood flow would appear to be unchanged in pregnancy [13] and no histological changes have been observed. Liver enzyme activity varies between species and between human individuals on a genetic basis, pregnancy itself producing inconsistent changes. Liver microsomal enzymes are susceptible to induction (that is, their activity is increased) by environmental agents such as smoking, anticonvulsants and some antibiotics. Progesterone is also an enzyme inducer, but oestrogens may compete with drugs for the enzymes involved in their breakdown. This anomaly can account for the inconsistent changes that have been detected in pregnancy, and the lower the oestrogen to progesterone ratio, the greater may be the enzyme induction [16,17].

Many studies of drug handling in pregnancy are uncontrolled and compare data obtained from pregnant women with those from non-pregnant women or men, obtained from the literature. Thus wide variations in results are reported for the same drug. In addition, some of the data supposedly for pregnant women are obtained at and after delivery, so for the majority of a terminal half-life calculation such subjects are not pregnant at all. However, some data now are available from patients studied throughout pregnancy and in the postpartum period, and provide convincing evidence of progressive pregnancy-associated changes in drug handling (see Figs 9.1, 9.3, 9.4 & 9.6).

A summary of the different types of change observed for a selection of drugs is given in Table 9.1. The elimination rates of drugs with high hepatic extraction ratios, being dependent upon hepatic blood flow, are unchanged in pregnancy, while those of drugs with extraction ratios less than 0.7 may be increased, decreased or unchanged. The more lipid soluble a drug, the more is its half-life likely to be prolonged in pregnancy, while the reverse is true for the less lipid soluble. Thus the $T_{1/2}$ of the polar benzodiazepine oxazepam, which is directly conjugated in the liver, is actually shortened in late pregnancy [18]. Pharmacokinetic studies in man, however, detect changes that are the resultant of alterations in drug absorption, distribution, protein binding and renal excretion, as well as hepatic breakdown, and so will be discussed later (p. 249).

If drug metabolism is impaired for any reason, then the effects may be serious for the fetus. For example, the fetal alcohol syndrome — where both physical and mental development of the fetus are grossly deranged—does not occur in all infants born to alcoholic mothers; Veghelyi and Osztovics [19] presented evidence that its occurrence is due not to alcohol but to high levels of

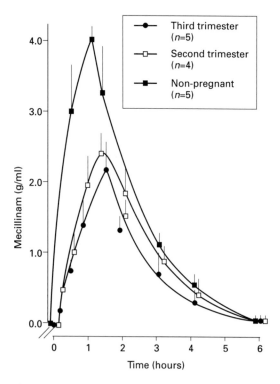

Fig. 9.3. Serum concentrations of mecillinam after a single oral dose of 400 mg of pivmecillinam. Mean and SE. Reproduced from Kjer and Ottesen [139], with permission.

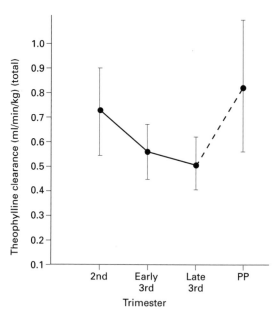

Fig. 9.4. Mean theophylline clearance based on total body weight, studied prospectively in eight asthmatic women. Clearance in the third trimester was significantly lower than postpartum ($P < 0.01$). Vertical bars: SD. Reproduced from Carter *et al.* [129], with permission. PP: postpartum.

acetaldehyde in mothers who have developed an impaired capacity to degrade it. A pregnant alcoholic taking disulphiram would similarly put her fetus at risk if she were to consume any alcohol.

Other sites of drug metabolism

Some drugs are sufficiently similar to endogenous compounds to be metabolized by specific enzymes; for example, sympathomimetic agents may be broken down by catechol-o-methyl transferase or monoamine oxidase. Antimetabolites may be broken down by xanthine oxidase and the muscle relaxant suxamethonium is hydrolysed by pseudocholinesterase in plasma. The concentration of pseudocholinesterase falls during pregnancy in about 30% of women [20]. In a small minority, the fall may be so great that they have an impaired ability to hydrolyse suxamethonium and may suffer prolonged paralysis after its administration in the usual anaesthetic doses.

Placenta

Almost all the drug-metabolizing reactions performed by the liver have been identified in placental tissue or homogenates, although there are certain exceptions, for example, pethidine is not demethylated by placental tissue [21]. The existence of these various metabolic capacities has suggested that the placenta has an important function in metabolizing drugs in pregnancy [22].

Extrapolation of research data to the clinical field must be made with some caution since estimates of the drug metabolizing capacity of the placenta have almost all been made *in vitro* on fractions of placental tissue. Certainly the protective effect of the placenta on the fetus in this respect cannot be relied upon. For example, though the placenta contains pseudocholinesterase, suxamethonium appears to cross the primate placenta in measurable amounts [23].

Though placental microsomal enzymes have little relevance to pharmacokinetics, they may be important in toxicology [24]. One interesting aspect of placental metabolism is the observation that the hydroxylation of benzpyrine by mixed function oxidases can be induced in animals by administration of a number of polycyclic aromatic hydrocarbons. Cigarette smoking markedly increases placental benzpyrine hydroxylase [25] in the second and third trimesters. This effect on placental enzymes is, however, one or two orders of magnitude lower than in corresponding liver preparations.

The fetus

Perinatal pharmacologists have repeatedly stressed the low capacity of the human newborn infant to metabolize drugs, for it eliminates many therapeutic substances much more slowly than adults [26,27]. It would be inappropriate for a fetus to be efficient at converting drugs to completely polar metabolites, such as conjugates, since they would not pass readily back across the placenta, and would therefore tend to become trapped in the fetal compartment, in amniotic fluid and gut lumen. Hence the well-known intolerance of the neonate to chloramphenicol, which in the adult is readily conjugated in the liver.

In contrast to many experimental animals, however, drug metabolism in the human fetal liver is relatively well advanced at term. Further, the liver obtained from human fetuses in early and mid-gestation is similarly able to perform a wide range of metabolic functions [28]. Human fetal tissues obtained in the second trimester of pregnancy contain concentrations of cytochrome P-450 comparable to those found in adult rat liver [29]. Human fetal liver microsomes also contain all the components necessary for drug hydroxylation reactions. These findings contrast with many studies in fetal animals where investigators have found no detectable cytochrome P-450 or P-450-dependent drug hydroxylation activity reactions in liver microsomes, even at comparatively late stages of gestation [30].

Electron microscopic studies of human fetal liver provide supporting evidence for drug-metabolizing activity within the liver early in pregnancy [31]. Before the third month of gestation, the endoplasmic reticulum of the human fetal liver consists of rough membranes but around the third month, complete differentiation of the hepatic cells occurs and smooth endoplasmic reticulum appears. This structure is associated with microsomal drug metabolizing activity in the adult. Furthermore, in experimental animals treated with inducing agents, an increase in smooth endoplasmic reticulum can be observed in the fetal liver.

Although drug metabolism by the fetus is quantitatively small in comparison with the mother, it is important because many carcinogenic and mutagenic compounds that might be supposed to be teratogens act via reactive intermediary products which are usually highly electrophilic. Such reactive metabolites are likely to be too unstable and non-diffusible to reach the fetus from the maternal circulation. The teratogenic potential of the parent compound therefore depends upon the ability of the fetus to carry out the appropriate metabolic processes. Evidence in mice suggests that genetically mediated induction of drug metabolizing enzymes may be associated with the production of birth defects from teratogens [32]. As constituents of tobacco smoke are powerful enzyme inducers, this would explain the increased frequency of congenital abnormalities in the offspring of mothers who smoke *and* take psychotropic drugs in pregnancy [33]. Moreover, it has been shown that only species who are able to convert thalidomide to a toxic epoxide metabolite are sensitive to its teratogenesis [34].

Excretion

As glomerular filtration rate increases by at least 50% [16], the elimination of drugs which depend on renal excretion is greatly enhanced in pregnancy (Fig. 9.3). Thus for polar compounds such as penicillins, cephalosporins, and pancuronium, clearance rate is increased and half-life is shortened (Table 9.1). Rather surprisingly, the renal clearances of both salbutamol and creatinine have been found to be reduced compared with the non-pregnant state, when the former agent is administered in premature labour [35]. Such an unusual change might be due to the premature labour.

Fetal drug exposure

Fetal drug exposure *in utero* is the product of duration of maternal administration and placental transfer. Because the principal trophoblast layer of the placenta is a syncytium, it is covered by a continuous lipid membrane. With respect to drug transfer, therefore, the placenta behaves like other lipid membranes such as the blood–brain barrier. Thus, lipid-soluble substances up to a molecular weight of 600 to 1000 can diffuse readily across the placenta, while water-soluble foreign molecules cross readily only up to a molecular weight of 100, above this level crossing much more slowly. Ions cross lipid membranes very slowly indeed, unless they are substrates for active transport, as is sodium, for example.

Thus drugs that affect the central nervous system, and can therefore cross the blood–brain barrier, also readily cross the placenta. Some drugs are weak electrolytes: for example, barbiturates, non-steroidal anti-inflammatory drugs, warfarin and anticonvulsants are weak acids while narcotic analgesics, local anaesthetics, tranquillizers, β-stimulants and blockers are weak bases. These substances all cross the placenta by non-ionic diffusion, and the non-ionized moiety equilibrates across the placenta with relative ease.

More highly polar compounds—certain penicillins, water-soluble contrast media, quaternary ammonium compounds (neuromuscular blocking drugs and old-fashioned ganglion blockers) and mannitol—cross the placenta slowly, such that equilibration across the placenta is never attained because fetal elimination is more rapid than transfer rate. The placenta is virtually impermeable to heparin, a large and highly polar molecule [36].

Flow-dependent transfer

In late pregnancy, the placental membrane separating maternal and fetal blood is only 2 μm thick where it directly overlies fetal capillaries, and offers no bar to diffusion of lipid soluble substances. Their rate of transfer is therefore dependent upon blood supply on either side of the placenta. Of these two elements, umbilical blood flow is probably the more important [37], since maternal blood flow is consistently greater. Such flow-dependent transfer has been demonstrated for anticonvulsants [38], narcotic analgesics [39], local anaesthetics [40] and ethanol [41]. During brief drug administration, such as general anaesthesia for caesarean section, the dose of anaesthetic received by a fit baby at elective section will be much greater than that in a distressed fetus at emergency section [37].

Permeability-dependent transfer

Polar substances cross the placenta at much slower rates that are dependent upon placental permeability rather than on blood flow. The transfer rates of water-soluble compounds such as urea, creatinine, erythrityl and mannitol fall as molecular weight increases [42]. At the dividing line between flow-limited and permeability-limited transfer is antipyrine, a popular pharmacologist's tool. It usually exhibits flow-dependent transfer but, at high flows or on first exposure, permeability limits its transfer but not that of more lipid soluble drugs [37,41,43]. The transfer of morphine also appears to be partly diffusion-limited [44]. Among borderline substances, transfer rate is dependent upon lipid solubility; thus, during early administration fetal/maternal ratios of polar drugs are low. For example, salbutamol crosses the placenta more slowly than does antipyrine [45], whereas terbutaline [46] and ritodrine [47] appear more diffusible.

Equilibrium ratios

Though lipophilic substances equilibrate readily across the placenta, concentrations on the two sides at equilibrium are not necessarily equal for all drugs. Disparities in affinity of maternal and fetal blood for drugs arise from two sources.
1   *Ion trapping.* Acidic drugs ionize more in the more alkaline maternal blood and basic drugs more in the baby. Because the non-ionized moiety tends to equilibrate across the placenta, the fetal/maternal free drug concentration ratio will be greater than 1 for bases and less than 1 for acids [48]. Thus, cord concentrations of

the basic drug dihydralazine are higher than those in the mother [49]. Also, when the fetus becomes acidotic, fetal/maternal ratios of basic drugs such as local anaesthetics actually increase [50,51].
2   *Protein binding.* Drugs do not cross the placenta in the protein-bound state, and inequalites in binding at the two sides of the membrane can lead to disparities in total drug concentrations at equilibrium. Fetal albumin concentrations may exceed maternal at term [14,52], thus the fetal/maternal ratio at equilibrium of a drug such as diazepam which is highly bound to albumin may be considerably greater than 1 [53]. Acid drugs that are albumin bound, such as thiopentone [54], which equilibrates across the placenta in a single circulation, and anticonvulsants [38] which are taken chronically, usually have fetal/maternal ratios near unity, since ion-trapping and binding disparities counterbalance one another. Fetal concentrations of α_1-acid glycoprotein are low and never exceed maternal [14], thus fetal/maternal ratios of drugs that are highly bound to this protein, such as bupivacaine [55], alfentanil [56] and oxprenolol [57] are consistently low, with a mean of 0.3 to 0.4. Although low fetal protein binding does not of course affect the active free concentration of drug in the fetal plasma, it nevertheless restricts total fetal dose and hence it reduces the stores in the new-born infant.

Equilibration

Highly lipid soluble drugs such as thiopentone and bupivacaine would appear to equilibrate rapidly across the placenta, since umbilical venous/maternal plasma concentrations do not rise with time. Equilibration of the entire fetal compartment, however, probably takes about 40 minutes [58; personal observation]. Fetal/maternal ratios of less lipid-soluble drugs such as terbutaline [46] and pethidine [59,60] have been noted to rise with time. It would appear that, following a single dose of pethidine, after an hour or so, when maternal concentration is falling, placental transfer is reversed. Slow accumulation of pethidine and active metabolites in fetal brain, however, results in more severe depression of babies born

3–4 hours after maternal pethidine administration than when dose–delivery interval is briefer [61].

Transfer of polar drugs such as penicillin, mannitol, quaternary ammonium compounds (neuromuscular blockers, ganglion blockers) and the angiotensin-converting enzyme inhibitor enalapril [62], is slow. After brief maternal administration, fetal/maternal ratios rise with time and may come to exceed unity as the drug disappears more rapidly from the maternal than the fetal compartment, and passes only slowly from fetus to mother. In steady state conditions, such as with continuous administration, fetal/maternal ratios remain low. This is because excretion by the fetal kidney of polar substances is more rapid than placental transfer, thus sink conditions apply. The result of such excretion is that amniotic fluid concentrations of penicillins, mannitol and hexamethonium ultimately exceed those in other compartments [63]. As the fetus drinks amniotic fluid, polar substances can be expected to concentrate in the fetal gut lumen, where they cannot be absorbed. When hexamethonium was given to women with hypertensive disease of pregnancy, not only did it inevitably fail to lower the blood pressure, it also resulted in paralytic ileus in the newborn. Figure 9.5 is a straight X-ray of a premature baby whose mother was investigated during pregnancy for hydronephrosis — the water-soluble X-ray contrast medium she received was visible in the baby's bowel for many days after birth.

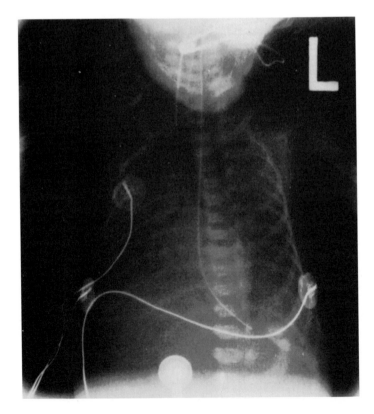

Fig. 9.5. Straight X-ray of a 4-day-old baby born at 27 weeks to a mother who had received water-soluble contrast medium for the investigation of a renal abnormality a week before delivery. Contrast medium is visible in the loop of bowel in the left hypochondrium.

Individual drugs

Antibiotics

Penicillins are acidic compounds with pK_a values of around 2 to 3; they are therefore more than 99.99% ionised at physiological pH. Such polar substances are rapidly excreted by the kidney. The pharmacokinetics of ampicillin has been the most extensively studied. Its clearance and distribution volume increase during pregnancy (Table 9.1), both overall and in relation to total body weight, and the half-life is shortened. The changes are more pronounced in the first and second trimesters than in the third [64]. Increased clearance during pregnancy has also been demonstrated for other penicillins, an example of which is given in Fig. 9.3. Thus following standard doses, plasma concentrations are reduced during pregnancy, but urinary concentrations are not. Placental transfer of the penicillins is slow but does occur, such a high degree of ionisation being only a slight bar to transfer across the human placenta. Transfer rates of *ampicillin* and *methicillin* are faster than those of the more polar *benzyl penicillin* and *dicloxacillin* [65,66]. After maternal administration of *ampicillin*, fetal plasma concentration rises slowly to exceed that in the mother after 1–3 hours. Amniotic fluid concentration remains low in early gestation, but in late gestation comes to exceed that in other compartments after 6–8 hours [65]. Excretion in human milk is limited. In the perfused human placenta clearance rates of both *ticarcillin* and clavulanic acid (the components of timentin) have been shown to be slow [67].

The *cephalosporin antibiotics* are also acidic compounds but, being less polar than the penicillins, their volume distribution has generally been found to be unchanged during pregnancy (Table 9.1). The total clearance of *cefuroxime* is increased during pregnancy and the half-life shortened [68]. Clearance of *cefoxitin* is not significantly altered in pregnancy, while serum concentrations of *moxalactam* and *ceftazidime* are 50% of the non-pregnancy values following a standard dose [69]. Their placental transfer has been studied in humans. Cefuroxime concentration in umbilical venous blood is about 50% of

maternal following an intravenous bolus given shortly before delivery, [70] while longer term treatment at around 30 weeks demonstrated effective concentrations in amniotic fluid and newborns [71]. Similarly penetration of ceftazidime into fetus and amniotic fluid has been found to be good in both early [72] and late pregnancy [73]. Long-term treatment with ceftizoxime may produce levels in amniotic fluid about two-fold those in fetal plasma, which are about two-fold those in maternal plasma [74].

Tetracyclines are relatively lipophilic and, because of their well recognised ability to penetrate fetal bones and teeth [75] and impair their development, are of course contraindicated in pregnancy.

Anti-epileptic drugs

The anticonvulsant *phenytoin* has been studied extensively. It is weakly acidic and highly bound to plasma albumin. It undergoes zero order elimination and therefore $T_{1/2}$ is not a constant that can be calculated. Most investigators agree that phenytoin clearance rises in late pregnancy, when dose increases may be necessary [12,76–78]. During pregnancy, protein binding may be reduced. As a result, the distribution volume can be expected to rise and hepatic clearance, being restrictive, to increase, while the proportion of phenytoin and its principal metabolite 5-*p*-hydroxyphenyl-5-phenylhydantoin (HPPH) does not change [13]. Another implication of altered protein binding is that the normal plasma monitoring is invalid. Knott *et al.* [12] have shown not only that phenytoin binding in pregnancy changes very unpredictably (Fig. 9.2) but also that clearance of unbound phenytoin may rise substantially in the third trimester in some patients while remaining within the normal range in others (Fig. 9.1). Phenytoin clearance is likely to show a substantial fall in the puerperium, many women requiring a dose reduction in this period to avoid toxicity.

Carbamazepine is neutral of albumin bound; plasma concentrations fall during pregnancy, while that of its principal (active) metabolite rises [79], indicating a general increase in the metabolism of this drug. Nau *et al.* [76] have shown the V_D and clearance of carbamazepine and *valproate* both rise in pregnancy, necessitating dose increases in some cases, while most workers find pharmacokinetics of phenobarbitone within the normal range in pregnancy [76,80].

As most anti-epileptic drugs are freely-diffusible and usually given long-term, they readily come into equilibrium across the placenta. Being neutral or weakly acidic and unbound or albumin-bound, fetal/maternal ratios at birth are usually ≤1 [81]. As valproate is rather more polar and has a short half-life, its transplacental distribution is variable.

It is important that anti-epileptic treatment continues throughout pregnancy, since the possibility of low-grade teratogenisis does not outweigh the risk to the fetus of anoxic damage which might result from a major fit. Breast feeding *must* be encouraged, since transfer of small amounts of drug to the newborn in the milk is an ideal means of gradual weaning from the full dose to which the fetus was exposed *in utero*.

Careful monitoring of anti-epileptic medication is clearly necessary in pregnancy and after delivery, particularly owing to great individual variability in the handling of these drugs. Moreover, an accurate indicator of unbound drug, such as saliva monitoring, is necessary for phenytoin.

Drugs used for pre-eclampsia

Antihypertensive drugs

The high incidence of pregnancy-induced hypertension and its proteinuric form, pre-eclampsia, means that an appreciable proportion of women will receive antihypertensive therapy, usually in the third trimester.

Antihypertensive drugs may affect the fetus:
1 if they cause maternal hypotension of rapid onset;
2 if they cross the placenta in sufficient amount to have a direct effect; this takes time.
Control of the cardiovascular system develops gradually and treatment regimes may thus have different effects at different gestations. Of particular theoretical importance is the need for an adequately functioning sympathetic nervous system to respond to hypoxia [82] and to the transition to extrauterine existence.

Although the hypertension of pre-eclampsia is not sympathetically mediated [83], β-blockers and α-methyldopa do have some anti-hypertensive effect in this condition, although they do not halt the disease progression. These agents differ widely in their water or fat solubility, their cardioselectivity and the way in which they are excreted. They are thus likely to have differing effects on the fetus. For example, *methyldopa* is a fat-soluble false neurotransmitter, which has been used for many years in obstetric practice. It lowers the maternal blood pressure, and evokes a tachycardia. It readily crosses the placenta and is excreted in the milk. Doppler haemodynamic studies suggest minimal deleterious effects on the fetus [84] and paediatric follow-up to four years has shown no significant effect [85].

Atenolol is a cardioselective β-blocker which is very poorly fat soluble and minimally protein bound (3%). Like methyldopa, it is almost entirely excreted via the kidneys. Thus excretion may be impaired in women with progressive renal failure in pre-eclampsia. It lowers maternal blood pressure, but at the cost of a bradycardia and significant effects on fetal haemodynamics [86].

A third type is the combined α- and β-blocking agent, *labetalol*. This is about 50% protein bound. Only 60% is excreted via the kidneys. Its kinetics are unchanged in pregnancy [87]. It is an effective antihypertensive agent, with minimal effects on maternal heart rate. It also has minimal effect on fetal heart rate and Doppler indices [88]. However, transient hypoglycaemia has been reported in the immediate neonatal period [89], especially in preterm infants [90].

Intracellular ionized calcium concentrations are major determinants of vascular smooth muscle contractility. These concentrations depend on the influx of extracellular calcium and the release of calcium from intracellular stores. Calcium channel blockers inhibit the influx of extracellular calcium. They are thus direct vasodilators and inhibitors of myometrial contractility and have been used as antihypertensive and tocolytic agents in pregnancy. Those mainly in current obstetric use are members of the 1,4-dihydropyridine family. The dihydropyridines most used have been *nifedipine, isradipine, nimodipine* and *nitrendipine*. These compounds differ markedly in their physiological effects and target vascular beds. For example, nimodipine appears broadly selective for the cerebral vasculature [91]. They are metabolized in the liver.

They all cross the placenta but fetal concentrations are less than maternal (e.g. 3.5 vs. 9.7 ng/ml for nimodipine, 2 hours after administration [91]). This may explain the consistent finding that maternal blood concentrations of calcium channel blockers which effectively lower maternal blood pressure are without significant adverse effect on fetal Doppler indices or heart nitrendipine [92], nifedipine [93]; nimodipine [91]; isradipine [94]). Adverse effects have, however, been reported when higher doses have been used experimentally in animals [95] and a case report linked severe fetal decelerations with the rapid lowering of maternal blood pressure after sublingual nifedipine [96]. Also the preterm fetal myocardium may be more sensitive to calcium channel blockers [97].

The maternal renin–angiotensin–aldosterone system is activated in normal pregnancy by progesterone-induced natriuresis [98]. The normal decrease in pressor response to angiotensin II (A II) is lost in women with established pregnancy-induced hypertension (PIH) or pre-eclampsia (PE) [99]. It might thus at first sight appear that angiotensin-converting enzyme inhibitors (ACEIs) could be a logical treatment for PIH/PE. These agents inhibit the conversion of the largely inactive angiotensin I to the highly active A II, and are increasingly used to treat hypertension outside pregnancy.

ACEIs are, however, clearly contraindicated in pregnancy, not on maternal grounds but on grounds of fetal well-being. The fetus appears to depend more on its renin–angiotensin–aldosterone system for cardiovascular homeostasis than does the adult [100]. ACEIs readily cross the placenta. Their main route of excretion is renal. Thus their administration to women with deteriorating renal function, as found in pre-eclampsia, will be associated with higher maternal and fetal blood concentrations. There are two distinct areas of concern.

Firstly, there is a series of case reports linking maternal ACEI intake during the period of organogenesis with a syndrome of hypocalvaria and renal tubular dysgenesis (summarized in [101] and [102]). Incomplete skull ossification and placental anomalies have also been reported in pups born to rats treated with *enalapril* [103]. However, inspection of available human data does suggest that a majority of women who conceive while taking ACEIs, but change therapy as soon as pregnancy is diagnosed, will have normal infants [101].

Secondly, there are abnormalities in fetal and neonatal renal function which, in susceptible individuals, lead to oliguria and consequent oligohydramnios. Since the ACEIs are excreted mainly through the kidney, this leads to a very long plasma half-life, even after birth [104], so that some infants require dialysis for 1–2 weeks after birth [101]. These infants are also very hypotensive.

Given the weight of data from animal studies and human case histories, there would appear to be no place for the use of ACEIs in obstetrics, given the wide-ranging actions of other antihypertensive agents. The specific angiotensin receptor blockers, recently introduced into clinical practice, should also be avoided.

Aspirin, a weak acid, with a pK_a of 3.5, is mainly present in its ionized form. It hydrolyses spontaneously to sodium salicylate, which has a much longer half-life in the blood than aspirin, 238 minutes vs. 15 minutes [105]. A conventional adult dose of 600 mg of aspirin blocks cyclooxygenase activity in both vascular endothelium and platelets, thereby inhibiting prostacyclin (PGI$_2$) and thromboxane (TxA$_2$) synthesis. In low dose, usually 75 mg per day, aspirin effectively blocks only platelet thromboxane, firstly because platelets within the portal system are exposed to the highest concentration of aspirin, while endothelial cells throughout the circulatory system are not, and secondly because platelets are unable to synthesize new thromboxane in their lifetime. The possibility therefore exists of manipulating the PGI$_2$/TxA$_2$ ratio, with little likelihood of either significant placental transfer of aspirin or its secretion into milk, since systemic concentrations will be very low.

The administration of 60 mg aspirin daily to

primigravidae from 16 weeks' gestation, in a placebo-controlled trial, was associated with significant falls in platelet aggregation induced by arachidonic acid and collagen, and in the release reaction. Aggregation not induced via the arachidonic acid cascade was unaltered. Serum concentrations of thromboxane B_2 (TxB_2), a major metabolite, were also lowered [106]. However, none of these parameters were lowered in the infants of these mothers [107]. Administration of a single dose of 100 mg aspirin during labour was associated with a significant fall in fetal serum TxB_2, but was otherwise without effect on fetal parameters [108]. As is now well-known, several large randomized trials have been unable to demonstrate any therapeutic benefit from low-dose aspirin in the prophylaxis of pre-eclampsia or intrauterine growth retardation [109–111].

Magnesium sulphate

Magnesium activates numerous enzyme systems in the body and acts as a physiological calcium antagonist. It has a tocolytic effect and in high concentration it produces presynaptic inhibition at the neuromuscular junction. *Magnesium sulphate* is most commonly used to prevent and treat eclamptic fits. It is not an anticonvulsant in the true sense. It appears to reverse cerebral vasospasm [112] and ameliorates the effects of cerebral ischaemia. Recent large-scale trials have shown convincingly that magnesium sulphate is effective in decreasing the recurrence of eclamptic fits [113] and in lessening their primary occurrence [114]. The trials demonstrated superiority over treatment with phenytoin and diazepam.

The main route for magnesium excretion is via the kidneys, with renal tubular reabsorption being the principal means of regulating plasma magnesium. The therapeutic range is narrow, with plasma concentrations in excess of 5 mmol/l causing muscle weakness. Plasma concentrations should be kept between 2 and 3.5 mmol/l; where rapid laboratory monitoring is not possible regular (15 minutes) assessment of the briskness of patellar reflexes may be used. Calcium gluconate is a rapid antidote when the therapeutic range and exceeded.

Just over 60% of total plasma magnesium is in the ionized form in the pregnant woman and 30% is protein bound. The binding protein is in lower concentration in the fetus, and a significantly higher proportion of magnesium (74%) is therefore ionized [115]. Neither serum concentrations nor percentage of ionized magnesium differ between normal pregnant and pre-eclamptic women [116]. Maternal therapeutic concentrations have been associated with decreased fetal heart rate (FHR) variability [117,118] and with blunted fetal responses to vibroacoustic stimulation [119]. These effects should be borne in mind when interpreting FHR traces during magnesium sulphate therapy. Moreover, magnesium given to mothers in preterm labour may be associated with an increase in neonatal mortality [120].

Drugs used for thyroid conditions

Thyroxine (T_4), and triiodothyronine (T_3) are synthesized in the thyroid gland, and in addition T_4 is converted in the periphery, principally the liver, to the more active T_3. They both have large molecules (T_4 molecular weight = 777) and are poorly soluble in water and lipid. In plasma both hormones are bound with high affinity principally to thyroid-binding globulin (TBG), T_4 about 99.97% and T_3 99.7%. Plasma TBG concentration rises in pregnancy, thus total plasma thyroid hormones may increase, but without a change in hormonal activity. If a woman becomes pregnant while on maintenance therapy, thyroxine dosage need not alter provided she was shown to be euthyroid before. Thyroxine does not cross the placenta, except possibly in the earliest weeks of gestation before the fetal production of thyroxine has started. Thyroid-stimulating hormones cannot cross the placenta but thyroid immunoglobulins do.

Carbimazole is probably the most commonly used anti-thyroid drug in the UK. It is moderately soluble in water and does not ionize but is hydrolysed and decarboxylated in the bloodstream into its active metabolite methimazole. This is available as a separate drug in Europe but not the UK [121]. It binds to plasma protein and has a half life of 5 hours, unaffected by the state of thyroid function. Carbimazole, as methimazole, crosses the placenta, and the drug can affect the fetal thyroid as it does the adult thyroid causing fetal hypothyroidism. *Propylthiouracil* is to be preferred in pregnancy, using the smallest dose which will maintain normal thyroxine and thyroid-stimulating hormone (TSH) levels.

Iodine is usually given in the form of potassium iodide. This is a highly ionized salt with a molecular weight of 166. Iodine passes rapidly across membranes, including the placenta, by an active transport process. Long-term treatment could result in hypothyroidism of the fetus but this does not preclude its use to cover thyroidectomy in pregnancy or in the rare thyrotoxic crises [122].

The radioisotope I131 should not be used in pregnancy. This too crosses the placenta readily carrying its radioactivity with it. It would be taken up by fetal thyroid tissue and could cause long-term damage.

Insulin

Insulin is a polypeptide hormone of 51 amino acids arranged in two chains linked by disulphide bridges. It has a molecular weight of about 5800 and, being a peptide, has low lipid solubility.

During pregnancy, fasting insulin concentration increases, though its kinetics are probably little altered. It does not cross the placenta in either direction.

Transfer of glucose across the placenta is not insulin-dependent. Glucose undergoes facilitated diffusion, a process that is saturable only at supradiabetic levels. Thus in diabetic mothers, hyperglycaemia results in massive glucose and free fatty acid transfer to the fetus, who responds by hyperinsulinism. Fetal glucose uptake, which is governed by fetal insulin and in part by placental lactogen, preserves the glucose gradient and enhances transfer. The result is fetal macrosomia. Oral hypoglycaemic agents cross the placenta and if given in pregnancy would catastrophically exacerbate fetal macrosomia. Thus good diabetic control with insulin to maintain normoglycaemia is crucial to successful diabetic pregnancy.

Folic acid

253

Folic acid is available pharmacologically as pteroyl monoglutamic acid in tablet or liquid form for oral use. After ingestion about 80% is absorbed into the body where it is distributed in plasma and extracellular fluid. From the plasma about 70% of the folate is passed into the cells. The folate is reduced by dihydrofolate reductase into tetrahydrofolate. Folic acid probably does not exist in the body but is the usual form of administration.

Randomized controlled trials have shown that adequate levels of folate in every pregnancy can reduce the incidence of neural tube defects (anacephaly and spina bifida) both among those with previous babies whose central nervous systems have been affected and among the total population [123]. Hence prophylactic folate should be started before pregnancy if possible to cover the time of neural tube closure (21–28 days).

Folate is also required in later pregnancy for it is involved with the acceptance and transfer of carbon atoms with DNA and RNA. Hence it is actively required in fetal growth and maternal haemopoiesis. Low levels are associated with megalobastic anaemia of pregnancy and the puerperium [124].

Folic acid has a molecular weight of 441. It is soluble in water particularly in a slightly alkaline pH and, as folate, passes across the placenta down a biological gradient from the higher concentration in maternal plasma to the lower one in fetal blood by facilitated transfer. The intracellular form has extra glutamic acid residues added to make folate pentaglutamate. This may be the way the active enzyme crosses the syncytiotrophoblast. It is reconverted to folate as it passes into the fetal plasma. In early pregnancy, the embryo has no stores of folate and if this vitamin is needed for the prevention of central nervous system abnormalities, it has to come from the mother continuously across the placental membranes. In late pregnancy, folate stores are built up but these will obviously be low in babies born well before term.

Ethyl alcohol

Ethanol is mainly metabolized in the liver, with over 90% being oxidized. It can inhibit the central release of oxytocin and was used to prevent preterm labour; better agents now exist. It passes across the placenta and rapidly reaches concentrations in the fetus equal to those of the mother. However, these concentrations fall more slowly than do the maternal ones when alcohol is being eliminated.

Alcohol affects fetal development on a dose-dependent fashion. Babies born to women consuming over 120 g of alcohol a week have growth retardation, mental hypoactivity and characteristic facial signs — the fetal alcohol syndrome [125].

Cocaine

Cocaine is an alkaloid derived from the coca leaf, and has been used medically as a paste or in solution as the hydrochloride salt to provide local anaesthesia to mucous surfaces. It has a sympathomimetic effect, producing vasoconstriction and central nervous system stimulation, not unlike the amphetamines. Though this vasoconstriction delays its absorption from mucous surfaces, it is more dangerous than modern local anaesthetics and is now rarely used in medicine. It remains a popular recreational drug however. Any drug with abuse potential inevitably crosses the blood–brain barrier and therefore also the placenta. Among regular cocaine abusers, it may be teratogenic [126]. Further, abuse is associated with higher rates of spontaneous miscarriage. The babies who survive pregnancy are small, both in length and head circumference, and they have a significant depression of interactive behaviour scores and response to stimuli [127]. However, more studies are needed to exclude the multi-variable negative factors also affecting the babies of such women—single motherhood, malnutrition, cigarette smoking, alcohol dependence and non-compliance with medical care programmes.

Xanthine derivatives

The uncontrolled study of theophylline kinetics carried out by Romero *et al.* [128] suggested that clearance was increased in pregnancy. However, an internally controlled study by Carter *et al.* [129] showed a progressive fall throughout gestation (Fig. 9.4) which the authors attributed to reduced hepatic metabolism.

By contrast, recorded changes in *caffeine* metabolism are consistent and moreover quite striking. Caffeine, with a molecular weight of 194 and a pK_a of 14, is a more lipid-soluble agent than theophylline, as witness its more pronounced central effects. Caffeine clearance also falls throughout gestation [130] (Fig. 9.6), moreover its $t_{1/2}$ is significantly prolonged compared to in the non-pregnant state [130,131] (Fig. 9.7) and reverts to normal in less than a month after delivery [132]. It has been postulated that this change might be due to a rise in pregnancy hormones [131] but there is no significant correlation between individual caffeine clearance values and oestriol, oestradiol or progesterone levels. Pregnant women are clearly more likely to experience caffeine toxicity if they drink a lot of coffee or strong tea but this change is not related to coffee aversion in early pregnancy [132].

Drugs used in labour

The kinetics of certain drugs that are commonly used in labour have been studied during parturition, in which circumstances the majority of measurements that make up the pharmacokinetic profile are inevitably made postpartum. Such patients are therefore not truly pregnant but this is nevertheless the relevant time to study such drugs. Pethidine kinetics would appear to be similar intrapartum and in the non-pregnant state [59] with no significant difference in the production of the primary metabolite, norpethidine [60]. By contrast, $t_{1/2}$ values for the much more lipid-soluble agents thiopentone [9,54], diazepam [133] and bupivacaine [134–136] are prolonged, though such studies were rarely internally controlled. Such kinetic changes do not necessarily indicate a dosage reduction, but should serve as a warning

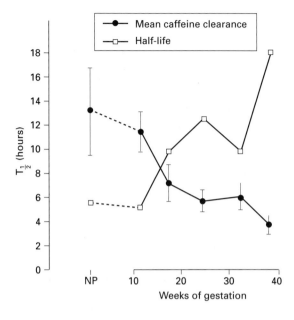
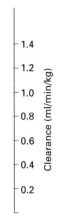

Fig. 9.6. Mean caffeine clearance and half-life. Data derived from the same subjects postpartum. Vertical bars: SE. From Aldridge *et al.* [130], with permission. NP: non-pregnant. Data obtained postpartum may not reflect the prepregnancy levels.

that residual effects of highly lipophilic drugs may be prolonged in the parturient.

Pethidine and all the more lipid soluble drugs readily come into equilibrium across the placenta in the non-ionized unbound state. If used in labour, pethidine depresses neonatal respiration and almost all neonatal neurobehavioural tests, including suckling, though the danger is negligible if given only within an hour of delivery. Modern opioids such as fentanyl are often given epidurally, and by this route are unlikely to depress the newborn. *Diazepam*, a very weak base that is bound to albumin, achieves high fetal levels and causes prolonged neonatal effects including hypothermia, hypotonia and hypoventilation. *Bupivacaine*, being unlikely to produce maternal systemic effects, produces little neonatal depression. *Thiopentone* produces only a transient effect on the mother, as it is given by intravenous bolus. When it is given only shortly before delivery, it has too little time to achieve a pharmacological level in fetal tissues. Neuromuscular blocking drugs are fully ionized and cannot achieve effective fetal concentrations when given to the mother for surgical relaxation.

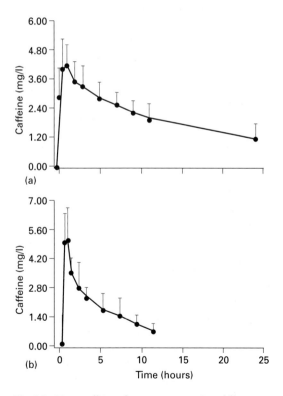

Fig. 9.7. Mean caffeine plasma concentrations following 150 mg caffeine taken orally (a) in eight women 30–40 weeks pregnant and (b) four women 4 days after delivery. Reproduced from Brazier *et al.* [131] with permission.

Conclusion

Maternal elimination of polar, non-lipid soluble drugs is generally more rapid in pregnant than that in non-pregnant individuals, such drugs being excreted unchanged by the kidney, whose function is enhanced in pregnancy. Moreover, concentrations of non-lipid soluble drugs are unlikely ever to rise to pharmacologically active levels in fetal plasma, though they may become concentrated in amniotic fluid and fetal gut lumen. Dose requirements of drugs of intermediate lipid-solubility, such as anticonvulsants, may also rise, though the increase is less when body weight changes are allowed for, and when free levels are measured. In some cases there is an increase in hepatic metabolism which may be accounted for by reduced protein binding. For such drugs, frequent monitoring of free drug concentration, which is best carried out on saliva, is mandatory. These drugs equilibrate, given time, in mother and fetus. Pharmacokinetics of many drugs in the intermediate category do not change significantly, particularly when body weight increase is allowed for. Maternal breakdown of the highly lipophilic drugs, however, is actually slower than in the non-pregnant state, while they readily distribute to the fetal compartment. The sojourn of lipophilic drugs is therefore prolonged in both mother and baby.

References

1 Coyle I.R., Wayner M.J. & Singer G. (1976) Behavioral teratogenesis: a critical evaluation. *Pharmacology, Biochemistry and Behavior* **4**, 191.

2 Lewis P.J. (1978) The effect of psychotropic drugs on the fetus. In *Mental Illness in Pregnancy and the Puerperium*. Ed. M. Sandler, p. 99. Oxford Medical Publications, Oxford.

3 Heinonen O.P., Slone D. & Shapiro S. (1977) *Birth Defects and Drugs in Pregnancy*. Publishing Sciences Group, Boston, Mass.

4 Forrest J.M. (1976) Drugs in pregnancy and lactation. *Medical Journal of Australia* **ii**, 138.

5 O'Sullivan G.M., Sutton A.J., Thompson S.A., Carrie L.E. & Bullingham R.E. (1987) Non-invasive measurement of gastric emptying in obstetric patients. *Anesthesia and Analgesia* **66**, 505.

6 Nimmo W.S., Wilson J. & Prescott L.F. (1975) Narcotic analgesics and delayed gastric emptying during labour. *Lancet* **i**, 890.

7 Ramsay R.E., Strauss R.G., Wilder B.J. & Willimore L.J. (1978) Status epilepticus in pregnancy: effect of phenytoin malabsorption on seizure control. *Neurology* **28**, 85.

8 Carter B.L., Garnett W.R., Pellock J.M., Stratton M.A. & Howell J.R. (1981) Effects of antacids on phenytoin bioavailability. *Therapeutic Drug Monitoring* **3**, 333.

9 Morgan D.J., Blackman G.L., Paull J.D. & Wolf L.J. (1981) Pharmacokinetics and plasma binding of thiopental. II. Studies at cesarean section. *Anesthesiology* **54**, 474.

10 McDonald-Gibson R.G., Young M. & Hytten F.E. (1975) Changes in plasma non-esterified fatty acids and serum glycerol in pregnancy. *British Journal of Obstetrics and Gynaecology* **82**, 460.

11 Krasner J.Y. & Yaffe S.J. (1975) Drug-protein binding in the neonate. In *Basic and Therapeutic Aspects of Perinatal Pharmacology*. Eds P.L. Morselli, F.I. Garattini & P. Sereni, p. 357. Raven Press, New York.

12 Knott C., Williams C.P. & Reynolds F. (1986) Phenytoin kinetics during pregnancy and the puerperium. *British Journal of Obstetrics and Gynaecology* **93**, 1030.

13 Dvorchik B.H. (1982) Drug disposition during pregnancy. *Biological Research in Pregnancy* **3**, 129.

14 Krauer B., Dayer P. & Anner R. (1984) Changes in serum albumin and α_1-acid glycoprotein concentrations during pregnancy: an analysis of feto-maternal pairs. *British Journal of Obstetrics and Gynaecology* **91**, 875.

15 Simpson P.J., Radford S.G. & Lockyer J.A. (1987) The influence of anaesthesia on the acute phase protein response to surgery. *Anaesthesia* **42**, 690.

16 Mucklow J.C. (1986) The fate of drugs in pregnancy. *Clinics in Obstetrics and Gynaecology* **13**, 161.

17 Nau H., Loock W., Schmidt-Gollwitzer M. & Kuhnz W. (1984) Pregnancy-specific changes in hepatic drug metabolism in man. In *Drugs and Pregnancy. Maternal drug handling — fetal drug exposure*. Eds B. Krauer, F. Krauer, F.E. Hytten & E. del Pozo, p. 45. Academic Press, London.

18 Tomson G., Lunell N.-O., Sundwall A. & Rane A. (1979) Placental passage of oxazepam and its metabolism in mother and newborn. *Clinical Pharmacology and Therapeutics* **25**, 74.

19 Veghelyi P.V. & Osztovics M. (1978) The alcohol syndromes: the intra-recombigenic effect of acetaldehyde. *Experientia* **34**, 195.

20 Shnider S.M. (1965) Serum cholinesterase activity during pregnancy, labor and the puerperium. *Anesthesiology* **26**, 335.

21 Van Petten G.R., Hirsch G.H. & Cherrington A.D. (1967) Drug-metabolizing activity of the human placenta. *Canadian Journal of Biochemistry* **46**, 1057.

22 Juchau M.R. (1976) Drug biotransformation in the placenta. In *Perinatal Pharmacology and Therapeutics*. Ed. B.L. Mirkin, p. 71. Academic Press, New York.

23 Drabkova J., Crul J.F. & Van Der Kleijn E. (1973) Placental transfer of ^{14}C labelled succinylcholine in

near-term Macaca mulatta monkeys. *British Journal of Anaesthesia* **45**, 1087.

24 Pelkonen O. (1984) Xenobiotic metabolism in the maternal–placental–fetal unit: implications for fetal toxicity. *Developmental Pharmacology and Therapeutics* **7** (Suppl. 1), 11.

25 Welch R.M., Harrison Y.E., Gommi B.W., Poppers P.J., Finster M. & Conney A.J. (1969) Stimulatory effects of cigarette smoking on the hydroxylation of 3,4-benzpyrene and the N-demethylation of 3-methyl-4-monomethylaminoazobenzene by enzymes in human placenta. *Clinical Pharmacology and Therapeutics* **10**, 100.

26 Cooper L.V., Stephen G.W. & Aggett P.J.A. (1977) Elimination of pethidine and bupivacaine in the newborn. *Archives of Diseases in Childhood* **52**, 638.

27 Horning M.G., Butler C.M., Nowlin J. & Hill R.M. (1975) Drug metabolism in the human neonate. *Life Sciences* **16**, 651.

28 Pelkonen O. (1973) Drug metabolism in human fetal liver: relationship to fetal age. *Archives internationales de pharmacodynamie et de therapie* **202**, 281.

29 Yaffe S.J., Rane A., Sjoqvist F., Boreus L.-O. & Orrenino S. (1970) The presence of a mono-oxygenase system in human fetal liver microsomes. *Life Sciences* **9**, 1189.

30 Rane A. & Sjoqvist F. (1972) Drug metabolism in the human fetus and newborn infant. *Pediatric Clinics of North America* **19**, 37.

31 Zamboni L. (1965) Electron microscopic studies of blood embryogenesis in humans. *Journal of Ultrastructure Research* **12**, 509.

32 Lambert G.H. & Nebert D.W. (1977) Genetically mediated induction of drug metabolizing enzymes associated with congenital defects in the mouse. *Teratology* **16**, 147.

33 Bracken M.B. & Holford T.R. (1981) Exposure to prescribed drugs in pregnancy and association with congenital malformation. *Obstetrics and Gynecology* **58**, 336.

34 Spielberg S.P. (1984) Pharmacogenetics and teratology. In *Drugs and Pregnancy. Maternal drug handling – fetal drug exposure*. Eds B. Krauer, F. Krauer, F.E. Hytten & E. del Pozo, p. 85. Academic Press, London.

35 Hutchings M.J., Paull J.D., Wilson-Evered E. & Morgan D.J. (1987) Pharmacokinetics and metabolism of salbutamol in premature labour. *British Journal of Clinical Pharmacology* **24**, 69.

36 Andrew M., Boneu B., Cade J., Cerskus A.L., Hirsh J., Jefferies A., Towell M.E. *et al.* (1985) Placental transfer of low molecular weight heparin in the pregnant sheep. *British Journal of Haematology* **59**, 103.

37 Hamshaw-Thomas A. & Reynolds F. (1985) Placental transfer of bupivacaine, pethidine and lignocaine in the rabbit: effect of umbilical flow rate and protein content. *British Journal of Obstetrics and Gynaecology* **92**, 706.

38 Knott C. & Reynolds F. (1986) Placental transfer of anticonvulsants in the rabbit: effect of maternal protein binding and fetal flow. *Placenta* **7**, 333.

39 Vella L.M., Knott C. & Reynolds F. (1986) Transfer of fentanyl across the rabbit placenta: effect of umbilical flow and concurrent drug administration. *British Journal of Anaesthesia* **58**, 49.

40 Hamshaw-Thomas A.H., Rogerson N. & Reynolds F. (1984) Transfer of bupivacaine, lignocaine and pethidine across the rabbit placenta: influence of maternal protein binding and fetal flow. *Placenta* **5**, 61.

41 Wilkening R.B., Anderson S., Martensson L. & Meschia G. (1982) Placental transfer as a function of uterine blood flow. *American Journal of Physiology* **242**, H429.

42 Illsley N.P., Hall S., Penfold P. & Stacey T.E. (1985) Diffusional permeability of the human placenta. *Contributions to Gynecology and Obstetrics* **13**, 92.

43 Wilkening R.B., Anderson S. & Meschia G. (1984) Non-steady state placental transfer of diffusible molecules. *Journal of Developmental Physiology* **6**, 121.

44 Szeto H.H., Umans J.G. & McFarland J. (1982) A comparison of morphine and methadone disposition in the maternal–fetal unit. *American Journal of Obstetrics and Gynecology* **143**, 700.

45 Nandakumaran M., Gardey C.L., Challier J.C., Richard M.-O., Panigel M. & Olive G. (1981) Transfer of salbutamol in the human placenta *in vitro*. *Developmental Pharmacology and Therapeutics* **3**, 88.

46 Bergman B., Bokström H., Borga O., Enk L., Hedner T. & Wangberg B. (1984) Transfer of terbutaline across the human placenta in late pregnancy. *European Journal of Respiratory Diseases* **65** (Suppl. 134), 81.

47 Gross T.L., Kuhnert B.R., Kuhnert P.M., Rosen M.G. & Kazzi N.J. (1985) Maternal and fetal plasma concentrations of ritodrine. *Obstetrics and Gynecology* **65**, 793.

48 Reynolds F. (1987) Transfer across membranes. In *Drugs in Anaesthesia: Mechanisms of Action*. Eds S.A. Feldman, G.F. Scurr & W. Paton, p. 63. Edward Arnold, London.

49 Franke G., Pietsch P., Schnieder T., Siegmund W., Grabow D. & Schutz H. (1986) Studies on the kinetics and distribution of dihydralazine in pregnancy. *Biological Research in Pregnancy and Perinatology* **7**, 30.

50 O'Brien W.F., Cefalo R.C., Grissom M.P., Viera S.F., Golden S.M., Uddin D.M. & Davies S.E. (1982) The influence of asphyxia on fetal lidocaine toxicity. *American Journal of Obstetrics and Gynecology* **142**, 205.

51 Kennedy R.L., Erenberg A., Robillard J.E., Merkow A. & Turner T. (1979) Effects of changes in maternal–fetal pH on the transplacental equilibrium of bupivacaine. *Anesthesiology* **51**, 50.

52 Krauer B., Nau H., Dayer P., Bischof P. & Anner R. (1986) Serum protein binding of diazepam and propanolol in the feto-maternal unit from early to late pregnancy. *British Journal of Obstetrics and Gynecology* **93**, 322.

53 Idänpään Heikkilä J.E., Jouppila P.I., Poulakka J.O. & Vorne M.S. (1971) Placental transfer and fetal metabolism of diazepam in early human pregnancy. *American Journal of Obstetrics and Gynecology* **109**, 1011.

258

54 Christensen J.H., Andreasen F. & Jansen J.A. (1981) Pharmacokinetics of thiopental in caesarian section. *Acta Anaesthesia Scandinavica* **25**, 174.

55 Piafsky K.M. & Knoppert D. (1978) Binding of local anaesthetics to α_1-acid glycoprotein. *Clinical Research* **26**, 836A.

56 Meuldermans W., Woestenborg R., Noorduin H., Camu F., Van Steenberge A. & Heykants J. (1986) Protein binding of the analgesics alfentanil and sufentanil in maternal and neonatal plasma. *European Journal of Clinical Pharmacology* **30**, 217.

57 Sioufi A., Hillion D., Lumbroso P., Wainer R., Olivier-Martin M., Schoeller J.P., Coluss D. *et al.* (1984) Oxprenolol placental transfer, plasma concentrations in newborns and passage into breast milk. *British Journal of Clinical Pharmacology* **18**, 453.

58 Dawes G.S. (1973) Theory of fetal drug equilibration. In *Fetal Pharmacology*. Ed. L. Boreus, p. 381. Raven Press, New York.

59 Tomson G., Garle R.I.M., Thalme B., Nisell H., Nylund L. & Rane A. (1982) Maternal kinetics and transplacental passage of pethidine during labour. *British Journal of Clinical Pharmacology* **13**, 653.

60 Kuhnert B.R., Kuhnert P.M., Prochaska A.L. & Sokol R.J. (1980) Meperidine disposition in mother, neonate and non-pregnant females. *Clinical Pharmacology and Therapeutics* **27**, 486.

61 Kuhnert B.R., Kuhnert P.M., Tu A.-S.L. & Lin D.C.K. (1979) Meperidine and normeperidine levels following meperidine administration during labor. II. Fetus and neonate. *American Journal of Obstetrics and Gynecology* **133**, 909.

62 Broughton Pipkin F. & Wallace C.P. (1986) The effect of enalapril (MK421), an angiotensin converting enzyme inhibitor, on the conscious pregnant ewe and her fetus. *British Journal of Pharmacology* **87**, 533.

63 Reynolds F. (1981) Distribution of drugs in amniotic fluid. In *Amniotic Fluid and its Clinical Significance*. Ed. M. Sandler, p. 261. Marcel Dekker, New York.

64 Kubacka R.T., Johnstone H.E., Tan H.S., Reeme P.D. & Myre S.A. (1983) Intravenous ampicillin pharmacokinetics in the third trimester of pregnancy. *Therapeutic Drug Monitoring* **5**, 55.

65 Nau H. Clinical pharmacokinetics in pregnancy and perinatology II. Penicillins. *Developmental Pharmacology and Therapeutics* **10**, 174.

66 Pacifici G.M. & Nottoli R. Placental transfer of drugs administered to the mother. *Clinical Pharmacokinetics* **28**, 235.

67 Fortunato S.J., Bawdon R.F., Swan K.F., Bryant E.C. & Sobhi S. Transfer of Timentin (ticarcillin and clavulanic acid) across the in vitro perfused human placenta: comparison with other agents. *American Journal of Obstetrics and Gynecology* **167**, 1595.

68 Philipson A. & Stiernstedt G. (1982) Pharmacokinetics of cefuroxime in pregnancy. *American Journal of Obstetrics and Gynecology* **142**, 823.

69 Giamarellou H., Gazis J., Petrikkos G., Antsaklis A., Aravantos D. & Daikos G.K. (1983) A study of cefoxitin, moxalactam, and ceftazidime kinetics in pregnancy. *American Journal of Obstetrics and Gynecology* **147**, 914.

70 Holt D.E., Broadbent M., Spencer J.A., de Louvois J., Hurley R. & Harvey D. The placental transfer of cefuroxime at parturition. *European Journal of Obstetrics, Gynecology and Reproductive Biology* **18**, 54; 177.

71 De Leeuw J.W., Roumen F.J., Bouckaert P.X., Cremers H.M. & Vree T.B. Achievement of therapeutic concentrations of cefuroxime in early preterm gestations with premature rupture of the membranes. *Obstetrics and Gynecology* **81**, 255.

72 Jorgensen N.P., Walstad R.A. & Molne K. The concentrations of ceftazidime and thiopental in maternal plasma, placental tissue and amniotic fluid in early pregnancy. *Acta Obstetrica et Gynecologica Scardinavica* **66**, 29.

73 Yamamoto T., Yasuda J., Kanao M. & Okada H. Fundamental and clinical studies on ceftazidime in the perinatal period. *Japanese Journal of Antibiotics* **39**, 2263.

74 Fortunato S.J., Bawdon R.E., Welt S.I. & Swan K.F. Steady-state cord and amniotic fluid ceftizoxime levels continuously surpass maternal levels. *American Journal of Obstetrics and Gynecology* **159**, 570.

75 Olanoff L.S. & Anderson J.M. Controlled release of tetracycline — III: A physiological pharmacokinetic model of the pregnant rat. *Journal of Pharmacokinetics and Biopharmaceuticals* **8**, 599.

76 Nau H., Kuhnz W., Egger H. J., Rating D. & Helge H. (1982) Anticonvulsants during pregnancy and lactation: transplacental, maternal and neonatal pharmacokinetics. *Clinical Pharmacokinetics* **7**, 508.

77 Lander C.M., Edwards V.E., Eadie M.J. & Tyrer J.H. (1977) Plasma anticonvulsant concentration during pregnancy. *Neurology* **27**, 128.

78 Lander C.M., Smith M.T., Chalk J.B., de Wytt C., Symoniw P., Livingstone I. & Eadie M.J. (1984) Bioavailability and pharmacokinetics of phenytoin during pregnancy. *European Journal of Clinical Pharmacology* **27**, 105.

79 Christiansen J., Mygind K., Munek O. & Dam M. (1977) Plasma levels of antiepileptic drugs in pregnancy. *Epilepsia* **18**, 295.

80 Luoma P.V., Heikkinen J.E. & Ylostalo P.R. (1982) Phenobarbital pharmacokinetics and salivary and serum concentration in pregnancy. *Therapeutic Drug Monitoring* **4**, 65.

81 Reynolds F. & Knott C. Pharmacokinetics in pregnancy and placental drug transfer. *Oxford Reviews of Reproductive Biology*. **11**, 389.

82 Walker D.W. (1994) Development of the autonomic nervous system, including adreno-chromaffin tissue. In *Textbook of Fetal Physiology*. Eds G.D. Thorburn & R. Harding, p. 287. Oxford Medical Publications, Oxford.

83 Assali N.S., Vergon J.M., Tada Y. & Garber S.T. (1952) Studies on autonomic blockade. VI. The mechanisms regulating hemodynamic changes in pregnant women and their relation to the hypertension of toxemia of pregnancy. *American Journal of Obstetrics and Gynecology* **63**, 978.

84 Montan S., Anandakumar C., Arulkumaran S., Ingemarsson I. & Ratnam S.S. (1993) Effects of methyldopa on uteroplacental and fetal hemodynamics in

pregnancy-induced hypertension. *American Journal of Obstetrics and Gynecology* **168**, 152.

85 Ounstead M.K., Moar V.A., Good F.J. & Redman C.W.G. (1980) Hypertension during pregnancy with and without specific treatment; the development of the children at the age of four years. *British Journal of Obstetrics and Gynaecology* **87**, 19.

86 Montan S., Ingemarrsson I., Marsal K. & Sjöberg N.-O. (1992) Randomised controlled trial of aten-olol and pindolol in human pregnancy: effects of fetal haemodynamics. *British Medical Journal* **304**, 946.

87 Rubin P.C., Butters L., Kelman A.W., Fitzsimons C. & Reid J.L. (1983) Labetalol disposition and concen-tration-effect relationships during pregnancy. *British Journal of Clinical Pharmacology*, **15**, 465.

88 Jouppila P. & Rasanen J. (1993) Effect of labetalol infusion on uterine and fetal hemodynamics and fetal cardiac function. *European Journal of Obstet-rics, Gynecology and Reproductive Biology* **51**, 111.

89 Macpherson M., Broughton Pipkin F. & Rutter N. (1986) The effect of maternal labetalol on the newborn infant. *British Journal of Obstetrics and Gynaecology* **93**, 539.

90 Hjertberg R., Faxelius G. & Lagercrantz H. (1993) Neonatal adaptation in hypertensive pregnancy: a study of labetalol vs hydralazine treatment. *Journal of Perinatal Medicine* **21**, 69.

91 Belfort M.A., Saade G.R., Moise K.J., Arcadia Cruz R.V.T., Adam K. *et al.* (1994) Nimodipine in the man-agement of preeclampsia: maternal and fetal effects. *American Journal of Obstetrics and Gynaecology* **171**, 417.

92 Allen J., Maigaard S., Forman A., Jacobsen P., Jespersen L.T. *et al.* (1987) Acute effects of nitrendip-ine in pregnancy-induced hypertension. *British Journal of Obstetrics and Gynaecology* **94**, 222.

93 Moretti M.M., Fairlie F.M., Sherif A., Khoury A.D. & Sibai B.M. (1990) The effect of nifedipine therapy on fetal and placental Doppler waveforms in preeclamp-sia remote from term. *American Journal of Obstet-rics and Gynaecology* **163**, 1844.

94 Wide-Svensson D.H., Ingemarsson I., Lunell N.-O., Forman A., Skajaa K. *et al.* (1995) Calcium channel blockade (isradipine) in treatment of hypertension in pregnancy: a randomized placebo-controlled study. *American Journal of Obstetrics and Gynaecology* **173**, 872.

95 Broughton Pipkin F. (1987) The effect of maternal drug therapy on the fetus. In *Hypertension in Preg-nancy*. Eds F. Sharp & E.M. Symonds, p. 305. Perina-tology Press, Ithaca, N.Y.

96 Hata T., Menabe A., Hata K. & Kitao M. (1995) Changes in blood velocities of fetal circulation in association with heart rate abnormalities: effect of sublingual administration of nifedipine. *American Journal of Perinatology* **12**, 80.

97 Agata N., Tanaka H. & Shigenobu K. (1994) Inotropic effects of ryanodine and nicardipine on fetal, neona-tal and adult guinea-pig myocardium. *European Journal of Pharmacology* **260**, 47.

98 Broughton Pipkin F. (1988) The renin–angiotensin system in normal and hypertensive pregnancies. In *Handbook of Hypertension, vol. 10. Hypertension during Pregnancy* Ed. P.C. Rubin, p. 118. Elsevier, Amsterdam.

99 Gant N.F., Daley G.L., Chand S., Whalley P.J. & MacDonald P.C. (1973) A study of angiotensin II pressor response throughout primigravid pregnancy. *Journal of Clinical Investigation* **52**, 2682.

100 Broughton Pipkin F. (1993) The fetal renin–angiotensin system. In *The Renin Angiotensin System*. Eds M.G. Nicholls & J.I.S. Robertson, p. 51.1. Gower Medical Publishing, London.

101 Anonymous (1989) Are ACE inhibitors safe in preg-nancy? Editorial. *Lancet* **ii**, 482.

102 Barr M. & Cohen M.M. (1991) ACE inhibitor fetopa-thy and hypocalvaria: the kidney–skull connection. *Teratology* **44**, 485.

103 Valdes G., Marinovic D., Falcon C., Chuaqui R. & Duarte I. (1992) Placental alterations, intrauterine growth retardation and teratogenicity associated with enalapril use in pregnant rats. *Biology of the Neonate* **61**, 124.

104 Bhatt-Mehta V. & Deluga K.S. (1993) Fetal exposure to lisinopril: neonatal manifestations and manage-ment. *Pharmacotherapy* **13**, 515.

105 Rowland M., Riegelman S., Harris P.A. & Sholkoff S. (1972) Absorption kinetics of aspirin in man follow-ing oral administration of an aqueous solution. *Journal of Pharmaceutical Sciences* **61**, 379.

106 Louden K.A., Broughton Pipkin F., Heptinstall S., Fox S., Mitchell J.R.A. *et al.* (1992) A randomized placebo-controlled study of the effects of low-dose aspirin on platelet reactivity and serum throm boxane B$_2$ production in non-pregnant women, in normal pregnancy and in gestational hypertension. *British Journal of Obstetrics and Gynaecology* **99**, 371.

107 Louden K.A., Broughton Pipkin F., Heptinstall S., Fox S.C., Tuohy P. *et al.* (1994) Neonatal platelet reactiv-ity and serum thromboxane B$_2$ production in whole blood: the effect of maternal low-dose aspirin. *British Journal of Obstetrics and Gynaecology* **101**, 203.

108 Ylikorkala O., Mäkilä U.-M., Kääpä P. & Viinikka L. (1986) Maternal ingestion of acetylsalicylic acid inhibits fetal and neonatal prostacyclin and throm-boxane in humans. *American Journal of Obstetrics and Gynecology* **155**, 345.

109 CLASP (Collaborative Low-dose Aspirin Study in Pregnancy) Collaborative group (1992) CLASP: a ran-domised trial of low-dose aspirin for the prevention and treatment of pre-eclampsia among 9364 pregnant women. *Lancet* **343**, 619.

110 Sibai B.M., Caritis S.N., Thom E. *et al.* (1993) Preven-tion of preeclampsia with low-dose aspirin in healthy, nulliparous pregnant women. *New England Journal of Medicine* **329**, 1213.

111 Caritis S., Sibai B., Hauth J., *et al.* (1998) Low-dose aspirin to prevent preeclampsia in women at high risk. *New England Journal of Medicine* **338**, 701.

112 Belfort M.A. & Moise K.J. (1992) Effect of magnesium sulfate on maternal brain blood flow in preeclampsia: a randomized, placebo-controlled study. *American Journal of Obstetrics and Gynaecology* **167**, 661.

113 The Eclampsia Trial Collaborative Group (1995) Which anticonvulsant for women with eclampsia?

260

Evidence from the Collaborative Eclampsia Trial. *Lancet* **345**, 1455.

114 Lucas M.J., Leveno K.J. & Cunningham F.G. (1995) A comparison of magnesium sulfate with phenytoin for the prevention of eclampsia. *New England Journal of Medicine* **333**, 202.

115 Handwerker S.M., Altura B.T., Jones K.Y. & Altura B.M. (1995) Maternal–fetal transfer of ionized serum magnesium during the stress of labor and delivery: a human study. *Journal of the American College of Nutrition* **14**, 376.

116 Handwerker S.M., Altura B.T. & Altura B.M. (1995) Ionized serum magnesium and potassium levels in pregnant women with preeclampsia and eclampsia. *Journal of Reproductive Medicine* **40**, 201.

117 Guzman E.R., Conley M., Stewart R., Ivan J., Pitter M. & Kappy K. (1993) Phenytoin and magnesium sulfate effects on fetal heart rate tracings assessed by computer analysis. *Obstetrics and Gynecology* **82**, 375.

118 Hiett A.K., Devoe L.D., Brown H.L. & Watson J. (1995) Effect of magnesium on fetal heart rate variability using computer analysis. *American Journal of Perinatology* **12**, 259.

119 Sherer D.M. (1994) Blunted fetal response to vibro-acoustic stimulation associated with maternal intravenous magnesium sulfate therapy. *American Journal of Perinatology* **11**, 401.

120 Mittendorf R., Covent R., Boman J., Khoshonood B., Lee K. & Ziegler M. Is tocolytic $MgSO_4$ associated with increased total paediatric mortality? *Lancet* **350**, 1517.

121 Cooper D.S., Bode H.H., Nath B., Saxe V., Maloof F. & Ridgeway E.C. (1984) Methimazole pharmacology in man. *Journal of Clinical Endocrinology and Metabolism* **58**, 473.

122 Melvin G. & Acetot Barlow J. (1978) Iatrogenic congenital goiter and hypothyroidism. *South Dakota Journal of Medicine* **31**, 15.

123 Department of Health (1992) *Folic Acid and Prevention of Neural Tube Defects*. HMSO, London.

124 Chanarin I. (1990) *The Megaloblastic Anaemias*. Blackwell Scientific Publications, Oxford.

125 Florey C. du V. (1992) Maternal alcohol consumption and its relation to the outcome of pregnancy. *International Journal of Epidemiology* **21** (Suppl. 1), p. 538.

126 Bingol N., Fuchs M., Diaz V., Stone R.K. & Gromisch D.S. (1987) Teratogenesis of cocaine in humans. *Journal of Pediatrics* **110**, 93.

127 Chasnoff I.J., Burns W.J., Schnoll S.H. & Burns K.A. (1985) Cocaine use in pregnancy. *New England Journal of Medicine* **313**, 666.

128 Romero R., Kadar N., Govea F.G. & Hobbins J.C. (1983) Pharmacokinetics of intravenous theophylline in pregnant patients at term. *American*

Journal of Perinatology **1**, 31.

129 Carter B.L., Driscoll C.E. & Smith G.D. (1986) Theophylline clearance during pregnancy. *Obstetrics and Gynecology* **68**, 555.

130 Aldridge A., Bailey J. & Neims A.G. (1981) The disposition of caffeine during and after pregnancy. *Seminars in Perinatology* **5**, 310.

131 Brazier J.L., Ritter J., Berland M., Khenfer D. & Faucon G. (1983) Pharmacokinetics of caffeine during and after pregnancy. *Developmental Pharmacology and Therapeutics* **6**, 315.

132 Knutti R., Rothweiler H. & Schlatter C. (1981) Effect of pregnancy on the pharmacokinetics of caffeine. *European Journal of Clinical Pharmacology* **21**, 121.

133 Moore R.G. & McBride W.G. (1978) The disposition kinetics of diazepam in pregnant women at parturition. *European Journal of Clinical Pharmacology* **13**, 275.

134 Belfrage P., Berlin A., Raabe N. & Thalme B. (1975) Lumbar epidural analgesia with bupivacaine in labor: drug concentration in maternal and neonatal blood at birth and during the first day of life. *American Journal of Obstetrics and Gynecology* **123**, 839.

135 Magno R., Berlin A., Karlsson K. & Kjellmer I. (1976) Anesthesia for cesarian section. IV. Placental transfer and neonatal elimination of bupivacaine following epidural analgesia for elective cesarian section. *Acta Anaesthesia Scandinavica* **20**, 141.

136 O'Sullivan G.M., Smith M., Morgan B., Brighouse D. & Reynolds F. (1988) H_2 antagonists and bupivacaine clearance. *British Journal of Anaesthesia* **43**, 93.

137 O'Hare M.F., Leahey W., Murnaghan G.A. & McDevitt D.G. (1983) Pharmacokinetics of sotalol during pregnancy. *European Journal of Clinical Pharmacology* **24**, 521.

138 Hogstedt S., Lindberg B. & Rane A. (1983) Increased oral clearance of metoprolol in pregnancy. *European Journal of Clinical Pharmacology* **24**, 217.

139 Kjer J.J. & Ottesen B. (1986) Pharmacokinetics of pivmecillinam hydrochloride in pregnant and non-pregnant patients. Letter. *Acta Pharmacologica et Toxicologica* **59**, 430.

140 Duvaldestin P., Demetriou M., Henzel D. & Desmonts J.M. (1978) The placental transfer of pancuronium and its pharmacokinetics during Caesarean section. *Acta Anaesthesia Scandinavica* **22**, 327.

141 Rayburn W., Shukla U., Stetson P. & Piehl E. (1986) Acetaminophen pharmacokinetics: comparison between pregnant and non-pregnant women. *American Journal of Obstetrics and Gynecology* **155**, 1353.

142 O'Hare M.F., Kinney C.D., Murnaghan G.A. & McDevitt D.G. (1984) Pharmacokinetics of propanolol during pregnancy. *European Journal of Clinical Pharmacology* **27**, 583.

PART 3

The Urogenital System

The Urinary System

CHRISTINE BAYLIS & J.M. DAVISON

The urinary system shares the widespread physiological upheaval of pregnancy, and a pregnant woman cannot be judged by the ordinary standards of renal function for a non-pregnant woman. The clinician must be familiar with normal changes because women with renal disease, a renal transplant or a history of a previous pregnancy complicated by severe hypertension may seek guidance on the advisability of conceiving or continuing a pregnancy already in progress. Although good advice consists of more than generalizations based on anecdotal experience, it must be realized that in clinical practice evidence-based information can be difficult to acquire because of limitations imposed by pregnancy. Consequently, animal models have been carefully developed to examine rigorously the mechanisms controlling the striking gestational renal alterations; this is a prerequisite for detection, understanding and management of renal problems in pregnant women. This chapter draws on the important classical publications and the most recent literature to present the key clinical facts, whilst highlighting underlying physiological principles.

Anatomical changes in the urinary tract

The kidneys of pregnant women enlarge because both vascular volume and interstitial space increase. Increased water content has been reported in the kidney of the pregnant rat, although others have also reported increased tissue weight [1,2]. Intravenous excretory urography performed immediately after delivery reveals that renal size is greater than that predicted by a standard height–weight nomogram and by 6 months post-delivery there is a decrease in renal length of 1 cm (Fig. 10.1) [3]. Ultrasound studies reveal that renal parenchymal volumes increase during pregnancy, by 70% at the beginning of the third trimester; a slight reduction then occurs during the first weeks postpartum [4]. Renal biopsy material obtained at caesarean section has shown that the microscopic structure of the kidney is similar in pregnant and non-pregnant subjects. Interestingly, however, the glomerular diameter in 27 autopsy cases was significantly greater than in non-pregnant controls [5]. Most of these autopsies were performed within 2 hours of death at Glasgow Royal Maternity Hospital (1935–1946) by Professor H.L. Sheehan, whose monograph (with Professor J.P. Lynch) focuses on the histology of the kidneys, liver and brains of women dying with pre-eclampsia and eclampsia.

The most striking anatomical change in the urinary tract is dilatation of the calyces, renal pelvis, and ureter (Fig. 10.2). These changes, invariably more prominent on the right side, can sometimes be seen in the first trimester and by the third trimester may be present in over 90% of women [6,7]. The cause of the dilatation may follow hormonal effects or be due to obstruction [8]. As pregnancy progresses, the supine or upright posture may cause partial ureteric obstruction as the enlarged uterus compresses the ureter at the pelvic brim. Ureteric dilatation terminates at the pelvic brim where the ureter crosses the iliac artery and at this point a filling defect termed the iliac sign can be seen in an excretory urogram (Fig. 10.2). There is increased tone in the upper ureter, hypertrophy of the ureteric smooth muscle and hyperplasia of its connective tissue, with no decrease in pacemaker activity for ureteral peristalsis, nor decrease in the frequency or amplitude of the ureteric contraction complex, so that it is erroneous to think of the ureters as toneless and floppy. Lastly, fetal pyelectasis (≥ 5 mm) is five to six times more likely to occur in fetuses of mothers with dilated collecting systems (with a similar temporal incidence), but the significance and/or the clinical applications are not yet clear [9].

Clinical implications of anatomical changes

Urine collection

Dilatation of the urinary tract may lead to collection errors in tests based on timed urine volume—for example, 24-hour creatinine clearance and/or protein excretion [2]. Errors are minimized if the pregnant woman is sufficiently hydrated for a high urine flow and/or if she lies down on her side for an hour before and at the end of the collection, precautions which stan-

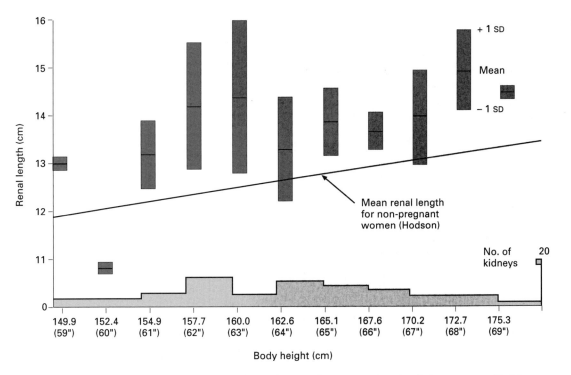

Fig. 10.1. Renal length, from excretion urograms taken in the immediate puerperium, in relation to maternal height. (Reproduced from Bailey and Rolleston [3], with permission.)

dardize the procedure and minimize dead-space errors.

Vesicoureteric reflux

Vesicoureteric reflux (VUR) occurs in at least 3% of pregnant patients at or near term. With advancing pregnancy, the enlarging uterus displaces the ureters laterally and the intravesical portions are shortened, passing through the muscular wall of the bladder perpendicularly rather than obliquely, rendering the junction functionally less competent. This is probably evident only when there is increased intravesical pressure such as during voiding and it has been suggested that a minimal intramural segment length of 10 mm may be critical in the prevention of VUR. As technical difficulties preclude the measurement of pressure differences between the bladder and the lower 5 cm of ureter, it has been difficult to document the loss of ureteric tone that would facilitate VUR.

Whatever the mechanism and consequences of VUR, the situation appears to be totally reversible with involution of the uterus. It remains to be confirmed if VUR encourages ascending urinary tract infection.

Acute hydronephrosis and hydroureter

The anatomical changes during pregnancy can be exaggerated with massive ureteral and renal pelvis distension (as well as slight reduction in cortical width) but this is usually without ill-effect [10]. Rarely, the changes may be extreme and precipitate the over-distension syndrome, hypertension [11] and renal failure [12]. Obstruction may occur at varying levels at or above the pelvic brim leading to only transient mild loin pain in some whilst others have recurrent episodes of severe loin pain or lower abdominal pain radiating to the groin [13]. Variation in symptoms with changes in posture and position are hallmarks of this condition. Urinalysis

266

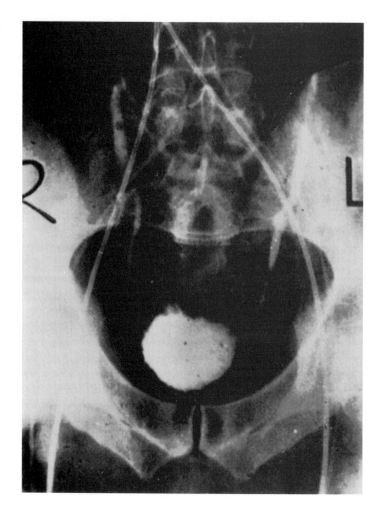

Fig. 10.2. Intravenous excretory urogram showing ureteral dilatation of pregnancy. The right ureter is abruptly cut off at the pelvic brim where it crosses the iliac artery (the so-called 'iliac sign').

shows few or no red cells and repeat midstream urine specimens are sterile. Diagnosis can be confirmed using limited excretory urography and/or ultrasound scanning (Fig. 10.3).

Non-traumatic rupture of the urinary tract

The overdistension syndrome of unremitting pain and haematuria upon the course of pyelonephritis suggests rupture of the urinary tract but rupture of the renal parenchyma, with haemorrhagic shock, formation of a flank mass and/or dissection of urinary tract contents intraperitoneally compels prompt surgical intervention, usually with nephrectomy [14].

Acute urinary retention

This rare symptom is caused by obstruction in and pressure around the lower urinary tract. The growing uterus may be involved, especially if retroverted, but urinary retention occurs in only about 1% of pregnant women with retroversion.

Interpretation of radiographs

Acceptable norms of kidney size should be increased by 1 cm if radiography is undertaken during pregnancy or immediately after delivery. Dilatation of the ureters may persist until the 16th postpartum week [15]. Ureteric dilation is

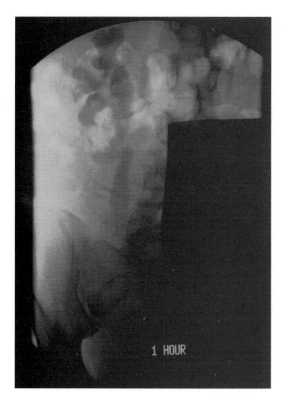

Fig. 10.3. Intravenous excretory urogram at 26 weeks' gestation showing a grossly dilated right-sided pelvic calcyceal system and a kinked ureter. This patient was originally diagnosed as having acute right-sided pyelonephritis unresponsive to antibiotics, with worsening loin pain radiating into her groin. Cystoscopy and ureteral stenting immediately resolved this situation. The stent was removed 4 weeks after normal delivery with no residual urinary tract problems.

permanent in up to 11% of parous women with no history of urinary tract infection and whether this is a harmless sequel of normal pregnancy or represents the residuum of missed infection is uncertain.

Renal haemodynamic alterations in human pregnancy

The perfect measurement of renal haemodynamics requires that the clinician must:
1   have knowledge of diet before the study,
2   control posture,
3   control volume and salt content of any infusion,
4   accept clearance values only if obtained during a period of stable urine flow and moderate diuresis, and
5   obtain control measurements before or after pregnancy [2].

The best studies in the normal pregnant woman have shown that effective renal plasma flow (ERPF) increases by some 50–80% between conception and midpregnancy (Fig. 10.4) [16] and then decreases during the third trimester (Fig. 10.5) [17–21] towards non-pregnant values [22–25]. There is a small increase during the first few days of the puerperium.

Glomerular filtration rate (GFR) increases less than ERPF during early pregnancy so that the ratio of GFR to ERPF, the filtration fraction, declines. In late pregnancy the filtration fraction increases to values similar to the non-pregnant norm [24]. The mechanism for this alteration is discussed later on p. 271.

Despite marked increases in renal haemodynamics, infusion of amino acids further increases ERPF and GFR, the increments being similar (10–18%) throughout gestation and postpartum [26]. Thus pregnancy does not attenuate so-called renal reserve.

Changes in creatinine clearance

Endogenous 24-hour creatinine clearance is a convenient, non-invasive method of assessing probable changes in GFR when infusion studies are impracticable (Fig. 10.6) [19]. Studies performed at weekly intervals after conception showed that 24-hour creatinine clearance increases by 25% 4 weeks after the last menstrual period and by 45% at 9 weeks (Fig. 10.4) [16]. During the third trimester a consistent and significant decrease towards non-pregnant values precedes delivery (Fig. 10.5) [17–21,23,27] and daily investigations have suggested a small increase during the first few days of the puerperium [28]. GFR values estimated from 24-hour creatinine clearances are consistently less than those obtained from clearances under infusion conditions of endogenous creatinine or inulin, due in part, to diurnal variation in GFR and in part to specific fluctuations in creatinine clearance. Caution must be exercised when interpreting renal function from creatinine clearance but

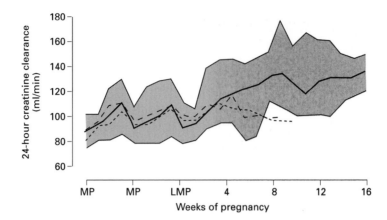

Fig. 10.4. Changes in 24-hour creatinine clearance measured weekly before conception and through to uncomplicated spontaneous abortion in two women (shown by dashed lines). Solid line represents the mean and the tinted area the range for nine women with successful obstetric outcome. (Reproduced from Davison and Noble [16], with permission.) MP: menstrual period; LMP: last menstrual period.

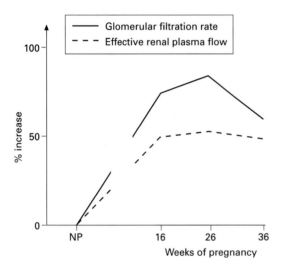

Fig. 10.5. Relative changes in renal haemodynamics during normal human pregnancy calculated from data given in Dunlop [17], Ezimokhai *et al.* [18], Davison [19,23]. NP: non-pregnant.

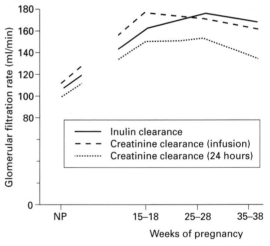

Fig. 10.6. Mean GFR in 10 healthy women during pregnancy and 8–12 weeks after delivery. (Reproduced from Davison [27], with permission.) NP: non-pregnant.

in clinical practice it is a valuable gauge in serial assessment.

Ultrasonic interrogation

A non-invasive method of serially or repetitively assessing the renal vasculature in pregnancy

would be as useful as it is in the non-pregnant population. Using combined B-mode imaging and duplex Doppler velocimetry, renal artery flow velocity waveforms have been analysed during normal pregnancy. Results vary from significant differences in indices (between pregnant and non-pregnant) to no effect of pregnancy

Table 10.1. Mean pulsatility index for right and left renal and intrarenal arteries in non-pregnant and pregnant women at varying stages of gestation. Values are means with standard deviations in parentheses. (From Sturgiss *et al.* [29].)

	Artery				
		Interlobar		Interlobular	
	Renal	Upper	Lower	Upper	Lower
Right kidney					
Non-pregnant (n = 8)	1.09 (0.19)	1.06 (0.14)	1.06 (0.19)	1.09 (0.18)	1.02 (0.13)
Pregnant					
Early (n = 8)	1.22 (0.15)	1.14 (0.20)	1.18 (0.15)	1.26 (0.15)	1.10 (0.27)
Mid (n = 11)	1.18 (0.22)	1.17 (0.19)	1.20 (0.23)	1.13 (0.18)	1.15 (0.21)
Late (n = 14)	1.12 (0.24)	1.09 (0.21)	1.12 (0.23)	1.07 (0.23)	1.04 (0.28)
Left kidney					
Non-pregnant (n = 8)	1.13* (0.13)	0.97 (0.07)	0.96 (0.14)	0.99 (0.12)	0.91 (0.08)
Pregnant					
Early (n = 8)	1.07 (0.25)	0.99 (0.13)	1.00 (0.13)	1.02 (0.16)	0.98 (0.16)
Mid (n = 11)	1.14 (0.23)	1.16 (0.23)	1.16 (0.19)	1.07 (0.26)	1.03 (0.15)
Late (n = 14)	1.07 (0.24)	0.99 (0.21)	1.07 (0.24)	0.94 (0.13)	1.01 (0.21)

*Significant ($P < 0.05$) versus left lower interlobular artery.

at all, possibly related to technical difficulties in visualizing the kidneys and renal hilus [2].

Colour flow mapping is better because a real-time map of the mean Doppler shift within blood vessels is displayed as a colour overlay on the B-mode image. When used in pregnancy to visualize renal arteries from a posterolateral approach, the positioning of the pulsed Doppler sample volume is optimized [29]. Furthermore, the position of the intrarenal arteries is revealed, allowing the analysis of waveform from the interlobar and interlobular arteries. Despite the use of this theoretically more precise technique, significant alterations between waveforms from pregnant and non-pregnant women were not found (Table 10.1) [29]. This lack of significant change was surprising, as the large increase in renal blood flow during pregnancy is thought to be due to reduced renal vascular resistance. It is likely, however, that waveform pulsatility reflects an interaction of several haemodynamic factors, many of which are altered during pregnancy. It is not yet possible to assess the individual effect on renal waveform variability of changes in maternal heart rate, stroke volume, blood pressure and blood flow because alterations of one variable affects the others.

Renal haemodynamic alterations in pregnant animal models

Gestational increases in GFR have been reported in a number of animal species including the rat, dog, rabbit, and sheep [1], with the rat being a particularly good animal model for both renal and systemic haemodynamic studies in pregnancy [30]. Most of the animal studies discussed below have been conducted in rats, although data from other species will be mentioned where appropriate.

Time course and magnitude of renal haemodynamic changes

As shown in Fig. 10.7a [31–33], GFR increases early in the conscious rat and has increased maximally by midpregnancy, to between 30 and 40% above the non-pregnant value. The elevated GFR is maintained throughout pregnancy, although close to term (22 days) there is a return towards the non-pregnant value [31]. A similar pattern of increase in GFR is also evident in the pregnant, anaesthetized volume-maintained rat prepared for micropuncture (Fig. 10.7b) [31–33], a preparation which allows measurement of the

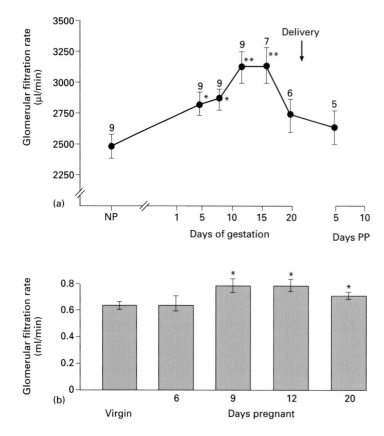

Fig. 10.7. (a) Magnitude and time course of the gestational change in GFR (for both kidneys) measured in the conscious, chronically catheterized Long-Evans rat by Conrad [31], with permission. (b) GFR (left kidney) measured in the anaesthetized, euvolaemic Munich-Wistar rat before and during pregnancy by Baylis [32–35], with permission. In both (a) and (b) data are shown as mean ± SE. A significant difference from the virgin value is denoted by *(P < 0.05) and **(P < 0.001). This composite is reproduced from Baylis [33], with permission. PP: postpartum

intrarenal mechanisms responsible for the renal haemodynamic changes in pregnancy.

Determinants of glomerular filtration

GFR is the product of the single nephron glomerular filtration rate (SNGFR) and the number of filtering glomeruli. There is no change in glomerular number in pregnancy; thus, increased GFR is due to increases in SNGFR. The net filtration pressure is a major determinant of SNGFR and as shown by the shaded area in Fig. 10.8, this is the difference between the glomerular hydrostatic pressure gradient, ΔP, favouring filtration and the glomerular oncotic pressure, $\Delta \pi$, opposing filtration. The other determinants are the filtration surface area and the water permeability of the glomerular capillary wall, which together can be calculated (from micropuncture measurements) as the glomerular capillary ultrafiltration co-efficient, K_f [34].

In normal non-pregnant rats, the net filtration pressure and the glomerular wall water permeability are high and filtration proceeds rapidly. Not all the available filtration surface area is utilized, i.e. the glomerular oncotic pressure (which increases along the length of the capillary as protein-free filtrate is removed) has increased to a value which equals (and opposes) the hydrostatic pressure gradient, somewhere before the end of the glomerulus (Fig. 10.8, curve A). This state is at filtration pressure equilibrium when SNGFR is highly dependent on glomerular plasma flow and any increase in plasma flow will elicit a proportional increase in filtration rate with no change in filtration fraction. This is achieved by increasing net filtration pressure will a shift in the glomerular oncotic pressure profile, e.g. from curve A to curve B

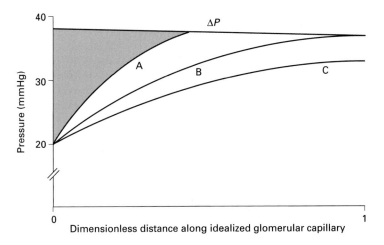

Fig. 10.8. Several possible profiles (curves A–C) of the intraglomerular oncotic pressure (Π) for a given hydrostatic pressure difference (ΔP) along an idealized glomerular capillary). Curves A and B are obtained at filtration pressure disequilibrium. The tinted area between ΔP and oncotic pressure curve A denotes the net ultrafiltration pressure obtained under these hypothetical conditions.

(see [34] for full explanation). In addition to plasma flow, hydrostatic pressure gradient and systemic oncotic pressure also control SNGFR by changing the net glomerular filtration pressure. Alterations in K_f will not influence SNGFR providing that filtration pressure equilibrium is maintained (Fig. 10.8, curve A). At filtration pressure disequilibrium, where a positive net ultrafiltration pressure persists over the entire length of the glomerular capillary (Fig. 10.8, curve C), SNGFR is influenced by changes in K_f [34]. Another consequence of filtration pressure disequilibrium is that filtration rate becomes less dependent on plasma flow; thus, an increase in plasma flow will produce some increase in filtration rate but proportionally less than the increased plasma flow, and hence filtration fraction falls. This may be the mechanism by which filtration fraction is reduced in the normal pregnant woman.

Glomerular haemodynamics in pregnancy in the rat

Micropuncture studies performed in the euvolaemic pregnant Munich-Wistar rat demonstrated increases of 30–40% in superficial cortical SNGFR by midpregnancy. As shown in Fig. 10.9 [35], the increase in SNGFR is the result exclusively of an increase in glomerular plasma flow rate, with the oncotic pressure of systemic blood (at the beginning of the glomerulus (π_A) and the glomerular hydrostatic pressure gradient (ΔP) unchanged by pregnancy [35]). Pregnant rats remain at filtration pressure equilibrium and K_f does not change markedly with pregnancy nor contribute to the gestational increase in SNGFR.

Plasma protein concentration, the albumin to globulin ratio and thence the systemic oncotic pressure are constant throughout the first part of pregnancy in the rat, with some reduction beyond around the 12th day [36]. This contrasts with pregnant women where plasma albumin concentration decreases early and remains low through to term [25]. Although a decline in systemic oncotic pressure (due to reduced plasma albumin) is predicted to increase GFR by lowering glomerular oncotic pressure, this effect is offset in practice since reductions in plasma protein concentration also lower K_f [37]. Thus, reduction in plasma protein concentration results in two offsetting changes in ultrafiltration determinants with little net change in GFR.

Micropuncture studies throughout pregnancy [30] reveal no sustained increase in glomerular

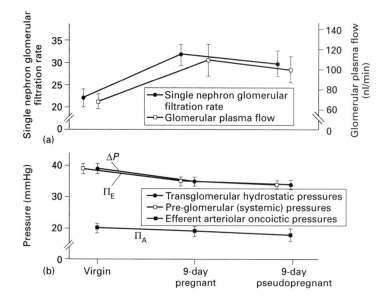

(a)

(b) Virgin   9-day   9-day
              pregnant   pseudopregnant

Fig. 10.9. (a) Determinants of glomerular filtration in the virgin 9-day pregnant and 9-day pseudopregnant Munich-Wistar rat studied under anaesthetized euvolaemic conditions. (b) The mean ultrafiltration pressures. Data given as mean ± SE, by Baylis [33,35].

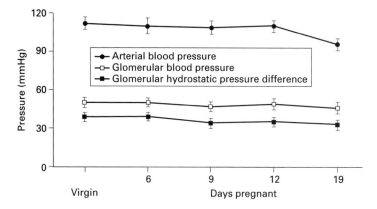

Fig. 10.10. Glomerular blood pressure, glomerular hydrostatic pressure difference and arterial blood pressure measured in virgin, 6-, 9-, 12- and 19/20-day pregnant, euvolaemic Munich-Wistar rats. Data shown as mean ± SE. Figure reproduced from Baylis [84], with permission.

capillary hydrostatic pressure (P_{GC}) at any time, despite gestational renal vasodilation, because there are proportional reductions in tone in the pre- and postglomerular resistance vessels, with increased plasma flow the sole determinant of the increased GFR (Fig. 10.10) [33]. Comparable human data are impossible to obtain but there are studies in women using neutral dextran sieving curves and mathematical modelling which, when combined with measured GFR, renal plasma flow (RPF) and plasma oncotic pressure provide indirect estimates of glomerular haemodynamics and membrane porosity. Serial data suggest that ΔP and K_f remain

unchanged throughout human pregnancy too, thus endorsing the exclusive role of increased RPF in the rise in GFR [25].

Long-term effects of augmented renal haemodynamics in normal pregnancy

Currently, clinicians worry about the possibility of prolonged periods of renal vasodilation damaging the glomerulus; it has been suggested that the primary damaging stimulus is the prolonged increase in P_{GC} which frequently attends renal vasodilation of the afferent arteriole in a variety of progressive glomerulopathies [38]. In pregnancy, chronic renal vasodilation, without sustained increments in P_{GC} or decrements of nephron number, is reversible [30].

In normal rats, five successive, closely spaced pregnancies (which represents prolonged renal vasodilation for approximately 6–7 months in a 1-year-old rat) had no adverse effects on glomerular or renal haemodynamics. In particular, there was no P_{GC} increment, proteinuria or morphological damage [39]. Thus, pregnancy *per se* does not lead to any acceleration in the nonspecific age-dependent deterioration in renal function. In humans, the evidence so far, albeit limited, also argues against glomerular injury resulting from normal pregnancy and reveals similar GFR increases in later compared with the first pregnancies [40] and with no obvious renal functional decline in the 23 years follow-up afterwards (J. Davison, unpublished data). Indeed, it is well known that women do not show any tendency for GFR to decline during the reproductive years and overall show far less of an age-dependent decline than men [41].

In summary, the gestational increase in GFR in rat is entirely due to renal vasodilation with consequent increases in RPF. Reductions in vascular tone in both pre- and postglomerular resistances are in proportion so that P_{GC} is constant in pregnancy. Similarly, increased GFR in the pregnant woman is the result of increased RPF with P_{GC} unchanged. The small reduction in filtration fraction, seen throughout most of the gestational period in the normal woman, is probably due to the development of filtration pressure disequilibrium because of the large increase in RPF (discussed above). The chronic renal vasodilation of pregnancy has no long-term kidney damaging effects.

Functional characteristics of the renal vasculature in pregnant animal models

Despite substantial plasma volume expansion and increased cardiac output, arterial blood pressure declines by midpregnancy, due to marked declines in total peripheral vascular resistance in both human and animal pregnancy [30,42]. There is no information currently available, from animal or human studies, to indicate how the gestational reduction in renal vascular resis-

tance is related to the decline in peripheral vascular resistance. The time courses, however, are different, since the maximal renal vasodilation is attained relatively early in pregnancy at a time when reduction in total peripheral vascular resistance has just begun.

Renal autoregulation during pregnancy

The kidney's ability to maintain blood flow and GFR over a range of blood pressures (i.e. to autoregulate) is dependent on variations in preglomerular arteriolar tone, which modulate RPF and P_{GC} [43]. Autoregulatory failure could present a problem in normal pregnancy both because of the decreased blood pressure and the chronic renal vasodilation. In midpregnancy, when renal blood flow and GFR are elevated, the autoregulation was the same in pregnant and virgin rats [44], with similar findings in the pregnant rabbit [45]; thus, gestational renal vasodilation does not alter the intrinsic renal autoregulatory ability (Fig. 10.11) [45]. In late-pregnant rats, however, where a gestational decrease in blood pressure has occurred, autoregulation of renal blood flow is intact but with some indication of a downward resetting in the 'threshold' possibly affording protection from periods of renal hypoperfusion [44]. Of note, however, is that autoregulation of renal blood flow in the ovine kidney may be impaired during pregnancy [46]. A tubuloglomerular feedback component as well as a myogenic component is involved in renal autoregulation [43], providing a mechanism whereby the rate of delivery of fluid (or some constituent of tubular fluid) controls the rate of filtration (SNGFR) at the glomerulus of the same nephron [47]. When fluid delivery in the early distal nephron increases (e.g. in response to an abrupt rise in blood pressure), this is sensed by the macula densa; a signal is sent to the parent glomerulus, which results in a vasoconstriction with a consequent reduction in SNGFR and restoration of early distal fluid delivery. In midpregnancy rats, tubuloglomerular feedback activity is normal, not suppressed, having reset to recognize the elevated SNGFR as normal [48]; thus, this component of the autoregulatory response is intact.

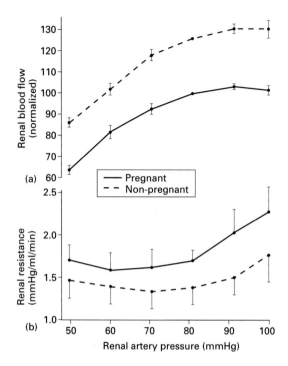

Fig. 10.11. (a) Renal blood flow and (b) renal vascular resistance during reduction in renal artery pressure in non-pregnant and late-pregnant rabbits. Renal blood flow expressed as percentage of flow at 80 mmHg in non-pregnant rabbits. Reproduced from Woods *et al.* [45], with permission.

Renal vasculature responsivity and vasodilatory capacity in pregnancy

In normal non-pregnant humans and experimental animals, a protein-rich meal or amino-acid infusion elicit substantial increases in GFR due to a selective renal vasodilation and increased renal plasma flow [49,50]. Interestingly, the pregnant rat responds to an acute amino-acid infusion with further substantial increases in both GFR and SNGFR, due solely to further increases in plasma flow [51], indicating extra significant reserve vasodilatory capacity despite chronic gestational renal vasodilation. To date, studies in normal women have been conflicting, since one group observed a substantial increase in endogenous creatinine clearance following a meat meal in the third trimester [52], whereas others have suggested that inulin and

p-aminohippurate clearances increase marginally, if at all, following a meat meal in normal pregnancy [53]. Recent work has suggested that chronic intake of dietary protein influences the renal response to acute protein feeding in pregnant women, which may explain the differences in the literature [54]. In response to intravenous amino acids, however, normal pregnant women show a marked renal vasodilatory response with GFR of 10–18% during pregnancy, similar to those postpartum [26].

Gestational renal vasodilation is still evident in the rat even after severe reduction of functional renal mass [55] and furthermore, in women with single kidneys (where compensatory renal hypertrophy has already occurred), pregnancy still causes a significant augmentation of renal haemodynamics. Increases are also evident in pregnancy in renal allograft recipients where, in addition to hypertrophy, the kidney is ectopic, at best partially innervated, possibly from an old, male donor, potentially damaged by previous ischaemia and immunologically different from both mother and fetus [22]. Surprisingly, the graft can usually augment function further in response to intravenous amino acids [56].

Mechanisms initiating the gestational increase in glomerular filtration rate

The first question, to determine whether the renal vasodilatory stimulus in pregnancy arises from the mother or from fetoplacental sources, has been easy to study in the rat. In pseudopregnancy, a state characterized by cessation of the œstrous cycle, rats exhibit identical changes in whole kidney and outer cortical single nephron function to those seen in pregnant rats. Also, the plasma volume expansion which attends normal pregnancy is evident in pseudopregnant rats [35]. These studies demonstrate that the fetoplacental unit is not necessary for the increase in GFR (or the volume expansion) of pregnancy and that some maternal stimulus must initiate these gestational changes. Although the placenta is not involved in the initiation of the gestational increase in GFR, there may be some role for placental factors in maintenance of the elevated GFR later in pregnancy, since removal of the placenta from midterm pregnant rats leads to reduction in GFR and renal plasma flow, later in the pregnancy [57].

Renin–angiotensin system and other vasoconstrictors

One possible explanation of the renal vasodilation of pregnancy is that the activity of an active vasoconstrictor system is reduced.

The renin–angiotensin II (A II) system is substantially modified during pregnancy and, although increases occur in plasma renin activity and plasma A II, a decreased responsivity to the vasopressor action of administered A II is also seen [42,58–61]. Whether this loss of sensitivity to the vasoconstrictor actions of A II extends to the renal resistance vessels and the glomerulus is not clear. In-vitro studies in pregnant rabbits and rats suggest down-regulation of glomerular A II receptors [62,63] but no difference in A II receptors in rabbit renal preglomerular vessels from pregnant and virgin animals [64]. Some studies report a mild blunting of the renal vasoconstrictor response to administered A II in pregnant rabbits [65] and rats [66], although others show normal renal vascular responsiveness to administered A II in pregnant rats, despite loss of pressor responsivity [67]. Also indirect, functional studies suggest that the glomeruli of midterm pregnant rats do not develop a reduced responsivity to A II, since the glomerulotoxic effects of gentamicin (mediated by A II) are not blunted by pregnancy [68].

Furthermore, since renal haemodynamics are not dependent on A II in the normal unstressed animal [69,70], loss of renal responsivity to endogenous A II cannot be the mechanism of the renal vasodilation of pregnancy. Also, studies in rats have indicated that A II-mediated renal vasoconstriction is unlikely to cause the close-to-term fall in GFR and renal plasma flow [69,71]. Vascular sensitivity to other vasoconstrictors is also influenced during pregnancy. Reduced peripheral responsiveness to administered noradrenaline and arginine vasopressin [42,66] occurs but there is uncertainty about reduced responsiveness to α-adrenergic agonists [72,73], although baroreflex-mediated bradycardia is enhanced [74,75]. Acute α_1-adrenoceptor

blockade has similar depressor and renal vasoconstrictor effects on virgin, midterm and late-pregnant, conscious rats [76], but acute blockade of the vascular arginine vasopressin (AVP) (V_1) receptor is without blood pressure or renal haemodynamic effect [77]. Thus, alterations in these systems are unlikely to contribute to the gestational renal vasodilation.

Prostaglandins

Prostaglandin (PG) could mediate the renal vasodilatation of pregnancy and increased urinary PGs in normal pregnant women, rats and rabbits and in pseudopregnant rats [66,78–80] has been assumed to reflect increased renal synthesis of these renal vasodilator hormones. Increased glomerular PG production in late-pregnant rats has been reported [81], which contrasts with studies showing no increased PG production by isolated glomeruli, cortical and papillary slices [82], despite a rise in urine PG excretion in pregnant rats. In-vitro studies in the rabbit show no difference in PG production by isolated glomeruli but increased levels in both cortical and papillary slices in late pregnant versus virgin rabbits [83]. Studies with acute cyclo-oxygenase inhibitors administered to the pregnant rat indicate that PGs are not the renal vasodilators of pregnancy, since there is no obliteration of the gestational rise in GFR in either anaesthetized rats or in the conscious, chronically catheterized preparation [66,84]. Chronic administration of cyclo-oxygenase inhibitors to pregnant rabbits (for 3 days) does not blunt the gestational rise in GFR [80]. The in-vitro data overall do not support increase in PGs as mediating the gestational rise in GFR.

Other vasodilator systems

Dopamine

Ths catecholamine produces selective renal vasodilation and could therefore be the gestational renal vasodilatory agent since elevated urinary dopamine excretion occurs during pregnancy [85]. At present, however, there is no evidence for a causal relationship between dopamine and the gestational renal vasodilation.

Atrial natriuretic peptide

Healthy women show increases in basal plasma atrial natriuretic peptide (ANP) during pregnancy with an increased metabolic clearance rate but apparently no attenuation of the natriuretic effect of infused ANP [86,87]. Since the glomerular haemodynamic mechanisms by which ANP can increase GFR are different to those of normal pregnancy, ANP is unlikely to be involved in the renal haemodynamic alterations of pregnancy and indeed infused ANP in human pregnancy produces no change in GFR (whilst reducing RPF) [88], akin to the effect in nonpregnant subjects [89]. In the rat, plasma ANP and vascular and renal haemodynamic responsiveness to ANP are unchanged during pregnancy [90–92].

Nitric oxide

The vasodilatory nitric oxide (NO) system, which acts via cyclic guanosine 3',5'-monophosphate (cGMP), is significantly involved in the regulation of blood pressure and renal function. Tonically produced NO controls peripheral resistance and blood pressure, both by direct vasodilatory actions and by blunting the responsiveness to vasoconstrictor factors [93,94].

A number of studies have investigated whether enhanced production and/or increased sensitivity to NO occurs in normal pregnancy [95,96]. Plasma and urinary levels of cGMP (the second messenger of NO) increase during pregnancy in rats and urinary cGMP increases in pseudopregnant rats [97], probably reflecting increased tissue cGMP production, since metabolic clearance rate is unaffected [97]. NO is unstable *in vivo* and is rapidly oxidized to NO_2 and NO_3 (NO_X) and the NO_X content of body fluids can be analysed, providing an index of NO production, after correction for dietary NO_X intake. As well as marked increments in 24-hour urinary NO_X excretion during pregnancy in the rat [98,99], plasma NO_X increased during pregnancy, with plasma and urinary NO_X correlating perfectly with increases in cGMP and not accountable for by increased dietary NO_X intake [98].

NO production in pregnant rats is resistant to NO synthesis inhibition [99], suggesting enhanced basal production. In-vitro studies in guinea pigs suggest enhancement of agonist-stimulated NO in pregnancy [100] and together with in-vivo studies suggest that NO is responsible for the pregnancy-associated refractoriness to administered vasoconstrictors [101,102]. Recent studies have shown that pregnancy increases mRNA levels for constitutive NOS in a variety of locations and oestrogen apparently provides the primary stimulus [103]. Normal pregnant rats exhibit signs of relative arginine deficiency since orotic acid excretion increases progressively during pregnancy [104] and plasma arginine levels are approximately 40% reduced in the basal state [105]. Whilst there is not complete agreement that increased NO plays a role in the normal falls in blood pressure in pregnancy [106,107], it probably has a role in the systemic cardiovascular responses to normal pregnancy.

Increased NO production may play a role in the renal vasodilation of pregnancy as it is certainly an important, physiological renal vasodilator [108]. Indeed, recent work in the conscious, pregnant rat suggests this to be the case: as shown in Fig. 10.12 [109], several doses of NO blockade, selectively abolish the mid-term rise in GFR, not shown by obliterating the gestational fall in renal vascular resistance [109]. Late-pregnant rats also exhibit an increased susceptibility to glomerular thrombosis, associated with a reduced NO response to lipopolysaccharide (LPS) because of arginine deficiency [105], presumably reflecting the increased utilization of L-arginine due to increased basal NO synthesis. Finally, chronic NO blockade during pregnancy leads to suppression of the normal peripheral and renal vasodilation, with falls in GFR, proteinuria, and increased maternal and fetal morbidity and mortality [29] in a pattern that closely resembles pre-eclampsia.

The available human data are controversial [96,110]. The 24-hour urinary excretion of cGMP increases in normal pregnancy [111] and is reduced in pre-eclampsia with $MgSO_4$ treatment of pre-eclamptics, restoring cGMP excretion to that of a normal late pregnancy [112]. Some report elevated plasma NO_X in normal pregnancy and reduction in pre-eclampsia [113] whereas others report no difference in values between non-pregnant, normal late-pregnant

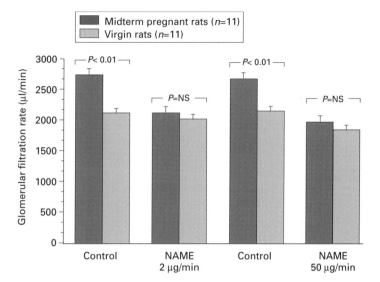

Fig. 10.12. Effect of two different doses of the NO synthesis inhibitor NAME on GFR in conscious chronically catheterized, midterm pregnant and virgin rats. Figure reproduced from Danielson and Conrad [109], with modifications.

and pre-eclamptic women for plasma NO_X [114] or 24-hour urinary NO_X excretion [115]. Of note, none of these studies employed a controlled low NO_X diet and there are substantial analytical pitfalls with clinical urinary NO_X measurements [116].

There is some evidence that arginine deficiency develops in normal pregnant women since maternal plasma arginine levels fall although cord blood levels are maintained [117] and orotic acid excretion increases markedly [118]. Information on the synthesis and responsivity of maternal blood vessels to NO is sparse but a recent in-vitro study showed no change in acetylcholine (ACh) stimulated relaxation in small subcutaneous arteries obtained from normal term pregnant and non-pregnant women [119]. Finally, observation that the circulating endogenous NO synthesis inhibitor asymmetric dimethyl arginine falls in pregnant women and is increased in pre-eclampsia [120] is noteworthy, perhaps suggestive of a permissive increase in NO synthesis in normals and a reduced NO synthesis in pre-eclamptics.

Influence of plasma volume expansion on gestational increases in glomerular filtration rate

Plasma volume expansion of sufficient magnitude will cause renal vasodilation with resultant

increases in renal plasma flow and GFR in non-pregnant rats. A cumulative volume expansion occurs during pregnancy in both humans and rats such that, close to term, plasma volume is enormously expanded [30,121]. There is, however, a dissociation between the plasma volume increase and the elevation in renal plasma flow and GFR in pregnancy, since the renal haemodynamic alterations are maximal quite early, before any substantial increase in plasma volume. Further, in acute plasma volume expansion of virgin rats by an amount equivalent to that retained by the 9th day of pregnancy, there are negligible effects on SNGFR or its determinants (Fig. 10.13) [122]. Thus, the plasma volume expansion of pregnancy is not the primary determinant of the gestational increase in GFR, although during pregnancy there may be altered sensitivity of the renal vasculature to the effects of volume expansion, such that it may play some role.

Renal tubular function in human and animal pregnancy

Although there are small decrements in many blood constituents during pregnancy, their filtered load will still increase due to increased GFR. These changes must be accompanied by parallel increments in tubular reabsorption otherwise massive depletion would ensue.

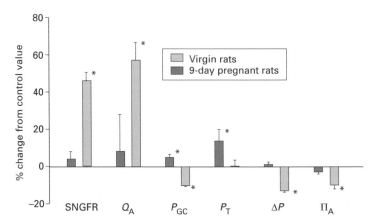

Fig. 10.13. SNGFR and its determinants are plotted as percentage change from control, during acute expansion of the plasma volume by 10–15% in virgins and for the 9-day pregnant rat in which plasma volume was chronically expanded by 10–15% compared with virgin controls. The asterisk (*) denotes a significant difference compared with the control value. Q_A: glomerular plasma flow; P_{GC}: glomerular capillary blood pressure; P_T: proximal tubule hydrostatic pressure; ΔP: mean glomerular hydrostatic pressure gradient; Π_A: pre-glomerular (systemic) oncotic pressure.

Renal handling of sodium

Renal sodium is the prime determinant of volume homeostasis and is discussed later (pp. 283–288).

Renal handling of uric acid

Uric acid, an endpoint of purine metabolism, is freely filterable at the glomerulus and cleared by the kidney at about 10% of the rate of inulin, implying that during its passage through the kidney most of that filtered is reabsorbed. Although a substantial proportion is reabsorbed in the proximal tubule, subsequent to this a balance between active secretion and further reabsorption regulates final excretion.

Serum uric acid concentration decreases by 25% during early pregnancy so that normal values range from 149–298 μmol/l with 298–327 μmol/l being an acceptable upper limit of normal. It has been suggested that this reflects alterations in the fractional excretion of uric acid (uric acid clearance/GFR) via a decrease in net tubular reabsorption [123]. The changes are greatest in early gestation because as pregnancy advances, the kidney appears to excrete a smaller proportion of the filtered uric acid load, and this increase in net reabsorption is associated with an increasing serum uric acid concentration.

There may be racial variations for the normal range as well as diurnal variations during pregnancy, with the highest values noted in the morning and lowest in the evening [124]. Also plasma levels tend to be higher in the presence of multiple fetuses [125]. As in the normal pregnant woman, uric acid excretion increases in the pregnant rat [126] but there are no data on tubular handling of uric acid in pregnancy.

Renal handling of glucose

Glucose excretion increases soon after conception and may exceed non-pregnant rates 10 times. The glycosuria varies markedly, both from day to day and within 24 hours, but the intermittency is unrelated to either blood sugar concentrations or gestational length. Normal non-pregnant values are re-established within a week of delivery.

Renal handling of glucose involves extensive proximal reabsorption of filtered load until the maximal reabsorptive capacity (TmG) is reached. In non-pregnant women, the TmG averages 1.6–1.9 mmol/min (300–350 mg/min), which, at normal glucose values, sufficiently exceeds filtered load to result in excretion of an almost glucose-free urine. The original concept of a fixed TmG is incorrect because trace quantities of glucose are always present in normal urine and TmG varies with changes in extracellular fluid volume and GFR [2,127].

Theoretically, glycosuria of pregnancy could be due to the inability of the renal tubules to cope with the increased filtered glucose load, a change in tubular reabsorption *per se*, or both. Serial studies of the renal handling of glucose under infusion conditions in women with varying degrees of glycosuria have shown that glucose reabsorption is less complete during pregnancy than when non-pregnant [127]. This is more so in pregnant women with obvious glycosuria, who, although no longer clinically glycosuric following pregnancy, still have incomplete reabsorption under infusion conditions when non-pregnant. All women, therefore, demonstrate variable decrements in the fractional reabsorption of glucose (T/F glucose) in pregnancy (Fig. 10.14) [128].

Animal studies have shown that glucose reabsorption depends on many factors including reabsorption of sodium and bicarbonate as well as changes in GFR and the regulation of the extracellular fluid volume [126]. Normal pregnant rats are glycosuric but this is not the result of diminished reabsorption from the proximal (reduced TmG) tubule but due to diminished net reabsorption from more downstream segments.

Renal handling of other sugars

The excretion of lactose, fructose, xylose, and fucose are increased in pregnancy, but not that of arabinose. Some oligosaccharides, which (similar to lactose) are presumably of mammary gland origin, appear in the urine of pregnant women.

Lactosuria is a benign condition of pregnancy of no clinical importance except as a possible source of confusion with glycosuria. It is easy to distinguish between glucose and lactose, since lactose does not react with glucose oxidase paper test strips.

Renal handling of water-soluble vitamins

Nicotinic acid, ascorbic acid, and folic acid are all excreted in increased amounts during pregnancy. In the case of folic acid, this is due to less efficient tubular reabsorption because plasma

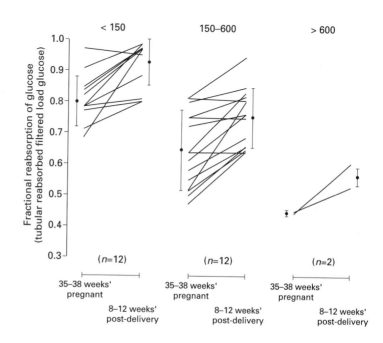

Fig. 10.14. Fractional reabsorption of glucose under infusion conditions (individual values and means ± SD) in 26 women studied during late pregnancy and after the puerperium. Women were divided into three groups according to their 24-hour glucose excretion (mg) during pregnancy (top). The within-groups significance (paired Student's t-test) for more than 150 mg/day, was $P > 0.001$; and for 150–600 mg/day, was $P < 0.001$. (Data were calculated from Davison and Hytten [128].)

folate declines in pregnancy and, despite the increase in GFR, the filtered load is unlikely to be increased.

Renal handling of amino acids

Urinary excretion of most, but not all, amino acids increases in pregnancy. There are three patterns of amino acid excretion [129]. Excretion of glycine, histidine, threonine, serine, and alanine increases in early pregnancy and remains elevated through to term. The excretion of lysine, cystine, taurine, phenylalanine, valine, leucine, and tyrosine also increases markedly in early pregnancy but thereafter tends to decline. Glutamic acid, methionine, and ornithine are excreted in slightly greater amounts than before pregnancy, isoleucine excretion is unchanged, and that of arginine tends to decrease. The reduction in arginine excretion is consistent with reduced arginine availability, discussed earlier in the context of increased NO production.

The increased excretion of most amino acids, together with reduced serum concentrations and the elevated GFR of pregnancy, point to the possibility of diminished tubular reabsorption. Based on 24-hour data, it has been calculated that for glycine the renal tubules may, on occasion, fail to reabsorb more than half the filtered. Overall, urinary amino-acid excretion during pregnancy may reach 2 g per day.

Potassium excretion

Even though aldosterone values are elevated and pregnancy urine is relatively alkaline, potassium excretion is *decreased* with a net potassium retention of approximately 350 mmol, most of which enters the enlarging tissues of mother and fetus. Furthermore, in contrast to non-pregnant subjects, pregnant women are resistant to the kaliuretic effects of a combination of exogenous mineralocorticoids and a high sodium intake. The gestational tendency to conserve potassium despite high concentrations of potent mineralocorticoids has been ascribed to the increased progesterone of pregnancy [47]. In normal man, desoxycorticosterone-induced

kaliuresis can be abolished by intramuscular progesterone [130] which in animal models also leads to a reduction in potassium excretion [131].

The tubular handling of potassium is complex, and micropuncture studies in the rat have shown that potassium delivery into the early distal tubule is reduced in pregnancy, due to increased reabsorption in the proximal tubule. Final urinary potassium excretion is *independent* of the filtered load of potassium and is determined largely by the magnitude of potassium secretion in the distal nephron [132]. Probably inhibition of potassium secretion in the collecting duct, and/or enhanced potassium recycling, provides the final mechanism of urinary potassium conservation by the gravid animal.

The resistance of pregnant women to the potassium-losing effects of steroids may benefit those with certain potassium losing diseases. Hypokalaemia is ameliorated during pregnancy in women with Conn's syndrome (primary aldosteronism) and Bartter's syndrome. On the other hand, renal resistance to kaliuretic stimuli in women with underlying disorders impairing potassium excretion could jeopardize pregnancy, as with sickle-cell anaemia [121].

Calcium excretion

Increased filtered calcium load inevitably accompanies the increased GFR of pregnancy. Although tubular reabsorption is enhanced, urinary calcium excretion still increases two- to threefold [133], possibly linked to the increased serum 1,25-dihydroxyvitamin D3 (calcitriol), which increases intestinal reabsorption of calcium and is known to cause hypercalciuria [134]. Calcitriol can suppress serum parathyroid hormone (directly and by increased serum calcium) such that renal calcium reabsorption is reduced at the level of the loop and the thick ascending limb of the loop of Henle.

Along with increased calcium excretion in pregnancy, urinary supersaturation is increased, predisposing to the formation of calcium stones. However, magnesium and citrate, known inhibitors of calcium kidney stones, also increase and must afford some protection against nephrolithiasis [134]. In addition, during pregnancy there is increased excretion of acidic glycoproteins, including Tamm–Horsfall protein (which originates within the cells of the nephron) and nephrocalcin [135], both of which inhibit calcium oxalate stone formation.

Renal regulation of acid–base balance

About 15 000 mmol of hydrogen ions are normally produced daily, which combine with bicarbonate to produce carbon dioxide to be excreted by the lungs. This would be a vast loss of body alkali but for the fact that most of the organic acid anions are further metabolized to generate new bicarbonate. Some 40–80 mmol of acid are produced daily whose anion is not further metabolized, either because it is lost in the urine or because it is inorganic. There represent the non-volatile acids and the bicarbonate lost in buffering them must be regenerated by the kidney. In pregnancy, the amount of acid to be eliminated might be increased due to an increased basal metabolism and greater food intake.

The renal regulation of acid–base ratio is altered in pregnancy [127]. The blood concentrations of hydrogen ions decrease by 2–4 mmol/l early in pregnancy, a decrement which is sustained until term. Thus, arterial (or arterialized venous) pH averages 7.44 in pregnant women, whereas it averages 7.40 in non-pregnant women. Simultaneously, plasma bicarbonate concentrations decrease by about 4 mmol so that values between 18 and 22 mmol/l are normal. This mild alkalaemia is believed to be respiratory in origin, since pregnant women normally hyperventilate and their arterial P_{CO_2} decreases from approximately 39 mmHg when non-pregnant to approximately 31 mmHg in pregnancy.

Renal bicarbonate reabsorption and hydrogen ion excretion appear unchanged by pregnancy but steady-state plasma bicarbonate and P_{CO_2} are less than in non-pregnant women [136]. Consequently, the pregnant woman is at a disadvantage when threatened by sudden metabolic acidosis, such as lactic acidosis in pre-eclampsia, diabetic ketoacidosis or acute renal failure.

Protein excretion

Protein excretion increases progressively throughout pregnancy. Approximately 4% of the total protein extracted is albumin. Many factors are involved including increased GFR, altered glomerular permselectivity and charge, as well as changes in tubular function. As mentioned in relation to calcium excretion, proteins which arise from the distal nephron (Tamm–Horsfall protein and nephrocalcin, for example) are also present in significant quantities. Proteins which normally undergo tubular reabsorption (retinol binding protein) and those which reflect altered tubular function (N-acetyl-β-glycosaminidase) are excreted in increased quantities, but the relative amounts of these tubular proteins are small [127].

Non-pregnant norms for total protein excretion and albumin excretion derived from early post-delivery data are greater than values at 6 months post delivery or pre-pregnancy. In fact, when pre-pregnancy norms are used, it is evident that both total protein excretion and albumin excretion increase in pregnancy, particularly in the third trimester. Even so, pregnancy norms have not been finally decided, especially near term, where changes may also relate to the onset of labour or a subclinical phase of pre-eclampsia [137].

Our unpublished observations, along with the better data from the literature, clarify the situation [22,138–142]. Both total protein excretion and albumin excretion are significantly elevated after 20 weeks in normal pregnancy. Figures 10.15 and 10.16 [141] reveal that in late pregnancy the means (and upper limits) for 24-hour total protein excretion and albumin excretion are 200 mg (260 mg) and 15 mg (30 mg), respectively. This agrees well with norms suggested for 24-hour means (and upper limits) of 117 mg (260 mg) for total protein excretion and 12 mg (29 mg) for albumin excretion [141], from a study where no normal pregnant women had significant albuminuria, defined as urinary albumin excretion of more than 30 mg/l.

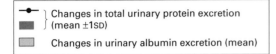

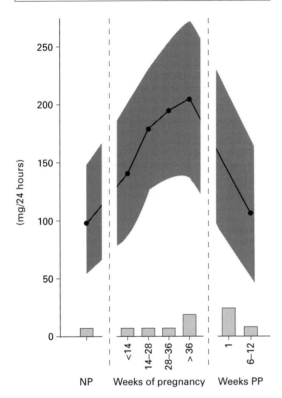

Fig. 10.15. Changes in total urinary protein excretion and urinary albumin excretion in eight women studied serially before, during and after pregnancy (unpublished personal data). NP: non-pregnant; PP: postpartum.

Osmoregulation in pregnancy

Very early in pregnancy women, plasma osmolality (P_{osm}) decreases to about 10 mosm/kg below the non-pregnant norm [143] due to a reduction in plasma sodium and associated anions (Fig. 10.17). This hypo-osmolality would inhibit antidiuretic hormone AVP release in non-pregnant individuals, leading to a state of continuous diuresis. This does not happen in pregnancy, however, because the osmotic thresholds for AVP release and thirst also decrease during the initial weeks of pregnancy (Fig. 10.18) [143–145]. The decrement in thirst threshold may precede that for hormone release, resulting in

mild transient polyuria early in pregnancy. The rat exhibits similar reductions in P_{osm} during pregnancy, while basal plasma AVP (P_{AVP}) and urinary concentrating and diluting capacity remain unchanged and the osmotic threshold for AVP release is reset to approximately 10 mosm/kg below that for virgins [146]. Significant reductions in P_{osm} also occur in Brattleboro rats with central diabetes insipidus; thus AVP is not necessary to evoke the decline in P_{osm} [53] and reductions in the thirst threshold must also play a key role.

Human chorionic gonadotrophin (hCG) may influence osmoregulation in pregnancy, since small increments in circulating hCG have been shown to decrease the osmotic thresholds for thirst and AVP secretion in non-pregnant women [145]. Furthermore, in a woman with a hydatidiform mole the osmotic thresholds were reduced and remained low for several weeks after evacuation, returning to normal only when hCG had decreased to the limit of detectability.

The metabolic clearance rate (MCR) of AVP (MCR_{AVP}) is similar to non-pregnant values in early pregnancy, but increases fourfold by the second trimester [147]. The blood of pregnant women contains a cystine aminopeptidase enzyme (vasopressinase) of placental origin, capable of inactivating large quantities of AVP *in vitro*. Whether or not this enzyme is active *in vivo* is unclear, but increments in the MCR_{AVP} correlate with the appearance and increase in plasma vasopressinase after midpregnancy [147]. Furthermore, the MCR of 1-desamino-(8-D-arginine) vasopressin (dDAVP), an AVP analogue resistant to in-vitro degradation by vasopressinase, does not increase during human gestation [148]. Further, the placenta can degrade AVP *in situ* and studies with in-vitro perfusion of term placentae suggest that this organ may be responsible for at least one-third of the increased hormonal disposal rates during pregnancy [149].

Volume status is a separate, non-osmotic determinant of AVP release [150]. Hypovolaemia stimulates and hypervolaemia blunts AVP secretion. Absolute blood volume increases significantly in pregnancy but how 'effective volume' is sensed is controversial. Hypovola-

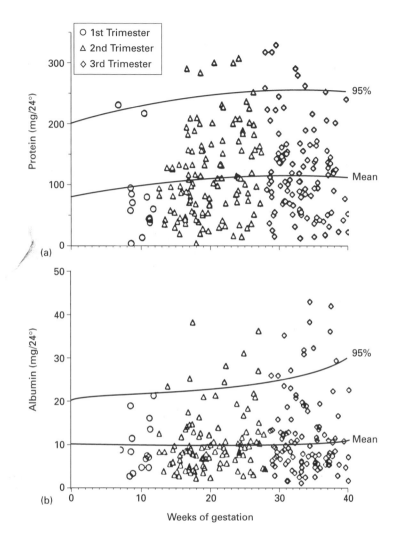

Fig. 10.16. Scatter plots of 270 women showing 24 hour urinary excretion of (a) total protein and (b) albumin by gestational age. Mean and 95% confidence limits are designated. Compiled from Figs 10.1, 10.2 and Higby *et al.* [168].

emia can diminish osmotic thresholds for AVP release and thirst and it has been postulated that the osmoregulatory changes are due to underfilling of the dilated intravascular compartment [151]. However, central volume expansion by water immersion in pregnancy has no effect on the reduced P_{osm} or the lowered osmotic thresholds [152]. In late pregnancy in the rat, where blood volume is almost twice normal, the relation between AVP secretion and percentage volume depletion, by graded haemorrhage, is similar to that in the virgin [153], indicating resetting of the non-osmotic release of AVP during pregnancy to sense the expanded volume as normal.

Body fluid homeostasis and renal function in pregnancy

As renal sodium handling is the prime determinant of volume homeostasis, it is appropriate to examine how changes in sodium and water handling influence extracellular fluid volume [154] (Table 10.2).

Renal handling of sodium

As well as the increase in total body weight, there is also accumulation of approximately 950 mmol of sodium distributed between the products of conception and the maternal extracellu-

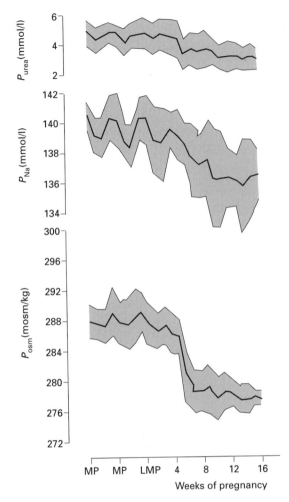

Fig. 10.17. Mean values (+ SD) for plasma (P$_{urea}$), sodium (P$_{Na}$) and osmolality (P$_{osm}$) measured at weekly intervals from before conception to the first trimester in nine women with successful obstetric outome. Reproduced from Davison *et al.* [143], with permission. MP: menstrual period; LMP: last menstrual period.

lar volume. This retention is gradual so that even in late pregnancy, the period of most rapid gain, it is only 3–4 mmol/day, usually too small for detection by conventional balance techniques.

The striking increment in renal haemodynamics is an important factor when considering renal sodium handling in pregnancy [121,155]. Even allowing for the 4–5 mmol/l gestational decrement in serum sodium, the filtered sodium

load still increases from non-pregnant levels of about 20 000 mmol/day to as much as 30 000 mmol/day. The extra 10 000 mmol to be reabsorbed is a quantity far greater than the expected salt-retaining effects of the antinatriuretic factors. Changes in glomerulotubular balance must ensure additional sodium is claimed daily for maternal and fetal stores.

Antinatriuretic factors

Several antinatriuretic hormones, mostly mineralocorticoids such as aldosterone and desoxycorticosterone, increase substantially during pregnancy [156]. The gestational increments in renin substrate, plasma renin activity, as well as plasma and urinary aldosterone are not due to subtle inadequate sodium intake. Furthermore, despite apparently high circulating levels, the renin–aldosterone system (RAS) responds appropriately when gravidas receive acute or chronic saline expansion or high salt diets, or when they are sodium restricted or receive diuretics and inhibition of aldosterone biosynthesis results in an inappropriate diuresis and subtle signs of volume depletion [60]. Thus, the activated RAS in pregnancy does not appear to function autonomously because the very high levels of aldosterone (which often exceed those in patients with primary aldosteronism), are appropriate and respond to homeostatic demands.

Natriuretic factors

The concentration of several potentially natriuretic hormones increases during pregnancy (e.g. oxytocin, vasodilating prostaglandins and melanocyte stimulating hormone) [121]. Of interest, elevated progesterone may also contribute to antinatriuresis, since it is a major source of increased desoxycorticosterone production, via extra-adrenal 21-hydroxylation [157]. Activity of the enzyme responsible for this conversion may be enhanced when oestrogen levels are increased, as in pregnancy, and renal steroid 21-hydroxylase activity may be particularly high in pregnancy so that substantial amounts of maternal desoxycorticosterone may be produced close to the renal receptor. Atrial natriuretic peptide (ANP) and its

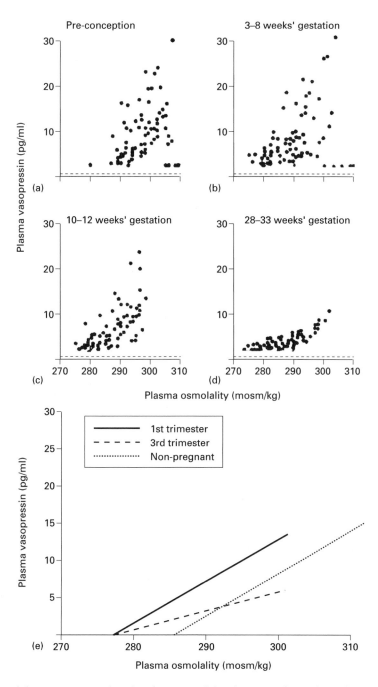

Fig. 10.18. Relation of plasma vasopressin (AVP) to plasma osmolality during serial 5% saline infusions in eight women commencing pre-pregnancy and continuing in pregnancy. Each point in a–d represents an individual plasma measurement. Highly significant mean regression lines from first and third trimesters and non-pregnant tests show the marked decrease in osmotic threshold for AVP release (abscissal intercept) during pregnancy. The osmotic thresholds for thirst (not shown) were always 2–5 mosm/kg above those for AVP release and were also 10 mosm/kg lower in pregnancy. From data given in Davison *et al*. [143–145].

Table 10.2. Factors determining sodium excretion during pregnancy. Net effect in normal pregnancy is gradual sodium retention of 950 mmol.

Antinatriuretic	Natriuretic	Uncertain or variable
Aldosterone	GFR	Filtration fraction
Angiotensin II	Progesterone	Prostaglandins
Oestrogen	ANP	AVP
Deoxycorticosterone	NO	Endothelin
Supine posture	DLIS	Cortisol
Upright posture		Human placental lactogen
		Placental 'shunting'
		Kinins
		Sympathetic nerves

metabolic clearance increase in human pregnancy although the plasma ANP increment is small relative to the marked intravascular volume expansion [87].

Transcellular sodium transport

The ouabain-sensitive Na+ K+-ATPase dependent pump is the main pathway for maintenance of sodium and potassium electrochemical gradients across most cell membranes and in the kidney this enzyme is involved in achieving sodium reabsorption. Pregnancy is associated with increased numbers of enzyme sites, both on circulating cells and in kidney [121] and enhanced enzyme function has also been demonstrated together with decrements in intracellular sodium, but the extent of increase in enzyme function appears to be significantly less than in enzyme numbers, suggesting relative enzyme inhibition [154,158,159]. Whether this is due to the elaboration of functionally inactive sites or to autoregulation by reduction in intracellular sodium is still uncertain but it does not appear to be due to a circulating sodium transport inhibitor. Nitric oxide, a potent natriuretic agent both by virtue of its direct inhibition of sodium resorption in the collecting duct and its renal vasodilatory effect, also increases in rat and possibly human pregnancy [96].

Effects of acute or chronic sodium loads

Studies of the effect of acute saline infusions on urinary sodium excretion have produced equivo-

cal results [154]. Where salt intake prior to the infusion was controlled, some reported no differences in the sodium excretory capacity in normal pregnancy compared to the non-pregnant state, while others suggested that both second- and third-trimester subjects respond with an enhanced natriuresis [160]. It has also been reported that pregnant women subjected to diets whose sodium content was as low as 10 mmol/day achieve urinary sodium balance as quickly as do non-pregnant controls, but these women actually lost weight so the data could be interpreted as suggesting that with extreme salt restriction gravidas manifest subtle salt wasting [60,121]. This is because sodium accumulation in late pregnancy should be in the range of 6–8 mmol/day and restricting intake to 10 mmol should reveal differences between the pregnant and non-pregnant state. Interestingly, in pregnant rat the cumulative 80% intravascular volume expansion and positive sodium balance achieved by late pregnancy is inhibited by sodium restriction at this time as is pregnancy outcome [161], whereas earlier in pregnancy zero sodium intake does not prevent expansion, which is presumably achieved by redistribution of fluid from other body fluid components [162].

Significance of body fluid volume and cardiovascular changes in pregnancy

Some basic facts concerning maternal physiological adaptation from early pregnancy onwards provide a starting point for discussion (Fig. 10.19):

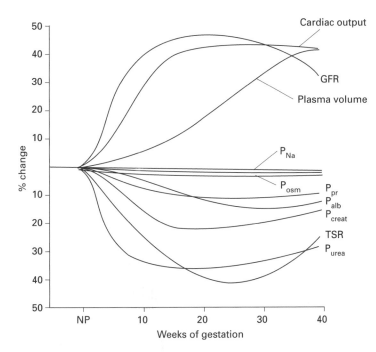

Fig. 10.19. Physiological changes induced by pregnancy, with increments and decrements in various parameters depicted in percentage terms relative to a non-pregnant (NP) baseline through to 40 weeks' gestation. GFR: glomerular filtration rate; P_{Na}: plasma sodium; P_{osm}: plasma osmolality; P_{pr}: plasma protein; P_{alb}: plasma albumin; P_{creat}: plasma creatinine; P_{urea}: plasma urea; TSR: total systemic resistance.

1 an increase in the capacity of the vascular system;

2 an increase in blood volume aimed at filling the enlarged vascular beds, particularly the venous capacitance system;

3 an increase in cardiac output, brought about by an increment both in the heart rate and the stroke volume;

4 a decrease in total systemic resistance as a consequence of peripheral vasodilatation and the new low-resistance shunt (the placenta), with the net haemodynamic effect of decreasing mean blood pressure;

5 changes in specific vascular beds, including the kidney, where haemodynamics are considerably augmented; and

6 adjustments reflected in the decrease in P_{osm} and solutes (mentioned above), which are not merely due to the expansion of plasma volume.

Reduced plasma volume expansion is associated with poor obstetric outcome and/or low birthweight but why maternal body fluid volumes increase during normal pregnancy is unclear, let alone the meaning and the chronological order of these physiological adaptations. Some postulate that the hypervolaemia is a sub-optimal response to the general vasodilation that accompanies pregnancy (the underfill theory), others consider it an epiphenomenon secondary to factors such as the marked increase in circulating mineralocorticoids (the overfill theory) and still others believe that there is continual resetting of volume sensing mechanisms as pregnancy progresses so that increments in absolute volume are sensed as normal (normal-fill).

The various arguments, analysed elsewhere [121,150,151,154,155,163–166] can be summarized as follows. Data supporting underfill include activation of the RAS, manifested not only by an increase in all its circulating components but also by observations that gravidas respond to small quantities of A II with a greater increase in aldosterone release than do non-pregnant subjects, and they experience exaggerated falls in blood pressure when treated with angiotensin-converting enzyme inhibitors. Serial haemodynamic studies of both women and baboons in early pregnancy also support the underfill hypothesis, as does the fact that adrenalectomy and/or sodium restriction is tolerated more poorly by pregnant rats than by non-pregnant controls.

Data supporting the overfill theory include absolute increments in extracellular volumes, high levels of circulating natriuretic factors and inhibitors of the membrane pump, increases in renal haemodynamics and increased sodium excretory capacity in response to saline infusions. The mean circulatory filling pressure measured in pregnant rodents has been described as either at the top limit of normal range or increased.

Data supporting the normal-fill hypothesis include animal experiments which probe relationships between intravascular volume depletion and AVP release as well as studies in rats and humans demonstrating that sodium and water reabsorption in the proximal nephron (determined by indices such as fractional lithium or free water clearances) is unaltered and in pregnancy urine is diluted normally when water loaded. These findings would be in accord with studies in the pregnant and non-pregnant states demonstrating similar sodium excretory responses to saline infusions.

The tubuloglomerular feedback system also functions as an intrarenal volume sensing and regulatory system, in which the delivery of tubule fluid is sensed by the macula densa (a specialized region in the early distal nephron). When fluid delivery increases, a signal is sent to the parent glomerulus, resulting in vasoconstriction with a consequent reduction in SNGFR and thus restoration of early distal fluid delivery. In some states of chronic volume expansion in the non-gravid animal, tubuloglomerular feedback activity is suppressed [47], an adaptation which allows the volume-expanded organism to excrete the excess volume load efficiently. In pregnancy, however, the tubuloglomerular feedback system is not suppressed but is reset to recognize the expanded volume and increased GFR as normal [48] (Fig. 10.20).

Clinical implications of functional changes

Creatinine and urea

Serum creatinine decreases from a non-pregnant value of 73 mmol/l to 65, 51 and 47 mmol/l, respectively, in successive trimesters of pregnancy; serum urea declines from non-pregnancy values of 4.3 mmol/l to pregnancy values of 3.5, 3.3 and 3.1 mmol/l, respectively. Familiarity with the changes is vital, because those normal values, in non-pregnant women, may signify decreased renal function in pregnancy. As a rough guide, values of serum creatinine and urea greater than 75 pmol/l and of 4.5 mmol/l, respectively, should alert the clinician to assess renal function further. Caution is necessary, however, when using serum creatinine levels alone, especially in the presence of renal disease, because even with a 50% loss of renal function, it is still possible for serum creatinine to be less than 130 µmol/l (Fig. 10.21).

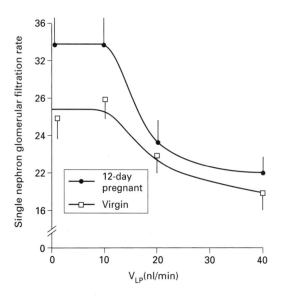

Fig. 10.20. Data (mean ± SE) given for SNGFR measured from early proximal sites during microperfusion of the late proximal segment of the same nephron, at rates (V_{LP}) of 0, 10, 20 and 40 nl/min for virgin rats and 12-day pregnant rats. Feedback curves are drawn as best fit through data points obtained for each group of rats.

Creatinine clearance

Although reciprocal or logarithmic levels of serum creatinine are often used to estimate GFR in relation to age, height and weight [167], this approach has been questioned [2] for pregnancy, because body weight or size do not reflect

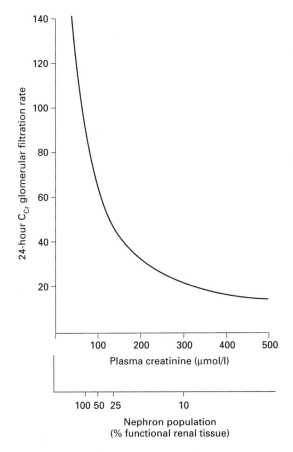

Fig. 10.21. Relation of clearance of creatinine (ml/min) to plasma creatinine concentration (μmol/l) and nephron population (%), assuming a constant creatinine excretion of about 1.2 g per day.

kidney size. Ideally, evaluation of renal function in pregnancy should be based on the clearance rather than the serum creatinine. To overcome such problems as washout from changes in urine flow and avoid difficulties caused by diurnal variations, 24-hour urine samples should be used for clearances.

Many methods of determining creatinine concentration in serum also measure non-creatinine chromogens, leading to overestimates that must be taken into account when calculating clearances. In addition, recent intake of cooked meat can increase serum creatinine by up to 16 μmol/l (because cooking converts preformed creatine into creatinine) and timing of blood sampling

during a clearance period should take this into account.

Uric acid

From the clinical viewpoint, it is of interest that serum uric acid and renal absorption are significantly greater in pregnancies complicated by pre-eclampsia or intrauterine growth retardation. Above a critical value of 350 mmol/l there is significant perinatal mortality in hypertensive patients and serial measurements can be used to monitor progress in pre-eclampsia [2]. It must be remembered that there is diurnal variation in serum levels, that variability is such that some healthy women have high levels without problems, that single random measurements are of no use clinically, and that levels tend to be higher with multiple pregnancy (see p. 278).

Glucose excretion

Glycosuria of pregnancy usually reflects alteration in renal function, not in carbohydrate metabolism [2]. Testing of random urine samples during pregnancy is unhelpful in diagnosis or control of diabetes mellitus and unrepresentative as to the degree of glycosuria present.

Proteinuria

As urine flow normally varies over a wide range from moment to moment, the protein concentration in a random specimen can give only a semiquantitative appraisal of the degree of proteinuria. Although this estimate recorded on an arbitrary scale (or as an approximate concentration) is valuable, more accurate quantitation is advisable. Proteinuria should not be considered abnormal until it exceeds 500 mg in 24 hours (twice the upper limit for normal pregnancy). Albumin excretion averages about 12 mg in 24 hours, with 29 mg in 24 hours as the upper limit of normal in pregnancy [141,168] (see also Figs 10.15 and 10.16).

Currently there are debates about the independent effect of pregnancy on long-term renal function (in health and disease) and about predictive tests for pre-eclampsia, using microalbuminuria to detect damage [2,30,40,137]. As discussed elsewhere in this chapter, the consensus is that pregnancy does not damage the kidney, and in any case, better markers are needed than albumin excretion alone.

Renal function tests in pregnancy

Routine tests for clinical practice include estimation of serum urea and electrolytes, creatinine clearance determination and urinary concentration and dilution assessment. Serial surveillance of 24-hour creatinine clearance and protein excretion should be performed and where possible compared with non-pregnant values.

If renal function deteriorates at any stage of pregnancy, reversible causes such as urinary tract infection or obstruction, subtle dehydration or electrolyte imbalance (perhaps secondary to inadvertent diuretic therapy) should be sought. Near term, a decrease in function of 15% (which affects serum creatinine minimally) is probably normal. If hypertension accompanies decreases in renal function, the outlook is usually more serious.

Disorders of water metabolism

Diabetes insipidus

The causes of diabetes insipidus antedating pregnancy are discussed in Chapter 12. Patients are rarely treated with synthetic forms of AVP, but if they are, the increment in hormone disposal rates will obviously require an increase in the AVP dosage. Currently, however, virtually all women with known central diabetes insipidus are managed with desmopressin (dDAVP), the MCR of which is not altered during pregnancy [149]. There are, however, reports of increased dDAVP requirements in pregnancy where symptoms associated with the threshold for thirst seem to have been misinterpreted as dDAVP escape. When such cases were appropriately studied, however, the preconception replacement dose has proved sufficient throughout gestation [150].

Nephrogenic diabetes insipidus

This is quite rare, although carriers of the X-linked variety may become polyuric in pregnancy. Diuretics, the mainstay of therapy in this disorder, work by depleting intravascular volume which results in increased proximal reabsorption of sodium and the delivery of less filtrate to the diluting site. The maintenance of hypovolaemia may not be optimal for pregnancy, but when the polyuria is massive, such agents may have to be used.

Transient diabetes insipidus

On occasion, polyuria and polydipsia may develop late in pregnancy, remitting postpartum. In these women the disorder might reflect massive in-vivo destruction of AVP by extremely elevated levels and/or exaggerated effects of vasopressinase [150]. Use of dDAVP, however, produces a concentrated urine. Another form of transient diabetes insipidus of pregnancy is where some women with partial central diabetes insipidus, asymptomatic when non-pregnant, manifest polyuria after midpregnancy coincident with the normal fourfold increase in MCR. In some women, transient diabetes insipidus only slowly remits postpartum, being resistant to both AVP and dDAVP.

Volume homeostasis and diuretics

In view of the mechanisms involved in the control of renal sodium reabsorption and the many haemodynamic and humoral alterations that occur during pregnancy, it is remarkable that problems related to sodium and water homeostasis do not constantly beset pregnant women. Admittedly, many pregnant women have asymptomatic oedema at some time during pregnancy but in the absence of pre-eclampsia, infants born to women with oedema of the hands and face actually weigh more at birth than do infants of non-oedematous women [169].

It remains to be established whether the increment in maternal extracellular fluid volume is required for optimal uteroplacental perfusion. It is interesting that in pre-eclampsia intravascular volume is decreased [154] with compromised placental perfusion and function, and the administration of a thiazide or frusemide can reduce placental function further.

Diuretics are sometimes given during pregnancy to prevent and to treat pre-eclampsia. Carefully controlled studies [170] have not confirmed the claim that prophylaxis with thiazides reduces the incidence of pre-eclampsia. Many diuretics affect the renal handling of uric acid and with few exceptions cause hyperuricaemia, which can obviously be confusing. Furthermore, diuretics are not without risk, causing maternal pancreatitis, severe hypokalaemia, neonatal electrolyte imbalance, cardiac arrhythmias and thrombocytopenia.

Renal dysfunction/insufficiency and pregnancy

An individual may lose approximately 50% of renal function and still maintain a serum creatinine level below 130 mmol/l (Fig. 10.20). If renal function is more severely compromised, however, small further decreases in GFR will cause serum creatinine to increase markedly. Nevertheless, a patient who has lost 75% of her nephrons may have lost only 50% of renal function and may have a deceptively normal serum creatinine due to hyperfiltration by the remaining nephrons. Evaluation of renal function is best based on the clearance of creatinine rather than on its serum (or plasma) concentration, or better still on measurement of GFR.

Patients with renal disease remain symptom-free until GFR declines to less than 25% of normal. Many serum constituents are frequently normal until a late stage of disease but, as renal function declines, the ability to conceive and to sustain a viable pregnancy decreases and degrees of functional impairment that do not cause symptoms or appear to disrupt homeostasis in non-pregnant individuals can jeopardize pregnancy [171–176].

Renal impairment and impact of pregnancy

Normal pregnancy is rare when renal function declines such that the non-pregnant plasma creatinine and urea exceed 275 mmol/l and 10 mmol/l, respectively.

Obstetric and long-term renal prognoses differ in women with different degrees of renal insufficiency, and the impact of pregnancy is best considered by categories of functional renal status prior to conception (Tables 10.3 and 10.4).

Preserved or mildly impaired renal function

Women with normal or slightly decreased pre-pregnancy renal function usually have a successful obstetric outcome, and pregnancy does

Table 10.3. Pre-pregnancy assessment: categories of renal functional status.

Category	Plasma creatinine (μmol/l)
Preserved/mildly impaired renal function	≤125
Moderate renal insufficiency	≥125
Severe renal insufficiency	≤250

Table 10.4. Renal disease and prospects for pregnancy: category of renal functional status, complications and outcome.

| Prospects | Category | | |
	Mild (%)	Moderate (%)	Severe (%)
Pregnancy complications	26	47	86
Successful obstetric outcome	96	90	51
Long-term sequelae	<3	25	53

Estimates based on 2370 women/3495 pregnancies (1973–1995) which attained at least 28 weeks gestation (SLE not included). (Davison J.M. & Baylis C., unpublished cumulative literature surveys). Very recent analyses of 125 pregnancies in 107 women with moderate and severe disease are important [176,179], revealing that whilst infant survival is now around 90% there is progress to endstage renal failure in about 16% of women within 1 year.)

not adversely affect the course of their disease [172,173]. Although true for most patients, some authors suggest that this statement should be tempered somewhat in lupus nephropathy, membranoproliferative glomerulonephritis, focal glomerulosclerosis, and perhaps IgA nephropathy and reflux nephropathy, which appear to be adversely influenced by intercurrent pregnancy. Most women with mild underlying renal disease show increments in RPF and GFR during pregnancy, although of smaller magnitude than those seen in normal pregnant women (Fig. 10.22) [177]. Importantly, however, hyperfiltration in these women is not accompanied by increments in P_{GC} (which could induce progression of the disease), nor is there evidence of permanent changes in membrane porosity [25] so the increased proteinuria of pregnancy usually resolves. Nevertheless, the increased protein excretion which occurs in 50% of pregnancies must not be neglected because a recent study [178] provides some evidence that pregnancies followed by an accelerated renal decline (n = 10) are especially seen where there is substantial proteinuria before and during pregnancy, compared to those where proteinuria was relatively stable (n = 20), i.e. 4.1 versus 1.7 g/24 hours (P < 0.005) and 3.6 versus 2.1 g/24 hours (P < 0.05), respectively.

Moderate renal insufficiency

Prognosis is more guarded when renal function is moderately impaired before pregnancy [179–181]. The major worries are serious renal deterioration (particularly early in pregnancy), uncontrolled hypertension and variable obstetric outcome, as well as an accelerated postpartum decline in renal function [171,176,181].

Severe renal insufficiency

Most women in this category have amenorrhoea and are anovulatory [182]. The likelihood of conception, let alone a normal pregnancy and delivery, is low but not, as some have been misled to believe, impossible [176,183–185]. The risk of severe maternal complications is much greater than the probability of a successful obstetric outcome.

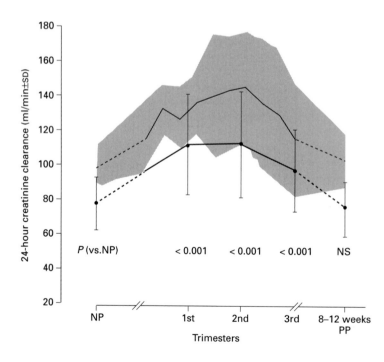

Fig. 10.22. Serial 24-hour creatinine clearances (mean ± 1 SD) during pregnancy complicated by chronic renal disease (solid line). Forty-three pregnancies of 18 women studied preconception, each trimester and 8–12 weeks after delivery [177]. Measurements from 10 healthy women (mean ± 1 SD) shown by shaded area. Data calculated from Davison [21]. PP: postpartum.

Renal functional surveillance in the presence of dysfunction

As emphasized earlier, serial data are mandatory to supplement routine antenatal observations (pp. 288–290). Specialized tests involving infusion procedures (to measure exactly GFR and renal blood flow) are usually not available and their use is primarily for clinical research. Tests that are available for use in routine clinical practice include the estimation of serum urea and electrolytes, creatinine clearance determination, urinary concentration and dilution assessment and the excretion of protein and albumin. To investigate a woman's renal function, serial tests should definitely be performed and where possible compared with her non-pregnant values.

Renal biopsy in pregnancy

Experience with renal biopsy in pregnancy is sparse, mainly because clinical circumstances rarely justify the risks. Biopsy is therefore usually deferred until after delivery. Reports of excessive bleeding and other complications in pregnant women have led some to consider pregnancy as a relative contraindication to renal biopsy [186] although others have not observed any increased morbidity [187]. When renal biopsy is undertaken immediately after delivery in women with well-controlled blood pressure and normal coagulation indices, the morbidity is certainly similar to that reported in non-pregnant patients.

A report on 111 preterm biopsies in pregnant women confirms and extends the impression that risks of the procedure resemble those in the non-pregnant population [188]. In fact, the incidence of transient gross haematuria (all patients undergoing biopsy have microscopic haematuria unless the kidney has been missed) was 0.9%, considerably less than in non-pregnant patients where it is 3–5%. Such excellent statistics no doubt reflect the experience and technical skills of the unit and careful prebiopsy evaluation of the patient; they should not be used to encourage inexperienced physicians to undertake biopsy in pregnant patients.

It is still important, however, to have specific indications for renal biopsy in pregnancy. Packham and Fairley [188] suggest that closed (percutaneous) needle biopsy should be undertaken more often, because they believe that certain glomerular disorders are adversely influenced by pregnancy and that specific therapy, such as antiplatelet agents, might be beneficial. The consensus, however, goes against such broad indications and reiterates that renal biopsy should be performed infrequently during pregnancy [189].

Long-term effects of pregnancy in renal disease in humans

Pregnancy does not cause any deterioration or otherwise affect the rate of progression of the disease beyond what might be expected in the non-pregnant state, provided that kidney dysfunction was minimal before pregnancy and hypertension is absent during pregnancy. An important factor in long-term prognosis could be the sclerotic effect that prolonged renal vasodilation might have in the residual intact glomeruli of the kidneys of these women. The situation may be worse in a single diseased kidney, with more sclerosis within the fewer intact glomeruli, where progressive loss of renal function could ensue in pregnancy. Although the evidence in healthy women and those with mild renal disease argues against hyperfiltration-induced damage in pregnancy [26,40,190], there is little doubt that in some women with moderate dysfunction there can be unpredicted, accelerated and irreversible renal decline in pregnancy or immediately afterwards [176].

Long-term effects of pregnancy on renal function in animal models

There is now considerable animal model evidence that prolonged periods of renal vasodilation may damage the glomerulus. Rats with experimentally induced diabetic nephropathy or extensive renal ablation develop increased filtration in remnant nephrons due to increases in plasma flow and P_{GC}, secondary to afferent arteriolar vasodilation, which precedes the appearance of glomerular injury [38]. A prolonged high intake of dietary protein accelerates the progression of these glomerular diseases in rats, while low levels of dietary protein are protective. Since high protein intake itself leads to chronic renal vasodilation and increases in renal plasma flow and glomerular filtration rate, the exacerbation due to high protein feeding may result from the imposition of an additional vasodilatory stimulus. In addition to animal studies, clinical observations have shown that dietary protein restriction is protective in a variety of progressive glomerular diseases although a recent, large multicentre trial has indicated that the benefit is slight [191]. It is believed that the primary damaging stimulus is the prolonged increase in glomerular blood pressure which frequently attends renal vasodilation [192]. It is certainly clear that systemic hypertension worsens glomerular injury in a range of diseases [193–195], presumably via increases in P_{GC} which exacerbate the underlying glomerular damage. In fact, in hypertensive states the degree of glomerular damage is directly related to P_{GC}, determined largely by the afferent arteriolar tone, rather than the systemic blood pressure [196,197]. Use of converting enzyme inhibitors or dietary protein restriction, both manoeuvres which reduce glomerular blood pressure, protect against the progression of new or established glomerular disease [198]. In the human, angiotensin converting enzyme inhibitions are strongly contraindicated in pregnancy.

As discussed earlier, pregnancy is also a state of increased filtration and chronic renal vasodilation, although unlike the situations cited above it is a physiological condition which occurs without loss of nephron number or underlying disease and is reversible. Also, *very importantly*, there is no sustained increase in P_{GC} during pregnancy since the renal vasodilation which attends pregnancy involves a near proportional reduction in tone, both at preglomerular sites and at efferent arterioles [30].

Underlying chronic renal vasodilation due to removal of renal mass

Studies where superimposition of five pregnancies on a state of chronic underlying renal vasodilation induced by uninephrectomy combined with high dietary protein feeding [199]

revealed elevation in P_{GC} in rats but there were no differences between repetitively pregnant rats and virgins. The cumulative long-term vasodilatory stimuli resulted in a greater SNGFR in the experimental animals than in two kidney age-matched controls. Although SNFGR was less in repetitively pregnant rats in their control state than in virgins, the presence of a substantial renal vasodilatory response to acute administration of intravenous amino acids suggests that these kidneys were not further damaged by the additional hyperfiltration stimuli of gestation/lactation. All uninephrectomized, high protein fed rats exhibited some morphological evidence of glomerular damage and elevated 24-hour protein excretion, compared with normal two kidney rats, but these signs of injury were not significantly worse in repetitively pregnant rats [199]. Perhaps the absence of glomerular hypertension in pregnancy is the reason for the lack of exacerbation of the underlying glomerular impairment due to long-term uninephrectomy with high dietary protein feeding. Studies in uninephrectomized rabbits with mild, underlying renal disease have also indicated that three repetitive consecutive pregnancies have no long-term injurious effects on the maternal kidney [200].

When comparing long-term effects of gestational renal vasodilation with other states of chronic vasodilation, it is significant that pregnancy occurs only in females who are more protected against the non-specific deterioration in renal function of the normal ageing process [201,202]. In male rats the kidney seems to be more at risk (than in females) from increases in glomerular blood pressure due to long-term effects of ablation and high protein induced renal vasodilation [199,203].

Experimentally induced glomerulonephritis

Antibasement membrane glomerulonephritis

Using specific antibodies, it has been possible to create specific lesions in male rats of varying severity which can be characterized with regard to effects on glomerular function, using micropuncture techniques [204]. Irrespective of the antibody employed, all workers report a marked reduction in K_f (sufficient to produce filtration pressure disequilibrium in all animals) and a substantial increase in P_{GC}. Because the alterations in K_f and P_{GC} are offsetting in terms of their influence on glomerular filtration, SNGFR and total GFR can remain relatively unchanged.

The effect of superimposition of pregnancy in rats with antiglomerular basement membrane glomerulonephritis [205] was associated with significant proteinuria and the glomerular haemodynamic changes in virgin females were similar to those reported previously for the male [204], i.e. high P_{GC} pressure and low K_f, with both SNGFR and total GFR maintained at near normal values. Remarkably, moderate gestational renal vasodilation occurred by midpregnancy, with increases in renal plasma flow despite dramatic alterations in P_{GC} and K_f, and furthermore, pregnancy did not aggravate the increase in P_{GC} due to the glomerulonephritis [205], nor exacerbate the glomerular disease in the short term. The degree of proteinuria and the glomerular morphology were similar in virgin and pregnant rats with glomerulonephritis, as were values of P_{GC} and K_f.

Fx1A antibody glomerulonephritis

Membranous glomerulonephritis is a major cause of nephrotic syndrome in adults and this model of membranous glomerulonephritis [206], is associated with massive proteinuria (>500 mg/24 hours), raised P_{GC} but normal systemic pressure [207]. With pregnancy, there are decreases in systemic blood pressure and P_{GC}, with an atypical increase in preglomerular arteriolar resistance [205]. As there is no acute worsening of the proteinuria or histologic evidence of injury, this model of membranous glomerulonephritis does not strictly resemble the situation in women with nephrotic syndrome where pregnancy can acutely exacerbate the disease. The short- and long-term effects of pregnancy on glomerular haemodynamics are quite variable in the presence of a renal disease and depend on the model. None of these models of normotensive renal disease are associated with a pregnancy-induced rise in P_{GC}. Thus, when pregnancy exacerbates glomerular damage in women it is unlikely to be via a haemodynamic mechanism.

It is known that a number of other factors are also involved in the pathogenesis of progressive glomerular disease, including hypertrophy of the glomerular tuft, which causes glomerular injury by increased intramural tension [208]. Mesangial expansion and matrix accumulation, which have a pathogenic role in immune-mediated and ablation-induced glomerular injury [209] are due to increased synthesis (in response to growth factors) and/or reduced rates of degradation [210]. Finally, defects in glomerular permeability to macromolecules cause proteinuria which leads to injury [211].

Renal changes in pregnancy with pre-eclampsia

Pre-eclampsia usually occurs after the 20th week of pregnancy and most frequently near term, being characterized by hypertension, proteinuria, oedema and at times coagulation abnormalities and liver dysfunction. The primary pathology, although unknown, is localized within the pregnant uterus because resolution always occurs after delivery. The crucial presence of trophoblast indicates that it has either an intrinsic abnormality or an abnormal relationship with the uterus. The multisystem sequelae or end organ pathologies are the actual maternal adaptations to the abnormality and are mediated by factors which enter the maternal circulation from the placenta.

Diagnostic dilemmas

The literature is confusing and controversial, largely because it is difficult to distinguish clinically between pre-eclampsia, essential hypertension, chronic renal disease and combinations of these separate entities. For example, certain women with undiagnosed essential hypertension show a decrement in blood pressure early in pregnancy and normal levels if first examined near midpregnancy. When frankly elevated blood pressures are recorded near term, they are then erroneously labelled pre-eclamptic. Furthermore, an accelerated phase of essential hypertension (albeit a rare event during pregnancy), certain forms of renal disease (glomerulonephritis and systemic lupus erythematosus)

296

Table 10.5. Renal pathology in 176 hypertensive gravidas diagnosed clinically as having pre-eclampsia. Modified from Fisher *et al.* [213].

Biopsy diagnosis	Number of patients	Primigravidas	Multiparas
*Pre-eclampsia	96	79	17
With nephrosclerosis	13	6	7
With renal disease	3	1	2
With both	2	1	1
Nephrosclerosis	19	3	16
With renal disease	4	2	2
Renal disease	31	12	19
Normal histology	8	0	8

*Glomerular capillary endotheliosis only evident on biopsy.

and phaeochromocytoma may all mimic pre-eclampsia [212].

The dilemmas are best illustrated when renal biopsy has been performed immediately after pregnancies complicated by hypertension. Table 10.5 shows the pathological diagnosis on postpartum renal biopsy of 176 patients biopsied because pregnancy was complicated by hypertension, proteinuria and oedema [213]. In most instances, the clinical diagnosis had been pre-eclampsia, but this was wrong in 25% of primiparas and more often than not in multiparas. Interestingly, a surprisingly large number of women had unsuspected parenchymal renal disease. Most suspect are series where many of the patients labelled pre-eclamptic were multiparous. In this respect, it has been suggested that some pregnant women with severe early onset pre-eclampsia may have another glomerular disease [214] or haemostatic or metabolic abnormalities associated with a vascular thrombosis tendency [215].

There is also the view that an increased risk of chronic hypertension exists many years after a pregnancy complicated by pregnancy-induced hypertension (37%) or pre-eclampsia (20%) compared with conditions after a normotensive pregnancy [216], but in the study groups, 35 and 33%, respectively, were multigravidae, as were 43% of controls. This contrasts with earlier work [217], which did not support the concept that pre-eclampsia was often due to underlying renal disease, since the incidence of pathological erythrocyte excretion rates in pregnancy did not differ between normotensive controls and pre-

eclamptic women. Lastly and reassuringly, women who have normotensive pregnancies have a lower incidence of subsequent hypertension than nulliparous women [213].

Anatomical changes

As part of the end organ pathology the glomeruli are diffusely enlarged and bloodless, due not to proliferation, but to hypertrophy of the intracapillary cells. These alterations, termed glomerular capillary endotheliosis, include hypertrophy of the cytoplasmic organelles in endothelial and occasionally mesangial cells, particularly the lysosomes, which undergo marked enlargement

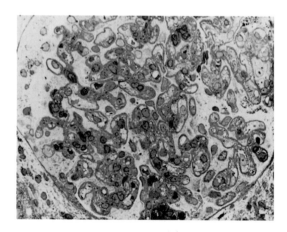

Fig. 10.23. An enlarged bloodless, so-called 'glomerular capillary endotheliosis', typical of pre-eclampsia: capillary lumina obstructed by hypertrophied intracapillary and mesangial cells (H&E × 350) (see Fig. 10.24).

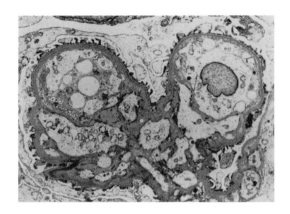

Fig. 10.24. Swelling and vacuolization of intracapillary cells causing obstruction of capillary lumina with intracytoplasmic droplet clusters but preservation of epithelial foot processes (EM × 6000).

and vacuolization, due to accumulation of free neutral lipids (Figs 10.23 and 10.24; see 212, 218 and 219 for reviews). Other lesions, observed occasionally, include subendothelial and mesangial electron-dense deposits, as well as interposition of mesangial cell cytoplasm or mesangial matrix. Glomerular endotheliosis is considered by most, but not all, to be virtually pathognomic of the disease and has a variable disappearance rate postdelivery [218]. The renal tubules are usually intact but occasionally, pre-eclampsia can cause both tubular and cortical necrosis.

Functional changes

Both GFR and ERPF decrease in the third trimester in pre-eclampsia, by approximately 25–35% in mild cases, remembering that the normal increase in pregnancy ranges between 40 and 50% above postpartum values. Thus, despite gross morphological changes, GFR in pre-eclampsia often remains above pre-pregnancy values and the pathological significance of the decrement may not be appreciated if one is not aware of pregnancy norms. The decrements in pre-eclampsia are usually mild or moderate and reverse rapidly after delivery [88], but an occasional patient may progress to acute tubular necrosis, especially when intervention or treatment is neglected or mishandled.

Uric acid clearance and renal reabsorption increase in pre-eclampsia. These changes may occur earlier (sometimes weeks before any other signs of the disease) and are more profound than GFR changes. There is increased serum uric acid and the level of hyperuricaemia correlates with the decrement in plasma volume that occurs in pre-eclampsia and indirectly with the plasma renin activity. Hyperuricaemia (>350 µmol/l) correlates with the severity of the pre-eclamptic lesion, as well as the poor fetal outcome.

Sodium excretion is decreased probably secondary to reduced GFR. Sodium balance is altered and pre-eclamptic women are avid salt retainers even during salt loading, behaving like sodium-depleted normotensive pregnant women. ANP levels are paradoxically elevated, partially accounted for by reduced ANP metabolic clearance and furthermore, the renal effects of infused ANP are augmented with GFR increments and exaggerated urinary sodium excretion [86,87]. There is little evidence to support a link between pre-eclampsia and elevated dietary sodium intake [154].

There is relative hypocalciuria, possibly due to low levels of 1,25-dihydroxyvitamin D, decreased intestinal calcium absorption, stimulation of parathormone and/or increased distal renal tubular reabsorption of calcium. It is not known how such changes relate to the widespread alterations in transmembrane calcium fluxes with elevation of intracellular calcium levels, which in vascular smooth muscle would enhance contractility, contributing to vasospasm. All these various functional changes, however, occur weeks or months prior to clinical recognition of the disease.

Abnormal proteinuria, which is non-selective, almost always accompanies pre-eclampsia. The diagnosis is suspect without this sign, even though glomerular endotheliosis has sometimes been described in the absence of increased protein excretion. Proteinuria may be minimal, moderate or severe (in the nephrotic range), the magnitude correlating with the severity of the morphological lesion. The consensus is that there does not appear to be a pre-warning phase of microalbuminuria undetected by the crude techniques of clinical screening [140,142]. Pre-eclampsia is the most common cause of nephrotic syndrome in pregnancy.

The mechanism of the proteinuria is ill-understood and the contributions of glomerular porosity (to different proteins), the haemodynamic determinants of GFR and the electrostatic properties of the glomerular wall are under review using neutral dextran sieving curves and mathematical modelling [26].

Renal function in pregnant animal models with pre-existing hypertension

Glomerular haemodynamics have been measured in non-pregnant (usually male) genetic and experimentally induced hypertension models, where in some P_{GC} is elevated along with arterial blood pressure, but in others, P_{GC} is near normal, due to high tone in the preglomerular resistance vessels. The magnitude of P_{GC} is important in terms of glomerular structure and function because sustained elevations in P_{GC} accelerate the rate of progression of underlying glomerular diseases, as discussed earlier. In addition, the extent of glomerular injury in hypertensive conditions may be dissociated from the absolute value of systemic blood pressure but is inversely related to pre-glomerular arteriolar resistance, which presumably implies a direct relation to P_{GC}.

Spontaneously hypertensive rat

Although the female spontaneously hypertensive rat develops hypertension and renal damage much more slowly than the male [220], virgin spontaneously hypertensive rat females of 1 year have an elevated mean arterial pressure and P_{GC} [68]. Three repetitive pregnancies have no long-term deleterious effects on glomerular function or structure, protein excretion, blood pressure and/or P_{GC}.

In the short term, midpregnant spontaneously hypertensive rats, most unusually, do not exhibit renal vasodilation [68], nor is GFR increased later in gestation [221]; thus, there is no reason to suspect that P_{GC} would rise further with pregnancy in this model. Although the kidney does not vasodilate, it is known that late pregnancy is profoundly antihypertensive in spontaneously hypertensive rats, indicative of peripheral vasodilation, possibly with increased NO production being responsible [222].

Hypertension induced by severe reduction of functional renal mass

Severe reduction of renal mass, by removal of five-sixths of the renal bulk, produces systemic and glomerular hypertension, secondary to preglomerular arteriolar vasodilation and a rapidly progressing glomerular injury to the remnant nephrons [190]. In virgin females, studied 4 weeks after five-sixths reduction of renal mass, systemic hypertension is evident together with high P_{GC} (~15 mmHg above normal) and proteinuria [55]. By midpregnancy, blood pressure is reduced and there is vasodilation of both pre- and postglomerular resistances and by late pregnancy blood pressure falls even further, the kidney remaining vasodilated and filtration and plasma flow elevated. Thus, despite severe reduction of renal mass, the remnant kidney is still capable of gestational renal vasodilation, and pre- and postglomerular resistances fall in parallel. Since blood pressure also falls, there is no change in P_{GC} and no acute worsening of proteinuria (U_PV). The glomerular pathology is also similar in the three groups; thus, acutely, pregnancy does not worsen the glomerular damage. Three closely spaced pregnancies result in no worsening of the glomerular pathology due to long term damage by pregnancy in this model [223].

Thus, in the spontaneously hypertensive rat and five-sixths renal reduction models of hypertension, pregnancy does not have an adverse stimulus either on blood pressure or the kidney, and may in fact be beneficial so that it has been difficult to reproduce the human situation where pregnancy sometimes has adverse effects when renal disease and hypertension are present.

Hypertension from chronic nitric oxide blockade

Blockade of NO synthesis in the male or non-pregnant rat leads to severe and progressive systemic hypertension with renal vasoconstriction and injury [70,224–227]. In pregnant rat in contrast to other hypertension models, chronic NO blockade in pregnancy results in suppression of the rises in GFR and RPF, suppression of the cumulative plasma volume expansion and development of high blood pressure and protein-uria close to term with increased maternal and fetal morbidity and mortality, resembling the situation in human pre-eclamptics. Therefore, this is a promising model to study the adverse interactions between pregnancy and underlying hypertension, with current data lending support to the hypothesis that NO deficiency plays a causal role in pre-eclamptic and/or other hypertensive complications of pregnancy.

Hypertension from adriamycin nephropathy

A single low dose of adriamycin produces slowly evolving hypertension and progressive glomerular disease. When pregnancy is superimposed early in the course of mild adriamycin nephropathy, the disease is accelerated and intensified, with increased blood pressure and urine protein excretion, suppression of the normal gestational rise in GFR and an adverse alteration in the glomerular eicosanoid ratio, with elevated thromboxane/prostaglandin: appearing close to term [228]. An augmented vascular sensitivity to administered vasoconstrictors also develops during pregnancy [229], reversible with thromboxane receptor antagonists, given from mid-pregnancy to term. Also, the hypertension is prevented and proteinuria attenuated with L-arginine supplementation (which stimulates NO synthesis), from midpregnancy to term [230], suggesting that a generalized endothelial dysfunction develops in pregnant rats with adriamycin nephropathy.

After two consecutive pregnancies, hypertension, proteinuria and glomerular damage were worsened compared with virgins (controls), suggestive of irreversible deterioration [231]. Thus, it is an excellent model for elucidating mechanisms whereby pregnancy sometimes exacerbates underlying renal disease, particularly in the presence of hypertension.

Renal function in human pregnancy with pre-existing hypertension

The most common hypertensive classification in the non-pregnant woman is essential hypertension, although this may itself be many diseases [121,211]. There have been several studies

on renal haemodynamics in non-pregnant women with essential hypertension, and in moderate uncomplicated hypertension, RPF and GFR are often close to normal. Many, not all, workers report an inverse relation between systemic blood pressure and RPF, but all agree that in severe hypertension RPF is reduced. There are several subdivisions within essential hypertension and importantly a subgroup of young hypertensives with increased RPF compared with normotensive controls, but generally as blood pressure increases RPF falls. There is, however, an accompanying rise in filtration fraction and GFR is relatively protected by elevation in P_{GC} but since clinical observations reveal little about GFR determinants, insights must be derived from animal models.

Studies in pregnancy are scanty but in the majority of cases pregnancy in essential hypertensives is viewed as a benign condition [210]. In third trimester essential hypertensives, RPF is variable but GFR is high, suggesting a gestational rise in GFR, but putting these data into context is difficult because some of these women were very large and also no pre-pregnancy or postpartum values were reported. In other studies, comparing normotensive women in the third trimester with women with essential hypertension (with glomerulonephritis or with pre-eclampsia), the essential hypertensives had lower GFR and RPF than the normotensives and were actually similar to women with pre-eclampsia and/or glomerulonephritis, but again there were no data on pre-pregnant women and there was a huge range in the values in the essential hypertensives, compared with the three other groups, giving credence to the likelihood of different subpopulations in this disease.

References

1 Conrad K.P. (1992) Renal changes in pregnancy. *Urology Annual* **6**, 313.
2 Sturgiss S.N., Dunlop W. & Davison J.M. (1994) Renal haemodynamics and tubular function in human pregnancy. *Clinical Obstetrics and Gynaecology (Baillière)* **8**, 209.
3 Bailey R.R. & Rolieston G.L. (1971) Kidney length and ureteric dilatation in the puerperium. *Journal of Obstetrics and Gynaecology of the British Commonwealth* **78**, 55.

300

4 Croce J.E., Signorelli P. & Chapparini I. (1994) Hydronephrosis in pregnancy: ultrasonographic study (in Italian). *Minerva Ginicologica* **46**, 147.

5 Sheehan H.L. & Lynch J.P. (1973) *Pathology of Toxaemia of Pregnancy.* Williams & Wilkins, Baltimore.

6 Cietak K.A. & Newton J.R. (1985) Serial quantitative nephronosonography in pregnancy. *British Journal of Radiology* **58**, 405.

7 Cietak K.A. & Newton J.R. (1985) Serial qualitative nephronosonography in pregnancy. *British Journal of Radiology* **58**, 399.

8 Rasmussen P.E. & Nielson F.R. (1988) Hydronephrosis during pregnancy: a literature survey. *European Journal of Obstetrics, Gynaecology and Reproductive Biology* **27**, 249.

9 Graif M., Kessler A., Hart S., Daitzchman M., Mashiach S., Boichis H. & Itzchak Y. (1992) Renal pyelectasis in pregnancy: correlative evaluation of fetal and maternal collecting systems. *American Journal of Obstetrics and Gynecology* **167**, 1304.

10 Brown M.A. (1990) Urinary tract dilatations in pregnancy. *American Journal of Obstetrics and Gynecology* **164**, 641.

11 Satin S.A., Seikin G.L. & Cunningham F.G. (1993) Reversible hypertension in pregnancy caused by obstructive uropathy. *Obstetrics and Gynecology* **81**, 823.

12 Brandes J.C. & Fritsche C. (1991) Obstructive acute renal failure by a gravid uterus: a case report and review. *American Journal of Kidney Disease* **18**, 398.

13 Eckford S.D. & Gingell J.C. (1991) Ureteric obstruction in pregnancy: diagnosis and management. *British Journal of Obstetrics and Gynaecology* **98**, 1137.

14 Meyers S.J., Lee R.V. & Munschauser R.W. (1985) Dilatation and non-traumatic rupture of the urinary tract during pregnancy: a review. *Obstetrics and Gynecology* **66**, 809.

15 Nielson F.R. & Rasmussen P.E. (1988) Hydronephrosis during pregnancy: four cases of hydronephrosis causing symptoms during pregnancy. *European Journal of Obstetrics, Gynaecology and Reproductive Biology* **27**, 245.

16 Davison J.M. & Noble M.C.B. (1981) Serial changes in 24-hour creatinine clearance during normal menstrual cycles and the first trimester of pregnancy. *British Journal of Obstetrics and Gynaecology* **88**, 10.

17 Dunlop W. (1976) Investigations into the influence of posture on renal plasma flow and glomerular filtration rate during late pregnancy. *British Journal of Obstetrics and Gynaecology* **83**, 17.

18 Ezimokhai M., Davison J.M., Philips P.R. & Dunlop W. (1981) Non-postural serial changes in renal function during the third trimester of normal pregnancy. *British Journal of Obstetrics and Gynaecology* **88**, 465.

19 Davison J.M. & Hytten F.E. (1975) Glomerular filtration during and after pregnancy. *Journal of Obstetrics and Gynecology of the British Commonwealth* **81**, 583.

20 Ezimokhai M., Davison J.M., Philips P.R. & Dunlop W. (1981) Non-postural serial changes in renal function during the third trimester of normal pregnancy.

British Journal of Obstetrics and Gynaecology **88**, 465.

21 Chapman A.B., Zamndio S., Woodmansee W., Merouani A., Osorio F., Johnson A., Moore L.G. et al. (1997) Systemic and renal hemodynamic changes in the luteal phase of the menstrual cycle mimic early pregnancy. *American Journal of Physiology* **273**, F777.

22 Chesley L.C. & Sloan D.M. (1964) The effect of posture on renal function in late pregnancy. *American Journal of Obstetrics and Gynecology* **189**, 754.

23 Davison J.M. (1985) The effect of pregnancy on kidney function in renal allograft recipients. *Kidney International* **27**, 74.

24 Roberts M., Lindheimer M.D. & Davison J.M. (1996) Alterations in glomerular hemodynamics and barrier function in normal pregnancy: assessment using neutral dextrans and heteroporous membrane modelling. *American Journal of Physiology* **220**, F338.

25 Chesley L.C. (1960) Renal functional changes in normal pregnancy. In *Clinical Obstetrics and Gynecology*, vol. 3, p. 349. PB Hoeber, New York.

26 Sturgiss S.N., Wilkinson R. & Davison J.M. (1996) Renal reserve during human pregnancy. *American Journal of Physiology* **271**, F16.

27 Davison J.M., Dunlop W. & Ezimokhai M. (1980) Twenty-four hour creatinine clearance during the third trimester of normal pregnancy. *British Journal of Obstetrics and Gynaecology* **87**, 106.

28 Davison J.M. & Dunlop W. (1984) Changes in renal haemodynamics and tubular function induced by normal human pregnancy. *Seminars in Nephrology* **4**, 198.

29 Sturgiss S.N., Martin K., Whittingham T.A. & Davison J.M. (1992) Assessment of renal circulation during pregnancy with color Doppler ultrasound. *American Journal of Obstetrics and Gynecology* **267**, 1250.

30 Baylis C. (1994) Glomerular filtration rate and volume regulation in gravid animal models. *Ballière's Clinical Obstetrics and Gynaecology* **8**, 235.

31 Conrad K.P. (1984) Renal hemodynamics during pregnancy in chronically catheterized conscious rats. *Kidney International* **26**, 24.

32 Baylis C. (1984) Renal hemodynamics and volume control during pregnancy in the rat. *Seminars in Nephrology* **4**, 208.

33 Baylis C. (1994) Glomerular filtration and volume regulation in gravid animal models. *Clinical Obstetrics and Gynaecology (Baillière)* **8**, 235.

34 Baylis C. (1986) Glomerular filtration dynamics. In *Advances in Renal Physiology*. Ed. C.J. Lote, p. 33. Croom Helm, London.

35 Baylis C. (1982) Glomerular ultrafiltration in the pseudopregnant rat. *American Journal of Physiology* **243**, F300.

36 Beaton G.H., Selby A.E. & Vene M.J. (1961) Starch gel electrophoresis of serum proteins: II. Slow a2-globulins and other serum proteins in pregnant, tumor bearing and young rats. *Journal of Biological Chemistry* **236**, 2005.

37 Baylis C., Ichikawa I., Willis W.T., Wilson C.B. &

Brenner B.M. (1977) Dynamics of glomerular ultra-filtration. IX. Effects of plasma protein concentration. *American Journal of Physiology* **232**, F58.

38 Meyer T.W., Anderson S., Rennke H.G. & Brenner B.M. (1987) Reversing glomerular hypertension stabilises glomerular injury. *Kidney International* **31**, 752.

39 Baylis C. & Rennke H.G. (1985) Renal hemodynamics and glomerular morphology in repetitively pregnant aging rats. *Kidney International* **28**, 140.

40 Davison J.M. (1988) The effect of pregnancy on long term renal function in women with chronic renal disease and single kidneys. *Clinical Experimental Hypertension* **B8**, 226.

41 Brown M.A., Sinosich M.J., Saunders D.M. & Gallery E.D.M. (1986) Potassium regulation and progesterone–aldosterone interrelationships in human pregnancy. *American Journal of Obstetrics and Gynecology* **155**, 349.

42 Paller M.S. (1984) Mechanism of decreased pressor responsiveness to ANG II, NE and vasopressin in pregnant rats. *American Journal of Physiology* **247**, H100.

43 Navar L.G. (1978) Renal autoregulation: perspectives from whole kidney and single nephron studies. *American Journal of Physiology* **234**, F357.

44 Reckelhoff J.F., Yokota S. & Baylis C. (1992) Renal autoregulation in mid-term and late pregnant rats. *American Journal of Obstetrics and Gynecology* **166**, 1546.

45 Woods L.L., Mizelle H.L. & Hall J.E. (1987) Autoregulation of renal blood flow and glomerular filtration rate in the pregnant rabbit. *American Journal of Physiology* **252**, R69.

46 Cha S.C., Aberdeen G.W., Mukaddam-Daher S., Quillen E.W. Jr & Nuwayhid B.S. (1993) Autoregulation of renal blood flow during ovine pregnancy. *Hypertension in Pregnancy* **12**, 71.

47 Blantz R.C. & Pelayo J.C. (1984) A functional role for the tubuloglomerular feedback mechanism. *Kidney International* **25**, 739.

48 Baylis C. & Blantz R.C. (1985) Tubuloglomerular feedback activity in virgin and pregnant rats. *American Journal of Physiology* **249**, F169.

49 Meyer T.M., Ichikawa I., Zatz R. & Brenner B.M. (1983) The renal hemodynamic response to amino acid infusion in the rat. *Transactions of the Association of American Physicians* **96**, 76.

50 Hostetter T.H. (1984) Human renal response to a meat meal. *American Journal of Physiology* **250**, F613.

51 Baylis C. (1988) Effect of amino acid infusion as an index of renal vasodilatory capacity in pregnant rats. *American Journal of Physiology* **254**, F650.

52 Brendolan A., Bragatini L., Chiaramonte S., Dell'Aquila R., Fabris A., Feriani M., Mentasti P. *et al.* (1985) Renal functional reserve in pregnancy. *Kidney International* **28**, 232A.

53 Barron W.M. & Lindheimer M.D. (1995) Effect of oral protein loading on renal hemodynamics in human pregnancy. *American Journal of Physiology.* **269**, R888.

54 Woods L.L. & Gaboury C.L. (1995) Importance of baseline diet in modulating renal reserve in pregnant women. *Journal of the American Society of Nephrology.*

55 Deng A. & Baylis C. (1995) Glomerular hemodynamic responses to pregnancy in rats with severe reduction of renal mass. *Kidney International* **48**, 39.

56 Davison J.M. (1994) Pregnancy in renal allograft recipients: problems, prognosis and practical management. *Clinical Obstetrics and Gynaecology (Baillière)* **8**, 501.

57 Matthews B.M. & Taylor D.W. (1960) Effects of pregnancy on inulin and para-aminolippmate clearances in the anaesthetised rat. *Journal of Physiology* **151**, 385.

58 Gant N.F., Daley G.L. Chand S., Whalley P.J. & MacDonald P.C. (1973) A study of angiotensin II pressor response throughout primigravid pregnancy. *Journal of Clinical Investigation* **52**, 2682.

59 Broughton-Pipkin R. (1988) The renin–angiotensin system in normal and hypertensive pregnancies. In *Handbook of Hypertension*, vol. 10. Ed. P.C. Rubin, p. 117. Elsevier, Amsterdam.

60 Bay W.H. & Ferris T.F. (1979) Factors controlling plasma renin and aldosterone during pregnancy. *Hypertension* **1**, 410.

61 Brown M.A., Broughton-Pipkin F. & Symonds E.M. (1988) The effects of intravenous angiotensin II upon blood pressure and sodium and urate excretion in human pregnancy. *Journal of Hypertension* **6**, 457.

62 Brown G.P. & Venuto R.C. (1986) Angiotensin II receptor alterations during pregnancy in rabbits. *American Journal of Physiology* **251**, E58.

63 Barbour C.J., Stonier C. & Aber G.M. (1990) Pregnancy-induced changes in glomerular angiotensin II receptors in normotensive and spontaneously hypertensive rats. *Clinical and Experimental Hypertension* **B9**, 43.

64 Brown G.P. & Venuto R.C. (1988) Angiotensin II receptors in rabbit renal preglomerular vessels. *American Journal of Physiology* **251**, E16.

65 Brown G.P. & Venuto R.C. (1991) Renal blood flow response to angiotensin II infusions in conscious pregnant rabbits. *American Journal of Physiology* **261**, F51.

66 Conrad K.P. & Colpoys M.C. (1986) Evidence against the hypothesis that prostaglandins are the vasodepressor agents of pregnancy. *Journal of Clinical Investigation* **77**, 236.

67 Masilamani S. & Baylis C. (1992) The renal vasculature does not participate in the peripheral refractoriness to administered angiotensin II in the late pregnancy rat. *Journal of the American Society of Nephrology* **3**, 566A.

68 Baylis C. (1989) Gentamicin-induced glomerulotoxicity in the pregnant rat. *American Journal of Kidney Disease* **13**, 108.

69 Baylis C. & Collins R.C. (1986) Angiotensin II inhibition on blood pressure and renal hemodynamics in pregnant rats. *American Journal of Physiology* **250**, F308.

70 Baylis C., Engels K., Harton P. & Samsell L. (1993) The acute effects of endothelial derived relaxing factor (EDRF) blockade in the normal conscious rat

302

are not due to angiotensin II. *American Journal of Physiology* **264**, F74.

71 Conrad K.P., Morganelli P.M., Brinck-Johnsen T. & Colpoys M.C. (1989) The renin–angiotensin system during pregnancy in chronically instrumented, conscious rats. *American Journal of Obstetrics and Gynecology* **161**, 1065.

72 McLaughlin M.K., Keve T.M. & Cooke R. (1989) Vascular catecholamine sensitivity during pregnancy in the ewe. *American Journal of Obstetrics and Gynecology* **160**, 47.

73 Pan Z.-R., Lindheimer M.D., Bailin J. & Barron W.M. (1990) Regulation of blood pressure in pregnancy: pressor system blockade and stimulation. *American Journal of Physiology* **258**, H1559.

74 Crandall M.E. & Heesch C.M. (1990) Baroreflex control of sympathetic outflow in pregnant rats: effects of captopril. *American Journal of Physiology* **258**, R1417.

75 Conrad K.P. & Russ R.D. (1992) Augmentation of baroreflex-mediated bradycardia in conscious pregnant rats. *American Journal of Physiology* **262**, R472.

76 Baylis C. (1995) Acute blockade of α-1-adrenoceptors has similar effects in pregnant and nonpregnant rats. *Hypertension in Pregnancy* **14**, 17.

77 Baylis C. (1993) Blood pressure and renal hemodynamic effects of acute blockade of vascular actions of AVP in normal pregnancy in the rat. *Hypertension in Pregnancy* **12**, 93.

78 Paller M.S., Gregorini G. & Ferris T.F. (1989) Pressor responsiveness in pseudopregnant and pregnant rats: role of maternal factors. *American Journal of Physiology* **257**, R866.

79 Hennessy A., Gillin A. & Horoath J. (1993) Cardiovascular research in pregnancy: the role of animal models. *Hypertension in Pregnancy* **12**, 413.

80 Venuto R.C. & Donker A.J.M. (1982) Prostaglandin E2, plasma renin activity and renal function throughout rabbit pregnancy. *Journal of Laboratory and Clinical Medicine* **99**, 239.

81 Gregoire I., Dupouy J.P., Fievet P., Sraer J.D. & Fournier A. (1987) Prostanoid synthesis by isolated rat glomeruli: effects of oestrous cycle and pregnancy. *Clinical Science* **73**, 641.

82 Conrad K.P. & Dunn M.J. (1987) Renal synthesis and urinary excretion of eicosinoids during pregnancy in the rat. *American Journal of Physiology* **253**, F1197.

83 Brown G.P. & Venuto R.C. (1988) In vitro renal eicosanoid production during pregnancy in rabbits. *American Journal of Physiology* **254**, E687.

84 Baylis C. (1987) Renal effect of cyclooxygenase inhibition in the pregnant rat. *American Journal of Physiology* **254**, F158.

85 Gregoire I., El Esper N., Goudry J., Boitte F., Fievet F., Makdassi R., Westeel F.P. *et al.* (1996) Plasma atrial natriuretic factor and urinary excretion of a ouabain displacing factor and dopaminine in normotensive pregnant women before and after delivery. *American Journal of Obstetrics and Gynecology* **162**, 71.

86 Castro L.C., Hobel C.J. & Gornbein J. (1994) Plasma levels of atrial natriuretic peptide in normal and hypertensive pregnancies: a meta-analysis.

American Journal of Obstetrics and Gynecology **171**, 1642.

87 Irons D.W., Baylis P.H. & Davison J.M. (1996) Effects of atrial natriuretic peptide on renal hemodynamics and sodium excretion during human pregnancy. *American Journal of Physiology* **271**, F239.

88 Irons D.W., Baylis P.H., Butler J.J. & Davison J.M. (1997) Atrial natriuretic peptide in pre-eclampsia: metabolic clearance, renal hemodynamics and sodium excretion. *American Journal of Physiology* **273**, F483.

89 Omer S., Mulay S., Cernacek P. & Varma D.R. (1995) Attenuation of renal effects of atrial natriuretic peptide during rat pregnancy. *American Journal of Physiology* **268**, F416.

90 Kristensen C.G., Nakagawa Y., Coe F.L. & Lindheimer M.D. (1986) Effect of atrial natriuretic factor in rat pregnancy. *American Journal of Physiology* **250**, R589.

91 Nadel A.S., Ballerman B.J., Anderson S. & Brenner B.M. (1988) Inter-relationships among atrial peptides, renin and blood volume in pregnant rats. *American Journal of Physiology* **254**, R793.

92 Masilamani S. & Baylis C. (1992) Pregnant rats are refractory to the natriuretic action of atrial natriuretic peptide. *American Journal of Physiology* **267**, R1611.

93 Moncada S., Palmer R.M.J. & Higgs E.A. (1991) Biosynthesis and endogenous roles of nitric oxide. *Pharmacological Reviews* **43**, 109.

94 Conrad K.P. & Whittemore S.L. (1992) NG-monomethyl-L-arginine and nitroarginine potentiate pressor responsiveness of vasoconstrictors in conscious rats. *American Journal of Physiology* **262**, R1137.

95 Poston L., McCarthy A.L. & Ritter J.M. (1995) Control of vascular resistance in maternal and feto-placental arterial beds. *Pharmacology and Therapeutics* **65**, 215.

96 Baylis C., Suto T. & Conrad K. (1996) Importance of nitric oxide in control of systemic and renal hemodynamics during normal pregnancy: studies in the rat and implications for pre-eclampsia. *Hypertension in Pregnancy* **15**, 147.

97 Conrad K.P. & Vernier K.A. (1989) Plasma levels, urinary excretion and metabolic production of cGMP during gestation in rats. *American Journal of Physiology* **257**, R847.

98 Conrad K.P., Joffe G.M., Kruszyna H., Rochelle L.G., Smith R.P., Chavez J.E. & Mosher M.D. (1993) Identification of increased nitric oxide biosynthesis during pregnancy in rats. *FASEB J* **7**, 566.

99 Engels K., Deng A., Samsell L., Hill C. & Baylis C. (1993) Increased nitric oxide (NO) production in normal pregnancy is resistant to inhibition. *Journal of American Society of Nephrology* **4**, 548A.

100 Weiner C., Liu K.Z., Thompson L., Herrig J. & Chestnut D. (1991) Effect of pregnancy on endothelium and smooth muscle: their role in reduced adrenergic sensitivity. *American Journal of Physiology* **261**, H1275.

101 Weiner C.P., Thompson L.P., Kang-Zhu L. & Herrig L.E. (1992) Endothelium-derived relaxing factor and indomethacin-sensitive contracting factor alter arterial contractile responses to thromboxane during

pregnancy. *American Journal of Obstetrics and Gynecology* **166**, 1171.

102 Molnar M. & Hertelendy F. (1992) Nw-nitro-L-arginine, an inhibitor of nitric oxide synthesis, increases blood pressure in rats and reverses the pregnancy-induced refractoriness to vasopressor agents. *American Journal of Obstetrics and Gynecology* **166**, 1560.

103 Weiner C.P., Lizasoain I., Baylis S.A., Knowles R.G., Charles I.G. & Moncada S. (1994) Induction of calcium-dependent nitric oxide synthases by sex hormones. *Proceedings of the National Academy of Science USA* **91**, 5212.

104 Milner J.A. & Visek W.J. (1978) Orotic aciduria in the female rat and its relation to dietary arginine. *Journal of Nutrition* **108**, 1281.

105 Raij L. (1994) Glomerular thrombosis in pregnancy: role of the L-arginine-nitric oxide pathway. *Kidney International* **45**, 775.

106 Umans J.G., Lindheimer M.D. & Barron W.M. (1990) Pressor effect of endothelium derived relaxing factor inhibition in conscious virgin and gravid rats. *American Journal of Physiology* **259**, F293.

107 St-Louis J. & Sicotte B. (1992) Prostaglandin- or endothelium-mediated vasodilation is not involved in the blunted responses of blood vessels to vasoconstrictors in pregnant rats. *American Journal of Obstetrics and Gynecology* **166**, 684.

108 Raij L. & Baylis C. (1995) Nitric oxide and the glomerulus (Editorial review). *Kidney International* **48**, 20.

109 Danielson L.A. & Conrad K.P. (1995) Nitric oxide mediates renal vasodilation and hyperfiltration during pregnancy in chronically instrumented, conscious rats. *Journal of Clinical Investigation* **96**, 482.

110 Morris N.H., Eaton B.M. & Dekker G. (1996) Nitric oxide, the endothelium, pregnancy and pre-eclampsia. *British Journal of Obstetrics and Gynaecology* **103**, 4.

111 Kopp L., Paradiz G. & Tucci J.R. (1977) Urinary excretion of cyclic 3',5'-adenosine monophosphate and cyclic 3',5'-guanosine monophosphate during and after pregnancy. *Journal of Clinical Endocrinology and Metabolism* **44**, 590.

112 Barton J.R., Sibai B.M., Ahokas R.S., Whybrew D. & Mercer B.M. (1992) Magnesium sulphate therapy in preeclampsia is associated with increased urinary cGMP excretion. *American Journal of Obstetrics and Gynecology* **167**, 931.

113 Seligman S.P., Buyon J.P., Clancy R.M., Young B.K. & Abramson S.B. (1994) The role of nitric oxide in the pathogenesis of preeclampsia. *American Journal of Obstetrics and Gynecology* **171**, 944.

114 Curtis N.E., Gude N.M., King R.G., Marriott P.J., Rook R.J. & Brennecke S.P. (1995) Nitric oxide metabolites in normal human pregnancy and pre-eclampsia. *Hypertension in Pregnancy* **14**, 339.

115 Brown M.A., Tibben E., Zammit V.C., Cario G.M. & Carlton M.A. (1995) Nitric oxide excretion in normal and hypertensive pregnancies. *Hypertension in Pregnancy* **14**, 319.

116 Baylis C. (1997) NO metabolism in normal and hypertensive pregnancy. *Nephrology* **3**, 141.

117 Domenech M., Gruppuso P.A., Nishino V.T., Susa J.B.

& Schwartz R. (1986) Preserved fetal plasma amino acid concentrations in the presence of maternal hypoaminoacidemia. *Pediatric Research* **20**, 1071.

118 Wood M.H. & O'Sullivan W.J. (1973) The orotic aciduria of pregnancy. *American Journal of Obstetrics and Gynecology* **116**, 57.

119 McCarthy A.L., Woolfson R.G., Raju S.K. & Poston L. (1993) Abnormal endothelial cell function of resistance arteries from women with preeclampsia. *American Journal of Obstetrics and Gynecology* **168**, 1323.

120 Fickling S.A., Williams D., Vallance P., Nussey S.S. & Whitley G.StJ. (1993) Plasma concentrations of endogenous inhibitor of nitric oxide synthesis in normal pregnancy and preeclampsia. *Lancet* **342**, 242.

121 Lindheimer M.D. & Katz A.I. (1992) Renal physiology and disease in pregnancy. In *The Kidney: Physiology and Pathophysiology* (2nd edn). Eds D.W. Seldin & G. Geibisch, p. 3371. Raven Press, New York.

122 Reckelhoff J.F., Samsell L. & Baylis C. (1989) Failure of an acute 10–15 per cent plasma volume expansion in the virgin female rat to mimic the increased glomerular filtration rate (GFR) and altered glomerular hemodynamics seen at midterm pregnancy. *Clinical and Experimental Hypertension* **B8**, 533.

123 Dunlop W. & Davison J.M. (1977) The effect of normal pregnancy upon the renal handling of uric acid. *British Journal of Obstetrics and Gynaecology* **84**, 13.

124 Barry C.I., Royle G.A. & Lake Y. (1992) Racial variation in serum uric acid concentration in pregnancy: a comparison between European, New Zealand Maori and Polynesian women. *Australian and New Zealand Journal of Obstetrics and Gynaecology* **32**, 17.

125 Fischer R.L., Bianculli K.W., Hediger M.L., Scholl T.O. (1995) Maternal serum uric acid levels in twin gestations. *Obstetrics and Gynecology* **85**, 60.

126 Atherton J.C. & Green R. (1994) Renal tubular function in the gravid rat. *Clinical Obstetrics and Gynaecology (Baillière)* **8**, 265.

127 Baylis C. & Davison J.M. (1998) The normal renal physiological changes which occur during pregnancy. In *Oxford Textbook of Clinical Nephrology* (2nd edn). Eds A.M. Davison, J.S. Cameron, J.-P., Grünfeld, D.N.S. Kerr & E. Ritz, Oxford University Press, Oxford, 2297.

128 Davison J.M. & Hytten F.E. (1975) The effect of pregnancy on the renal handling of glucose. *Journal of Obstetrics and Gynaecology of the British Commonwealth* **82**, 374.

129 Hytten F.E. & Cheyne G.A. (1972) The aminoaciduria of pregnancy. *Journal of Obstetrics and Gynaecology of the British Commonwealth* **79**, 424.

130 Lindheimer M.D., Richardson D.A., Ehrlich E.N. & Katz A.I. (1987) Potassium homeostasis in pregnancy. *Journal of Reproductive Medicine* **32**, 517.

131 Mujais S.K., Nora N.A. & Chen Y. (1993) Regulation of the renal Na:K pump: role of progesterone. *Journal of the American Society of Nephrology* **3**, 1488.

132 Giebisch G., Malnic G. & Berliner R.W. (1986) Renal transport and control of potassium excretion. In *The*

304

Kidney (3rd edn). Eds B.M. Brenner & F.C. Rector Jr, p. 177. W.B. Saunders, Pennsylvania.

133 Howarth A.T., Morgan D.B. & Payne R.B. (1977) Urinary excretion of calcium in late pregnancy and its relation to creatinine clearance. *American Journal of Obstetrics and Gynecology* **239**, 499.

134 Maikranz P., Lindheimer M. & Coe F. (1994) Nephrolithiasis in pregnancy. *Clinical Obstetrics and Gynaecology (Baillière)* **8**, 375.

135 Davison J.M., Shiells E.A., Philips P.R., Barron W.M. & Lindheimer M.D. (1993) Metabolic clearance of vasopressin and an analogue resistant to vasopressinase in human pregnancy. *American Journal of Physiology* **264**, F348.

136 Lim V.S., Katz A.I. & Lindheimer M.D. (1976) Acid-base regulation in pregnancy. *American Journal of Physiology* **231**, 1764.

137 Bar J., Hod M., Erman A., Friedman S. & Ovadia Y. (1995) Microalbuminuria: prognostic and therapeutic implications in diabetic and hypertensive pregnancy. *Diabetic Medicine* **12**, 649.

138 Lopez-Espinoza I., Dhar H., Humphreys S. & Redman C.W.G. (1986) Urinary albumin excretion in pregnancy. *British Journal of Obstetrics and Gynaecology* **93**, 176.

139 Wright P.S., Bennet J.B., Watts G. & Polak A. (1987) The urinary excretion of albumin in normal pregnancy. *British Journal of Obstetrics and Gynaecology* **94**, 413.

140 Musiani R., Marchesi D. & Tiraboschi G. (1991) Urinary albumin excretion in normal pregnancy and pregnancy induced hypertension. *Nephron* **59**, 416.

141 Higby K., Suiter C.R., Phelps J.Y., Siler-Khodr T. & Langer O. (1994) Normal values of urinary albumin and total protein excretion during pregnancy. *American Journal of Obstetrics and Gynecology* **171**, 984.

142 Douma C.E., van der Post J.A.M., van Acker B.A.C., Boer K. & Koopman M.G. (1995) Circadian variation of urinary albumin excretion in pregnancy. *British Journal of Obstetrics and Gynaecology* **102**, 107.

143 Davison J.M., Vallotton M.B. & Lindheimer M.D. (1981) Plasma osmolality and urinary concentration and dilution during and after pregnancy: evidence that lateral recumbency inhibits maximal urinary concentrating ability. *British Journal of Obstetrics and Gynaecology* **88**, 472.

144 Davison J.M., Gilmore E.A., Durr J., Robertson G.L. & Lindheimer M.D. (1984) Altered osmotic thresholds for vasopressin secretion and thirst in human pregnancy. *American Journal of Physiology* **246**, F105.

145 Davison J.M., Shiells E.A., Phillips P.R. & Lindheimer M.D. (1988) Serial evaluation of vasopressin release and thirst in human pregnancy: the role of chorionic gonadotrophin in the osmoregulatory changes of gestation. *Journal of Clinical Investigation* **81**, 798.

146 Lindheimer M.D. & Barron W.M. (1994) Water metabolism and vasopressin secretion during pregnancy. *Clinical Obstetrics and Gynaecology (Baillière)* **8**, 311.

147 Davison J.M., Shiells E.A., Baron W.M., Robinson A.G. & Lindheimer M.D. (1989) Changes in the metabolic clearance of vasopressin and in plasma vasopressinase throughout human pregnancy. *Journal of Clinical Investigation* **83**, 1313.

148 Davison J.M., Shiells E.A., Philips P.R., Barron W.M. & Lindheimer M.D. (1989) Metabolic clearance rates (MCR) of arginine vasopressin (AVP) and 1-deamino-81D-AVP (DPAVP) in human pregnancy (P): evidence that placental enzymes increase MCRs of AVP in gestation. *Clinical Research* **37**, 596A.

149 Landon M.J., Copas D.K., Shiells E.A. & Davison J.M. (1988) Degradation of radiolabelled arginine vasopressin (I-AVP) by the human placenta perfused *in vitro*. *British Journal of Obstetrics and Gynaecology* **95**, 488.

150 Lindheimer M.D. & Davison J.M. (1995) Osmoregulation, the secretion of arginine vasopressin and its metabolism during pregnancy (Minireview). *European Journal of Endocrinology* **132**, 133.

151 Davison J.M., Shiells E.A. & Lindheimer M.D. (1989) The influence of humoral and volume factors on the altered osmoregulation of normal human pregnancy. *American Journal of Physiology* **258**, F900.

152 Schrier R.W. (1988) Pathogenesis of sodium and water retention in high-output and low-output cardiac failure, nephrotic syndrome, cirrhosis and pregnancy. *New England Journal of Medicine* **319**, 1127.

153 Barron W.M., Stamoutsos B.A. & Lindheimer M.D. (1984) Role of volume in the regulation of vasopressin secretion during pregnancy in the rat. *Journal of Clinical Investigation* **73**, 923.

154 Brown M.A. & Gallery E.D.M. (1994) Volume homeostasis in normal pregnancy and pre-eclampsia: physiology and clinical implications. *Clinical Obstetrics and Gynaecology (Baillière)* **8**, 287.

155 Duvekott J.J. & Peeters L.H.H. (1994) Maternal cardiovascular haemodynamic adaptions to pregnancy. *Obstetrical and Gynecological Survey* **49**, 51.

156 August P. & Lindheimer M.D. (1995) Pathophysiology of preeclampsia. In *Hypertension: Pathophysiology, Diagnosis and Management* (2nd edn). Eds J.H. Laragh & B.M. Brenner, p. 2407.

157 Trolifors B., Alestig K. & Jagenburg R. (1987) Prediction of glomerular filtration rate from serum creatinine, age, sex and body weight. *Acta Medica Scandinavica* **221**, 495.

158 Gallery E.D.M., Rowe J., Brown M.A., Boyce E.S., Ross M., Grigg R. & Gyory A.Z. (1986) Erythrocyte electrolyte transport in normal and hypertensive pregnancy. *Proceedings of the 5th International Congress for the International Society for the Study of Hypertension in Pregnancy* **8A**.

159 Macphail S., Thomas T.H., Wilkinson R., Dunlop W. & Davison J.M. (1991) Erythrocyte hydration in normal human pregnancy. *British Journal of Obstetrics and Gynaecology* **98**, 1205.

160 Graves S.W., Cook S.L. & Seely E.W. (1995) Fluid and electrolyte handling in normal pregnancy. *Journal of the Society for Gynecological Investigation* **2**, 291.

161 Kirksey A. & Pike R.L. (1962) Some effects of high and low sodium intakes during pregnancy in the rat. I. Food consumption, weight gain, reproductive performance, electrolyte balances, plasma total protein

and protein fraction in normal pregnancy. *Journal of Nutrition* **77**, 33.

162 Baylis C. & Munger K. (1990) Persistence of maternal plasma volume expansion in midterm pregnant rats maintained on a zero sodium intake: evidence that early gestational volume expansion does not rely on renal sodium retention. *Clinical and Experimental Hypertension* **B3**, 237.

163 Phippard A.F., Horvath J.S. & Glynn E.M. (1986) Circulatory adaptation to pregnancy: serial studies of haemodynamics, blood volume, renin and aldosterone in the baboon (Papio Hamadryas). *Journal of Hypertension* **4**, 773.

164 Schrier R.W. & Dürr J.A. (1987) Pregnancy: an overfill or underfill state. *American Journal of Kidney Disease* **9**, 284.

165 Schrier R.W. & Briner V.A. (1991) Peripheral arterial vasodilation hypothesis of sodium and water retention in pregnancy: implications for pathogenesis of pre-eclampsia-eclampsia. *Obstetrics and Gynecology* **77**, 632.

166 Duvekot J.J. & Peeters L.L.H. (1994) Maternal cardiovascular hemodynamic adaptations to pregnancy. *Obstetric and Gynecological Survey* **49**, S1.

167 Trolifors B., Alestig K. & Jagenburg R. (1987) Prediction of glomerular filtration rate from serum creatinine, age, sex and body weight. *Acta Medica Scandinavica* **221**, 495.

168 Higby K., Suiter C.R. & Siler-Khodr T. (1995) A comparison between two screening methods for detection of microproteinuria. *American Journal of Obstetrics and Gynecology* **173**, 1111.

169 Davison J.M. (1997) Edema in pregnancy. *Kidney International* **51**, 590.

170 Collins R., Yusuf P. & Peto R. (1985) Overview of randomised trials of diuretics in pregnancy. *British Medical Journal* **290**, 17.

171 Cunningham F.G., Cox S.M. Harstad T.W,. Mason R.A. & Pritchard J.A. (1990) Chronic renal disease and pregnancy outcome. *American Journal of Obstetrics and Gynecology* **163**, 453.

172 Lindheimer M.D. & Katz A.I. (1994) Gestation in women with kidney disease: prognosis and management. *Clinical Obstetrics and Gynaecology (Baillière)* **8**, 387.

173 Jungers P., Houillier P., Forget D., Labrunie M., Skkiri H., Giatras I. & Descamps-Latscha B. (1995) Influence of pregnancy on the course of primary chronic glomerulonephritis. *Lancet* **346**, 1122.

174 Abe S. (1996) Pregnancy in glomerulonephritic patients with decreased renal function. *Hypertension in Pregnancy* **15**, 305.

175 Holley J.L., Barnardini J., Quadri K.H.M., Greenberg A. & Laifer S.A. (1996) Pregnancy outcomes in a prospective metched control study of pregnancy and renal disease. *Clinical Nephrology* **45**, 77.

176 Jones D.C. & Hayslett J.P. (1996) Outcome of pregnancy in women with moderate or severe renal insufficiency. *New England Journal of Medicine* **335**, 226.

177 Katz A.I., Davison J.M., Hayslett J.P., Singson E. & Lindheimer M.D. (1980) Pregnancy in women with kidney disease. *Kidney International* **18**, 192.

178 Hemmelder M.H., de Zeeuw D., Fidler V. & de Jong P.E. (1995) Proteinuria: a risk factor for progeny-related renal function decline in primary glomerular disease? *American Journal of Kidney Diseases* **26**, 187.

179 Jungers P., Chauveau D., Choukroun G., Moynot A., Skhiri H., Houillier P., Forget D. et al. (1997) Pregnancy in women with impaired renal function. *Clinical Nephrology* **47**, 281.

180 Hou S. (1994) Peritoneal dialysis and hemodialysis in pregnancy. *Clinical Obstetrics and Gynaecology (Baillière)* **8**, 481.

181 Jungers P. & Chauveau D. (1997) Pregnancy in renal disease. *Kidney International* **52**, 871.

182 Imbasciati E. & Ponticelli C. (1991) Pregnancy and renal disease: predictors for fetal and maternal outcome. *American Journal of Nephrology* **11**, 353.

183 Imbasciati E., Pardi G., Capetta P., Ambroso G., Bozzetti P. & Pagliari B. (1986) Pregnancy in women with chronic renal failure. *American Journal of Nephrology* **6**, 193.

184 Malik G.H., Al-Wakeel J.S., Shaikh J.F., Al-Mohoya S., Dohami H., Kechrid M. & El Gamal H. (1997) Three successive pregnancies in a patient on haemo dialysis. *Nephrology Dialysis Transplantation* **12**, 1991.

185 Hou S. (1997) Pregnancy in women treated with dialysis. *Saudi Journal of Kidney Disease and Transplantation* **8**, 3.

186 Schewitz L.J., Friedman E.A. & Pollak V.E. (1965) Bleeding after renal biopsy in pregnancy. *Obstetrics and Gynecology* **26**, 295.

187 Lindheimer M.D., Fisher K.A., Spargo B.H. & Katz A.I. (1981) Hypertension in pregnancy: a biopsy study with long term follow up. *Contributions to Nephrology* **25**, 71.

188 Lindheimer M.D. & Davison J.M. (1987) Renal biopsy during pregnancy: 'To b or not to b'. *British Journal of Obstetrics and Gynaecology* **94**, 932.

189 Packham D.K. & Fairley K.F. (1987) Renal biopsy: indications and complications in pregnancy: *British Journal of Obstetrics and Gynaecology* **94**, 935.

190 Roberts M, Lindheimer M.D. & Davison J.M. (1997) Glomerular dynamics and membrane porosity in pregnant women with pre-existing glomerular disease. *Hypertension in Pregnancy* **16**, 17.

191 Klahr S., Level A.S. & Beck G.J. (1994) The effects of dietary protein restriction and blood pressure control on the progression of chronic renal disease: modification of diet in renal disease study group. *New England Journal of Medicine* **330**, 877.

192 Brenner B.M. (1985) Nephron adaptations to renal injury or ablation. *American Journal of Physiology* **249**, F324.

193 Goldstein R.S., Tarloff J.B. & Hook J.B. (1988) Age-related nephropathy in laboratory rats. *FASEB J* **2**, 2241.

194 Larochelle P. (1991) Glomerular capillary pressure and hypertension. *American Heart Journal* **122**, 1228.

195 Levi M. & Rowe J.W. (1992) Renal function and dysfunction in aging. In *The Kidney: Physiology and Pathophysiology*. Eds D.W. Seldin & G. Giebisch, p. 3433. Raven Press, New York.

306

196 Olsen J.L., Wilson S.K. & Heptinstall R.H. (1986) Relation of glomerular injury to pre-glomerular resistance in experimental hypertension. *Kidney International* **29**, 849.

197 Dworkin L.D., Feiner H.D. & Randazo J. (1987) Glomerular hypertension and injury in desoxycorticosterone-salt rats on antihypertensive therapy. *Kidney International* **31**, 718.

198 Bjorck S., Mulech H., Johnsen S.A., Norden G. & Aurell M. (1992) Renal protective effect of enalapril in diabetic nephropathy. *British Medical Journal* **304**, 343.

199 Baylis C. & Wilson C.B. (1989) Sex and the single kidney. *American Journal of Kidney Disease* **13**, 290.

200 Packham D.K., Hewitson T.D., Whitworth J.A. & Kincaid Smith P.S. (1991) Physiological and biochemical effects of pregnancy in uninephrectomised rabbits. *Clinical and Experimental Hypertension in Pregnancy* **B10**, 35.

201 Meyer B.R. (1991) Renal function in aging. *Journal of the American Geriatrics Society* **37**, 791.

202 Silbiger S.R. & Neugarten J. (1995) The impact of gender on the progression of chronic renal disease. *American Journal of Kidney Disease* **25**, 515.

203 Lombet J.R., Adler S.G., Anderson P.S., Nast C.C., Olsen D. & Glassock R.J. (1988) Sex vulnerability in the subtotal nephrectomy (NX) model of glomerulosclerosis. *Kidney International* **33**, 3784.

204 Wilson C.B. & Blantz R.C. (1985) Nephroimmuno-pathology and pathophysiology. *American Journal of Physiology* **248**, F319.

205 Baylis C., Reese K. & Wilson C.B. (1989) Glomerular effects of pregnancy in a model of glomerulonephritis in the rat. *American Journal of Kidney Disease* **14**, 452.

206 Couser W.G. & Abrass C.K. (1988) Pathogenesis of membranous nephropathy. *Annual Review of Medicine* **29**, 517.

207 Baylis C., Deng A. & Couser W.G. (1995) Glomerular hemodynamic effects of late pregnancy in rats with experimental glomerulonephropathy. *Journal of American Society of Nephrology* **6**, 1197.

208 Daniels B.S. & Hostetter T.H. (1990) Adverse effect of growth factors in the glomerular microcirculation. *American Journal of Physiology* **258**, F1409.

209 Floege J., Alpers C.E. & Burns M.W. (1992) Glomerular cells, extracellular matrix accumulation and the development of glomerular sclerosis in the remnant kidney model. *Laboratory Investigation* **66**, 485.

210 Davies M., Coles G.A., Thomas G.J., Martin J. & Lovett D.H. (1990) Proteinases and the glomerulus: their role in glomerular diseases. *Klinika Wochenschrift* **68**, 1145.

211 Remuzzi G. & Bertani T. (1990) Is glomerulosclerosis a consequence of altered glomerular permeability to macromolecules? *Kidney International* **38**, 384.

212 Gaber L.W., Spargo B.H. & Lindheimer M.D. (1994) Renal pathology in pre-eclampsia. *Clinical Obstetrics and Gynaecology (Baillière)* **8**, 443.

213 Fisher K.A., Luger A., Spargo B.H. & Lindheimer M.D. (1981) Hypertension in pregnancy: clinical–pathological correlations and late prognosis. *Medicine* **60**, 267.

214 Ihle B.U., Long P. & Oats J. (1987) Early onset pre-eclampsia: recognition of underlying renal disease. *British Medical Journal* **294**, 79.

215 Dekker G.A., deVries J.I.P., Doelitzsch P.M. *et al.* (1995) Underlying disorders associated with severe early onset preeclampsia. *American Journal of Obstetrics and Gynecology* **173**, 1042.

216 Nisell H., Lintu H., Lunell N.O., Möllerstrom G., Petterson E. (1995) Blood pressure and renal function seven years after pregnancy complicated by hypertension. *British Journal of Obstetrics and Gynaecology* **102**, 876.

217 Gallery E.D.M., Ross M. & Györy A.Z. (1993) Urinary red blood cells and cast excretion in normal and hypertensive human pregnancy. *American Journal of Obstetrics and Gynecology* **168**, 67.

218 Naicker T., Randeree G.H., Moodley J., Khedun S.M., Ramsaroop P. & Seedat S.K. (1997) Correlation between histological changes and loss of anionic change of the glomerular basement membrane in early-onset pre-eclampsia. *Nephron* **75**, 201.

219 Suzuki S., Gejyo F., Ogino S., Maruyama Y., Ueno M., Nishi S., Kimura H. *et al.* (1997) Postpartum renal lesions in women with pre-eclampsia. *Nephrology, Dialysis and Transplantation* **12**, 2488.

220 Feld L.G., Brentjens J.R. & Van Liew J.B. (1981) Renal injury and proteinuria in female spontaneously hypertensive rats. *Renal Physiology* **4**, 46.

221 Baylis C. (1989) Immediate and longterm effects of pregnancy on glomerular function the SHR. *American Journal of Physiology* **257**, F1140.

222 Ahokas R.A., Mercer B.M. & Sibai B.M. (1991) Enhanced EDRF activity in pregnant, spontaneously hypertensive rats. *American Journal of Obstetrics and Gynecology* **165**, 801.

223 Leaker B., Becker G.J., El-Khatib M., Hewitson T.D. & Kincaid Smith P.S. (1992) Repeated pregnancy does not accelerate glomerulosclerosis in rats with subtotal renal ablation. *Clinical and Experimental Hypertension in Pregnancy* **B11**, 1.

224 Baylis C., Heaton P. & Engels K. (1990) Endothelial derived relaxing factor (EDRF) controls renal hemodynamics in normal rat kidney. *Journal of the American Society of Nephrology* **1**, 875.

225 Baylis C., Mitsuka B. & Deng A. (1992) Chronic blockade of nitric oxide synthesis in the rat produces systemic hypertension and glomerular damage. *Journal of Clinical Investigation* **90**, 275.

226 Deng A. & Baylis C. (1993) Locally produced EDRF controls preglomerular resistance and the ultrafiltration coefficient. *American Journal of Physiology* **264**, F212.

227 Romero J.C., Lahera V., Salom M.G. & Biondi M.L. (1992) Role of EDRF nitric oxide on renal function. *Journal of the American Society of Nephrologists* **2**, 1371.

228 Podjarny E., Bernheim J.L., Rathaus M. & Pomeranz M. (1992) Adriamycin nephropathy: a model to study the effects of pregnancy on renal disease in rat. *American Journal of Physiology* **263**, F711.

229 Bernheim J., Podjarny E., Pomeranz A., Feldman V., Gonen O. & Rathaus M. (1994) Pregnancy induced hypertension in rats with early adriamycin nephropathy. *Nephrology, Dialysis, Transplantation* **3**, 13.

230 Podjarny E., Pomeranz M., Bernheim J.L. & Rathaus M. (1993) Effects of L-arginine treatment in pregnant rats with adriamycin nephropathy. *Hypertension in Pregnancy* **12**, 517.

231 Pomeranz M., Podjarny E., Bernheim J., Rathaus M. & Green J. (1995) Effect of recurrent pregnancies on the evolution of adriamycin nephropathy. *Nephrology Dialysis Transplantation* **10**, 2049.

The Genital System

P.J. STEER & M.R. JOHNSON

The uterus

Like most other smooth muscle, the uterus is spontaneously contractile. It is able to perform considerable mechanical work when required to expel the shedding endometrium during menstruation or to deliver the fetus at term. At other times it must remain quiescent, to allow implantation of the blastocyst and growth of the fetus. Thus, it is important to understand not only how the uterus contracts during menstruation and labour, but how it is prevented from contracting during pregnancy.

Structure

The smooth muscle cells of the uterus are grouped into bundles separated by thin sheets of connective tissue composed of collagen, elastic fibres, fibroblasts and mast cells. The collagenous connective tissue probably serves two functions: a support for the muscle fibres and a transmission network for the tension developed by contraction of the smooth muscle elements.

The arrangement of the smooth muscle bundles in the human uterus appears complex, being different in different layers (Fig. 11.1) [1]. There are apparently three or four distinct layers, with an innermost layer of longitudinal fibres, then a layer containing a vascular supply with bundles running in all directions, and finally an outermost layer of circular spiral and longitudinal bundles, continuous at least in part with the other ligamentous supports of the uterus and with the cervix.

Ultrastructural studies reveal that the uterine smooth muscle cell is spindle shaped and between 20 and 600 μm long, and 2 and 10 μm in diameter, depending on its functional state; it is largest at the end of pregnancy.

The nerve supply

The uterus is innervated predominantly from the autonomic nervous system [2], through the inferior hypogastric or uterovaginal plexus in the base of the broad ligament. The nerves follow the blood vessels, particularly the uterine

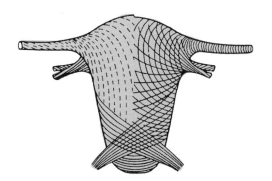

Fig. 11.1 Diagrammatic representation of the principal muscle fibre arrangements of the human uterus. Longitudinal fibres are shown at top left with clockwise and counter-clockwise spirals of circular fibres on the right. Note integration with supporting ligaments of the uterus. (Courtesy of S.R.M. Reynolds and Paul Hoeber Inc.)

and vaginal arteries (see Fig. 11.2); those to the cervix form a plexus with several small paracervical ganglia, one, the uterine cervical ganglion, being larger. Uterine nerves pass upwards with the uterine arteries and communicate with the nerves from the ovarian plexus. The preganglionic or sympathetic fibres which supply the uterus come from the T12 and L1 segments of the spinal cord while the preganglionic parasympathetic fibres arise in the second, third and fourth sacral segments of the cord relaying at the paracervical ganglia. The sympathetic nerves produce both vasoconstriction and uterine contraction while the para-sympathetic nerves stimulate vasodilatation and uterine relaxation; these effects are strongly modulated by hormonal effects. The dilation of the cervix is responsible for the majority of the pain of labour and its afferent pain fibres have their origin in the dorsal roots of the upper sacral nerves. Pain fibres from the body of the uterus pass in sympathetic nerves through the superior hypogastric plexus and the lumbar splanchnic nerves to cells in the dorsal roots of the lower thoracic and upper lumbar spinal cord.

The mechanism of myometrial contraction
(Fig. 11.3)

The contractile ability of muscle is dependent on the interaction between two contractile proteins, actin and myosin [3]. Arrays of thick filaments containing myosin interdigitate with arrays of thin filaments containing actin. Interaction occurs through cross-bridges protruding from the myosin filament and binding reversibly with the actin filament. The energy for contractions comes from adenosine triphosphate (ATP). The events leading to uterine muscle contraction start at the cell membrane with a stimulus, either electrical or hormonal, which usually (not invariably) initiates an action potential. An action potential results from a reciprocal flow of various charged ions, notably sodium, potassium, and calcium, through ion channels.

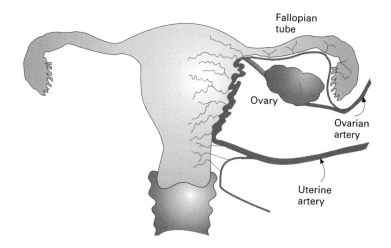

Fallopian tube

Ovary

Ovarian artery

Uterine artery

Fig. 11.2. The blood supply of the uterus.

The pregnant human myometrium has spontaneous electrical activity which is generated from pacemaker cells and which is transmitted over the uterus as a whole during a uterine contraction. The ability of myometrial cells to contract depends on the distribution of ions across the plasma membrane. The higher concentrations of sodium and calcium outside the cell and of potassium within the cell set up a resting membrane potential. As pregnancy advances, the resting potential of myometrial cells falls. Thus, an action potential is generated and propagated more easily. The generation of an action potential is dependent on the influx of sodium and calcium ions, repolarization occurs as a result of the efflux of potassium ions through fast (voltage dependent) and slow (calcium regulated) channels. The former (voltage dependent), open with cell depolarization, and the latter are receptor regulated, i.e. dependent on an agonist binding to the receptor. In the human, two forms of the fast type have been identified, each activated at different membrane potentials.

Myometrial cell contraction occurs with the rise of intracellular calcium and is terminated with the fall in calcium ion concentration. There is then an associated change in the intracellular calcium concentration. Normally this lies in the region of 10^{-7}–10^{-8} mmol/l but when it rises to 10^{-6} mmol/l the actin/myosin filaments interact. Myosin consists of four polypeptide chains, two heavy and two light. In the presence of the increased calcium concentration the 20 000 molecular weight myosin light chain is phosphorylated by the enzyme myosin light-chain kinase. This requires the presence of a protein called calmodulin, which forms a complex with calcium. This complex has a high affinity for myosin light-chain kinase. The binding of the complex to the myosin light-chain kinase allows the kinase to carry out the phosphorylation of myosin light chain which then interacts with the actin filament to produce an overall shortening of the fibril (Fig. 11.3). Calcium is undoubtedly a key ion in the contraction process. A substantial part of the calcium needed for contraction comes from the extracellular fluid, where its concentration (10^{-3} mol/l) is some 10 000 times higher than in the myometrial cell (10^{-7} mol/l). At rest, the cell membrane has a low permeability for calcium, but calcium can enter the cell through ion channels following a contraction. A major class of drugs, the calcium channel blockers, act by binding to the cell membrane within these channels, blocking them. Such drugs include the dihydropyridines nitrendipine, nicardipine and nifedipine. In clinical use, nifedipine has been shown to reduce uterine activity in women with dysmenorrhoea [4] and in preterm labour [5]. There do appear to be other calcium channels which can be opened by noradrenaline, but these are of lesser potency in the stimulation of myometrial contraction [3].

In addition to calcium from outside the cell, calcium released from the sarcoplasmic reticulum also plays an important role in initiating contractions [3]. The sarcoplasmic reticulum is a system of tubules originating from the cell wall and permeating the cytoplasm. It accounts for about 5% of the cell volume. Recent evidence suggests that the action potential is conducted from the membrane down the sarcoplasmic reticulum, allowing the rapid release of calcium deep in the cell. Even if the cell is bathed in a calcium-free solution, the release of calcium from the reticulum is sufficient to produce contraction. The reticulum also provides an efficient mechanism for producing relaxation because in the presence of ATP it continually sequesters calcium, thus reducing intracellular calcium concentrations.

In vitro, myometrial contraction is optimal at an extracellular calcium concentration of 2.5 mmol/l, an increase or decrease in the concentration inhibits the generation of spontaneous contractions. This reflects the dual roles played by calcium ions; the initial influx of calcium ions is excitatory, but the increased intracellular concentration of calcium stimulates potassium efflux and the stabilization of the membrane. When extracellular calcium ions are too low, the initial rise is insufficient, and when too high, the increased activity of the potassium channel hyperpolarizes the membrane. Sodium plays an important role in the human uterus, possibly in cell-to-cell conduction and in the regulation of spontaneous myometrial activity. However, the exact mechanisms underlying these effects are uncertain and await clarification. The efflux of potassium ions terminates an action poten-

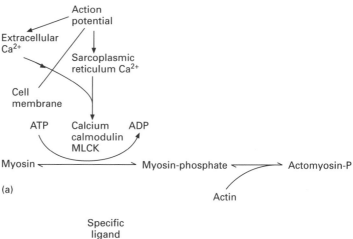

(a)

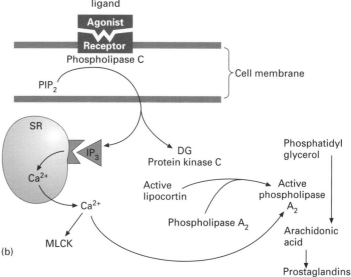

Fig. 11.3. (a) Physiology of uterine smooth muscle contraction. (b) Possible actions of second messengers in the initiation of uterine contractions. ADP: adenosine diphosphate; ATP: adenosine triphosphate; DG: diacylglycerol; IP_3: inositol 1,4,5-triphosphate; MLCK: myosin light chain kinase; PIP_2: phosphatidylinositol 4,5-bisphosphate; SR: Sarcoplasmic reticulum.

(b)

tial, and the resting membrane potential is dependent on the membrane permeability to potassium. The latter determines the ease of initiation of an action potential and hence myometrial contractility. There appear to be three types of potassium channels in animal myometrium, fast, intermediate and slow, the prevalence of each varying depending on the reproductive state. Calcium itself has been shown to activate potassium channels directly, these channels may be linked to β-adrenergic receptors. Potassium conductance determines the length of the plateau phase of the contraction and hence of the duration of the contraction itself.

Second messengers

In recent years, the important role of second messengers in regulating uterine contractility has become apparent. Second messengers transduce a stimulus at the outside of the cell membrane into an action in the cytoplasm. Hormones stimulating (or suppressing) uterine activity bind to specific receptors on the outside of the cell membrane. Cyclic monophosphates form an important component of these receptors, although their roles are still indeterminate. Activation of cyclic guanosine monophosphate (cGMP) was at one time thought to cause uterine contraction, but recently cGMP generation has been linked to myometrial relaxation through its ability to lower intracellular calcium levels. Agents such as nitric oxide have been suggested to work via cGMP. With advancing gestation cGMP generation is reduced and this is thought to underlie the diminished myometrial response to nitric oxide. Some ligands probably work through their interaction with phosphoinositides (a component of all cell membranes) [6–9]. The phosphoinositides are components of the cell membrane. Structurally, they have a glycerol backbone, with a fatty acid in position 1, arachidonic acid in position 2, and inositol in position 3. In a proportion of phosphoinositides, the inositol group is further phosphorylated at positions 4 and 5. The current view is that the binding of specific ligands to their receptors activates phospholipase C (PLC), resulting in hydrolysis of phosphoinositol-4,5-bisphosphonates to diacylglycerol and inositol 1-4,5-trisphosphate (IP_3). Although five different forms of PLC have been identified, it appears that a single isoform is active in the human amnion at term [10]. IP_3 binds to specific receptors linked to calcium channels on the sarcoplasmic reticulum and stimulates calcium release. IP_3 binding to its receptor is inhibited by calcium and its action terminated when it is metabolized by specific phosphomonoesterases to IP_2, IP_1 and inositol (see Fig. 11.3b).

Diacylglycerol has actions independent of IP_3. These include:

1 The activation of protein kinase C (PKC) which in turn activates phospholipase A (PLA) which releases arachidonic acid.

2 Inhibition of acyl transferase, which increases the levels of available arachidonic acid.

3 Its conversion to phosphatidic acid which may be involved in the later effects of receptor activation and in the mobilization of calcium.

4 Acting as a source of arachidonic acid for further prostaglandin (PG) production.

Cyclic adenosine monophosphate (cAMP) is currently thought to play an important role as a second messenger in myometrial relaxation by activating protein kinase A (PKA), which in turn phosphorylates myosin light-chain kinase. This decreases its affinity for the calcium–calmodulin complex and so reduces the phosphorylation of myosin. PKA may also reduce intracellular calcium concentrations by promoting its uptake into the sarcoplasmic reticulum and inhibiting the formation of IP_3.

Another important group of second messengers are the G-proteins. Guanine nucleotide-binding proteins link receptor activation to intracellular response. G-proteins consist of three main subunits, α, β, and γ, but multiple forms of each of the subunits exist. These proteins are linked to enzymes (adenylate cyclase,

Fig. 11.4. High magnification micrograph of a gap junction. Note seven-lined appearance. ×250 000. Reproduced from Chard and Grudzinskas [311], with permission.

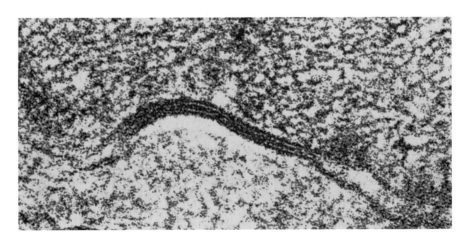

Table 11.1. The factors which influence myometrial contractility during pregnancy in the human. All of these hormones act through second messengers which alter the ion balance across the membrane and hence its resting potential.

Negative (produce relaxation)	Positive (produce contraction)	Variable
Progesterone	Oestrogen	PGE
Relaxin	Oxytocin	Relaxin/PG interaction
β_2-adrenergic stimulants	$PGF_{2\alpha}$	Corticotrophin releasing hormone (CRH)
Nitric oxide	Endothelin	
Adrenaline	Noradrenaline	Catecholamines

phospholipase C) and ion channels and amplify the initial response to receptor occupation through these linkages. Each of the subunits may be linked to an intracellular response. G-proteins may either stimulate (G_s) or inhibit (G_i) adenyl cyclase (see below). Pregnancy suppresses the link between G-proteins and phosphoinositide hydrolysis, which may contribute to the maintenance of myometrial quiescence.

Co-ordination of contracting muscle

To achieve an effective uterine contraction, the myometrium has to contract synchronously. This may be achieved in part by the inherent pattern of contraction and relaxation observed in isolated myometrial strips, but its co-ordination across the whole organ, in the absence of any specialized conduction tissue, is likely to be due to the presence of gap junctions between myometrial cells [10]. Gap junctions connect the interiors of two cells; each may contain thousands of channels (Fig. 11.4). These channels offer low resistance connections between cells which allow the rapid propagation of electrical activity. Structurally, they are made of bundles of the protein connexin [11]. They appear around the time of the onset of labour, whether at term or before [12] and their formation appears to be inhibited by progesterone and enhanced by both oestrogen and PGs [13,14].

Myometrial quiescence is promoted by reductions in pacemaker activity, cell excitability and cell connections. Thus, agents which promote calcium and potassium efflux, increase cAMP levels and close gap junctions such as β_2-agonists and relaxin promote quiescence. Many

hormones/chemicals affect uterine contractility (see Table 11.1). They include:

Endothelin

This group of peptides (endothelin 1-3 [ET-1,2,3]), better known for their effect on vascular tone, have several potential roles in the female reproductive tract. In the non-pregnant state, endothelin may be involved in menstruation and in the regulation of trophoblast invasion at the time of implantation [15]. During pregnancy, maternal circulating levels probably gradually increase and are even higher during labour [16]. Fetal levels are higher than those in the maternal circulation, but although they also rise with labour, there appears to be no relationship between the two compartments [16]. Amniotic fluid levels are highest of all, and like those in the maternal circulation, these rise with the onset of labour, whether at term or before, although whether this is a primary or secondary event is uncertain [17].

Endothelin receptors are widely expressed and have been reported to be present in myometrium, placenta, decidua and chorion, but not amnion [18]. Myometrial sensitivity to ET has been reported to increase with the onset of labour in the rat, and there is an associated increase in receptor expression [19]; however, there is no evidence in the human of a similar process [20]. Indeed, whether ET has a role in the onset of labour is disputed, but its decidual secretion is modulated by oxytocin (OT) [21], and pre-treatment of myometrial strips *in vitro* with ET enhances their response to OT [22], suggesting that the two inotropic agents may interact to increase myometrial contractility. Both

314 ET and OT act through the same pathway, to generate IP$_3$ and increase intra-cellular calcium levels [23,24].

Nitric oxide

Nitroglycerin and sodium nitroprusside were shown to inhibit myometrial contractions before they were recognized to be nitric oxide donors [25]. Animal studies have shown that L-arginine, sodium nitroprusside and nitric oxide itself inhibits spontaneous myometrial activity *in vitro*, and that this effect is reduced by an inhibitor of guanylate cyclase [26], suggesting that a nitric oxide-cGMP system may modulate myometrial activity. However, the inhibition of Nitric oxide synthase (NOS) *in vivo* does not alter myometrial activity [27]. Thus, nitric oxide may play a role in the maintenance of myometrial quiescence during pregnancy [28,29], but it does not appear to be essential under normal circumstances. For a more extensive review, the reader is referred to the review by Morris *et al.* [29]. However, one short report has suggested that nitric oxide donors may inhibit preterm labour in the human [30]; the results of several large randomized studies currently in progress are awaited with interest.

Catecholamines

Stimulation of α-receptors is excitatory, while β$_2$-receptor activation is inhibitory. The α effect is probably mediated both through increased chloride conductance, which depolarizes the membrane, and prolongs the plateau part of the action potential by increased calcium conductance. The β$_2$ effect is due to membrane stabilization through increased potassium conductance and increased cAMP production [31].

The cervix

The contrast between the quiescence of the uterus during pregnancy and its activity during labour is enormous; the contrast between the function of the cervix during the antepartum period and during labour is equally great. Its function changes from that of a firm, almost cartilaginous, structure to that of an elastic organ which can stretch to a diameter of 10 cm or more during labour, and then return almost to its original dimensions.

The recognition that the cervix is a collagenous tissue quite different from the main body of the uterus is primarily attributable to the work of Danforth [32]. Amino acid analysis indicates that as much as 80% of the total protein of the non-pregnant cervix is collagen [33]. Histology shows a highly organized arrangement of collagen fibres with few cellular elements [34,35] and electron microscopy demonstrates that in the first trimester of pregnancy the collagen fibres are arranged in bundles within a regular matrix (Fig. 11.5). This presumably accounts for the structural rigidity of cervical tissue.

Tissue distensibility is governed primarily by the interfibrillar ground substance, composed predominantly of glycosaminoglycans. Present evidence suggests that hormones which act upon the cervix do so largely by acting upon the ground substance. It is important to recognize that the uterus cannot be simply divided into a muscular portion, comprising the fundus-corpus and a fibrous structure, the cervix. There is a gradual fall in the smooth muscle content from the fundus to the cervix, shown by histological analysis [36]. The isthmus, from which the lower segment is formed, has a lower muscle content than the corpus and this morphological arrangement of tissues must be correlated with function. There is a marked difference in the smooth muscle to collagen ratio between different regions of the cervix, as measured by actomyosin content, the muscle content being highest at the uterine end, and the collagen content being highest at the distal end [35] (Fig. 11.6). It is probable that changes in the collagen content of the cervix are necessary before normal human birth can take place. Studies have shown that women in oxytocin-augmented labour with failure of the cervix to dilate have higher collagen levels and lower collagen solubility measures than women in normally progressive labour [37]. Serum collagenase levels support this hypothesis; at term, levels are double those of the non-pregnant state, even when the cervix remains unripe [38]. The levels are quadrupled when the cervix ripens, and in labour, levels are twice as high in women progressing normally compared with women progressing slowly.

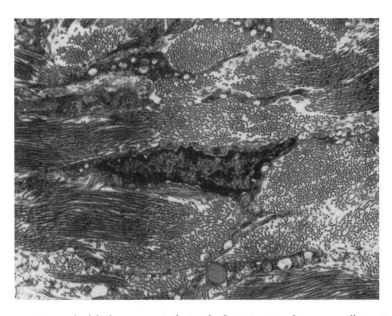

Fig. 11.5. An electron micrograph of the human cervix during the first trimester of pregnancy, illustrating the highly organized collagen fibrillar arrangement. A fibroblast, with long cytoplasmic projections can be seen in the centre of the field (Parry, Johnstone & Ellwood, unpublished work). ×8500.

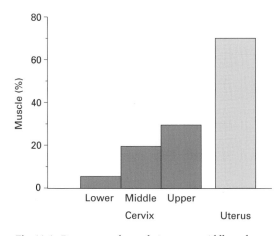

Fig. 11.6. Percentage of muscle in upper, middle and lower regions of the cervix, and the uterus, as estimated by histology. Measurement of actomyosin content also reveals this gradual reduction in cervical muscle.

Although collagen makes up 10–15% of the wet weight of the cervix, the proteoglycans, which constitute only about 0.2%, are probably very important because of their extraordinary ability to hold water [39]. For example, 1 g of hyaluronan can bind almost 1 l of water. The proteoglycans are made up of a variety of protein cores (varying in size from 5000 to 600 000 Da), to which from one to 100 glycosaminoglycans are attached. Various domains on the molecules attach to matrix macromolecules such as fibronectin and cytokines such as epidermal growth factor. The probable primary role of the proteoglycans is to attract water into the interstices of the collagen and matrix macromolecule framework, distending it and giving it a tense structure. Breakdown of the matrix structure induced, for example, by oestrogens, prostaglandins, hyaluronidase or collagenase, releases the pressure, allowing the tissue to become flexible, distensible and elastic. It has also been suggested that these substances change the ratio of proteoglycan small 1 (PG-S1) to PG-S2, which in turn changes the organization and mechanical properties of collagen.

Recent work has implicated a bewildering variety of cytokines and enzymes which may also be implicated in cervical ripening. For example, recent work has shown up to fourfold increases in the mRNA levels of insulin-like growth factor-1 (IGF1) in the cervix as term approaches [40], a phenomenon which in the rat appears to be under oestrogenic control. IGF1 may initiate a signalling cascade resulting in collagenase release. Vaginal fluid contains a wide range of bacteria, and it has long been known that the cervix is heavily infiltrated with granulocytes, especially when there is premature rupture of membranes. It has been assumed that this is simply a response to potential infection, but the demonstration of steadily increasing amounts of granulocyte elastase in the cervix as term approaches suggests that this may be one way in which infection promotes preterm labour [41].

The cervix has a small but significant muscle component which has been estimated by histological methods at approximately 10% [42]. There has been considerable controversy over the exact arrangement of this muscle and the accuracy of the method of analysis [43]. The functional significance of cervical smooth muscle is unclear and this question has provoked considerable discussion. The cervix will exhibit spontaneous contractile activity both *in vivo* [44] and *in vitro* [45] and is reactive to certain pharmacological agents, particularly ergometrine and prostaglandins. Hughesdon's observations on the arrangement of muscle at the level of the internal os may suggest an anatomical basis for a functional sphincter [34], although there is great individual variation in the degree of muscle organization. This author, however, does suggest that the sparse cervical muscle may become functionally more significant as the connective tissue framework loses structural rigidity during softening, and he concludes that the external muscular layers could influence the extent of cervical dilatation. More recent studies of the muscular properties of the non-pregnant cervix and myometrium have shown that contractile strength is 40 times higher at the fundus than at the distal cervix, weight for weight. It is 30 times higher in the isthmus and five times higher in the proximal cervix [46]. None the less, the studies of Olah and colleagues [47,48] have shown that in early labour, it appears that the muscular activity of the cervix is sufficient that the cervix actually constricts with contractions in early labour (before and up to 4 cm dilatation only). It may be that cervical contractions have an important role in maintaining cervical integrity during Braxton Hicks contractions in pregnancy before the onset of labour, and they may also have a part to play in remodelling the cervix during the latent phase of labour.

In summary, it is important to appreciate that the tissues which make up the uterus are not the same for all regions. In the main body of the uterus and the cervix there are smooth muscle and connective tissue components, with predominance of a different component in each structure. Whether the muscular and fibrous elements can be influenced by the same control mechanisms is considered later. However, these basic differences in structure must be taken into consideration if we are to understand the factors controlling the function of the whole organ.

Hormonal control of early pregnancy
(see Fig. 11.7)

Ovarian function, the corpus luteum and progesterone

The beginning of pregnancy is timed differently in fetus and mother. For the fetus, pregnancy starts at the moment of fertilization, but maternal recognition of pregnancy probably occurs several days later when the the blastocyst in the fallopian tube first starts secreting substances which are likely to have an effect on maternal tissues. Experiments using cultured trophoblast suggest that such signals could include corticotrophin-releasing hormone (CRH), β-endorphin, melanocyte-stimulating hormone, and dynorphin A (all secretions also produced in the hypothalamus) (see also Chapter 17). In addition, gonadotrophin-releasing hormone (GnRH) and inhibin are secreted, and they may act in a local paracrine way to regulate human chorionic gonadotrophin (hCG) secretion. GnRH initiates events which transform the corpus luteum of the menstrual cycle, from which the ovum and blastocyst were derived, into the corpus luteum of pregnancy. The lifespan of the corpus luteum (which begins to regress about 8 weeks after ovulation if pregnancy does not occur), is thus prolonged.

The cyclical nature of ovarian function is arrested and the endocrine conditions essential

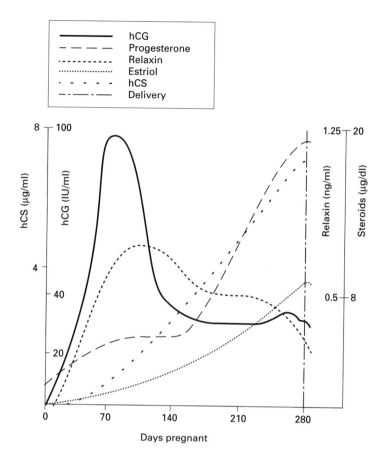

Fig. 11.7. Hormonal changes in early pregnancy. From Ganong [312].

for the pregnancy to continue are maintained. The corpus luteum secretes mainly the steroid hormone progesterone, which has been identified in ovarian venous blood throughout human pregnancy [49], although the levels at term are only just detectable, and very much lower than the levels in the first half of pregnancy.

The essential role of the corpus luteum in the maintenance of early human pregnancy has been recognized since the early years of this century through studies on the effects of its surgical removal. In recent times there has been debate about the earliest stage of pregnancy at which removal of the corpus luteum no longer leads to spontaneous abortion (see also Chapter 17). Tulsky and Koff [50] removed corpora lutea between the 35th day and 77th day of pregnancy in 14 patients; two women aborted spontaneously having had their operations on the 39th and 41st day of pregnancy. The patient operated

on at 35 days continued her pregnancy until it was terminated artificially on the 44th day; the other pregnancies also continued until terminated 1–2 weeks later. Csapo et al. [51] did not fully substantiate these findings in 12 patients who had total removal of luteal tissue in the first trimester either by local excision or by osophorectomy. The group of seven patients who aborted had a mean ± SEM length of pregnancy of 49 ± 2 days (range, 42–57 days) at operation; the other five patients who did not abort averaged 61 ± 4 days at operation (range, 52–74 days). These findings therefore suggest that the corpus luteum is essential for the maintenance of human pregnancy until somewhere between days 50 and 60 (calculated from the last menstrual period) when the placenta becomes the main progesterone-producing organ. It has been suggested that the discrepancy between the two studies could be due to a failure of the sur-

318

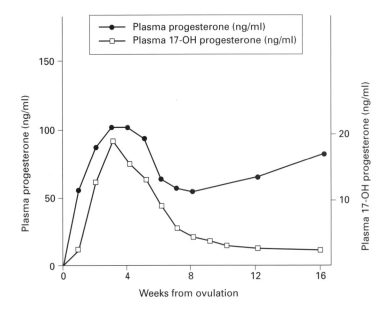

Fig. 11.8. Plasma levels of progesterone and 17α-hydroxyprogesterone in early pregnancy. Ovulation induced by human menopausal gonadotrophins and chorionic gonadotrophin. Redrawn from Shearman [54].

geon to recognize the presence of accessory corpora lutea (found in five of the 24 patients in one series [52]). Biochemical evidence is in general agreement with this timing of the luteal–placental shift in progesterone production.

The ability of the corpus luteum to synthesize steroid hormones is best reflected in early pregnancy by measurement of circulating concentrations of the progesterone metabolite 17α-hydroxyprogesterone [53], since the placenta has either no, or a very limited, capacity for 17α-hydroxylation (measurement of progesterone concentrations will reflect both corpus luteum and placental function). The hormonal transition from dependence on the corpus luteum to placental steroid productions is illustrated in Fig. 11.8 [54] by the dip in peripheral progesterone levels 6–8 weeks after ovulation, followed by a secondary rise; 17α-hydroxyprogesterone levels reach their peak 3–4 weeks after ovulation and then fall without a subsequent increase. The secondary rise in progesterone levels is accompanied by a secondary rise in oestradiol-17β levels [55,56], indicating rapidly increasing steroid production by the trophoblast 8–10 weeks after ovulation. The pattern of peripheral plasma progesterone and 17α-hydroxyprogesterone levels found in pregnancy following ovulation induction is similar to that in spontaneous pregnancies, although levels are

several-fold lower in the latter [55–57]. Csapo and his colleagues clearly showed that progesterone from the corpus luteum is indispensable for the maintenance of early human pregnancy [51,52] by demonstrating a continuous fall in circulating progesterone levels along with development of increasingly powerful uterine activity in patients who abort following luteectomy. This is in contrast to excision of the corpus luteum without abortion when there is a transient decrease followed by a rise of progesterone levels with no change in uterine activity. In addition, progesterone replacement therapy for 7 days (200 mg intramuscularly daily in oil) apparently prevented abortion in a group of seven patients who had a surgical excision of the corpus luteum; they showed increased plasma progesterone and maintained oestradiol levels on treatment, whereas surgery alone led to abortion in seven of 11 other patients not given progesterone. Replacement therapy with oestradiol-17β did not prevent abortion in yet another group of women after excision. The essential contribution of the corpus luteum to circulating progesterone levels and to the prevention of expulsion of the embryo from the uterus in the early weeks of human pregnancy seems unequivocal.

What prolongs the lifespan of the corpus luteum and stimulates progesterone secretion until the conceptus has reached a stage of development when it becomes autonomous? Classically, hCG was assigned this essential role and there is a good deal of evidence that hCG may be luteotrophic or at least be part of a luteotrophic complex. Evidence includes observations that injections of hCG will prolong the luteal phase of the menstrual cycle [58–61], although in most cases by no more than several days. Thus, it does not mimic the much greater prolongation of activity of the corpus luteum of pregnancy. The endocrine conditions of early pregnancy, however, are very difficult to replicate. Human pituitary luteinizing hormone (LH) given to women during the luteal phase of the cycle will also postpone menstruation in a similar way to hCG [60], both hormones lengthening the cycle by 8–9 days. Human chorionic gonadotrophin and LH treatment also raise plasma progestagen levels two to three times higher than in control cycles, suggesting that both are capable of stimulating progesterone synthesis by the normal corpus luteum *in vivo* [60].

If hCG is luteotrophic, then it must be produced in advance of the expected time of regression of the corpus luteum. Both bioassays and immunoassays (e.g. ELISA tests) detect the appearance of hCG in the peripheral plasma and the urine often by 7 days after ovulation, that is before the initiation of implantation of the blastocyst. The site of production of hCG is probably the trophoblast and it has been suggested that hCG may act synergistically with other placental hormones such as human placental lactogen (hPL). The reason why the human corpus luteum regresses in early pregnancy, at a time when both hCG and hPL levels are rising, remains puzzling [53,55,56]. On the other hand, biochemical and morphological studies of the corpus luteum in pregnancy suggest that it continues to function until term. Although the size of the corpus luteum at term is only half that achieved during the luteal phase of the menstrual cycle [62], it secretes progesterone throughout pregnancy [49,63] and follicular growth and atresia continue until term [64,65]. Follicular growth can be stimulated by administration of exogenous gonadotrophins near term [66] but whether hCG plays any part in maintaining the function of the corpus luteum throughout pregnancy remains unknown.

Another mechanism which may be important in maintaining early pregnancy is the apparent suppression of prostaglandin concentrations in decidual tissue [67,68]. In the presence of a conceptus, both prostaglandin F (PGF) and prostaglandin E (PGE) concentrations in the decidua of early pregnancy are lower than those measured in the endometrium at any stage of the normal menstrual cycle. In the midsecretory phase of the menstrual cycle, increased production of oestradiol and progesterone is associated with, and may be causally related to, increased concentrations of PGF in the endometrium. The expected similar effect of increased steroid hormone production in early pregnancy on decidual prostaglandin concentration seems to be inhibited by some factor or factors originating from the conceptus. The prostaglandin inhibitory factor has yet to be defined, but current evidence suggests that it may be a glycoprotein called lipocortin [69].

Relaxin

The hormone relaxin, a polypeptide of low molecular weight whose major source is the corpus luteum of the sow, has been identified as a secretory product of the human corpus luteum in early and late pregnancy [70]. Although there have been claims that relaxin may be produced by the decidua, it appears in the human to be solely produced by the corpus luteum (circulating relaxin levels disappear following luteectomy in late pregnancy). It is accordingly suggested that relaxin is the only hormone in the peripheral circulation that can be used as an index of the function of the corpus luteum in pregnancy. In view of its myometrial inhibitory properties in some species, relaxin may play a role in the maintenance of early human pregnancy, although this is speculative at present, and the true function of this hormone has yet to be clarified. The relaxin receptor has recently been identified on human myometrial cells and in fetal membranes [71,72], but the postreceptor effects remain unclear. Relaxin may exert an effect through several potential postreceptor mechanisms; these include cAMP generation, the opening of membrane potassium channels and a reduction in intracellular calcium levels. Relaxin has been shown to generate cAMP in several situations, but the time course of cAMP generation appears to follow that of mechanical relaxation of the uterus and so its specific role is difficult to dissect out from the global changes occurring in this situation [73,74]. Indeed, *in vivo*, despite producing myometrial relaxation as effectively as β_2-agonists, cAMP levels increased relatively little [75]. However, relaxin does inhibit myosin light-chain kinase activity suggesting that some of its action is mediated through cAMP. However, other mechanisms must be responsible for its acute myometrial effects. Relaxin may open potassium channels and hyperpolarize the plasma membrane, but the evidence for this is conflicting [76]. Relaxin has been shown to increase calcium efflux and antagonize oxytocin-induced increases in intracellular calcium and IP_3 levels in animal studies [77,78]. Thus, relaxin does cause myometrial relaxation, but the exact mechanisms involved are uncertain and the physiological importance of this inhibition, certainly in the human, are unproved.

Maintenance of pregnancy

Maintenance of pregnancy can occur only if the uterus can accommodate the growing products of conception by expansion. To do this, the uterine muscle grows enormously, becomes more compliant and uncoils its spiralling muscle bundles.

During pregnancy, the growth in weight of the uterus is spectacular. Its mean weight increases from about 50 to 1100 g at term, a 20-fold increase [79]. Myometrial growth is probably almost entirely due to hypertrophy of muscle cells although there may be hyperplasia in early pregnancy. The growing conceptus is a powerful stimulus to myometrial growth and evidence from animals suggests that distension alone can maintain both the function and the synthesis of the contractile proteins of the myometrium. Although hormones, notably oestrogens, can also have a growth-promoting effect and can regulate actomyosin synthesis, stretch induced by the enlarging uterine contents seems to be a major stimulus to growth. Clinical evidence of uterine size in women with an extrauterine pregnancy supports these findings, King [80] reporting that, with a full-term living fetus in the extrauterine cavity, the size of the uterus was equivalent to that of a 3-month intrauterine pregnancy.

The greater compliance of pregnant myometrium compared with non-pregnant myometrium [81] means that pregnant muscle can be stretched much more than non-pregnant muscle, without losing the ability to develop maximal active tension. This property may depend more on changes in the connective tissue component of the uterus than in alteration in the properties of the contractile protein elements.

The hormonal stimulus to increased growth and compliance of the uterine muscle in pregnancy probably results mainly from the interaction between oestrogens and progesterone which are derived initially from the corpus luteum but later largely from placental synthesis. In general, oestrogen affects growth through effects on the synthesis of the proteins of the contractile mechanism and the enzymes concerned in energy provision. Progesterone is involved during early pregnancy in the preparation of the endometrium for implantation of the ovum and then throughout most of pregnancy with the maintenance of a quiescent myometrium, this block on myometrial excitability being exercised through the excitation and conduction mechanisms of the muscle cells.

Changes in the oestrogen to progesterone ratio and absolute reductions in the circulating levels of progesterone have long been thought to be important in the genesis of labour. Early reports of falling progesterone levels in the circulation prior to the onset of labour have not been confirmed [82–85]; however, there is a rise in the saliva oestriol to progesterone (E3/P) ratio (which has been shown to reflect the unbound unconjugated or free levels in the circulation) in around 70% of women before the onset of labour at term [84], and this rise occurs inappropriately in at least 50% of women in preterm labour with intact membranes. Two studies have suggested that exogenous progesterone may inhibit preterm labour [86,87]. Furthermore, the ability of the progesterone antagonist, mifepristone (previously known as RU486), to induce labour supports the notion that progesterone acts to maintain human pregnancy [88,89]. It has been demonstrated that, at least in part, this effect is due to accelerated ripening (increased distensibility) of the cervix [90]. The in-vitro effects of mifepristone suggest that progesterone not only inhibits prostaglandin synthesis, but also enhances prostaglandin dehydrogenase activity.

The rise in the salivary E3/P ratio does not occur in women who continue their pregnancy post-term and require induction. Animal studies suggest that oestrogens promote oxytocin and oxytocin receptor mRNA expression, prostaglandin synthesis, and gap junction formation, which would tend to promote the onset of labour [91]. However, controversy surrounds the question of whether oestrogen, given intravenously or topically, is able to induce labour. Some studies report cervical ripening, an increase in uterine activity and increased responsiveness to oxytocin, while others do not [92,93]. In-vitro studies, using human tissue, confirm the suggested role of progesterone in the maintenance of pregnancy [94]. They also suggest that progesterone metabolites are even more potent supressors of myometrial activity and that they may act through the release of γ-aminobutyric acid [95]. Oestrogens appear also to inhibit myometrial contractility, by inhibiting receptor-operated calcium channels and the release of calcium from intracellular stores [94]. It has been suggested that progesterone and oestrogen may act in a paracrine manner, such that tissue changes are not apparent systemically. According to this theory, there is local progesterone withdrawal and increased oestrogen synthesis, occurring with or before the onset of labour [96]. Currently, the role of oestrogen and progesterone in human pregnancy remains unclear. Although the weight of evidence supports the idea of progesterone maintaining pregnancy, the place of oestrogen in the onset of labour is uncertain.

Measurement of uterine activity

Perhaps the most useful characteristic of uterine activity to measure would be the tension in the myometrium itself; unfortunately, this has proved impossible in the human as the techniques required would be unacceptably invasive. Alternative measures have included electromyography and amniotic fluid pressure (intrauterine pressure [IUP]) measurement; the latter has proved to be the most valuable. The history of IUP measurement was reviewed by Bell in 1952 [97]. It was first performed successfully by Schatz in 1872 using a bag inserted into the uterus and connected by tubing to a pressure manometer. In 1952, Williams and Stallworthy replaced the bag and tubing by a fluid-filled, open-ended polythene catheter [98]. In due course, the mercury manometers and smoked drums used to record contractions as late as the 1960s gave way to electrical strain-gauge transducers connected to ink pen chart recorders, but the next major advance was the introduction of catheter-tipped intrauterine pressure transducers by Steer et al. in the mid-1970s [99]. The safety and simplicity of this technique has led to a resurgence of interest in IUP measurement and the physiology of uterine action.

Even using modern techniques, however, the measurement of IUP cannot give a precise assessment of uterine action in terms which can be related directly to uterine muscle tension. Caldeyro-Barcia et al. [100] measured uterine wall tension using both intramyometrial balloon catheters and external tocodynamometers, and compared the values with IUP. They concluded that the relation was complex, and depended upon the co-ordination of the various parts of the uterus and the efficiency with which the presenting part of the fetus sealed the cervix. Even the measurement of IUP itself has uncertainties; Knoke et al. [101] have reported a difference of up to 20% in peak contraction pressure recorded via two simultaneously recording intrauterine catheters, a finding corroborated by Arulkumaran et al. [102] and Chua et al. [103]. The reasons for this are not clear; it has been speculated that the catheters/transducers might be in two separate fluid compartments in the uterus, that fluid-filled catheters might become blocked with vernix, or that direct pressure on one or both of the intrauterine transducers might produce artefactual readings. Whatever the cause, it appears to be random, because cumulative measures of uterine active pressure area vary little between catheters (<5%) despite the large variations between one contraction and the next.

322   However, even if we knew the intrauterine pressure exactly, we could still not deduce precisely the uterine muscle tension being developed. This is because the system often leaks; if the presenting part is not a water-tight fit with the cervix, fluid will escape during a contraction, lowering the pressure developed and leading to an underestimation of the muscle wall tension being developed. Even if there is a water-tight seal, differences in cervical compliance will modulate the relationship between the uterine muscle wall tension and the IUP developed, as has been elegantly demonstrated by Gee *et al.* [104] (when the uterus contracts, the cervix gives way to differing degrees; the more it gives way, the lower is the rise in IUP for a given rise in wall tension).

Recently, it has been shown that measuring the force between the presenting part and the cervix is a better predictor of the eventual mode of delivery than the measurement of IUP [105–107]. Force between two (more or less) solid objects, the head and cervix, is unlike that in a fluid, such as amniotic fluid. Force in a fluid is transmitted in all directions (as 'pressure') but between two solids, the local pressure is exerted only at right angles to the surface of the solid. It therefore has a direction (vector) and hence is described as a vector quantity. The transducers used are pins (like little mushrooms) pressing on miniature strain gauges and mounted at 2 cm intervals along a moulded polyurethane strip 40 cm long, 1.4 cm wide and 0.5 cm thick. This strip is passed through the cervix and lies between the fetal head and the cervix/lower segment of the uterus (Fig. 11.9). The pins face the cervix and measure the force with which the fetal head is being pushed onto the cervix. As they are measuring this push (force) and not pressure (transducers record only about 5 g force for each 100 mmHg pressure in the fluid around them; forces up to 100 g weight can be recorded in labour), the transducers record the effect not only of the rise in intra-amniotic pressure pushing the head down onto the cervix, but also the direct transmission of force down the trunk of the baby and the direct traction of the fundal muscle on the lower segment and cervix, neither of which are reflected in changes in the intrauterine pressure. Not only is the absolute value of the head to cervix force more closely related to the rate of cervical dilatation than the

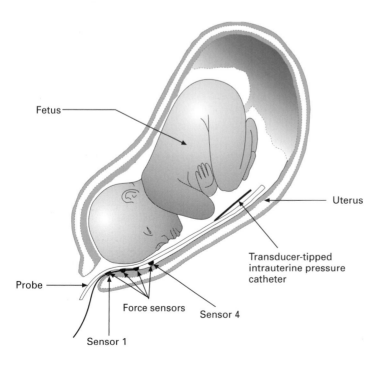

Fetus

Uterus

Transducer-tipped intrauterine pressure catheter

Probe

Force sensors   Sensor 4

Sensor 1

Fig. 11.9. Diagrammatic view of the head-to-cervix force probe within the uterus and the relative position of the sensors.

intra-amniotic pressure, but the ratio between the force and pressure (the higher the force for a given intra-uterine pressure, the better the progress) and the spread of forces (the wider the better) also give useful information about how the head to cervix interaction is working. The relationships between these forces and the biochemical changes in the cervix during labour are currently being investigated.

Evolution of uterine activity during pregnancy

There is a gradual evolution of uterine activity (as assessed by IUP measurement) throughout pregnancy. As early as 7 weeks, the uterus displays some activity, with contractions of very high frequency (about 2 per minute) but very low intensity (about 1–1.5 kPa) [108]. This pattern continues until about 20 weeks [109]

but thereafter the uterine contractions increase both in frequency and amplitude until term, the increase being most rapid in the last 6–8 weeks of pregnancy [108–110] (Fig. 11.10). This change is thought to be mediated by the appearance of gap junctions within the myometrium [4]. The appearance of gap junctions seems to depend on a complex interaction of the changes in oestrogen, progesterone and prostaglandin levels which occur in late pregnancy. The appearance of low frequency but high pressure contractions is often appreciable to the mother and they are clinically termed Braxton Hicks contractions. Although they may be as strong as labour contractions, they are not normally painful, as the cervix does not yet dilate appreciably during each contraction. The pain of labour is associated with cervical dilatation, and depends therefore on the increase in cervical compliance referred to clinically as ripening.

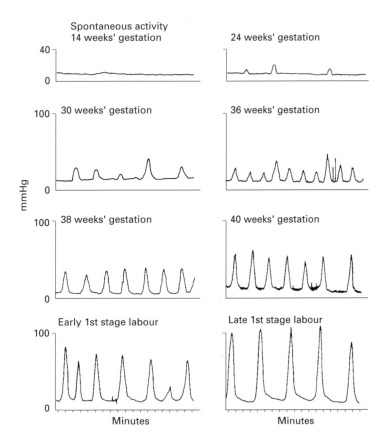

Fig. 11.10. The evolution of spontaneous uterine activity in human pregnancy. Recordings of intrauterine pressure changes showing development of contractions of increasing frequency and intensity throughout gestation and in labour. Modified from data of Csapo and Sauvage [108].

Sensitivity of the uterus to oxytocin and prostaglandins

Uterine sensitivity to oxytocin is dependent on both gestational age and the level of spontaneous uterine activity [110–113]. Accordingly, the uterus is normally very insensitive to oxytocin up to midpregnancy, and very high infusion rates of oxytocin (up to 128 mU/min) may have to be administered to stimulate uterine contractions in order, for example, to induce abortion. However, by 30 weeks' gestation, uterine sensitivity has increased markedly and the infusion rate of oxytocin required has fallen to as little as 8 mU/min; by 40 weeks, 4 mU/min is usually sufficient to increase uterine activity to levels similar to those seen in spontaneous labour [114]. At this latter gestation, there is some correlation between cervical ripeness and the infusion rate of oxytocin required to reproduce uterine activity [115], but considerable individual variation remains. Thus, when any individual woman is given oxytocin for therapeutic reasons, the infusion rate cannot be calculated *a priori* but must be determined by measurement of uterine activity and titration to find the most effective dose.

In contrast to the very variable sensitivity of the uterus to oxytocin at different stages of pregnancy, prostaglandins E2 and F2$_\alpha$ will induce contractions at any gestational age [116]. This supports the concept that prostaglandins represent the final mediator of uterine contractions by direct action on muscle cells either through effects on myometrial cAMP or through intracellular effects on calcium mobilization [117].

Cervical changes before labour

As uterine activity builds up during pregnancy, the cervix gradually softens and the canal dilates. Cervical softening seems to take place at an early stage of pregnancy, followed, in general, by some dilatation of the external os which is clinically detectable by about 24 weeks, and opening of the internal os in one-third of primigravidae by 32 weeks [118] (Fig. 11.11). Effacement is usually a late phenomenon, occurring mainly in the last few weeks. These gradual

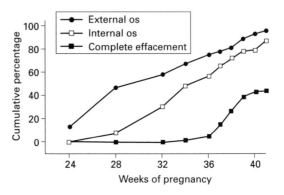

Fig. 11.11. Cumulative percentage of primigravid patients (*n* = 77) in whom an index finger could be passed through the external or internal cervical os or in whom the cervix was fully effaced from 24 weeks of pregnancy until the onset of labour.

changes in pregnancy seem peculiar to the human cervix, as the cervix of most animals studied remains firm and closed until shortly before delivery. The changes observed in the human cervix may reflect a continuing hormonal influence, and correlate well with the gradual rise in circulating levels of oestrogens.

The definition of abnormality of cervical function during pregnancy poses problems since we understand so little of the physiological changes. In late pregnancy there is remarkable variation in the clinical changes in the cervix between patients. Labour may start in one patient with a long, firm, undilated cervical canal, whereas another patient may have had a fully effaced, soft, dilating cervix for several weeks before labour starts. The clinical state of the cervix is thus a poor indicator of the gestation at which labour will start. Further studies are required to identify the factors which contribute to cervical malfunction during pregnancy, and, in particular, any hormonal basis for the observed changes.

Control of onset of labour

The timing of the onset of labour in humans would appear to be less precise than in many other species. Analysis of the length of gestation in almost 50 000 women in Amsterdam [119] who began labour spontaneously and delivered a single living fetus showed a reasonably Gaussian distribution, slightly skewed to the left, with a mean length of 39.6 weeks (Fig. 11.12). The majority of births occurred within 2 weeks of the mean (81.2%, with 12.6% before 38 weeks and 6.2% after 42 weeks). This span of 6 weeks around term when most human births occur is in agreement with data calculated from the likely date of conception according to basal body temperature charts. In two series it was suggested that most spontaneous term deliveries occur 250–285 days [120] or 241–288 days [121] after presumed ovulation. This wide range of the normal duration of pregnancy is of importance when we come to consider the controlling mechanisms for initiating labour at term; it then becomes obvious that we are not looking for a timing mechanism which imposes a high degree of precision on the process.

Fetal influences at the onset of labour

This timing mechanism might reside in the fetal brain, as suggested by the findings of Honnebier and Swaab [119] in human anencephaly without hydramnios and where labour began spontaneously. The distribution of gestation in 29 such pregnancies with an anencephalic fetus was very different from controls, although the mean gestational length was identical in the two groups (Fig. 11.13) with as many births in anencephaly occurring several weeks before as after term. These findings are similar to the wide distribution of gestational length observed in experimentally produced anencephalic fetal rhesus monkeys [122] but were different from earlier reports [123–126] which had concentrated on the association between anencephaly and prolonged pregnancy. However, it would appear that, in the absence of the fetal brain, precise control over gestational length is lost, although mechanisms for initiating labour seem to be intact in many anencephalics.

Despite these data casting doubt on any hypothesis that the human fetal brain might trigger the onset of labour, the concept (attributed to Hippocrates) that the mammalian fetus might play an active role in initiating its own birth has attracted a vast amount of animal experimental work in the past 35 years. That the activity of the fetal pituitary might initiate parturition seemed possible from evidence of the extreme prolongation of pregnancy in cattle,

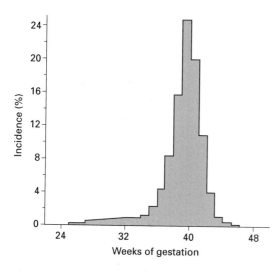

Fig. 11.12. Frequency distribution of gestational length for a group of 50 000 pregnant women with spontaneous onset of labour.

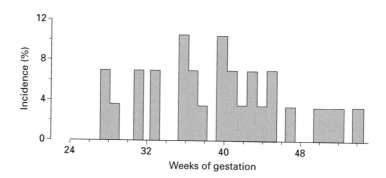

Fig. 11.13. Frequency distribution of gestational length for a group of 29 women with an anencephalic fetus, no hydramnios and spontaneous onset of labour.

326 sheep and humans where the fetus had a congenital malformation affecting the hypothalamohypophysial area. Liggins' elegant experimental work [127] on sheep during the 1960s established that fetal hypophysectomy *in utero* prevented parturition in that species and subsequent work by several groups described the sequence of endocrine events that preceded the onset of labour in sheep [128]. In summary, parturition in sheep is initiated by a surge of cortisol secretion by the fetal adrenal cortex which acts on placental enzymes to activate the biosynthetic pathway from progesterone through to oestrogens. Thus, placental secretion of progesterone falls as it is increasingly metabolized to oestrogens whose secretion rises. This rapid change in the steroid hormone environment stimulates release of prostaglandins both from the placenta and myometrium, increases the sensitivity of the myometrium to oxytocin and initiates uterine contractions which become powerful enough to expel the fetus — provided that softening and dilatation of the cervix has occurred.

The situation is much less clear in the human fetus, however, and we are still uncertain whether or not the human fetal adrenal gland plays any role in the initiation of labour. Most of the evidence now suggests that, if it is involved, it is unlikely that increased secretion of the glucocorticoid, cortisol, plays a major part. Labour can certainly start where there is congenital absence of the fetal adrenals [129] and, although there can be prolongation of pregnancy with congenital idiopathic adrenal hypoplasia and normal pituitary function [130], labour does begin. Another approach has been to measure cortisol levels in the umbilical circulation at birth; support can be found both for and against cord cortisol levels being higher after spontaneous than after induced labour. Murphy was the first to suggest that cortisol levels in cord blood were significantly higher if labour had started spontaneously than if it was induced [131], and she subsequently showed higher umbilical arterial than venous levels after spontaneous labour—suggesting cortisol secretion by the fetus [132]. These and the many studies that followed can all be criticized on the grounds that labour itself (spontaneous or induced) may have

caused the changes in fetal cortisol levels rather than that the raised levels preceded labour, and subsequent evidence suggested that this might indeed be the case [133]. In addition, cord levels of cortisone at delivery may merely reflect maternal cortisone levels and the maternal stress of labour, since the human placenta possesses the enzyme 11β-hydroxysteroid dehydrogenase [134] which would convert maternal cortisol to cortisone on its transplacental passage [135,136].

Similar criticisms can be made of the interpretation that the rising levels of cortisol in amniotic fluid in late pregnancy reflect increasing fetal adrenal cortisol secretion [137], since maternal cortisol levels are also increasing at this time. One study overcame these criticisms by obtaining serial samples of fetal scalp blood through an amnioscope starting at 2 cm cervical dilatation [133]; there was no difference in mean plasma cortisol concentrations in fetal blood obtained early in spontaneous or induced labour (Fig. 11.14) although there was a continuous rise in fetal plasma cortisol as labour advanced, the

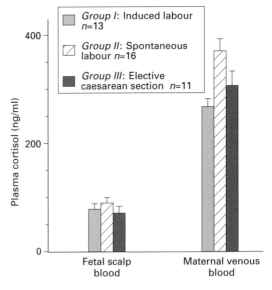

Fig. 11.14. Mean (SEM) plasma cortisol concentrations in simultaneously obtained fetal scalp blood and maternal venous blood at induction of labour and early in spontaneous labour compared to cortisol concentrations in arterial cord blood and maternal venous blood at elective caesarean section. From Gennser *et al.* [313].

rise being more rapid in spontaneous labour. This study measured total unconjugated cortisol but other studies suggest that there may be an increase in unbound cortisol [138]. The only criticism of the scalp blood cortisol study [133] would be of the methodology which did not include chromatography; and cortisol levels measured by the Swedish authors at elective caesarean section [133] were three to four times higher than those measured after chromatography by Murphy [131], suggesting lack of specificity in the Swedish workers' cortisol assay. Despite this criticism, that study produced the most convincing evidence that spontaneous onset of labour is not likely to be preceded by any dramatic rise in total cortisol in the fetal circulation.

Further evidence against increased glucocorticoid activity initiating human labour comes from studies where exogenous corticosteroid has been given to the mother or injected into the amniotic fluid at or after term. Maternal administration of betamethasone or dexamethasone in large doses in late pregnancy seems to have no effect on the length of gestation, although there is a dramatic reduction in maternal plasma oestrogen and cortisol levels [139] (Fig. 11.15) and in cord cortisol levels [140] — but without effect on progesterone. Betamethasone crosses the human placenta and is likely to suppress both fetal and maternal adrenal steroid hormone synthesis. In particular, it suppresses dehydroepiandrosterone sulphate (DHAS), the major precursor of placental oestrogen synthesis, so that circulating oestrogen levels in the mother fall, but this seems to have no effect on placental progesterone synthesis. In the human placenta, glucocorticoids do not induce the enzymes produced at term in the sheep placenta and which lead to the fall in progesterone and rise in oestrogens in the maternal circulation in that species. The biosynthetic pathway for oestrogen synthesis in late pregnancy is thus very different in the two species, being a predominantly placental event at parturition in the sheep but involving both fetal and maternal adrenal cortex as well as placenta in human pregnancy. This may go some way to explaining the differences in the efficacy of glucocorticoids in initiating labour in sheep and humans. But glucocorticoids injected into the amniotic fluid in post-term human pregnancy do seem to have effects on uterine activity [141–143] and induce labour more quickly than control saline injection (Fig. 11.16). This piece of evidence therefore implicates glucocorticoids in the control of uterine activity although whether the dose used can be considered physiological is questionable and the mechanism of action of intra-amniotic glucocorticoid is not clear.

Another fetal adrenal steroid hormone which could be involved in triggering labour is DHAS, a major circulating steroid in the fetus at birth with concentrations significantly higher in umbilical arterial than venous plasma [144], which supports the idea of fetal production. DHAS is the principal fetal precursor for placental oestradiol and oestrone synthesis and, as such, along with maternally derived DHAS, could play a major role in the increasing production with advancing pregnancy of biologically active oestrogen which may be necessary for uterine contractility. The rapid fall in DHAS levels in the neonate during the first few weeks of life [145,146] suggests an intrauterine role for this adrenal steroid; this decrease in neonatal DHAS levels correlates with the known regression of the fetal zone of the adrenal cortex in the first month of extrauterine life [147]. The fetal zone of the fetal adrenal cortex lies next to the medulla, occupies almost 80% of the cortex at birth [148] and is responsible for the relatively large size of the human adrenal gland at birth. The remainder of the fetal adrenal cortex, which will give rise to the zona glomerulosa, zona fasciculata and zona reticularis, is called the definitive or adult cortex.

Some studies have suggested that the fetal and definitive zones of the human fetal adrenal gland have different functional capacities. When superfused in vitro in midpregnancy, corticosteroids were found to be secreted primarily by the definitive zone, whereas DHAS was found to be the main secretory product of the fetal zone [149]. An understanding of the control of these two zones and of the steroids secreted by them is of obvious importance and attention was focused on the possible regulatory role of fetal anterior pituitary hormones and of placental hormones such as hCG. An explanation is

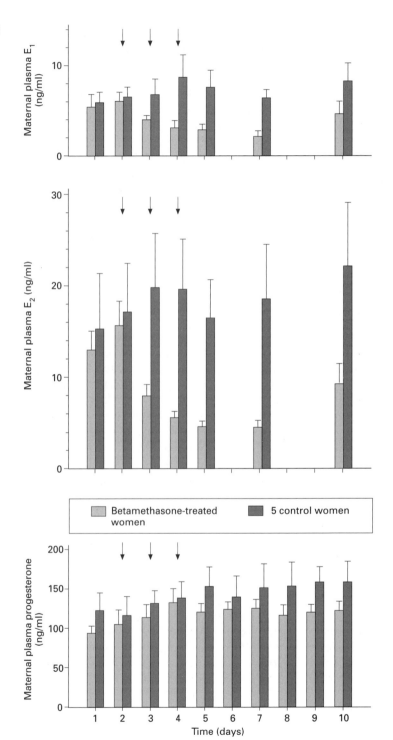

Fig. 11.15. Maternal peripheral venous plasma concentrations of oestrone (E_1), oestradiol (E_2) and progesterone in eight to 10 betamethasone-treated women and five controls. Betamethasone phosphate 6 mg and betamethasone acetate 6 mg were given daily for 3 days as indicated by arrows.

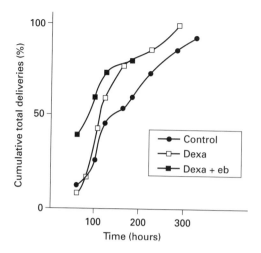

Fig. 11.16. Cumulative percentage of deliveries in 45 women at 41 weeks or more of pregnancy who were given intra-amniotic injection of dexamethasone 20 mg (dexa), dexamethasone 20 mg + oestradiol benzoate 20 mg (dexa + eb) or vehicle (control). From Liggins [142].

needed for fetal zone atrophy after birth in the presence of a functional pituitary and for normal growth up to midpregnancy of the fetal zone in anencephaly [150] with an absent hypothalamus and likely deficiencies of pituitary hormones. It could be that in midpregnancy, hCG is a trophic hormone for the fetal zone [148,151], regulating DHAS production. Adrenocorticotrophic hormone (ACTH) can stimulate in vitro lung maturation in the human but appears to have no role in the onset of labour. It is of interest that, in the sheep, the surge of cortisol in the fetus at the end of pregnancy not only initiates parturition but also stimulates final maturation of many fetal organs over the course of a few days. It may be biologically more sensible that, in human pregnancy, these two vital functions come under different control mechanisms, for in the human fetus maturation of, for example, lung function normally precedes the initiation of labour by 4–6 weeks. Hence, for most human infants, survival is the rule, even if labour is initiated up to 6 weeks before term; whereas in some species, such as the sheep, premature birth even in the last week or two of pregnancy may be fatal for the newborn if the endocrine events initiating parturition are bypassed. This would make sense in the context of an evolutionary trend to earlier birth in the human than in other primates, to resolve the conflict of increasing brain (and therefore head) size in association with decreasing pelvic size (to enhance adaptation to the upright posture). This problem gives rise to a much higher rate of obstructed labour in humans than other mammals, and can only be resolved (in the absence of caesarean section) by babies being smaller at birth.

Over the last 5 million years the human pelvis has narrowed (an adaptation to bipedal gait) and over the last 500 000 years the human brain has grown by 500% [152]. This has given rise to the human problem of obstructed labour (which kills one in 15 first-time mothers in sub-Saharan Africa). The narrow African pelvis, well-suited to sprinting, is not so suitable for labour. One solution is progressive neotonization of the human fetus, i.e. it is being born at an earlier stage of development. Already, African babies are born lighter, at an earlier gestation, but with more mature lungs, than European babies [152]. An alternative strategy is growth restriction, resulting in human babies being born at a smaller proportion of their adult weight than other mammals, allowing for the variation in the length of gestation. It was established by Walters and Hammond in experiments crossing Shetland ponies with Shire horses that with reduced maternal constraint, babies with the same genetic endowment will grow to a much larger proportion of their adult weight at birth if their mother is large rather than small [153]. That the same applies to humans was first reported by Brooks et al., who analysed the results of ovum donation and showed that babies whose genetic mothers were small and whose incubating mother was large had significantly greater birth weights than their genetic siblings born to their natural mother [154]. Thus it might be argued that all human fetuses are growth restricted to a degree; only when this is severe is an increased rate of catch-up growth after birth insufficient to compensate.

Posterior pituitary

Another component of the fetal hypothalamic-pituitary axis which may play a role in the initiation of labour is the posterior pituitary gland with its active peptides, oxytocin and vasopressin.

Since the ability of posterior pituitary extracts to stimulate labour became apparent almost 100 years ago, oxytocin has been linked with the onset of labour. Oxytocin acts through specific cell-surface receptors to increase intracellular calcium by inhibiting the extrusion of calcium by the calcium pump, opening calcium channels, and stimulating the release of IP_3 (via phospholipase C) [155]. The overall effect is to increase the frequency of action potential generation, to promote their propagation and to potentiate myometrial contraction by prolonging the plateau phase of the contraction. The measurement of circulating oxytocin levels during pregnancy is complicated by the presence of placentally produced oxytocinase. However, data derived from studies using assays with an extraction step suggest that oxytocin levels rise minimally during pregnancy, but that with the onset of labour the frequency of oxytocin pulses increases [156]. In addition, with advancing gestation, myometrial oxytocin receptor expression and hence myometrial sensitivity to oxytocin increase [157,158]. Thus, there is no need for the circulating levels of oxytocin to increase for myometrial contractility to be enhanced.

Oxytocin is also synthesized in the decidua and may act locally to stimulate myometrial contractility [159]. Changes in the local oestrogen to progesterone ratio may be important in the regulation of the synthesis of oxytocin [160] and the expression of the oxytocin receptor [161]. Coincident with increases in myometrial receptor expression, decidual and fetal membrane oxytocin receptor mRNA expression is also increased [162].

Oxytocin binding to these membranes results in prostaglandin synthesis and release [163,164]. There are higher concentrations of both vasopressin and oxytocin in the umbilical circulation than in the maternal circulation with an arteriovenous difference for both peptides, suggesting that fetal secretion may have a role [165]. Fetal administration of oxytocin can stimulate contractions of the uterus in sheep and in human anencephaly [166] but whether this has any functional significance is unknown. The source of oxytocin circulating in the fetus is not entirely clear. However, all authors who have studied fetal oxytocin concentrations have found that after spontaneous labour, the concentration of oxytocin in arterial cord blood is markedly higher than in venous cord blood. This implies that the fetus has been secreting considerable amounts of oxytocin [165,167]. Since it is well established that oxytocin can cross the placenta, these results suggest a transfer of oxytocin from fetus to mother at a rate of 1–3 mU/min, sufficient to promote uterine activity in many women at term. Indeed, plasma concentrations of oxytocin measured during induction of labour by intravenous infusion of oxytocin at 1–5 mU/min correspond well with the plasma levels found in very early labour [167].

Thus, the evidence favours a role for oxytocin in the onset and progression of labour. This is supported by reports of the successful use of oxytocin antagonists in preterm labour [168,169]. The role of vasopressin in the onset of labour is even less clear than the role of oxytocin. Evidence that vasopressin is even more active than oxytocin in stimulating phosphoinositide metabolism in human decidua cells [170] suggests that it may well have a role, because the hydrolysis of cellular phospholipid and the accompanying release of unesterified arachidonic acid is of primary importance in regulating the production of prostaglandins, the final mediators of the uterine contraction, but whether fetal levels of vasopressin are actually high enough to invoke this metabolic pathway has yet to be established.

The control of the initiation of labour by the fetal endocrine system thus remains enigmatic. Undoubtedly there is activation of various components of the fetal hypothalamus–pituitary–adrenal axis at birth as shown by the high concentrations of its various secretory products in the umbilical circulation; but at least some of the evidence suggests this may occur as a result of labour rather than be the initiating event.

Fetal death

An argument against an essential fetal role in the initiation of labour is that labour almost invariably follows fetal death, albeit after varying intervals of time. The interval between fetal death and the onset of labour is apparently inversely related to the gestational age of the fetus at the time of death [171] — varying from 37% undelivered within a week if death occurred before 32 weeks, to 18% if the fetus died between 38 and 42 weeks. There also seems to be a correlation between placental damage at the time of fetal death and the interval to labour. When placental abruption causes fetal death, labour ensues rapidly (within 48 hours in 47 of 55 cases reported by Grandin and Hall [171], whereas in rhesus incompatibility the average interval between fetal death and delivery was 14 days [171]. Csapo [172] interpreted these findings as supporting the idea that placental endocrine function is responsible for timing delivery, and that the role of the fetus in pregnancy maintenance far outweighs its role in pregnancy termination. An alternative interpretation is that, if the final endocrine event controlling the myometrium is the release of intrauterine prostaglandins, then with a dead fetus this could be achieved by a mechanism bypassing the usual physiological events. It is likely that, when massive haemorrhage occurs behind the placenta or when the fetus has been dead for several days and intrauterine tissue death takes place, prostaglandins could be released—their release possibly being promoted by a dramatic or gradual fall in progesterone secretion from the placenta as shown in sheep experiments [173].

Influence of the placenta

The main placental hormones implicated in the onset of labour are progesterone and oestradiol, but their exact role in the control of parturition remains obscure and controversial.

Progesterone

The withdrawal of the progesterone block on the myometrium at the end of pregnancy, a hypothesis put forward by Csapo over 30 years ago, has been difficult to prove or disprove in pregnant women. Csapo was originally intrigued by the report that a woman had delivered twins 6 weeks apart, which suggested to him that the

mechanism initiating labour must be controlled locally within the uterus. Subsequent experimental work convinced him that progesterone, secreted by the placenta throughout pregnancy, could inhibit myometrial contractility by direct passage from its site of synthesis without entering the maternal systemic circulation. This local inhibitory effect of placental progesterone could be reduced late in pregnancy because increasing uterine volume would mean that the placenta influenced a relatively smaller and smaller area of the uterine wall. However, attempts to reproduce this local effect clinically by injecting large doses of progesterone directly into the myometrium did not produce convincing inhibition of uterine activity and, although for the uterus in midpregnancy the concentration of progesterone in the myometrium is highest in areas underlying the placenta and lowest in the areas furthest from placental attachment [174], this is not so at term [175]. Other clinical attempts — giving huge doses of progesterone to women to prolong labour at term, to postpone preterm labour or to prevent early abortion—have all been relatively unsuccessful [174], leading to scepticism in accepting the progesterone block hypothesis. In addition, measurement of progesterone concentrations in the maternal peripheral circulation has, in the main, not supported the idea of any withdrawal of progesterone at the end of the human pregnancy. Most studies, too numerous to refer to here, show rising concentrations of progesterone up to the onset of labour while others do not. Unlike the findings in animal studies where a decline in progesterone levels is clearly associated with the onset of labour, in the human no clear picture has emerged. Two studies [176,177], both on young primigravidae, show a decline in mean progesterone concentrations in the peripheral circulation before the onset of labour at term (Fig. 11.17) and in the uterine vein, and one study reported that progesterone concentrations were higher at elective caesarean section than at caesarean section performed early in spontaneous labour [172]. However, measurement of plasma progesterone not bound to plasma proteins and considered physiologically active showed that levels continue to rise with advancing pregnancy [178], and in fact form

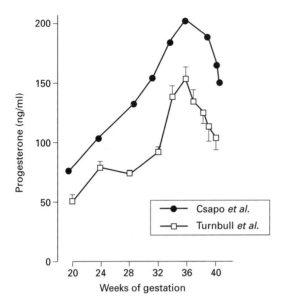

Fig. 11.17. Mean concentrations of peripheral plasma progesterone measured serially throughout pregnancy in two published studies. Redrawn from Csapo et al. [176] and Turnbull et al. [177]. All patients were primigravid and went into labour spontaneously at term.

a greater proportion of the total (bound plus unbound) progesterone in the plasma at 40 weeks (13%) than at 24 weeks (6%). Alteration in maternal peripheral levels of progesterone may not be of importance for parturition if the hormone acts locally on the myometrium. At term, there appears to be no correlation between peripheral blood and myometrial progesterone concentrations [175], but alterations in the binding of the hormone to receptors in uterine muscle could occur.

Oestrogens

Placental production of oestrogens increases throughout pregnancy with some evidence of an acceleration in the rate of increase in the latter weeks as measured by urinary excretion of oestrogens (oestriol in particular) and of plasma concentrations of oestradiol-17β and oestrone sulphate [179] (Fig. 11.18). Although oestriol is quantitatively the most important oestrogen produced by the placenta in pregnancy, oestradiol-17β is considered to be the most relevant in terms of biological activity. It is now well estab-

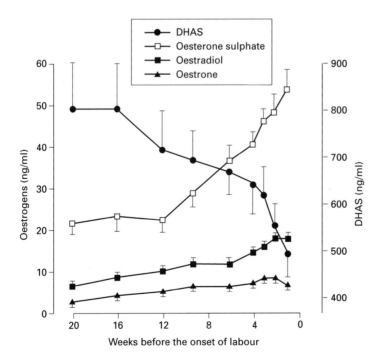

Fig. 11.18. Concentrations (mean ± SEM) of DHAS, oestradiol, oestrone and oestrone sulphate in maternal peripheral plasma measured serially up to the onset of spontaneous labour.

lished that DHAS of both fetal and maternal adrenal origin contributes to oestrogen biosynthesis by the placenta, probably in approximately equal proportions [180] (see Chapter 14). The ability of the placenta to take up and metabolize DHAS to oestrogens is reflected in the increased metabolic clearance rate for DHAS in pregnancy [181,182] which, in turn, causes a progressive decrease in DHAS concentration, falling rapidly in the last few weeks of pregnancy [179,183] (Fig. 11.16). Turnbull *et al.* [179] agreed that, since women can go into labour without concentrations of oestradiol rising (although mean concentrations rise rapidly in the last few weeks before labour), this would argue for a facilitatory rather than a causative role for oestradiol in the initiation of labour. There is certainly no dramatic increase in oestradiol concentrations in plasma in association with the onset of labour at term.

The effects of oestradiol administration on uterine contractility in women in late pregnancy are consistent with a postulated facilitatory effect. Oestradiol appears to stimulate a transient increase in uterine activity and reduce the oxytocin threshold of the uterus but does not generally stimulate powerful enough uterine contractions to lead to delivery [184–186]. It should be remembered, however, that labour can be initiated when maternal plasma oestradiol concentrations are low, as occurs following administration of large doses of synthetic glucocorticoid to the mother [139]. On the other hand, patients with placental sulphatase deficiency (associated with male sex-linked ichthyosis) and extremely low circulating levels of oestradiol-17β [187,188] may have prolonged gestation (particularly in a first pregnancy) and may encounter difficulties with induction of labour leading to the need for delivery by caesarean section [189–192].

Thus there is no clear evidence that placental production of progesterone or oestradiol alters dramatically at the onset of labour to initiate powerful uterine contractions. Rather, there are changing concentrations of these two hormones in the maternal peripheral circulation for several weeks before labour, which may facilitate increasing uterine activity but seem unlikely to be critical for labour initiation.

Influence of fetal membranes

The steroid hormones and prostaglandins must be considered.

Steroid hormones

One way in which the myometrium could be affected by intrauterine progesterone production or metabolism, without any significant alteration in placental production or in maternal plasma concentrations of the hormone, is through the fetal membranes, which are known to contain a relatively high concentration of progesterone [193]. Some studies support the idea that metabolic events occurring in the fetal membranes near term play a central role in the initiation of human labour [194,195]. It has been shown, for example, that both chorion laeve and amnion contain enzymes responsible for breakdown of progesterone, although there is a decreased rate of metabolism of progesterone in the fetal membranes several weeks before term. In addition, the cytoplasm of both amnion and chorion contains a protein which binds progesterone as well as cortisol, and which appears to increase at the end of pregnancy before labour [196]. Such a binding protein could produce an effective local progesterone withdrawal in the membranes and hence in the myometrium, assuming that a hormone produced in the membranes can reach the uterine muscle without first being transported to the maternal peripheral circulation. Since the fetal membranes appear avascular [197], however, it is difficult to envisage the means by which a hormone can reach the myometrium from amnion or chorion, other than by diffusion.

The fetal membranes, in particular chorion, also contain other steroid-metabolizing enzymes (such as sulphatases) which can cleave DHAS to DHA [198] and oestrone sulphate to oestrone [199]; these could have important implications for the control of intrauterine oestrogen synthesis. Another chorionic enzyme which may be important for parturition is the 11β-hydroxysteroid dehydrogenase which can interconvert cortisol and cortisone. As gestation progresses, the activity of this enzyme in fetal membranes favours increased cortisol produc-

333

334   tion [199,200], and is therefore a potential source of the rising concentrations of cortisol found in amniotic fluid with increasing gestational age [134,184]. The functional significance of these steroid enzymes in the fetal membranes is not clear. They could be more important for such membrane functions as transport or formation and turnover of amniotic fluid than for control of myometrial function; however, the discovery that the membranes might represent a potentially important control mechanism for steroid hormones inside the uterus has opened up new areas for research.

Prostaglandins

The contractile effects of PGE_2 and $F_{2\alpha}$ are mediated through their ability to increase intracellular calcium. The effect on intracellular calcium levels is mediated through both cell surface and sarcoplasmic reticulum receptors. It is unclear whether prostaglandins affect potassium channel conductance, although arachidonic acid and its products have been reported to modulate their function [201]. Electrically, the effect of prostaglandins appears to be to prolong the plateau part of the action potential [202]. The first suggestion that prostaglandins may play a role in the initiation of labour came from Karim [203] who reported the presence of PGE_1, PGE_2, $PGF_{1\alpha}$ and $PGF_{2\alpha}$ in amniotic fluid; levels of amniotic fluid $PGF_{1\alpha}$ and $PGF_{2\alpha}$ were subsequently found to be higher during than before labour. These findings, along with the known stimulatory effect of prostaglandins on the human uterus, led to the supposition that these compounds were involved in the onset of labour. There is still good reason to believe that this is so, although whether prostaglandins initiate labour or are more involved in the maintenance of labour is debatable. Furthermore, most of the early evidence for involvement of prostaglandins in labour, based on measurements in tissues or in blood, is now known to be fallacious. Because prostaglandins may be formed as a result of trauma when tissue samples are collected or handled, by platelets when a blood sample is taken, or by storage of plasma for a few weeks even at low temperatures, valid measurements of prostaglandins are extremely difficult.

Measurement in amniotic fluid is more attractive because of lack of enzymes which would synthesize or metabolize [204] prostaglandins but, even in that fluid, early measurements [203] were probably not reliable. Keirse and his colleagues [205,206] found, for example, that amniotic fluid prostaglandins were probably exclusively PGE_2 and $PGF_{2\alpha}$ rather than PGE_1 and $PGF_{1\alpha}$, corresponding to the predominance of arachidonic acid (the precursor of PGE_2 and $PGF_{2\alpha}$) over dihomo-γ-linolenic acid (precursor of PGE_1 and $PGF_{1\alpha}$) in intrauterine tissues. The source of amniotic fluid PGE_2 and $PGF_{2\alpha}$ may be the fetal membranes, since evidence has accumulated in recent years that the membranes contain the necessary enzymes for synthesis of these prostaglandins.

Evidence from measurements in plasma from the maternal uterine vein and radial artery has supported the view that the prostaglandins involved in labour onset are $F_{2\alpha}$, 13,14-dihydro-15-keto-$F_{2\alpha}$ and E_2 [207]. In contrast, changes in peripheral levels of oestrogen, progesterone, prolactin and prostacyclin (inferred from the measurement of the metabolite 6-keto-prostaglandin $F_{1\alpha}$ metabolite) were not evident when prelabour values were compared to those obtained in labour.

The obligatory precursor of PGE_2 and PGF_2 is the essential fatty acid, arachidonic acid, present in most tissues in esterified form, although it is only the unesterified or free form which leads to the synthesis of prostaglandins. Arachidonic acid is derived almost entirely from glycerophospholipids, a step probably under the control of the enzyme phospholipase A_2 which catalyses the release of free precursor fatty acids and which is presumed to be rate-limiting for prostaglandin biosynthesis. The conversion of arachidonic acid to prostaglandins proceeds in several stages and is accomplished by an enzyme complex, prostaglandin synthetase [208,209]. The first step converts arachidonic acid into the cyclic endoperoxides prostaglandins G_2 and H_2 involving the enzyme cyclo-oxygenase. These intermediate endoperoxides are relatively unstable, with a half-life of about 5 minutes. PGH_2 is in turn converted to the primary prostaglandins PGE_2 and PGF_2 by specific enzymes, an isomerase and reductase respectively. PGE$_2$ and PGF$_2$ can then be metabolized, first through oxidation of the 15-hydroxyl group to the 15-keto derivative, under the influence of the enzyme 15-hydroxyprostaglandin dehydrogenase, then to the 13,14-dihydro compound by the reductase enzyme. This latter metabolite of PGF$_{2\alpha}$, 14-dihydro-15-keto-PGF$_{2\alpha}$, is a stable degradation product and measurement of its concentration in peripheral plasma has been preferred to that of the primary compound, not only because of its stability on storage but also because of its higher endogenous concentrations and the fact that it is likely in pregnancy to reflect intrauterine prostaglandin production [210]. Although in the past it was thought that only PGE$_2$, PGF$_2$ and PGD$_2$ were the main and biologically significant products of a prostaglandin synthetase reaction, it is now known that there are other biologically important pathways from the cyclic endoperoxides [209].

Both PGG$_2$ and PGH$_2$ can be metabolized to prostacyclin (PGI$_2$) and thromboxane A$_2$ (TXA$_2$) which in turn break down to 6-keto-PGF$_{1\alpha}$ and TXB$_{2\alpha}$ respectively. In relation to parturition, prostacyclin may have effects on the smooth muscle of the uterus, but there is no evidence for thromboxane being involved in myometrial activity. Thromboxane and prostacyclin possess potent platelet aggregatory and antiaggregatory effects respectively and may be of importance in the control of, for example, the fetal ductus

arteriosus, or of haemostasis after delivery of the placenta rather than uterine contractility. A simplified scheme for the pathways from arachidonic acid is shown in Fig. 11.19.

Aspirin-like drugs (prostaglandin synthetase inhibitors) affect prostaglandin biosynthesis by inhibiting the cyclo-oxygenase enzyme and the first step in arachidonic acid metabolism. Thus, these drugs will prevent production of the cyclic endoperoxides and all their derivatives including prostacyclin, thromboxane A$_2$ and the primary prostaglandins, PGE$_2$ and PGF$_{2\alpha}$.

Many studies indicate that the fetal membranes may be involved in the synthesis and metabolism of prostaglandins in late pregnancy. The membranes contain significant amounts of esterified arachidonic acid [211], and also of the enzyme phospholipase A$_2$ [212,213], which may account for the free arachidonic acid in amniotic fluid in late pregnancy [214]. There is no evidence, however, that phospholipase A activity differs in fetal membranes taken during, as opposed to before, the onset of labour [213]; hence, the increased free arachidonic acid concentrations in amniotic fluid in labouring women [214] cannot be explained on the basis of increased phospholipase A activity in fetal membranes, decidua or myometrium [213].

Further evidence that the membranes may be involved in production of prostaglandins comes from studies by in-vitro incubation techniques

Fig. 11.19. Metabolic pathway of arachidonic acid.

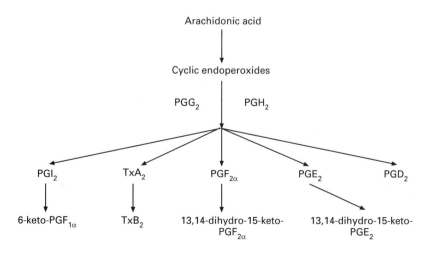

336 showing the capacity of the membranes in late gestation for prostaglandin synthesis [215,216], and of the amnion in particular for PGE_2 production in an in-vitro superfusion system [217]. In addition, the membranes possess both 15-hydroxyprostaglandin dehydrogenase and 13,14-prostaglandin reductase enzymes [216] responsible for the initial steps in the degradation of prostaglandins; these enzymes appear much more active in the chorion than amnion. Again, there was no difference in the ability of chorion to metabolize prostaglandins before or after the onset of labour [218].

The evidence presented thus far suggests the fetal membranes as a potential source of the primary prostaglandins PGE_2 and $PGF_{2\alpha}$ and of 13,14-dihydro-15-keto-$PGF_{2\alpha}$ found in amniotic fluid before and after labour [205,206,219]. The amnion has the greatest capacity to synthesize prostaglandins and it increases markedly towards term [220]. The synthesis of cycloxygenase-2 (COX-2) increases markedly with the onset of labour [221,222]. In order for the synthetic capacity of the amnion to be realized, there must be an increase in arachidonic acid availability. The sources of arachidonic acid in the fetal membranes are phosphatidylethanolamine and phosphatidylinositol; both are the substrates for phospholipases A_2 and C. In-vitro studies suggest that PLA_2 and PLC activity increase in the amnion with advancing gestation. However, steady state mRNA levels for PLA_2 are less in the amnion and chorion than in the placenta, and while the levels increase in the placenta with the onset of labour, there is no such increase in the fetal membranes. These data suggest that COX-2 availability rather than PLA_2 may be the rate-limiting step in prostaglandin synthesis in the fetal membranes [223]. In-vitro studies have suggested that prostaglandin production may be modulated by vasopressin, epidermal growth factor, amines and catecholamines. These factors may modulate prostaglandin production either by altering arachidonic acid availability or COX-2 activity.

Accepting that the amnion has increased substrate and the capacity to synthesize increased amounts of prostaglandins with advancing gestation and the onset of labour, it is unclear whether these prostaglandins have access to the myometrium or whether they are metabolized as they cross the amnion and chorion [224,225]. Indeed, the chorion is rich in prostaglandin dehydrogenase, and may be an effective barrier to prostaglandin transfer, but some cells lack this enzyme and may allow the transfer of prostaglandins to the myometrium [226]. There appears to be no change in the expression of prostaglandin receptors with advancing gestation [3], and whether there are high and low affinity receptors is uncertain, although the affinity of the PGE receptor seems to be 10–20 times that of the $PGF_{2\alpha}$ receptor. However, the increased levels of prostaglandins may be sufficient in the absence of any change in receptor expression.

Influence of the decidua

The first evidence that the decidua may be a major site of intrauterine prostaglandin synthesis in late pregnancy came from the work of Karim and Devlin [227]. Subsequent work has supported this to some extent. At term, the concentrations of PGE_2 and $PGF_{2\alpha}$ are higher in decidua (and myometrium) than in amnion, chorion or placenta [68], but there may have been more trauma to the tissues with the highest concentrations of prostaglandins. In addition, tissues with the lowest concentrations, i.e. chorion and placenta, have the highest rates of metabolism of prostaglandins [204,215]. Certainly the decidua contains enzymes necessary for the synthesis of prostaglandins, in particular phospholipase A_2 [210,213,228], but there is no evidence of any increased activity of decidual phospholipase A after the onset of labour [211].

An attractive hypothesis relating decidual prostaglandin production to parturition has come from Gustavii [229,230]. He proposes that a key role is played by the lysosomes of decidual cells which are known to contain phospholipase A_2 [231] and which are said to be extremely fragile. Because oestrogens can labilize the membrane of the lysosomes and there is evidence of degeneration of decidual cells in late pregnancy [230], Gustavii suggests that rising oestrogen concentrations and falling progesterone concentrations at the end of pregnancy would act as lysosomal labilizers. A chain of reactions would occur, leading to release of lysosomal enzymes—phospholipase A_2 in particular, which act on membrane phospholipids to release arachidonic acid, which in turn is converted to the primary prostaglandins PGE_2 and $PGF_{2\alpha}$ as described earlier. Gustavii's hypothesis is proposed not only to explain the onset of labour at term, but to explain the mechanism of midtrimester abortion following intra-amniotic inaction of hypertonic saline, a procedure which induces release of prostaglandins into the amniotic fluid [232]. Missed abortion is also explained by Gustavii in terms of his hypothesis, with continuing progesterone production and falling oestrogen production delaying the rate of decidual regression and thereby suppressing prostaglandin synthesis [232]. Yet extra-amniotic injection of physiological saline will readily induce effective uterine contractions in most cases of missed abortion [232]. A hypothetical scheme for labour based on Gustavii's hypothesis is shown in Fig. 11.20.

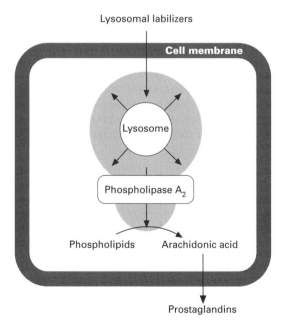

Fig. 11.20. A scheme for the synthesis of prostaglandins.

Decidua or membrane control of labour?

In support of decidua rather than fetal membranes controlling the onset of labour is evidence from abdominal pregnancies cited by Gustavii [232]. There are several reports that labour starts at term in women with an extrauterine pregnancy, painful uterine contractions being experienced [232]. In that situation, there are no fetal membranes in the uterine cavity although there is a decidual lining. Thus, the only way the myometrium could be influenced by metabolic events occurring in the fetal membranes is through the maternal circulation; these clinical reports must cast some doubt on local prostaglandin control of uterine activity being sited in the membranes or placenta rather than in the decidua. The same arguments could, of course, be levelled against placental or membrane steroid hormones directly influencing the myometrium when the fetus develops in the abdominal cavity.

Influence of amniotic fluid

Amniotic fluid may give a better reflection of intrauterine production of some hormones than the peripheral plasma. This is especially so for prostaglandins because of the lack of prostaglandin synthesizing or metabolizing enzymes in amniotic fluid [137]. In this fluid there is no evidence of increased production of PGF in the latter weeks of pregnancy if samples taken by amniocentesis [233,234] or amniotomy [233] are considered separately (Fig. 11.21). Levels of PGF and its major metabolite, 13,14-dihydro-15-keto-PGF (PGFM), are significantly higher in amniotic fluid obtained by amniotomy as opposed to that of amniocentesis in late gestation [233]; this supports the idea of a local control mechanism for prostaglandin production. This may relate to disruption of the membranes or the decidua as discussed earlier, or to rapid release of prostaglandins in response to stimulation of the vagina or cervix during the procedure of amniotomy [210] (Fig. 11.22). Failure to appreciate these influences on amniotic fluid prostaglandin concentrations may have led earlier workers [235,236] to suggest that there was a progressive rise in prostaglandin

338

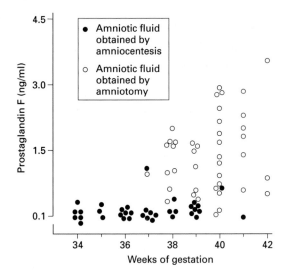

Fig. 11.21. Concentrations of PGF in amniotic fluid obtained by amniocentesis and amniotomy before the onset of labour. From Mitchell *et al.* [233].

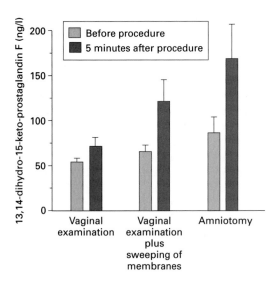

Fig. 11.22. Mean (SEM) peripheral plasma concentrations of 13,14-dihydro-15-keto-PGF in women in late pregnancy before and 5 minutes after vaginal examination, vaginal examination plus sweeping of the membranes and amniotomy.

levels in amniotic fluid after 36 weeks' gestation if the concentration of fluid obtained at amniocentesis and amniotomy were not considered separately. PGE levels in amniotic fluid appear to increase sharply at 36 weeks, without much

change thereafter to term [234] and this may help to promote the increasing uterine activity and cervical changes in the last few weeks of pregnancy. At the onset of labour, if amniotic fluid samples taken by amniotomy are considered, there is a significant difference in PGF levels in samples taken in late pregnancy before labour compared to levels early in spontaneous labour [179]. These data suggest an increased release of prostaglandins in association with the onset of labour, but whether this release precedes labour and is responsible for its initiation is unknown.

A basic assumption is that the rate-limiting step in prostaglandin synthesis is the availability of substrate, arachidonic acid. But amniotic fluid [237], as well as many intrauterine tissues [238], contains a vast excess of arachidonic acid in relation to PGE and PGF levels and it seems unlikely that substrate availability is limiting in prostaglandin synthesis within the uterus. On the other hand, intra-amniotic injection of arachidonic acid has been shown to induce abortion in midpregnancy and labour in later pregnancy in the presence of a dead fetus [214], although there were no controls in that study.

The rise in prostaglandin in amniotic fluid at the onset of labour provides one of the few clues that prostaglandins may be involved in the onset of labour — although their exact role remains an enigma. That they are likely to play a role, however, is suggested by evidence [239,240] that women who ingest a prostaglandin synthetase inhibitor (aspirin) during pregnancy have prolonged pregnancies compared with controls, although the degree of prolongation is not great (about 7 days in one observational study [239].

Other prostaglandin synthetase inhibitors such as indomethacin also suppress uterine contractions effectively in the short term, although their longer term use has been avoided because of the possibility of adverse fetal effects, notably premature closure of the ductus arteriosus [241].

Corticotrophin-releasing hormone and the hypothalamic–pituitary–adrenal axis

Work in the sheep model defined the importance of ACTH and cortisol in the onset of labour [242–244]. However, in the human, such a role for the fetal adrenal axis has not been identified. Rather, there is increasing evidence that placental corticotrophin-releasing hormone (CRH) may play an important role in the timing of the onset of labour. CRH was first reported to be present in the placenta in 1982 [245]. It is synthesized in the syncytiotrophoblast and secreted into the maternal circulation [246]. It is detectable in the maternal blood from 20 weeks rising steadily to 35 weeks when levels increase markedly to term [247]. It is present in the fetal circulation, but at about 10% of the maternal levels [248]. Maternal levels of CRH have been reported to be elevated in several pathological types of pregnancy, pre-eclampsia, preterm labour, intra-uterine growth retardation and twin pregnancies [249–251]. The role of, and the factors inducing, the increased levels of CRH in these states are unknown, although corticosteroids have been shown to enhance CRH production [252].

CRH activity in both the maternal and fetal circulations is modulated by CRH-binding protein (CRHBP). Synthesized in the liver, placenta and brain, its circulating levels are in excess of those of CRH, such that most of the circulating CRH is likely to be bound. However, towards term, when the levels of CRH are rising, those of the CRHBP are declining, resulting in increasing free levels of circulating CRH [248]. This also occurs in pregnancies complicated by pre-eclampsia and preterm labour, where CRH levels are elevated and CRHBP levels are reduced [248].

At the end of pregnancy, the elevated levels of maternal CRH may have several different roles, but the overall effect appears to be the promotion of the onset of labour. The CRH receptor appears to exist in three states during pregnancy [253]. Initially, it is of low affinity and uncoupled from adenylate cyclase, with advancing gestation, and possibly coincident with the increased availability of CRH in late pregnancy, the receptor switched to being high affinity (greater than that of the CRHBP) and linked to adenylate cyclase and cyclo-oxygenase [254]. These linkages result in increased intracellular levels of cAMP and PGE_2, both of which inhibit myometrial contractions. Finally, around the time of the onset of labour, the receptor changes back to

a low affinity, uncoupled state [255]. This occurs probably both as a result of the lower expression of $G_{\alpha s}$ [256] and in response to the combined activity of oxytocin and CRH, thus promoting the action of oxytocin and $PGF_{2\alpha}$.

In addition to its direct effects on the myometrium, CRH has several paracrine effects, it dilates the fetoplacental circulation [257], enhances the release of placental ACTH which may be important locally and/or in the activation of the fetal adrenal [258], and increases the production of PGE_2 and $PGF_{2\alpha}$ by the trophoblast and fetal membranes [259]. The last may be important in the promotion of the onset of labour, as prostaglandins have been shown to enhance placental production of CRH, again establishing another positive feedback loop [260]. The importance of these roles is uncertain, but the latter may be important or have local paracrine effects within the placenta or fetal membranes altering the production of other factors.

In the fetus, it has been shown that CRHBP behaves in a similar fashion to that described above; thus, fetal CRH is increasingly active approaching term. It has been suggested that increased CRH activates the fetal pituitary–adrenal axis, increasing the circulating levels of glucocorticoids which in turn are known to enhance placental CRH production [252]. Thus, a positive feedback loop is established, with the putative roles of CRH being (i) the maturation of the fetal lungs via the increased circulating levels of glucocorticoids, and (ii) the stimulation of the onset of labour, either via the increased fetal glucocorticoids or directly through the direct actions of CRH on the placenta and myometrium.

Maternal influences

Influences of the myometrium

The ethical problems associated with obtaining samples of human myometrium in late pregnancy mean that there is limited information on synthesis or metabolism of hormones considered to be important for parturition. There are some data, however, suggesting that the uterine muscle may be capable of controlling its hormonal environment without invoking control-

340 ling mechanisms from elsewhere. For example, although intracellular binding proteins for both oestradiol and progesterone are present in human myometrium, there appears to be no information about their activities in relation to the onset of labour. Receptors for oxytocin [261] and for prostaglandins [262] have also been identified in human pregnant myometrium; their functional significance is unknown. Murphy [263] has suggested that her findings of a dramatic increase in late pregnancy in the ability of uterine muscle to convert cortisone to cortisol might serve to explain the stabilization of lysosomes and prevention of the synthesis of prostaglandins until the onset of labour or might play a role in immunological mechanisms. Another important aspect is the development of gap junctions as pregnancy progresses [264]. Junctions between smooth muscle cells can be identified by electron microscopy as seven layers or bands of alternating electron-opaque and electron-transparent material; the central electron-transparent gap (hence gap junction) appears continuous with the extracellular space. The outer leaves of the gap junction membranes are separated by a 2 nm gap. Garfield *et al.* [264] propose that the absence of gap junctions before labour may be important for the maintenance of pregnancy and their appearance in labour may be necessary for the development of effective uterine contractions leading to delivery.

Influences of the endocrine system

The ovaries are not necessary for the initiation of labour since, as discussed earlier, they are dispensable, as far as maintenance of pregnancy is concerned during the first trimester. Similarly, other maternal endocrine organs do not seem vital for the onset of labour, although the data are sometimes difficult to interpret. Hypophysectomized women [265] and women with diabetes insipidus [266] usually go into labour at term but, as Hytten and Leitch point out [79], oxytocin may be secreted by the hypothalamus even when the posterior pituitary has been removed. From the work of Chard [267] there is no evidence of an acute release of oxytocin before the onset of labour and the conclusion is that maternal oxytocin plays little, if any, part in the initiation of human parturition. Adrenalectomized women on corticosteroid maintenance therapy can go into labour spontaneously, although women with Addison's disease have, on average, a greater length of pregnancy than controls but with a wide range, from 252 to 312 days [268].

Autonomic nervous system

The physiological significance of the innervation of the human uterus is unknown. Because parturition can occur after complete spinal transection, central neural connections do not seem essential for labour (for a review, see Bell [269]. Fluorescent histochemistry has demonstrated both adrenergic and cholinergic fibres in the human uterus with an increasing density of fibres from the body of the uterus to the cervix. The adrenergic innervation of the uterine muscle includes both α-excitatory and β-inhibitory receptors, and the relative dominance of these receptors is altered by the hormonal status. While the non-pregnant uterus contracts in response both to noradrenaline and adrenaline, at term only noradrenaline causes contractions [270], adrenaline producing relaxation [271,272]. α-Receptor blocking drugs such as phentolamine cause a decrease in uterine activity when infused into women in late pregnancy, and inhibit the increased uterine activity produced in response to noradrenaline [271]. Adrenaline-like drugs, much favoured in clinical practice to suppress the uterine contractions of preterm labour, produce an inhibitory effect on uterine activity which does not occur in the presence of a β-blocking agent such as propranolol [270]. Propranolol itself causes significant enhancement of uterine activity when infused intravenously in late pregnancy [273]. The development of adrenaline-like drugs with a high affinity for uterine β-receptors has helped to reduce the unwanted cardiovascular side-effects of these drugs in obstetric practice, but unwanted effects on cardiac β-receptors still occur.

The evidence for the presence of α- and β-receptors in the human uterus is fairly conclusive but the involvement of the autonomic system in the initiation of labour remains uncertain and the relations between endocrine and nervous mechanisms are undoubtedly complex.

Other maternal factors affecting the onset of labour

Investigators over the last 10 years have increasingly realized the potential importance of cytokines, which can be released from the cervix or fetal membranes in response to stretching or bacterial activity. Vaginal fluid contains microorganisms, bacterial toxins and cytokines such as interleukin-1β, to which the fetal membranes are exposed as the cervix gradually ripens and dilates. This could initiate a cascade effect, resulting in the observed escalation of prostaglandin production, and also in the production of endothelin-1, a potent uterotonic which is found in amniotic fluid in concentrations 10–100 times greater than in plasma [17], which doubles at the onset of labour, and the concentration of which correlates highly significantly with that of the uterotonic prostaglandins. Histamine may also be involved as a local regulator of phospholipase A_2 and $PGF_{2\alpha}$, interacting with interleukin-1 [274].

Control of uterine activity in labour

There is increasing evidence that prostaglandins are likely to be important for the maintenance of progressive labour although there may be reservations (discussed earlier) about their role in its initiation. Effective labour involves the development of frequent, powerful and coordinated uterine contractions so that the fetal presenting part descends gradually through the pelvis and the cervix progressively softens, effaces and dilates. Whether prostaglandins alone can effect such a complex sequence of events is not known and several mechanisms may be involved.

With the onset of labour there is a statistically significant increase in the amniotic fluid concentrations of PGE [205,234], PGF [206,237, 275] and 13,14-dihydro-15-keto-PGF (PGFM) [207,219] as cervical dilatation progresses (Fig. 11.23). That this increase is not merely an effect of uterine contractility is shown by the findings

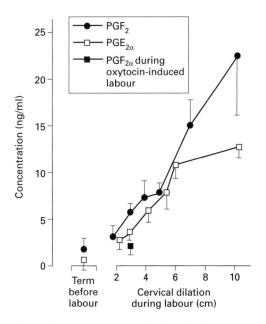

Fig. 11.23. Concentrations of PGE_2 and $PGF_{2\alpha}$ in amniotic fluid during late pregnancy and spontaneous labour. Concentrations of $PGF_{2\alpha}$ in samples obtained during oxytocin-induced labour are also shown.

that concentrations of PGF are higher in early spontaneous labour than if labour is induced by intravenous oxytocin infusion [206] (see Fig. 11.23). In addition, several hours of artificially stimulated uterine activity are necessary before PGF concentrations begin to rise [275]. Further evidence of increased intrauterine prostaglandin production during labour is seen in the rising concentrations of PGFM in the peripheral plasma [276,277], and the increased excretion in urine of the major urinary metabolite of PGF [278].

One situation where there may be a deficiency of intrauterine prostaglandins is in anencephaly, since this fetal abnormality appears to be associated with very low levels of prostaglandins in amniotic fluid during labour [179]. Despite this, the first stage of labour is not significantly prolonged in mothers with an anencephalic fetus and no hydramnios, although the second stage is twice as long as in controls with a normal fetus. These data have been interpreted as suggesting that the fetal brain is necessary for the normal completion of delivery, but not for the earlier

342 stage of labour [279]. An alternative hypothesis is of course the simpler one that the lack of an effective dilation of the vagina in the second stage (due to the lack of a large distending head) leads to a failure of the Ferguson reflex. The fetal neurohypophysis is considered the likely area of importance since anencephalic fetuses do not seem to produce the posterior lobe hormones, oxytocin and vasopressin [279].

Maternal, as well as fetal, oxytocin may be important for the final stages of labour since the frequency of a 'spurt' release of oxytocin measured in the maternal circulation increases as labour progresses and reaches a maximum at the time of delivery [267]. On the other hand, some reports suggest that women with diabetes insipidus are able to labour normally [266], although there are also reports of delayed parturition in these women [79]. Indirect evidence for the involvement of oxytocin in labour is that the administration of ethanol (which depresses posterior pituitary activity) can suppress labour, although ethanol may also have a direct action on uterine smooth muscle [280].

The release of both oxytocin and prostaglandins in labour could be under the control of a neuroendocrine reflex arising from the genital tract, the Ferguson reflex [281]. This proposes the release of oxytocin secondary to vaginal distension, which has the secondary effect of raising prostaglandin levels—as in sheep. Alternatively, increasing prostaglandin production may in itself release oxytocin [282]. It is an attractive hypothesis that increasing cervical dilatation during labour and distension of the upper vagina in second stage labour, could, by reflex action, release powerful oxytocics like prostaglandins and oxytocin in order to stimulate effective uterine contractions for delivery of the fetus. Certainly vaginal examination in late human pregnancy and in labour raises circulating levels of prostaglandins [210], but there is no conclusive evidence that it does so through reflex release of oxytocin [283]. In addition, epidural analgesia in labour, which would block the spinal part of the reflex and hence oxytocin release, does not prolong established first-stage labour [284] but does suppress the uterine contractions induced by artificial cervical dilation [285]. The mechanism whereby stimulation of the upper genital tract in late human pregnancy and labour causes local release of prostaglandin is therefore uncertain but appears not to involve oxytocin as in some other species studied. The evidence [286] that orgasm during pregnancy can cause painful uterine contractions and that the incidence of orgasm after 32 weeks' gestation was significantly higher in patients who delivered preterm than at term, might relate to release of prostaglandins during intercourse, again by stimulation of the upper vagina [210] or through release of prostaglandins from seminal fluid. On the other hand, there is no evidence of raised levels of primary prostaglandins or of PGFM in the circulation of women in unexplained early preterm labour [277], although prostaglandin synthetase inhibitor drugs such as indomethacin will inhibit premature uterine contractions [287].

Control of cervical changes in labour

The co-ordination of myometrial contractility and cervical dilatation is a prerequisite of normal labour and a description of the control mechanisms of parturition must include adequate explanations of both processes. It is an attractive hypothesis that the endocrine control of parturition involves the functional activity of these two distinct parts of the uterus. In active labour, the contracting myometrium exerts its influence on the cervix via the fetal presenting parts and Lindgren has studied this aspect of cervical dilatation exhaustively [288]. But uterine contractions alone cannot cause the cervix to soften, and dramatic changes must occur within the rigid cervical tissue to permit the work of uterine contractions to be expressed as cervical dilatation. In many patients it is recognized that cervical softening may precede labour to a large extent but it seems appropriate to discuss the possible mechanisms at this point.

There is unfortunately no complete description available of the tissue changes which underlie cervical softening. Danforth has stated that the process must be explained in terms of dramatic alteration in the collagen framework of the tissue. His work has revealed a fall in the proportion of collagen at term [42], and a corresponding increase in the hexosamine-containing ground substance components, the glycosaminoglycans (GAGs) [289]. An activation of collagenolytic enzyme systems probably underlies the gross morphological changes observed [37,38,290]. Von Maillot and Zimmermann [291] have demonstrated a dramatic increase in the soluble fraction of cervical collagen during active dilatation. Their data do not, however, differentiate between a change in the collagen fibril, and a permissive change in GAGs allowing increased extraction of collagen from the tissue. There are reports available of changes in GAGs at term, including the appearance of species not present in the tissue during pregnancy [292,293]. A complete characterization of connective tissue changes is still required before our understanding of this process can increase.

Another area in which our knowledge is scanty is the complex relation between GAGs and collagen fibrillar organization. Histological studies of cervical tissue during pregnancy and parturition have been quite extensive [42,294], and reveal a disorganization of fibre bundles during softening. Ultrastructural studies have failed to reveal any dramatic change in the fibrillar arrangement, although the possibility remains that a change in the GAGs permits increased distortion of the tissue by altering fibrillar mobility within the collagenous framework.

There is now evidence accumulating for direct hormonal effects on the cervix. Oestradiol-17β, administered either intravenously [295] or by local extra-amniotic application [296], can produce changes in the cervical state. Prostaglandins — usually given in a viscous gel either extra-amniotically [297] or, more commonly, vaginally [298] — are now used widely to ripen the cervix prior to the induction of labour, if the cervix is unfavourable. There has, however, been some controversy over a proposed local action on the cervix of these substances, for it has yet to be shown that the cervical changes can occur in the absence of uterine activity which may be induced by the prostaglandin. In addition to this, a definite causal role for these hormones must be established by elucidating the mechanism of cervical changes, in terms both of connective tissue activation and smooth muscle relaxation.

A possible role for prostaglandins merits further discussion, as both PGE and PGF have been as agents for cervical ripening [299,300]. In-vitro observations have shown that PGE is relaxant on non-pregnant human cervical strips [45]. PGF is, in contrast, a constrictor *in vitro*, while observations *in vivo* have shown a constrictor action of both PGE and PGF on the pregnant cervix [301]. These oxytocic actions on the cervix are almost certainly an action on cervical smooth muscle, and the conflicting reports are not necessarily relevant to the problem of cervical softening during dilatation [302]. A direct local action of PGE on the cervix, which must be explained in terms of connective tissue mechanisms, has been reported by Conrad and Ueland [303]. Both oral administration of PGE for induction of labour and in-vitro incubation with PGE will reduce the stretch modulus of cervical tissue strips, demonstrating an increase in distensibility. An additional observation which these workers made was that induction of labour with oxytocin, as opposed to PGE, did not reduce the stretch modulus of the tissue [304]. Studies of pregnant sheep have demonstrated that cervical tissue itself is a source of PGE, and both in-vitro and in-vivo observations confirm a significant increase in PGE production by the cervix during dilatation [305]. In contrast, there is no apparent increase in the ability of cervical tissue to synthesize PGF. There is also a significant increase in 6-oxo-$PGF_{1\alpha}$ production, reflecting increased prostacyclin synthesis [306]. These observations have formed the basis of a theory for involvement of locally synthesized prostaglandins in the mechanism of cervical softening. Observations on human cervical tissue have demonstrated an increased capacity for prostaglandin production by the tissue during active dilatation, although this increase is not specific for PGE [307] (Fig. 11.24). The hypothesis that PGE is important in cervical softening through a direct local action on cervical connective tissue is also supported by the clinical observations that PGE is a far more potent agent than PGF for ripening the unfavourable cervix [298].

The unfavourable cervix at term, and its associated likelihood of a prolonged labour and difficulties inducing labour with oxytocin, is a

344

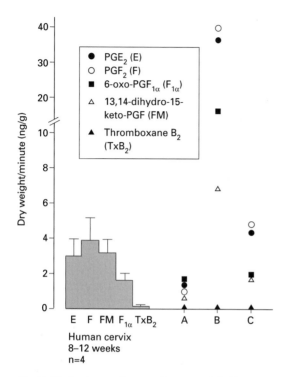

Fig. 11.24. In-vitro production of prostanoids by the human cervix: production rates of PGF₂, PGE₂, 13,14-dihydro-15-keto-PGF, 6-oxo-PGF₁α and thromboxane B₂ have been measured by superfusion of cervical tissue taken after emergency caesarean section (C/S) followed by hysterectomy. Comparison with production rates obtained for the 1st trimester cervix reveals that active dilatation may be associated with increased prostanoid production. A: 37 weeks elective C/S; B: 34 weeks emergency C/S, 6–7 cm dilatation; C: 40 weeks emergency C/S at full dilatation.

clinical problem which has been solved to some extent in recent years by local prostaglandin application. But our lack of understanding of the normal mechanisms of cervical softening still hinders our attempts to mimic the normal tissue changes using drugs.

Uterine involution

In the few days immediately following parturition, the uterus regresses rapidly, the cervix reforms and the cervical canal gradually closes. Within a few weeks of birth the uterus has returned to near its non-gravid dimensions. One of the few studies on human uterine involution

[310] showed the rapid decrease in tissue mass, with total weight reduced by about 50% within 7 days of parturition. Total uterine weight, water, muscular protein, collagen and hexosamine were all shown to decrease in the same proportions. There was not evidence of degenerative or necrotic changes in the uterus in the puerperium. The exact mechanisms involved in uterine involution are the subject of debate but they may be hormonal and relate to withdrawal of placental hormones. Electron microscopy studies in postpartum guinea pigs [311] suggest that smooth muscle cells, macrophages and the endothelial cells of myometrial vessels may all participate in involution. There is autodigestion of cytoplasmic organelles, thus reducing the contents of the cytoplasm, and degradation of extracellular collagen and ground substance. These processes seem to be carried out by an increase in the number of lysosomes and in the activity of their hydrolytic enzymes. It is tempting to speculate that prostaglandins are likely to be released in these circumstances, but further investigation is necessary to clarify the role of hormones in the process of postpartum uterine involution.

References

1 Schwalm H. & Dubrauszky V. (1966) The structure of the musculature of the human uterus — muscles and connective tissue. *American Journal of Obstetrics and Gynecology* **94**, 391.

2 Davies D.V. & Davies F. (eds) (1964) *Gray's Anatomy*, 3rd edn. Longman, London.

3 Carsten M.E. & Miller J.D. (1987) A new look at uterine muscle contraction. *American Journal of Obstetrics and Gynecology* **157**, 1303.

4 Andersson K.-E. & Ulmsten U. (1978) Effects of nifedipine on myometrial activity and lower abdominal pain in women with primary dysmenorrhoea. *British Journal of Obstetrics and Gynaecology* **85**, 142.

5 Andersson K.-E. (1977) Inhibition of uterine activity by the calcium antagonist nifedipine. In *Pre-term Labour*. Eds A. Anderson, R. Beard, J.M. Brudenell & P.M. Dunn, p. 101. Royal College of Obstetricians and Gynaecologists, London.

6 Schrey M., Read A. & Steer P. (1986) Oxytocin and vasopressin stimulate inositol phosphate production in human gestational myometrium and decidua cells. *Bioscience Reports* **6**, 613.

7 Schrey M., Read A. & Steer P. (1987) Stimulation of phospholipid hydrolysis and arachidonic acid mobilization in human uterine decidua cells by phorbol ester. *Biochemical Journal* **246**, 705.

8 Schrey M., Cornford P., Read A. & Steer P. (1988) A role for phosphoinositide hydrolysis in human smooth muscle during parturition. *American Journal of Obstetrics and Gynecology* **159**, 964.

9 Liggins G. & Wilson T. (1989) Phospholipases in the control of human parturition. *American Journal of Perinatology* **6**, 153.

10 Bleasdale J.E., Bala G.A. & Thakur N.R. (1990) Characterization of the major phosphoinositide-specific phospholipase C of human amnion. *Biology of Reproduction* **43**, 704.

11 Garfield R.E., Kannan M.S. & Daniel E.E. (1980) Gap junction formation in myometrium: control by estrogens, progesterone, and prostaglandins. *American Journal of Physiology* **238**, C81.

12 Beyer E.C., Kistler J., Paul D.L. & Goodenough D.A. (1989) Antisera directed against connexin 43 peptides react with a 43-kD protein localised to gap junctions localised to myocardium and other tissues. *Journal of Cell Biology* **108**, 595.

13 Garfield R.E. & Hayashi R.H. (1981) Appearance of gap junctions in the myocardium of women during labour. *American Journal of Obstetrics and Gynecology* **140**, 254.

14 MacKenzie L.W. & Garfield R.E. (1985) Hormonal control of gap junctions in the myometrium. *American Journal of Physiology* **248**, C296.

15 Lockwood C.J. & Schatz F. (1996) A biological model of the regulation of peri-implantation hemostasis and menstruation. *Journal of the Society of Gynaecological Investigation* **3**, 159.

16 Hakkinen L.M., Vuolteenaho O.J., Leppaluoto J.P. & Laatikainen T.J. (1992) Endothelin in maternal and umbilical cord blood in spontaneous labor and at elective caesarean delivery. *Obstetrics and Gynecology* **80**, 72.

17 Casey M.L., Brown C.E., Peters M. & MacDonald P.C. (1993) Endothelin levels in human amniotic fluid at mid-trimester and at term before and during spontaneous labor. *Journal of Clinical Endocrinology and Metabolism* **76**, 1647.

18 Hasegawa M., Sagawa N., Itoh H., Inamori K., Mori T., Yano J., Ogawa Y. *et al.* (1995) Endothelin receptors in the human amnion, chorion laeve, decidua vera and placenta. *Reproduction, Fertility and Development* **7**, 1585.

19 Yallampalli C. & Garfield R.E. (1994) Uterine contractile responses to endothelin-1 and endothelin receptors are elevated during labor. *Biology of Reproduction* **51**, 640.

20 Maggi M., Vannelli G.B., Fantoni G., Baldi E., Magini A., Peri A., Giannini S. *et al.* (1994) Endothelin in the human uterus during pregnancy. *Journal of Endocrinology* **142**, 385.

21 Neulen J. & Breckwoldt M. (1994) Placental progesterone, prostaglandins and mechanisms leading to initiation of parturition in the human. *Experimental and Clinical Endocrinology* **102**, 195.

22 Valenjela G.L., Hewitt C.W. & Ducsay C.A. (1995) Endothelin potentiates the in vitro contractile response of pregnant human myometrium to oxytocin. *American Journal of Obstetrics and Gynecology* **172**, 1573.

23 Izumi H., Byam-Smith M. & Garfield R.E. (1995) Gestational changes in oxytocin- and endothelin-1-induced contractility of the pregnant rat myometrium. *European Journal of Pharmacology* **278**, 187.

24 Molnar M. & Hertelendy F. (1995) Signal transduction in rat myometrial cells: Comparison of the actions of endothelin-1, oxytocin and prostaglandin F2 alpha. *European Journal of Endocrinology* **133**, 467.

25 Diamond J. (1983) Lack of correlation between cyclic GMP elevations and relaxation of non-vascular smooth muscle by nitroglycerin, nitroprusside, hydroxylamine and sodium azide. *Journal of Pharmacological Experimental Therapy* **225**, 422.

26 Yallampalli C., Izumi H., Byam-Smith M. & Garfield R.E. (1994) An L-arginine: nitric oxide system exists in the uterus and inhibits contractility during pregnancy. *American Journal of Obstetrics and Gynaecology* **170**, 175.

27 Yallampalli C. & Garfield R.E. (1993) Inhibition of nitric oxide produces signs similar to pre-eclampsia. *American Journal of Obstetrics and Gynaecology* **169**, 1316.

28 Morris N., Sooranna S., Eaton B. & Steer P. (1995) Exhaled NO concentration and amniotic fluid nitrite concentration in pregnancy. *European Journal of Clinical Investigation* **25**, 138.

29 Morris N., Eaton B.M. & Dekker G. (1996) Nitric oxide, the endothelium, pregnancy and pre-eclampsia. *British Journal of Obstetrics and Gynaecology* **103**, 4.

30 Lees C., Campbell S., Jauniaux E., Brown R., Ramsay B., Gibb D., Moncada S. *et al.* (1994) Arrest of preterm labour and prolongation of gestation with glyceryl trinitrate, a nitric oxide donor. *Lancet* **343**, 1325.

31 Bulbring E. & Tomita T. (1987) Catecholamine action on smooth muscle. *Pharmacology Reviews* **39**, 49.

32 Danforth D.N. (1947) The fibrous nature of the uterine cervix, and its relation to the isthmic segment in gravid and non-gravid uteri. *American Journal of Obstetrics and Gynecology* **53**, 541.

33 Danforth D.N. & Buckingham J.C. (1973) In *Biology of the Cervix*. Eds R.J. Blandau & K. Moghissi, p. 351. University of Chicago Press, Chicago.

34 Hughesdon P.E. (1952) The fibromuscular structure of the cervix and its changes during pregnancy and labour. *Journal of Obstetrics and Gynaecology of the British Commonwealth* **59**, 763.

35 Rorie D.K. & Newton M. (1967) Histological and chemical studies of the smooth muscle in the human cervix and uterus. *American Journal of Obstetrics and Gynecology* **99**, 466.

36 Schwalm H. & Dubrauszky V. (1966) The structure of the musculature of the human uterus—muscles and connective tissue. *American Journal of Obstetrics and Gynecology* **94**, 391.

37 Granstrom L., Ekman G. & Malmstrom A. (1991) Insufficient remodelling of the uterine connective tissue in women with protracted labour. *British Journal of Obstetrics and Gynaecology* **98**, 1212.

38 Granstrom L., Ekman G., Malmstrom A., Ulmsten U. & Woessner J.F. (1992) Serum collagenase levels in

346

relation to the state of the human cervix during pregnancy and labor. *American Journal of Obstetrics and Gynecology* **167**, 1284.

39 Uldbjerg N. & Malmstrom A. (1991) The role of proteoglycans in cervical dilatation. *Seminars in perinatology* **15**, 127.

40 Stjernholm Y., Sahlin L., Akerberg S., Elinder A., Eriksson H., Malmstrom A. & Ekman G. (1996) Cervical ripening in humans: Potential roles of estrogen, progesterone and insulin-like growth factor-I. *American Journal of Obstetrics and Gynecology* **174**, 1065.

41 Kanayama N. & Terao T. (1991) The relationship between granulocyte elastase-like activity of cervical mucus and cervical maturation. *Acta Obstetrica et Gynecologica Scandinavica* **70**, 29.

42 Danforth D.N., Buckingham J.G. & Roddick J.W. (1960) Connective tissue changes incident to cervical effacement. *American Journal of Obstetrics and Gynecology* **80**, 939.

43 Danforth D.N. (1954) The distribution and functional activity of cervical musculature. *American Journal of Obstetrics and Gynecology* **68**, 1261.

44 Schild H.O., Fitzpatrick R.J. & Nixon W.C.W. (1951) Activity of the human cervix and corpus uteri: Their response to drugs in early pregnancy. *Lancet* **i**, 250.

45 Najak Z., Hillier K. & Karim S.M.M. (1970) The action of prostaglandins on the human isolated non-pregnant cervix. *Journal of Obstetrics and Gynaecology of the British Commonwealth* **77**, 701.

46 Petersen L., Oxlund H., Uldbjerg N. & Forman A. (1991) In vitro analysis of muscular contractile ability and passive biomechanical properties of uterine cervical samples from non-pregnant women. *Obstetrics and Gynecology* **77**, 772.

47 Olah K., Gee H. & Brown J. (1993) Cervical contractions: the response of the cervix to oxyxtocic stimulation in the latent phase of labour. *British Journal of Obstetrics and Gynaecology* **100**, 635.

48 Olah K., Gee H. & Brown J. (1994) The effect of cervical contractions on the generation of intrauterine pressure during the latent phase of labour. *British Journal of Obstetrics and Gynaecology* **101**, 341.

49 Mikhail G. & Allen W.M. (1967) Ovarian function in human pregnancy. *American Journal of Obstetrics and Gynecology* **99**, 308.

50 Tulsky A.S. & Koff A.K. (1957) Some observations on the role of the corpus luteum in early human pregnancy. *Fertility and Sterility* **8**, 118.

51 Csapo A.I., Pulkkinen M.O., Ruttner B., Sauvage J.P. & Wiest W.G. (1972) The significance of the human corpus luteum in pregnancy maintenance. I. Preliminary studies. *American Journal of Obstetrics and Gynecology* **112**, 1061.

52 Csapo A.I., Pulkkinen M.O. & Wiest W.G. (1973) Effects of luteectomy and progesterone replacement therapy in early pregnant patients. *American Journal of Obstetrics and Gynecology* **115**, 759.

53 Yoshimi T., Strott C.A., Marshall J.R. & Lipsett M.B. (1969) Corpus luteum function in early pregnancy. *Journal of Clinical Endocrinology and Metabolism* **29**, 225.

54 Shearman, R.P. (Ed.) *Human Reproductive Physiology* (1972) Blackwell Scientific Publications, Oxford, p. 174.

55 Mishell D.R., Thorneycroft I.H., Nagata Y., Murata T. & Nakamura R.M. (1973) Serum gonadotropin and steroid patterns in early human gestation. *American Journal of Obstetrics and Gynecology* **117**, 631.

56 Hertogh R. De., Thomas K., Bietlot Y., Vanderheyden I. & Ferin J. (1975) Plasma levels of unconjugated estrone, estradiol and estriol and of HCS throughout pregnancy in normal women. *Journal of Clinical Endocrinology and Metabolism* **40**, 93.

57 Corker C.S., Michie E., Hobson B. & Parboosingh J. (1976) Hormonal patterns in conceptual cycles and early pregnancy. *British Journal of Obstetrics and Gynaecology* **83**, 489.

58 Brown W.E. & Bradbury J.T. (1947) A study of the physiologic action of human chorionic hormone: The production of pseudo-pregnancy in women by chorionic hormones. *American Journal of Obstetrics and Gynecology* **53**, 749.

59 Browne J.S.L. & Venning E.H. (1938) The effect of intramuscular injection of gonadotropic substances on the corpus luteum phase of the human. *American Journal of Physiology* **123**, 26.

60 Hanson F.W., Powell J.E. & Stevens V.C. (1971) Effects of hCG and human pituitary LH on steroid secretion and functional life of the human corpus luteum. *Journal of Clinical Endocrinology and Metabolism* **32**, 211.

61 Segaloff A., Sternberg W.H. & Gaskill C.J. (1951) Effects of luteolytic doses of chorionic gonadotropin in women. *Journal of Clinical Endocrinology* **11**, 936.

62 Gillman J. & Stein H. (1941) Human corpus luteum of pregnancy. *Surgery, Gynecology and Obstetrics* **72**, 129.

63 Weiss G., O'Byrne E.M. & Steinetz B.G. (1976) Relaxin: Product of human corpus luteum of pregnancy. *Science* **194**, 948.

64 Nelson W.W. & Greene R.R. (1958) Some observations on the histology of the human ovary during pregnancy. *American Journal of Obstetrics and Gynecology* **76**, 66.

65 Dekel N., David M.P., Yedwab G.A. & Kraicer P.F. (1977) Follicular development during late human pregnancy. *International Journal of Fertility* **22**, 24.

66 White C.A. & Bradbury J.T. (1965) Ovarian theca lutein cysts: Experimental formation in women prior to repeat cesarean section. *American Journal of Obstetrics and Gynecology* **92**, 973.

67 Maathuis J.B. & Kelly R.W. (1978) concentrations of prostaglandins F_{2a} and E_2 in the endometrium throughout the human menstrual cycle, after the administration of clomiphene or an oestrogen-progestogen pill and in early pregnancy. *Journal of Endocrinology* **77**, 361.

68 Willman E.A. & Collins W.P. (1976) Distribution of prostaglandin E_2 and F_{2a} within the foetoplacental unit throughout pregnancy. *Journal of Endocrinology* **69**, 413.

69 Wilson T. (1988) Lipocortins and their possible role in the onset of labour. *Prostaglandin Perspectives* **4**, 1.

70 Schwabe C., Steinetz B., Weiss G., Segaloff A., McDonald J.K., O'Byrne E., Hochman J. *et al.* (1978)

Relaxin. In *Recent Progress in Hormone Research* vol. 34. Ed. R.O. Greep, p. 123. Academic Press, New York.

71 Oscheroff P.L. & King K.L. (1995) Binding and cross-linking of ^{32}P-labeled human relaxin to human uterine cells and primary rat atrial cardiomyocytes. *Journal of Clinical Endocrinology and Metabolism* **136**, 4377.

72 Garibay-Tupus J.L., Maaskrant R.A., Greenwood F.C. & Bryant-Greenwood G.D. (1995) Characteristics of the binding of ^{32}P-labeled human relaxins to the human fetal membranes. *Journal of Endocrinology* **145**, 441.

73 Sanborn B.M., Kuo H.S., Weisbrodt N.W. & Sherwood O.D. (1980) The interaction of relaxin on the rat uterus. I. Effect of cyclic nucleotide levels and spontaneous contractile activity. *Endocrinology* **106**, 1210.

74 Kemp B. & Niall H.D (1981) Effect of relaxin on the cAMP-dependent protein kinase in rat uterus. In *Relaxin*. Eds G.D. Bryant-Greenwood, H.D. Niall & F.C. Greenwood, p. 273. Elsevier/North Holland, New York.

75 Downing S.J., McIlwrath A. & Hollingsworth M. (1992) Cyclic adenosine 3'5'-monophosphate and the relaxant action of relaxin in the rat uterus in vivo. *Journal of Reproduction and Fertility* **96**, 857.

76 Downing S.J. & Hollingsworth M. (1993) Uptake of relaxin in the uterus and cervix of the rat in vivo: influence of ovarian steroids and tolerance. *Journal of Reproduction and Fertility* **99**, 121.

77 Ginsburg F.W., Rosenberg C.R., Schwartz M., Colon J.M. & Goldsmith L.T. (1988) The effect of relaxin on calcium fluxes in the rat uterus. *American Journal of Obstetrics and Gynecology* **159**, 1395.

78 Anwer K., Hovington J.A. & Sanborn B.M. (1989) Antagonism of contracts and relaxants at the level of intracellular calcium and phosphoinositide turnover in the rat uterus. *Endocrinology* **124**, 2995.

79 Hytten F.E. & Leitch I. (1971) *The Physiology of Human Pregnancy*, 2nd edn, p. 333. Blackwell Scientific Publications, Oxford.

80 King G. (1954) Advanced extrauterine pregnancy. *American Journal of Obstetrics and Gynecology* **67**, 712.

81 Schofield B.M. & Wood C. (1964) Length-tension relation in rabbit and human myometrium. *Journal of Physiology* **175**, 125.

82 Turnbull A.C., Patten P.T., Flint A.P.F., Keirse M.J.N.C., Jeremy J.Y. & Anderson A.B.M. (1974) Significant fall in progesterone and rise in oestradiol levels in human peripheral plasma before the onset of labour. *Lancet* **i**, 101.

83 Bibby J.G. (1980) Studies in human pregnancy and parturition with particular reference to the role of prostaglandins and steroid hormones. MD thesis, University of Otago, Dunedin, New Zealand.

84 Darne J., McGarrigle H.H.G. & Lachelin G.C.L. (1987) Saliva oestriol, oestradiol, oestrone and progesterone levels in pregnancy; spontaneous labour at term is preceded by a rise in the saliva oestriol : progesterone ratio. *British Journal of Obstetrics and Gynaecology* **94**, 227.

85 Lewis P.R., Galvin P.M. & Short R.V. (1987) Salivary oestriol and progesterone concentrations in women during late pregnancy, parturition and the puerperium. *Journal of Endocrinology* **115**, 177.

86 Erny R., Pigne A., Prouvost C., Gamerre M., Malet C., Serment H. & Barrat J. (1986) The effects of oral administration of progesterone for premature labour. *American Journal of Obstetrics and Gynaecology* **154**, 525.

87 Noblot G., Audra P., Dargent D., Faquer F. & Mellier G. (1991) The use of micronised progesterone in the treatment of menace of preterm delivery. *European Journal of Obstetrics, Gynecology and Reproduction* **40**, 203.

88 Cameron I. & Baird D. (1988) Early pregnancy termination: A comparison between vacuum aspiration and medical abortion using prostaglandin (16, 16 dimethyl-trans-gamma2-PGE1 methyl ester) or the antiprogestogen RU 486. *British Journal of Obstetrics and Gynaecology* **95**, 271.

89 El-Rafaey H. & Templeton A. (1994) Early abortion induction by a combination of mifepristone and oral misoprostol: A comparison between two dose regimens of misoprostol and their effect on blood pressure. *British Journal of Obstetrics and Gynaecology* **101**, 792.

90 Carbonne B., Brennand J.E., Maria B., Cabrol D. & Calder A. (1995) Effects of gemeprost and mifepristone on the mechanical properties of the cervix prior to first trimester termination of pregnancy. *British Journal of Obstetrics and Gynaecology* **102**, 553.

91 Fuchs A. & Fuchs F. (1984) Endocrinology of parturition: a review. *British Journal of Obstetrics and Gynaecology* **91**, 948.

92 Gordon A. & Calder A. (1977) Oestradiol applied locally to ripen the unfavourable cervix. *Lancet* **2**, 1319.

93 Flint A.P.F. (1979) Role of progesterone and oestrogens in the control of the onset of labour in man: A continuing controversy. In *Human Parturition. New Concepts and Developments*. Eds M.J.N.C. Keirse, A.B.M. Anderson & J.B. Gravenhorst, p. 85. University Press, Leiden.

94 Kostrzewska A., Laudanski T. & Batra S. (1993) Effect of ovarian steroids and diethylstilboestrol on the contractile responses of the human myometrium and intramyometrial arteries. *European Journal of Pharmacology* **233**, 127.

95 Putnam C.D., Brann D.W., Kolbeck R.C. & Mahesh V.B. (1991) Inhibition of uterine contractility by progesterone and progesterone metabolites: Mediation by progesterone and gamma amino butyric acid receptor systems. *Biology of Reproduction* **45**, 266.

96 Mitchell B.F., Challis J.R. & Lukash L. (1987) Progesterone synthesis by human amnion, chorion, and decidua at term. *American Journal of Obstetrics and Gynaecology* **157**, 349.

97 Bell G.H. (1952) Abnormal uterine action in labour. *Journal of Obstetrics and Gynaecology of British Empire* **59**, 617.

98 Williams E.A. & Stallworthy J.A. (1952) A simple method of internal tocography. *Lancet* **i**, 330.

348

99 Steer P.J., Carter M.C., Gordon A.J. & Beard R.W. (1978) The use of catheter-tip pressure transducers for the measurement of intrauterine pressure in labour. *British Journal of Obstetrics and Gynaecology* **85**, 561.

100 Caldeyro-Barcia R., Alvarez H. & Reynolds S.R.M. (1950) A better understanding of uterine contractility through simultaneous recording with an internal and a seven channel external method. *Surgery, Gynecology and Obstetrics* **91**, 641.

101 Knoke J.D., Tsao L.L., Neuman M.R. & Roux J.F. (1976) The accuracy of measurements of intrauterine pressure during labour: A statistical analysis. *Computers and Biomedical Research* **9**, 177.

102 Arulkumaran S., Yang M. & Ratnam S.S. (1991) Reliability of intrauterine pressure measurements. *Obstetrics and Gynecology* **78**, 800.

103 Chua S., Arulkumaran S., Yang M., Ratnam S. & Steer P. (1992) The accuracy of catheter-tip pressure transducers for the measurement of intrauterine pressure in labour. *British Journal of Obstetrics and Gynaecology* **99**, 186.

104 Gee H., Taylor E. & Hancox R. (1988) A model for the generation of intrauterine pressure in the human parturient uterus which demonstrates the critical role of the cervix. *Journal of Theoretical Biology* **133**, 281.

105 Gough G.W., Randall N.J., Genevier E.S., Sutherland I.A. & Steer P.J. (1990) Head to cervix forces and their relationship to the outcome of labor. *Obstetrics and Gynecology* **75**, 613.

106 Allman A.C.J., Genevier E.S.G., Johnson M.R. & Steer P.J. (1996) Head-to-cervix force: an important physiological variable in labour. 1. The temporal relationship between head-to-cervix force and intrauterine pressure during labour. *British Journal of Obstetrics and Gynaecology* **103**, 763.

107 Allman A.C.J., Genevier E.S.G., Johnson M.R. & Steer P.J. (1996) Head-to-cervix force: an important physiological variable in labour. 2. Peak active force, peak active pressure and mode of delivery. *British Journal of Obstetrics and Gynaecology* **103**, 769.

108 Csapo A.I. & Sauvage J.P. (1968) The evolution of uterine activity during human pregnancy. *Acta Obstetricia et Gynecologica Scandinavica* **47**, 181.

109 Anderson A.B.M. & Turnbull A.C. (1968) Spontaneous contractility and oxytocin sensitivity of the human uterus in mid-pregnancy. *Journal of Obstetrics and Gynaecology of the British Commonwealth* **75**, 271.

110 Caldeyro-Barcia R. & Peiros J.J. (1959) Oxytocin and contractility of the pregnant human uterus. *Annals of the New York Academy of Science* **75**, 813.

111 Turnbull A.C. & Anderson A.B.M. (1968) Uterine contractility and oxytocin sensitivity during human pregnancy in relation to the onset of labour. *Journal of Obstetrics and Gynaecology of the British Commonwealth* **75**, 278.

112 Theobald G.W., Robards M.F. & Suter P.E.N. (1969) Changes in myometrial sensitivity to oxytoxin in man during the last six weeks of pregnancy. *Journal of Obstetrics and Gynaecology of the British Commonwealth* **76**, 385.

113 Poseiro J.J. & Noriega-Guerra L. (1961) Dose response relationships in uterine effects of oxytocin infusions. In *Oxytocin*. Eds R. Caldeyro-Barcia and H. Heller. Pergamon Press, Oxford.

114 Seitchik J. & Castillo M. (1983) Oxytocin augmentation of dysfunctional labour. II. Uterine activity data. *American Journal of Obstetrics and Gynecology* **145**, 526.

115 Embrey M.P. & Anselmo J.F. (1962) the effects of intravenous oxytocin on uterine contractility. II. Induction of labour with oxytocin: correlation of uterine response in late pregnancy with clinical events. *Journal of Obstetrics and Gynaecology of the British Commonwealth* **69**, 918.

116 Embrey M.P. (1975) *Prostaglandins in Reproduction*. Churchill-Livingstone, Edinburgh.

117 Carsten M.E. (1977) Can hormones regulate myometrial calcium transport? In *The Biochemistry of Smooth Muscle*. Ed. N.L. Stephens, p. 617. University Park Press, Baltimore.

118 Anderson A.B.M. & Turnbull A.C. (1969) Relationship between length of gestation and cervical dilatation, uterine contractility, and other factors during pregnancy. *American Journal of Obstetrics and Gynecology* **105**, 1207.

119 Honnebier W.J. & Swaab D.F. (1973) The influence of anencephaly upon intrauterine growth of fetus and placenta and upon gestation length. *Journal of Obstetrics and Gynaecology of the British Commonwealth* **80**, 577.

120 Stewart H.L. (1952) Duration of pregnancy and postmaturity. *Journal of American Medical Association* **148**, 1079.

121 Guerrero R. & Florez P.E. (1969) The duration of pregnancy. *Lancet* **ii**, 268.

122 Novy M.J., Walsh S.W. & Kitsinger G.W. (1977) Experimental fetal anencephaly in the rhesus monkey: Effect on gestational length and fetal and maternal plasma steroids. *Journal of Clinical Endocrinology and Metabolism* **45**, 1031.

123 Malpas P. (1933) Postmaturity and malformations of the foetus. *Journal of Obstetrics and Gynaecology of the British Empire* **40**, 1046.

124 Comerford J.B. (1965) Pregnancy with anencephaly. *Lancet* **i**, 679.

125 Milic A.B. & Adamson K. (1969) The relationship between anencephaly and prolonged pregnancy. *Journal of Obstetrics and Gynaecology of the British Commonwealth* **76**, 102.

126 Anderson A.B.M., Laurence K.M. & Turnbull A.C. (1969) The relationship in anencephaly between the size of the adrenal cortex and the length of gestation. *Journal of Obstetrics and Gynaecology of the British Commonwealth* **76**, 196.

127 Liggins G.C., Kennedy P.C. & Holm L.W. (1967) Failure of initiation of parturition after electrocoagulation of the pituitary of the fetal lamb. *American Journal of Obstetrics and Gynecology* **98**, 1080.

128 Liggins G.C., Fairclough R.J., Grieves S.A., Forster C.S. & Knox B.S. (1977) Parturition in the sheep. In *The Fetus and Birth*, Ciba Foundation Symposium 47, p. 5. Elsevier/Excerpta Medica/North Holland, Amsterdam.

129 Pakravan P., Kenny F.M., Depp R. & Allen A.C. (1974) Familial congenital absence of adrenal glands: Evaluation of glucocorticoid, mineralocorticoid and estrogen metabolism in the perinatal period. *Journal of Pediatrics* **84**, 74.

130 Laverty C.R.A., Fortune D.W. & Beischer N.A. (1973) Congenital idiopathic adrenal hypoplasia. *Obstetrics and Gynecology* **41**, 655.

131 Murphy B.E.P. (1973) Does the human fetal adrenal play a role in parturition? *American Journal of Obstetrics and Gynecology* **115**, 521.

132 Leong M.K.H. & Murphy B.E.P. (1976) Cortisol levels in maternal venous and umbilical cord arterial and venous serum at vaginal delivery. *American Journal of Obstetrics and Gynecology* **124**, 471.

133 Ohrlander S., Gennser G. & Eneroth P. (1976) Plasma cortisol levels in human fetus during parturition. *Obstetrics and Gynecology* **48**, 381.

134 Osinski P.A. (1960) Steroid 11β-ol dehydrogenase in human placenta. *Nature* **187**, 777.

135 Beitins I.Z., Bayard F., Ances I.G., Kowarski A. & Migeon C.J. (1973) The metabolic clearance rate, blood production, interconversion and transplacental passage of cortisol and cortisone in pregnancy near term. *Pediatric Research* **7**, 509.

136 Murphy B.E.P., Clark S.J., Donald I.R., Pinsky M. & Vedady D. (1974) Conversion of maternal cortisol to cortisone during placental transfer to the human fetus. *American Journal of Obstetrics and Gynecology* **118**, 538.

137 Murphy B.E.P., Patrick J. & Denton R.L. (1975) Cortisol in amniotic fluid during human gestation. *Journal of Clinical Endocrinology and Metabolism* **40**, 164.

138 Talbert L.M., Pearlman W.H. & Downing Potter H. (1977) Maternal and fetal serum levels of total cortisol and cortisone, unbound cortisol and corticosteroid-binding globulin in vaginal delivery and cesarean section. *American Journal of Obstetrics and Gynecology* **129**, 781.

139 Ohrlander S., Gennser G., Batra S. & Lebech P. (1977) Effect of betamethasone administration on estrone, estradiol-17β, and progesterone in maternal plasma and amniotic fluid. *Obstetrics and Gynecology* **49**, 148.

140 Gennser G., Ohrlander S. & Eneroth P. (1976) Cortisol in amniotic fluid and cord blood in relation to prenatal betamethasone load and delivery. *American Journal of Obstetrics and Gynecology* **124**, 43.

141 Nwosu U.C., Wallach E.E. & Bolognese R.J. (1976) Initiation of labour by intra-amniotic cortisol instillation in prolonged human pregnancy. *Obstetrics and Gynecology* **47**, 137.

142 Liggins G.C. (1977) Discussion. In *The Fetus and Birth*, Ciba Foundation Symposium 47. p. 421. Elsevier/Excerpta Medica/North Holland, Amsterdam.

143 Mati J.K.G., Horrobin D.F. & Bramley P.S. (1973) Induction of labour in sheep and in humans by single doses of corticosteroids. *British Medical Journal* **ii**, 149.

144 Chang R.J., Buster J.E., Blakeley J.L., Okada D.M., Hobel C.J., Abraham G.E. & Marshall J.R. (1976) Simultaneous comparison of Δ5-3β-hydroxysteroid levels in the fetoplacental circulation of normal pregnancy in labour and not in labour. *Journal of Clinical Endocrinology and Metabolism* **42**, 744.

145 Reiter E.O., Fuldauer V.G. & Root A.W. (1977) Secretion of the adrenal androgen, dehydroepiandrosterone sulfate during normal infancy, childhood, and adolescence, in sick infants, and in childbirth with endocrinologic abnormalities. *Journal of Pediatrics* **90**, 766.

146 De Peretti E. & Forest M.G. (1978) Pattern of plasma dehydroepiandrosterone sulfate levels in humans from birth to adulthood: Evidence for testicular production. *Journal of Clinical Endocrinology and Metabolism* **47**, 572.

147 Tähkä H. (1951) On the weight and structure of the adrenal glands and the factors affecting them, in children of 0–2 years. *Acta Paediatrica Scandinavica* **40** (Suppl. 81).

148 Johannisson E. (1968) The foetal adrenal cortex in the human: Its ultrastructure at different stages of development and in different functional states. *Acta Endocrinologica* **58** (Suppl. 130) p. 7.

149 Serón-Ferré M., Lawrence C.C., Siiteri P.K. & Jaffé R.B. (1978) Steroid production by definitive and fetal zones of the human fetal adrenal gland. *Journal of Clinical Endocrinology and Metabolism* **47**, 603.

150 Benirschke K. (1956) Adrenals in anencephaly and hydrocephaly. *Obstetrics and Gynecology* **8**, 412.

151 Serón-Ferré M., Lawrence C.C. & Jaffé R.B. (1978) Role of hCG in regulation of the fetal zone of the human fetal adrenal gland. *Journal of Clinical Endocrinology and Metabolism* **46**, 834.

152 Johanson D.C., Edey M.A. (1981) *Lucy — the beginnings of humankind.* Penguin, London.

153 Walters A. & Hammond J. (1938) The maternal effects on growth and conformation in Shire horse–Shetland pony crosses. *Proceedings of the Royal Society* **125**, 311.

154 Brooks A.A., Johnson M.R., Steer P.J., Pawson M.E. & Abdalla H.I. (1995) Birth weight: Nature or nurture? *Early Human Development* **42**, 29.

155 Kao, C.Y. (1989) Electrophysiological properties of uterine muscle. In *The Biology of the Uterus*. Eds R.M. Wynn & W.P. Jollie, p. 403. Springer, London.

156 Fuchs A.R., Romero R., Keefe D., Parra M., Oyarzun E. & Behnke E. (1991) Oxytocin secretion and human parturition: Pulse frequency and duration increase during spontaneous labor in women. *American Journal of Obstetrics Gynaecology* **165**, 1515.

157 Takahashi K., Diamond F., Bieniarz J., Yen H. & Burd L. (1980) Uterine contractility and oxytocin sensitivity in preterm, term and post-term pregnancy. *American Journal of Obstetrics Gynaecology* **136**, 774.

158 Fuchs A.R., Fuchs F., Husslein P. & Soloff M.S. (1984) Oxytocin receptors in pregnant human uterus. *American Journal of Obstetrics Gynaecology* **150**, 734.

159 Miller F.D., Chibbar R. & Mitchell B.F. (1993) Synthesis of oxytocin in amnion, chorion and decidua: A potential paracrine role for oxytocin in the onset of human parturition. *Regulatory Peptides* **45**, 247.

160 Richard S. & Zingg H.H. (1990) The human oxytocin gene promoter is regulated by estrogens. *Journal of Biological Chemistry* **265**, 6098.

161 Maggi M., Magini A., Fiscella A., Giannini S.,

350

Fantoni G., Toffoletti F., Massi G. *et al.* (1992) Sex steroid modulation of neurohypophysial hormone receptors in human nonpregnant myometrium. *Journal of Clinical Endocrinology and Metabolism* **74**, 385.

162 Takemura M., Kimura T., Nomura S., Makino Y., Inoue T., Kikuchi T., Kubota Y. *et al.* (1994) Expression and localisation of human oxytocin receptor mRNA and its protein in chorion and decidua during parturition. *Journal of Clinical Investigation* **93**, 2319.

163 Fuchs A.R., Husslein P. & Fuchs F. (1981) Oxytocin and the initiation of human parturition. II. Stimulation of prostaglandin production in human decidual cells by oxytocin. *American Journal Obstetrics Gynaecology* **141**, 694.

164 Moore J.J., Moore R.M. & Vander Kooy D. (1988) Protein kinase C activation is required for oxytocin induced prostaglandin production in human amnion cells. *Journal of Endocrinology* **72**, 1073.

165 Chard T., Hudson C.N., Edwards C.R.W. & Boyd N.R.H. (1971) Release of oxytocin and vasopressin by the human foetus during labour. *Nature* **234**, 352.

166 Honnebier W.J., Jösis A.C. & Swaab D.F. (1974) The effect of hypophysial hormones and human chorionic gonadotrophin (hCG) on the anencephalic fetal adrenal cortex and on parturition in the human. *Journal of Obstetrics and Gynaecology of British Commonwealth* **81**, 423.

167 Husslein P. (1987) The role of oxytocin in the onset of pre-term labour. *Prostaglandin Perspectives* **3**, 40.

168 Akerlund M., Hauksson A., Lundin S., Melin P. & Trojanar J. (1987) Vasotocin analogues which competitively inhibit vasopressin stimulated contractions in healthy women. *British Journal of Obstetrics and Gynaecology* **93**, 22.

169 Goodwin T.M., Paul R. & Silver H. (1994) The effect of the oxytocin anatagonist atosiban on preterm uterine activity in the human. *American Journal of Obstetrics Gynaecology* **170**, 474.

170 Schrey M.P., Read A.M. & Steer P.J. (1987) Stimulation of phospholipid hydrolysis and arachidonic acid mobilization in human decidua cells by phorbol ester. *Biochemical Journal* **246**, 705.

171 Grandin D.J. & Hall R.E. (1960) Fetal death before the onset of labor: An analysis of 407 cases. *American Journal of Obstetrics and Gynecology* **79**, 237.

172 Csapo A.I. (1977) The 'see-saw' theory of parturition. In *The Fetus and Birth*, Ciba Foundation Study Group 47, p. 159. Elsevier/Excerpta Medica/North Holland, Amsterdam.

173 Mitchell M.D. & Flint A.P.F. (1977) Progesterone withdrawal: Effects on prostaglandins and parturition. *Prostaglandins* **14**, 611.

174 Runnebaum B. & Zander J. (1971) Progesterone and 20α-dihydroprogesterone in human myometrium during pregnancy. *Acta Endocrinologica* **66** (Suppl.), 150.

175 Batra S. & Bengtsson L.P. (1978) 17β-Estradiol and progesterone concentrations in myometrium of pregnancy and their relationships to concentrations in peripheral plasma. *Journal of Clinical Endocrinology and Metabolism* **46**, 622.

176 Csapo A.I., Knobil E., Van der Molen H.J. & Wiest W.G. (1971) Peripheral plasma progesterone levels during human pregnancy and labor. *American Journal of Obstetrics and Gynecology* **110**, 630.

177 Turnbull A.C., Patten P.T., Flint A.P.F., Keirse M.J.N.C., Jeremy J.Y. & Anderson A.B.M. (1974) Significant fall in progesterone and rise in oestradiol levels in human peripheral plasma before the onset of labour. *Lancet* **i**, 101.

178 Batra S., Bengtsson L.P., Grundsell H. & Sjöberg N.-O. (1976) Levels of free and protein-bound progesterone in plasma during late pregnancy. *Journal of Clinical Endocrinology and Metabolism* **42**, 1041.

179 Turnbull A.C., Anderson A.B.M., Flint A.P.F., Jeremy J.Y., Keirse M.J.N.C. & Mitchell M.D. (1977) Human parturition. In *The Fetus and Birth*, Ciba Foundation Symposium 47, p. 427. Elsevier/Excerpta Medica/North Holland, Amsterdam.

180 Siiteri P.K. & MacDonald P.C. (1963) The utilisation of circulating dehydroepiandrosterone sulfate for oestrogen synthesis during human pregnancy. *Steroids* **2**, 713.

181 Gant N.F., Hutchinson H.T., Siiteri P.K. & MacDonald P.C. (1971) Study of the metabolic clearance rate of dehydroisoandrosterone sulfate in pregnancy. *American Journal of Obstetrics and Gynecology* **111**, 555.

182 Madden J.D., Siiteri P.K., MacDonald P.C. & Gant N.F. (1976) The pattern and rates of metabolism of maternal plasma dehydroisandrosterone sulfate in human pregnancy. *American Journal of Obstetrics and Gynecology* **125**, 915.

183 Nieschlag E., Walk T. & Schindler A.E. (1974) Dehydroepiandrosterone (DHA) and DHA-sulfate during pregnancy in maternal blood. *Hormone and Metabolic Research* **6**, 170.

184 Pinto R.M., Votta R.A., Montuori E. & Baleiron H. (1964) Action of estradiol 17β on the activity of the pregnant human uterus. *American Journal of Obstetrics and Gynecology* **88**, 759.

185 Pinto R.M., Fisch L., Schwarcz R.L. & Montuori E. (1964) Action of estradiol 17β upon uterine contractility and the milk-ejecting effect in the pregnant woman. *American Journal of Obstetrics and Gynecology* **90**, 99.

186 Pinto R.M., Leon C., Mazzocco N. & Scasserra V. (1967) Action of estradiol 17β at term and at onset of labor. *American Journal of Obstetrics and Gynecology* **98**, 540.

187 Oakey R.E., Cawood M.L. & MacDonald R.R. (1974) Biochemical and clinical observations in a pregnancy with placental sulphatase and other enzyme deficiencies. *Clinical Endocrinology* **3**, 131.

188 Osathanondh R., Canick J., Ryan K.J. & Tulchinsky D. (1976) Placental sulfatase deficiency: A case study. *Journal of Clinical Endocrinology and Metabolism* **43**, 208.

189 France J.T. & Liggins G.C. (1969) Placental sulfatase deficiency. *Journal of Clinical Endocrinology and Metabolism* **29**, 138.

190 Fliegner J.R.H., Schindler I. & Brown J.B. (1972) Low urinary oestriol excretion during pregnancy associated with placental sulphatase deficiency or congeni-

tal adrenal hypoplasia. *Journal of Obstetrics and Gynaecology of the British Commonwealth* **79**, 810.

191 France J.T., Seddon R.J. & Liggins G.C. (1973) A study of a pregnancy with low estrogen production due to placental sulfatase deficiency. *Journal of Clinical Endocrinology and Metabolism* **36**, 1.

192 Tabei T. & Heinrichs W.L. (1976) Diagnosis of placental sulfatase deficiency. *American Journal of Obstetrics and Gynecology* **124**, 409.

193 Pulkkinen M.O. & Enkola K. (1972) The progesterone gradient of the human fetal membranes. *International Journal of Gynaecology and Obstetrics* **10**, 93.

194 Milewich L., Gant N.F., Schwarz B.E., Prough R.A., Chen G.T., Athey B. & MacDonald P.C. (1977) Initiation of human parturition. VI. Identification and quantification of progesterone metabolites produced by the components of human fetal membranes. *Journal of Clinical Endocrinology and Metabolism* **45**, 400.

195 Milewich L., Gant N.F., Schwarz B.E., Chen G.T. & MacDonald P.C. (1977) Initiation of human parturition. VIII. Metabolism of progesterone by fetal membranes of early and late human gestation. *Obstetrics and Gynecology* **50**, 45.

196 Schwarz B.E., Milewich L., Johnston J.M., Porter J.C. & MacDonald P.C. (1976) Initiation of human parturition. V. Progesterone binding substance in fetal membranes. *Obstetrics and Gynecology* **48**, 685.

197 Bourne G. (1965) *The Human Amnion and Chorion.* Year Book Medical Publishers, Chicago.

198 Gant N.F., Milewich L., Calvert M.E. & MacDonald P.C. (1977) Steroid sulfatase activity in human fetal membranes. *Journal of Clinical Endocrinology and Metabolism* **45**, 965.

199 Murphy B.E.P. (1977) Chorionic membrane as an extra-adrenal source of foetal cortisol in human amniotic fluid. *Nature* **266**, 179.

200 Tanswell A.K., Worthington D. & Smith B.T. (1977) Human amniotic membrane corticosteroid 11-oxidoreductase activity. *Journal of Clinical Endocrinology and Metabolism* **45**, 721.

201 Kurachi Y., Ito H., Sugimoto T., Shimuzu T., Miki I. & Ui M. (1989) Arachidonic acid metabolites as intracellular modulators of the G protein-gated cardiac K+ channel. *Nature* **337**, 555.

202 Kawarabayashi T. & Sugimori H. (1985) Effects of oxytocin and prostaglandin F2α on pregnant human myometrium recorded by the single sucrose-gap method: Comparison of an in-vitro experiment and an in vivo trial. *Asia-Oceania Journal of Obstetrics and Gynaecology* **11**, 247.

203 Karim S.M.M. (1966) Identification of prostaglandins in human amniotic fluid. *Journal of Obstetrics and Gynaecology of the British Commonwealth* **73**, 903.

204 Keirse M.J.N.C. & Turnbull A.C. (1975) Metabolism of prostaglandins within the pregnant uterus. *British Journal of Obsetetrics and Gynaecology* **82**, 887.

205 Keirse M.J.N.C. & Turnbull A.C. (1973) E prostaglandins in amniotic fluid during late pregnancy and labour. *Journal of Obstetrics and Gynaecology of the British Commonwealth* **80**, 970.

206 Keirse M.J.N.C., Flint A.P.F. & Turnbull A.C. (1974) F prostaglandins in amniotic fluid during pregnancy and labour. *Journal of Obstetrics and Gynaecology of the British Commonwealth* **81**, 131.

207 Davidson B.J., Murray R.D., Challis J.R.G. & Valenzuela G.J. (1987) Estrogen, progesterone, prolactin, prostaglandin E_2, prostaglandin $F_{2\alpha}$, 13,14-dihydro-15-keto-prostaglandin $F_{2\alpha}$, and 6-keto-prostaglandin F_α gradients across the uterus in women in labor and not in labor. *American Journal of Obstetrics and Gynecology* **157**, 54.

208 Pace-Asiak C.R. (1977) Oxidative biotransformations of arachidonic acid. *Prostaglandins* **13**, 811.

209 Vane J.R. (1978) Inhibitors of prostaglandin, prostacyclin and thromboxane synthesis. In *Advances in Prostaglandin and Thromboxane Research*, vol. 4. Eds F. Coceani & P.M. Olley, p. 27. Raven Press, New York.

210 Mitchell M.D., Flint A.P.F., Bibby J., Brunt J., Arnold J.M., Anderson A.B.M. & Turnbull A.C. (1977) Rapid increases in plasma prostaglandin concentrations after vaginal examination and amniotomy. *British Medical Journal* **ii**, 1183.

211 Schwarz B.E., Schultz F.M., MacDonald P.C. & Johnston J.M. (1975) Initiation of human parturition. III. Fetal membrane content of prostaglandin E_2 and $F_{2\alpha}$ precursor. *Obstetrics and Gynecology* **46**, 564.

212 Schultz F.M., Schwarz B.E., MacDonald P.C. & Johnston J.M. (1975) Initiation of human parturition. II. Identification of phospholipase A_2 in fetal chorioamnion and uterine decidua. *American Journal of Obstetrics and Gynecology* **123**, 650.

213 Grieves S.A. & Liggins G.C. (1976) Phospholipase A activity in human and ovine uterine tissues. *Prostaglandins* **12**, 229.

214 MacDonald P.C., Schultz M., Duenhoelter J.H., Gant N.F., Jimenez J.M.L., Pritchard J.A., Porter J.C. *et al.* (1974) Initiation of human parturition. I. Mechanism of action of arachidonic acid. *Obstetrics and Gynecology* **44**, 629.

215 Keirse M.J.N.C. & Turnbull A.C. (1976) The fetal membranes as a possible source of amniotic fluid prostaglandins. *British Journal of Obstetrics and Gynaecology* **83**, 146.

216 Duchesne M.J., Thaler-Dao H. & Crastes de Paulet A. (1978) Prostaglandin synthesis in human placenta and fetal membranes. *Prostaglandins* **15**, 19.

217 Mitchell M.D., Bibby J., Hicks B.R. & Turnbull A.C. (1978) Specific production of prostaglandin E_2 by human amnion *in vitro*. *Prostaglandins* **15**, 377.

218 Keirse M.J.N.C., Hanssens M.C.A.J.A., Hicks B.R. & Turnbull A.C. (1976) Prostaglandin metabolism in placenta and chorion before and after the onset of labor. *European Journal of Obstetrics and Gynecology and Reproductive Biology* **6**, 1.

219 Keirse M.J.N.C., Mitchell M.D. & Turnbull A.C. (1977) Changes in prostaglandin F and 13,14-dihydro-15-keto-prostaglandin F concentrations in amniotic fluid at the onset and during labour. *British Journal of Obstetrics and Gynaecology* **84**, 743.

220 Okazaki T., Casey M.L., Okita J.R., MacDonald P.C. & Johnston J.M. (1981) Initiation of human parturition. XIII. Phospholipase A2 and diacylglycerol lipase activities in fetal and decidua vera tissues from

352

early and late gestation. *Biology of Reproduction* **25**, 103.

221 Smieja Z., Zakar T., Walton J. & Olson P. (1993) Prostaglandin endoperoxide synthase kinetics in human amnion before and after labor at term and following preterm labor. *Placenta* **14**, 163.

222 Slater D., Berger L., Newton R., Moore G.E. & Bennett P.R. (1994) The relative abundance of type 1 to type 2 cyclo-oxygenase mRNA in human amnion at term. *Biochemical and Biophysical Research Communication* **198**, 304.

223 Aitkin M.A., Rice G.E. & Brennecke S.P. (1990) Gestational tissue phospholipase A2 mRNA content and onset of spontaneous labour in humans. *Reproduction, Fertility and Development* **2**, 575.

224 Nackla S., Skinner K., Mitchell B.F. & Challis J.R.G. (1986) Changes in prostaglandin transfer across human fetal membranes following spontaneous labour. *American Journal of Obstetrics Gynaecology* **155**, 1337.

225 Roseblade C.K., Sullivan M.F., Khan F., Lumb M.R. & Elder M.G. (1990) Limited transfer of prostaglandin E2 across fetal membranes before and after labour. *Acta Obstetrica et Gynaecologica Scandinavica* **69**, 399.

226 Challis J.R.G., Riley S.C. & Yang K. (1991) Endocrinology of labour. *Fetal Medicine Reviews* **3**, 47.

227 Karim S.M.M. & Devlin J. (1967) Prostaglandin content of amniotic fluid during pregnancy and labour. *Journal of Obstetrics and Gynaecology of the British Commonwealth* **74**, 230.

228 Åkesson B. & Gustavii B. (1975) Occurrence of phospholipase A_1 and A_2 in human decidua. *Prostaglandins* **9**, 667.

229 Gustavii B. (1973) Studies on the mode of action of intra-amniotically and extra-amniotically injected hypertonic saline in therapeutic abortion. *Acta Obstetricia et Gynaecologica Scandinavica* suppl. **25**, 1.

230 Gustavii B. (1975) Release of lysosomal acid phosphatase into the cytoplasm of decidual cells before the onset of labour in humans. *British Journal of Obstetrics and Gynaecology* **82**, 177.

231 Schwarz B.E., Schultz F.M., MacDonald P.C. & Johnston J.M. (1976) Initiation of human parturition. IV. Demonstration of phospholipase A_2 in the lysosomes of human fetal membranes. *American Journal of Obstetrics and Gynecology* **125**, 1089.

232 Gustavii B. (1977) Human decidua and uterine contractility. In *The Fetus and Birth*, Ciba Foundation Symposium 47, p. 343. Elsevier/Excerpta Medica/North Holland, Amsterdam.

233 Mitchell M.D., Anderson A.B.M., Keirse M.J.N.C. & Turnbull A.C. (1977) Evidence for a local control of prostaglandins within the pregnant human uterus. *British Journal of Obstetrics and Gynaecology* **84**, 35.

234 Dray F. & Frydman R. (1976) Primary prostaglandins in amniotic fluid in pregnancy and spontaneous labour. *American Journal of Obstetrics and Gynecology* **126**, 13.

235 Salmon J.A. & Amy J.J. (1973) Levels of prostaglandin $F_{2\alpha}$ in amniotic fluid during pregnancy and labour. *Prostaglandins* **4**, 523.

236 Hibbard B.M., Sharma S.C., Fitzpatrick R.J. & Hamlett J.D. (1974) Prostaglandin $F_{2\alpha}$ concentrations in amniotic fluid in late pregnancy. *Journal of Obstetrics and Gynaecology of the British Commonwealth* **81**, 35.

237 Keirse M.J.N.C., Hicks B.R., Mitchell M.D. & Turnbull A.C. (1977) Increase of the prostaglandin precursor, arachidonic acid, in amniotic fluid during spontaneous labour. *British Journal of Obstetrics and Gynaecology* **84**, 937.

238 Filshie G.M. & Anstey M.D. (1978) The distribution of arachidonic acid in plasma and tissues of patients near term undergoing elective or emergency Caesarean section. *British Journal of Obstetrics and Gynaecology* **85**, 119.

239 Lewis R.B. & Schulman J.D. (1973) Influence of acetylsalicyclic acid, an inhibitor of prostaglandin synthesis, on the duration of human gestation and labour. *Lancet* **ii**, 1159.

240 Collins E. & Turner G. (1975) Maternal effects of regular salicylate ingestion in pregnancy. *Lancet* **ii**, 335.

241 Creasy R.K. (1987) Inhibition of preterm labour. *Prostaglandin Perspectives* **3**, 38.

242 Liggins G.C. (1968) Premature parturition after infusion of corticotrophin or cortisol into foetal lambs. *Journal of Endocrinology* **42**, 323.

243 Liggins G.C. (1973) The physiological role of prostaglandins in parturition. *Journal of Reproduction and Fertility* **18** (Suppl.), 143.

244 Wintour E.M., Bell R.J., Carson R.S., MacIssac R.J., Tregear G.W., Vale W. & Wang X.M. (1986) Effect of long-term infusion of ovine corticotrophin-releasing factor in the immature ovine fetus. *Journal of Endocrinology* **111**, 469.

245 Shibasaki T., Odagiri E., Shizume K. & Ling N. (1982) Corticotrophin-releasing factor-like activity in human placental extracts. *Journal of Clinical Endocrinology and Metabolism* **55**, 384.

246 Riley S.C. & Challis J.R.G. (1991) Corticotrophin-releasing hormone production by the placenta and fetal membranes. *Placenta* **12**, 105.

247 Sasaki A., Liotta A.S., Luckey M.M., Margioris A.N., Suda T. & Krieger D. (1984) Immunoreactive corticotrophin-releasing factor is present in human maternal plasma during the third trimester of pregnancy. *Journal of Clinical Investigation* **76**, 2026.

248 Perkins A.V., Linton E.A., Eben F., Simpson J., Wolfe C.D.A. & Redman C.W.G. (1995) Corticotrophin-releasing hormone and corticotrophin-releasing hormone binding protein in normal and pre-eclamptic human pregnancies. *British Journal of Obstetrics and Gynaecology* **102**, 118.

249 Wolfe C.D.A., Patel S.P., Linton E.A., Campbell E.A., Anderson J., Dornhorst A., Lowry P.J. *et al.* (1988) Plasma corticotrophin-releasing factor (CRF) in abnormal pregnancy. *British Journal of Obstetrics and Gynaecology* **95**, 1003.

250 Goland R.S., Jozak S., Warren W.B., Conwell I.M., Stark R.I. & Tropper P.J. (1993) Elevated levels of umbilical cord plasma corticotrophin-releasing hormone in growth retarded fetuses. *Journal of Clinical Endocriology and Metabolism* **77**, 1174.

251 Warren W.B., Goland R.S., Wardlaw S.L., Stark R.I.,

Fox H.E. & Conwell I.M. (1990) Elevated maternal plasma corticotrophin-releasing hormone levels in twin gestation. *Journal of Perinatal Medicine* **18**, 39.

252 Robinson B.G., Emanuel R.L., Frim D.N. & Majzoub J.A. (1988) Glucocorticoid stimulates the expression of corticotrophin-releasing hormone-gene in human placenta. *Proceedings of the National Academy of Sciences of the USA* **85**, 5244.

253 Hillhouse E.W., Milton N., Grammatopoulos D. & Quartero H.W.P. (1993) The identification of a human myometrial corticotrophin-releasing hormone receptor that increases in affinity during pregnancy. *Journal of Clinical Endocrinology and Metabolism* **76**, 736.

254 Grammatopoulos D., Milton N. & Hillhouse E.W. (1994) The human myometrial CRH receptor: G proteins and second messengers. *Cellular and Molecular Endocrinology* **76**, 245.

255 Grammatopoulos D., Stirrat G.M., Williams S.A. & Hillhouse E.W. (1996) The biological activity of the corticotrophin-releasing hormone receptor-adenylate cyclase complex in human myometrium is reduced. *Journal of Clinical Endocrinology and Metabolism* (in press).

256 Europe-Finer G.N., Phaneuf S., Tolkovosky A.M., Watson S.P. & Lopez-Bernal A. (1994) Down-regulation of gas in human myometrium in term and preterm labour: A mechanism for parturition. *Journal of Clinical Endocrinology and Metabolism* **79**, 1835.

257 Clifton V.L., Read M.A., Leitch I.M., Boura A.L.A., Robinson P.J. & Smith R. (1994) Corticotrophin-releasing hormone-induced vasodilatation in the human fetal placental circulation. *Journal of Clinical Endocrinology and Metabolism* **79**, 666.

258 Petragalia F., Sawchenko P.E., Rivier J. & Vale W. (1987) Evidence for the local stimulation of ACTH-secretion by coticotrophin-releasing factor in human placenta. *Nature* **328**, 717.

259 Jones S.A. & Challis J.R.G. (1989) Local stimulation of prostaglandin production by corticotrophin releasing hormone in fetal membranes and placenta. *Biochemical and Biophysical Research Communication* **159**, 964.

260 Petragalia F., Sutton S. & Vale W. (1989) Neurotransmitters and peptides modulate the release of immunoreactive CRH from cultured human placental cells. *Journal of Obstetrics and Gynaecology* **160**, 247.

261 Soloff M.S., Swartz T.L. & Steinberg A.H. (1974) Oxytocin receptors in human uterus. *Journal of Clinical Endocrinology and Metabolism* **38**, 1052.

262 Wakeling A.E. & Wyngarden L.J. (1974) Prostaglandin receptors in human, monkey, and hamster uterus. *Endocrinology* **95**, 55.

263 Murphy B.E.P. (1977) Conversion of cortisol to cortisone by the human uterus and its reversal in pregnancy. *Journal of Clinical Endocrinology and Metabolism* **44**, 1214.

264 Garfield R.E., Rabideau S., Challis J.R.G. & Daniel E.E. (1979) Ultrastructural basis for maintenance and termination of pregnancy. *American Journal of Obstetrics and Gynecology* **133**, 308.

265 Little B., Smith D.W., Jessiman A.G., Selenkow H.A., Van T'Hoff W., Eglin J.M. & Moore D.F. (1958) Hypophysectomy during pregnancy in a patient with cancer of the breast: Case report with hormone studies. *Journal of Clinical Endocrinology and Metabolism* **18**, 425.

266 Hendricks C.H. (1954) The neurohypophysis in pregnancy. *Obstetrical and Gynecology Survey* **9**, 323.

267 Chard T. (1973) The posterior pituitary and the induction of labour. In *Endocrine Factors in Labour*. Eds A. Klopper & J. Gardner, p. 61. Cambridge University Press, Cambridge.

268 Osler M. (1962) Addison's disease and pregnancy. *Acta Endocrinologica* **41**, 67.

269 Bell C. (1972) Autonomic nervous control of reproduction: Circulatory and other factors. *Pharmacological Reviews* **24**, 657.

270 Wansbrough H., Nakanishi H. & Wood C. (1968) The effect of adrenergic receptor blocking drugs on the human uterus. *Journal of Obstetrics and Gynaecology of the British Commonwealth* **75**, 189.

271 Bourne A. & Burn J.H. (1927) The dosage and action of pituitary extract and the ergot alkaloids on the uterus in labour with a note on the action of adrenalin. *Journal of Obstetrics and Gynaecology of the British Empire* **34**, 249.

272 Wansbrough H., Nakanishi H. & Wood C. (1967) Effect of epinephrine on human uterine activity *in vitro* and *in vivo*. *Obstetrics and Gynecology* **30**, 779.

273 Barden T.P. & Standar R.W. (1969) The effects of propranolol on uterine activity in term human pregnancy. *Journal of Reproductive Medicine* **2**, 188.

274 Schrey M.P., Hare A.L., Ilson S.L. & Walters M.P. (1995) Decidual histamine release and amplification of prostaglandin F2 alpha production by histamine in interleukin-1 beta-primed decidual cells: potential interactive role for inflammatory mediators in uterine function at term. *Journal of Clinical Endocrinology & Metabolism* **80**, 648.

275 Hillier K., Calder A.A. & Embrey M.P. (1974) Concentrations of prostaglandin $F_{2\alpha}$ in amniotic fluid and plasma in spontaneous and induced labours. *Journal of Obstetrics and Gynaecology of the British Commonwealth* **81**, 257.

276 Gréen K., Bygdeman M., Toppozada M. & Wiqvist N. (1974) The role of prostaglandin $F_{2\alpha}$ in human parturition. Endogenous levels of 15-keto-13,14-dihydroprostaglandin $F_{2\alpha}$ during labor. *American Journal of Obstetrics and Gynecology* **120**, 25.

277 Mitchell M.D., Flint A.P.F., Bibby J., Brunt J., Arnold J.M., Anderson A.B.M. & Turnbull A.C. (1978) Plasma concentrations of prostaglandins during late human pregnancy: influence of normal and pre-term labour. *Journal of Clinical Endocrinology and Metabolism* **46**, 947.

278 Hamberg M. (1974) Quantitative studies on prostaglandin synthesis in man. III. Excretion of the major urinary metabolites of prostaglandin $F_{1\alpha}$ and $F_{2\alpha}$ during pregnancy. *Life Sciences* **14**, 247.

279 Swaab D.F., Boer K. & Honnebier W.J. (1977) The influence of the fetal hypothalamus and pituitary on the onset and course of parturition. In *The Fetus and Birth*, Ciba Foundation Symposium 47,

354

p. 379. Elsevier/Excerpta Medica/North Holland, Amsterdam.

280 Fuchs F., Fuchs A.-R., Poblete V.F. & Risk A. (1967) Effect of alcohol on threatened premature labor. *American Journal of Obstetrics and Gynecology* **99**, 627.

281 Ferguson J.K.W. (1941) A study of the motility of the intact uterus at term. *Surgery, Gynecology and Obstetrics* **73**, 359.

282 Gillespie A., Brummer H.C. & Chard T. (1972) Oxytocin release by infused prostaglandin. *British Medical Journal* **i**, 543.

283 Fisch L., Sala N.L. & Schwarcz R.L. (1964) Effect of cervical dilatation upon uterine contractility in pregnant women and its relation to oxytocin secretion. *American Journal of Obstetrics and Gynecology* **90**, 108.

284 Matadial L. & Cibils L.A. (1976) The effect of epidural anesthesia on uterine activity and blood pressure. *American Journal of Obstetrics and Gynecology* **125**, 846.

285 Sala N.L., Schwarcz R.L., Althabe O., Fisch L. & Fuente O. (1970) Effect of epidural anesthesia upon uterine contractility induced by artificial cervical dilatation in human pregnancy. *American Journal of Obstetrics and Gynecology* **106**, 26.

286 Goodlin R.C., Keller D.W. & Raffin M. (1971) Orgasm during pregnancy: Possible deleterious effects. *Obstetrics and Gynecology* **38**, 916.

287 Zuckerman H., Reis U. & Rubinstein I. (1974) Inhibition of human premature labour by indomethacin. *Obstetrics and Gynecology* **44**, 787.

288 Lindgren L. (1973) In *Biology of the Cervix*. Eds R.J. Blandau & K. Moghissi, p. 385. University of Chicago Press.

289 Danforth D.N., Veiss A., Breen M., Weinstein H.G., Buckingham J.C. & Manalo P. (1974) The effect of pregnancy and labor on the human cervix: Changes in collagen, glycoproteins and glycosaminoglycans. *American Journal of Obstetrics and Gynecology* **120**, 641.

290 Ito A., Naganeo K., Mori Y., Hirakawa S. & Hayashi M. (1977) PZ-Peptidase activity in human uterine cervix in pregnancy at term. *Clinica Chimica Acta* **78**, 267.

291 Von Maillot K. & Zimmermann B.K. (1976) The solubility of collagen of the uterine cervix during pregnancy and labour. *Archiv für Gynäkologie* **220**, 275.

292 Karube H., Kanke Y. & Mori Y. (1975) Increase of structural glycoprotein during dilatation of human cervix in pregnancy at term. *Endocrinologica Japonica* **22**, 445.

293 Von Maillot K. & Greiling H. (1977) Der Glykosaminoglykan-Gehalt der Cervix Uteri während Schwangerschaft und Geburt. *Archiv für Gynäkologie* **224**, 220.

294 Ichijo M., Shimizu T. & Sasai Y. (1976) Histological aspects of cervical ripening. *Tohoku Journal of Experimental Medicine* **118**, 153.

295 Pinto R.M., Wenceslao R. & Votta R.A. (1965) Uterine cervix ripening in term pregnancy due to the action of estradiol 17β. *American Journal of Obstetrics and Gynecology* **92**, 319.

296 Gordon A.J. & Calder A.A. (1977) Oestradiol applied locally to ripen the unfavourable cervix. *Lancet* **ii**, 1319.

297 Calder A.A., Embrey M.P. & Tait T. (1977) Ripening of the cervix with extra-amniotic prostaglandin E_2 in viscous gel before induction of labour. *British Journal of Obstetrics and Gynaecology* **84**, 264.

298 MacKenzie I.Z. & Embrey M.P. (1978) The influence of pre-induction vaginal prostaglandin E_2 gel upon subsequent labour. *British Journal of Obstetrics and Gynaecology* **85**, 657.

299 MacLennan A.H. & Green R.C. (1979) Cervical ripening and induction of labour with intravaginal prostaglandin $F_{2\alpha}$. *Lancet* **i**, 117.

300 MacKenzie I.Z. & Embrey M.P. (1979) A comparison of PGE_2 and $PGF_{2\alpha}$ vaginal gel for ripening the cervix before induction of labour. *British Journal of Obstetrics and Gynaecology* **86**, 167.

301 MacKenzie I.Z. (1976) The effect of oxytocics on the human cervix during mid-trimester pregnancy. *British Journal of Obstetrics and Gynaecology* **83**, 780.

302 Hillier K. (1976) The effect of prostaglandins. In *The Cervix*. Eds J.A. Jordan & A. Singer, p. 236. W.B. Saunders, Philadelphia.

303 Conrad J.T. & Ueland K. (1976) Reduction of the stretch modulus of human cervical tissue by prostaglandin E_2. *American Journal of Obstetrics and Gynecology* **126**, 218.

304 Conrad J.T. & Ueland K. (1979) The stretch modulus of human cervical tissue in spontaneous, oxytocin-induced and prostaglandin E_2-induced labour. *American Journal of Obstetrics and Gynecology* **133**, 11.

305 Ellwood D.A., Mitchell M.D., Anderson A.B.M. & Turnbull A.C. (1979) A significant increase in *in vitro* production of PGE by the ovine cervix at delivery. *Journal of Endocrinology* **81**, 133P.

306 Ellwood D.A., Mitchell M.D., Anderson A.B.M. & Turnbull A.C. (1980) Specific changes in the *in vitro* production of prostanoids by the ovine cervix at parturition. *Prostaglandins* **19**, 479.

307 Ellwood D.A., Mitchell M.D., Anderson A.B.M. & Turnbull A.C. (1980) The *in vitro* production of prostanoids by the human cervix during pregnancy: Preliminary observations. *British Journal of Obstetrics and Gynaecology* **87**, 210.

308 Montfort I. & Pérez-Tamayo R. (1961) Studies on uterine collagen during pregnancy and puerperium. *Laboratory Investigation* **10**, 1240.

309 Dessouky A.D. (1971) Myometrial changes in postpartum uterine involution. *American Journal of Obstetrics and Gynecology* **110**, 318.

310 Ganong W.F. (Ed.) *Review of Medical Physiology*, 16th edn (1993) Prentice-Hall International, London.

311 Chard T. & Grudzinskas J.G. (eds) (1994) *The Uterus*, p. 66. Cambridge Reviews in Human Reproduction, Cambridge University Press, Cambridge.

312 Ganong W.F. (ed.) (1993) *Review of Medical Physiology*, 16th edn. Prentice-Hall International, London.

313 Gennser G., Ohrlander S. & Eneroth P. (1977) Fetal cortisol and the initiation of labour in the human. In *The Fetus and Birth*. Elsevier/Excerpta Medica/North Holland, Amsterdam.

PART 4

The Endocrine System

The Hypothalamus and Pituitary Gland

MARY L. FORSLING

The hypothalamus

The hypothalamus is the region where co-ordination of endocrine and neural control occurs. As well as controlling endocrine, behavioural and autonomic nervous system functions, it is a site for immune neuro-endocrine reactions. This region of the brain makes up the ventral half of the diencephalon and forms the lateral walls of the third ventricle. It is below and anterior to the thalamus from which it is separated by the hypothalamic sulcus. The posterior limits are defined by the mammillary bodies, while the anterior boundaries are provided by the optic chiasma which is a useful landmark. It consists of several fairly distinct subdivisions (Fig. 12.1) but may be considered to be divided anteroposteriorly into the following main regions, the chiasmatic (supraoptic) lying above the chiasma, the tuberal (infundibulotuberal) connected with the hypophyseal stalk and the posterior (mammillary). Mediolaterally are the periventricular, the intermediate (medial) and lateral zones [1]. The hypothalamus controls the maintenance of the internal environment, namely the restorative and reproductive functions and the readiness of the body to respond to external stimuli. It is able to do this as it receives input from all areas of the periphery and has massive connections with the limbic system which provide it with processed information concerning external stimuli. In addition, there are receptors located within its structures, namely thermoreceptors, important in evoking compensatory mechanisms as core temperature alters; osmoreceptors, important in controlling thirst and fluid excretion; and possibly glucose receptors, important in controlling food intake. Outputs from the hypothalamus control the pituitary gland and the activity of the sympathetic and parasympathetic systems. Although Sherrington concluded that the hypothalamus is the head ganglion of the autonomic nervous system, it has not yet been possible to identify conclusively by what routes control is achieved.

Microstructure of the pituitary gland

By contrast, the control of the pituitary gland is well defined. The gland acts to control many endocrine functions in the body via six hormones: the glycoproteins, luteinizing hormone (LH), follicular-stimulating hormone (FSH) and thyroid-stimulating hormone (TSH), and the polypeptide and peptide hormones, growth hormone, prolactin and adrenocorticotrophic hormone (ACTH). Because of its central role in the control of endocrine function, it has been termed 'the conductor of the endocrine orchestra', but in view of the work of Harris [2] and his successors, it is probably more correct to apply this term to the hypothalamus and describe the pituitary as the leader of the orchestra. The pi-

357

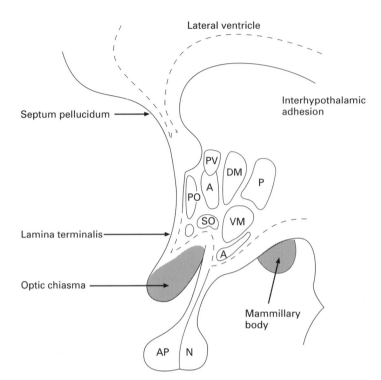

Fig. 12.1. Principal nuclei of the human hypothalamus. PV: paraventricular; PO: preoptic; A: anterior; DM: dorsomedial; P: posterior; SO: supraoptic; VM: ventromedial; A: arcuate. The pituitary gland is indicated by AP (anterior pituitary) and N (posterior pituitary). From Forsling and Grossman [16], with permission of the authors and publishers.

tuitary comprises an anterior and a posterior lobe and, in some species, but not humans, a clearly defined intermediate lobe between the two.

The two parts of the pituitary have different embryological origins. The anterior pituitary derives from an upgrowth of the buccal cavity named Rathke's pouch, while the pituitary stalk and the posterior pituitary develop as a downgrowth of the neural tissue which forms the floor of the third ventricle. The posterior pituitary thus comprises glial cells and nerve terminals, the cell bodies lying in two hypothalamic nuclei: the supraoptic and paraventricular nuclei. The adult hypothalamo-neurohypophyseal system undergoes reversible neuronal glial and synaptic changes in response to physiological stimulation. Thus, during parturition and lactation, when increased oxytocin secretion occurs, there is reduced coverage of the oxytocinergic somata and dendrites so that their surfaces become directly juxtaposed. In the neurohypophysis there is enlargement and multiplication of neurosecretory terminals together with retraction of glial processes [3].

In contrast, the anterior pituitary has no nerve supply, the control being hormonal. Anterior pituitary cells were originally classified according to their staining properties, the chromophils, which can be subdivided into acidophils and basophils, and chromophobe cells. However, they are now named after their specific secretory products. The acidophil-staining cells are the somatotrophs, producing growth hormone and the lactotrophs, producing prolactin. The somatotrophs are the largest and most abundant class of chromophils, normally forming over 50% of the adenohypophyseal cells [4]. The lactotrophs are randomly distributed through the pituitary and in non-pregnant women and men contain evenly dense granules about 200 nm in diameter or irregular granules resulting from fusion. Because of their glycoprotein product, the thyrotrophs and the gonadotrophs are basophilic, as are the corticotrophs. Numerically, the thyrotrophs are the least common type, forming less than 5% of the parenchymal cells of the anterior pituitary.

In non-pregnant women, the pituitary gland has been found to be about 20% heavier than in men [5]. Gland size increases during pregnancy [6]; estimates vary, but the weight is greater by 30% during the first pregnancy and in subsequent pregnancies by 50%. This increase in weight essentially results from an increase in size of the anterior pituitary, in particular the mammotrophs which become dominant in pregnancy and hypertrophy in lactation [7]. The secretory granules become about 600nm in diameter and are the largest in any hypophyseal cell [8]. By 11 months postpartum the regression of lactotroph hyperplasia is incomplete [9]. The proportion of somatotrophs is said to fall during pregnancy and there is recruitment of inhibited somatotrophs, namely those with reduced growth hormone (GH) mRNA, to become mammosomatotrophs [9]. These changes in pituitary microstructure are reflected in the circulating concentrations of the hormones. The number of gonadotrophs also falls and LH release is suppressed to the extent that by delivery the pituitary content of LH is less than 1% of normal [10]. While the circulating concentrations of ACTH and TSH are known to increase during pregnancy, the thyrotroph and corticotroph populations remain unchanged [11]. By magnetic resonance, the stalk remains in the midline, but the neurohypophysis is not visualized during the third trimester [12].

An increase in the size of the pituitary during pregnancy is clinically significant in women with existing pituitary tumours. If the adenoma fills the space in the fossa or if the adenoma increases in size, then the pituitary may expand through the dura and upwards. As is the case, for example, in acromegaly, the patient then experiences headache and visual field defects or, more rarely, a cavernous sinus syndrome. Even if no treatment is given the signs and symptoms generally remit following delivery and there are no permanent neurological consequences [13].

Blood supply to the pituitary

The arterial blood supply to the posterior pituitary comes directly from the inferior hypophyseal artery, a branch of the intracavernous internal carotid artery. The anterior pituitary, however, has no direct arterial blood supply. Nutrients and hormones arrive via the portal vessels (Fig. 12.2) which arise from a primary plexus in the median eminence which lies at the start of the stalk [14]. The rate of blood flow is high in this plexus which derives from the internal carotid artery via the superior hypophyseal artery, which joins with arteries from the circle of Willis. Reduced blood flow to the pituitary, associated with post-partum haemorrhage, was in the past the commonest cause of hypopituitarism (Sheehan's syndrome [15]). The mechan-

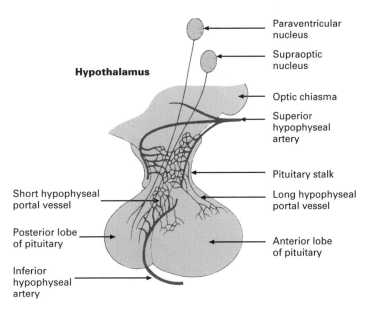

Fig. 12.2. The human pituitary gland and surrounding region showing the portal circulation. From Stanier and Forsling [123], with permission of the authors and publishers.

Hypothalamus

Paraventricular nucleus

Supraoptic nucleus

Optic chiasma

Superior hypophyseal artery

Pituitary stalk

Long hypophyseal portal vessel

Anterior lobe of pituitary

Short hypophyseal portal vessel

Posterior lobe of pituitary

Inferior hypophyseal artery

ism underlying the ischaemia is not clear, but during pregnancy the pituitary gland is probably more sensitive to hypoxaemia because of its increased metabolic requirements and may be more susceptible to vasoconstrictor influences. Furthermore, any swelling associated with the necrosis might compromise blood supply further. It has been estimated that if more than about 30% of the gland is preserved, the condition is asymptomatic. Sheehan observed that even when massive necrosis occurred, residual tisssue remained at the pars tuberalis and in the two lateral poles of the pituitary, but these are not perfused by hypothalamo–hypophyseal portal blood and may not therefore be exposed to hypothalamic hormones. In contrast to other pituitary conditions, the prolactin concentrations are low and an initial feature may be a failure to lactate, with subsequent amenorrhoea.

Control of pituitary hormone secretion

Control of anterior pituitary function is summarized in Fig. 12.3. The hormones controlling anterior pituitary function are synthesized in the tuberoinfundibular neurones which have small cell bodies, being described as parvicellu-

lar neurones. They lie in a region also termed the hypophysiotrophic area and terminate directly on the capillaries of the portal vessels. Most hypothalamic hormones are stimulatory, hormones from the peripheral target organs providing a generally inhibitory effect. Growth hormone and prolactin with no specific target endocrine gland are additionally controlled by inhibitory hormones, respectively somatostatin, produced largely in the arcuate nucleus and prolactin inhibiting hormone, although insulin-like growth factor (IGF1) does have a negative feedback effect on growth hormone secretion. Separate releasing hormones have not been found for LH and FSH, there being only the one gonadotrophin releasing hormone, GnRH, produced in the periventricular and arcuate nuclei. With the exception of prolactin-inhibiting hormone, which is believed to be dopamine, all the hypothalamic hormones are peptides.

Release of these hormones is controlled by inputs from higher centres as well as by feedback from peripheral target organs [16]. There is also, as in the case of growth hormone, a short feedback loop involving the anterior pituitary hormone secretion [17]. Secretion of the anterior pituitary hormones and presumably of the releasing hormones is pulsatile. Secretion, as in

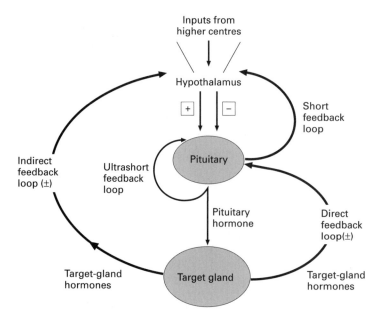

Fig. 12.3. Feedback loops in the control of anterior pituitary secretion. Growth hormone and prolactin do not have specific target gland feedback, nor have all pathways been proved for every hormone. From Stanier and Forsling [123], with permission of the authors and publishers.

the case of ACTH, may show a circadian rhythm, the concentrations being highest in the early morning and lowest at midnight. Secretion of other hormones such as growth hormone, prolactin and TSH is sleep related, circulating hormone concentrations reaching a peak during sleep. The model for control of the hypothalamo–pituitary–target gland axis is regularly modified as new discoveries are made, as, for example, the finding of binding proteins for growth hormon and corticotrophin-releasing hormone (CRH) [18,19]. The principal growth hormone-binding protein (GHBP), which has a high affinity, but low capacity, represents the extracellular domain of the growth hormone receptor. Continuous exposure to growth hormone increases the concentrations of GHBP, which in turn alters the pattern of growth hormone to which the receptors are exposed as well as altering their sensitivity to growth hormone. In this way not only the amount and pattern of growth hormone secretion, but also the responsiveness of peripheral target tisssues, may be regulated by the endocrine hypothalamus [20]. Posterior pituitary secretions are controlled mainly by signals to the hypothalamic nuclei, but can be modified by inputs to the terminals in the pituitary. The main factor controlling vasopressin release is total body water, the stimuli being an increase in osmolality or a fall in circulating blood volume [21]. Oxytocin release in women occurs primarily during parturition and lactation [22].

Maternal pituitary support of pregnancy

Although the microanatomy of the pituitary gland as well as its secretory activity show clear changes during pregnancy, impaired function does not usually jeopardize the pregnancy. Indeed, pregnancies resulting from induction of ovulation in women with hypopituitarism follow a normal course and even hypophysectomy performed as early as at 12 weeks of gestation does not usually result in fetal loss; neither does primary pituitary hyperfunction in the mother affect the fetus. Compared with that in other species, human pregnancy shows little dependence on the pituitary–ovarian axis and the maternal pituitary hormones have little

effect on the pregnancy after implantation [23]. The conceptus produces human chorionic gonadotrophin (hCG), which maintains the corpus luteum and progesterone production, and after 1–5 weeks it is also producing the steroid hormones required for pregnancy. Overall, the placenta produces large quantities of steroid and peptide hormones which directly or indirectly produce the wide variety of physiological adaptations seen in maternal systems. Amongst the proteins and peptides produced by the placenta are hormones with structural and biological similarities to those of the anterior pituitary. In addition to a gonadotrophin, these include placental lactogen (chorionic somatomammotrophin), placental growth hormone variant, chorionic TSH and chorionic ACTH. The releasing hormones chorionic CRH [24], chorionic GnRH [25,26] and chorionic somatostatin [27,28] have also been described. Despite the large amounts of some of these hormones entering the circulation, there is relatively little effect on the maternal hypothalamus–pituitary axis.

The steroid hormones produced by the placenta have a direct effect on the secretion of certain pituitary hormones. Potentially, the elevated oestrogen concentrations could alter feedback on the pituitary and hypothalamus through an increase in the concentration of hormone binding globulins for the target organ secretions. Thyroxine binding, cortisol binding-globulin and sex hormone-binding globulin are all elevated resulting in an increase in the total and bound amounts of the hormones. Free hormone concentrations, however, are relatively little affected [29]. The destruction or removal of any endocrine organ leads to compensatory changes in other organs and systems and delivery of the infant and placenta causes both immediate and long-term adjustments to the loss of pregnancy hormones. This includes an effect on the hypothalamus–pituitary axis, the activity of which is further influenced in women who breast feed.

Anterior pituitary secretion

Even though the maternal pituitary does not play a central role in the endocrine control of pregnancy, there are, as would be predicted from the morphological changes, altered profiles of hormone secretion [30].

Prolactin

The increase in lactotrophs in the pituitary over the course of pregnancy is reflected in an increase in the pituitary content of the hormone. It is the increased oestrogen produced during pregnancy which stimulates DNA synthesis and mitotic activity of the lactotrophs as well as increasing prolactin mRNA and hormone synthesis [31]. In non-pregnant women, oestrogen produces relatively small increases in prolactin concentrations, but the raised progesterone levels in pregnancy will also stimulate prolactin secretion [32]. Prolactin is the only pituitary hormone exhibiting a progressive rise in plasma concentrations throughout pregnancy. As shown in Fig. 12.4, they start to rise within a few days of conception, a rise which continues until at term values of up to 200 ng/ml may be obtained, some 10–20 times higher than in non-pregnant women [33]. Prolactin is also synthesized by the decidual tissue, although little of this material appears in the maternal circulation. The placenta also synthesizes placental lactogen [34], which is believed to exert an inhibitory effect on prolactin production, effectively mimicking the ultrashort feedback loop. Evidence in support of this comes from work on molar pregnancies in which placental lactogen concentrations are low and this inhibitory effect would not occur [35]. For any

given gestational age, the prolactin concentrations in such pregnancies are higher than normal. Although plasma prolactin is elevated, the normal pulsatile pattern of secretion persists [36] and the nocturnal and food-induced increases are still seen. This indicates that the normal neuroendocrine regulatory mechanisms are intact, consistent with the observation that the dopamine agonist bromocriptine inhibits prolactin secretion during pregnancy [13]. However, there is relatively little information available on the control of prolactin during pregnancy because of the obvious limitations to the administration of drugs at this time.

During pregnancy, prolactin plays an important role in breast development. In conjunction with oestrogen it causes primarily ductal, but also lobuloalveolar, growth and in the presence of progesterone its effect on alveolar growth is greatly enhanced. There is also evidence that prolactin can stimulate pancreatic β-cell production and may facilitate the production of insulin in pregnancy. In general, prolactin seems to promote the activities of other hormones and throughout pregnancy it may have widespread effects in addition to synergistic actions with ovarian and adrenal steroids. The prolactin produced by the decidua, while having no effect on the mother, produces high concentrations in the amniotic fluid where its role may be to regulate salt and water transport across the extraembryonic membranes [34].

With the onset of labour, prolactin concentrations fall. Delivery is associated with a surge in prolactin release, which is followed by a fall

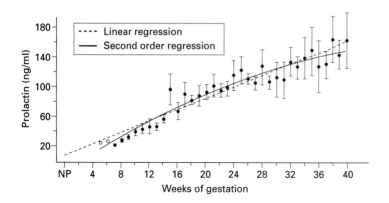

Fig. 12.4. Serial prolactin concentrations in the serum of non-pregnant and pregnant women throughout gestation. From Rigg *et al.* [33], with permission of the authors and publishers. $Y = 9.847 + 3.588\,X$. Correlation coefficient = 0.956. $P < 0.00005$.

both in women who breast feed and in those who do not, presumably as a result of the withdrawal of the oestrogen produced by the fetoplacental unit. Variable patterns of secretion are seen, depending upon whether lacation is maintained. In non-nursing mothers, prolactin concentrations return to basal within 30 days [37], remaining significantly above basal in mothers who feed their infants, so that concentrations may be elevated for up to 2 years. The normal sleep-associated increase in prolactin is evident 10 days after delivery [38]. The act of suckling produces a five- to tenfold increase in circulating concentrations via a neuroendocrine reflex, the afferent input originating in receptors in the nipple. Tactile sensitivity of the nipple is markedly reduced during pregnancy, but rapidly increases in the first few days following delivery [39]. The neuroendocrine reflex is believed to be modulated by oestrogen since anti-oestrogen preparations such as tamoxifen block the suckling-induced release of prolactin and impair milk production while leaving basal prolactin concentrations unchanged [40].

Prolactin is essential for milk production, but insulin and adrenal steroids are also necessary. They are, for example, required for casein mRNA production by mouse mammary epithelial cells in response to prolactin [41]. Lactation does not occur during pregnancy because of the blocking effect of the high concentrations of placental steroids and indeed does not commence until non-conjugated oestrogens fall to non-pregnant levels at about 36–48 hours postpartum. Lactation is accompanied by a large increase in the number of prolactin receptors in the mammary gland and, like the growth hormone receptors, there appears to be autorgulation by the pituitary hormone [42]. Milk production is therefore maintained, despite the attenuated reponse to suckling as lactation progresses. The importance of the increased sensitivity of the breast to prolactin is illustrated by the report of normal lactation in a woman who had previously undergone hypophysectomy for a pituitary tumour and who had impaired prolactin release during suckling [43]. In the early puerperium, the amount of milk produced is positively correlated with the amount of prolactin released. Milk secretion is also dependent on the additional stimulus of emptying of the breast, which is aided by oxytocin release.

Growth hormone

Secretion of growth hormone differs in men and women, the secretory rates in premenopausal women being higher than in men. In a study of 24-hour profiles of growth hormone secretion, it was found that the 24-hour integrated growth hormone concentration correlated with oestradiol, but not testosterone [44]. It appears that the late follicular concentrations of oestradiol may enhance circulating growth hormone via an amplitude-modulated, rather than a frequency-modulated, effect on the endogenous growth hormone pulse. Progesterone may blunt this oestrogen-associated effect. In view of the effect of oestrogen, it is rather surprising that during the second half of gestation, the pituitary secretion falls. A blunting to such stimuli of growth hormone release as arginine infusion [45] and insulin hypoglycaemia [46] has also been reported. These observations result from the production of a growth hormone variant by the syncytiotrophoblastic epithelium of the placenta. This does not show the same patterns of release as growth hormone of pituitary origin and is presumed to have a negative feedback effect on pituitary secretion.

The growth hormone genes GH-N (growth hormone-normal gene) and GH-V (growth hormone-variant gene, placental growth hormone) belong to a family of closely related genes. The products of these two genes differ by 13 amino acids that are dispersed throughout the polypeptide chain. During the first 22 weeks of gestation, growth hormone is synthesized in the maternal pituitary by the expression of the GH-N gene. From 22 weeks of gestation to term, circulating concentrations of growth hormone continue to increase, the increase in the latter half of pregnancy being due to expression of the GH-V gene in the placenta [47]. Growth hormone production by the placenta is non-pulsatile and does not respond to growth hormone-releasing hormone [48]. The role of the growth hormone variant is not clear, but it is known to have a slightly different profile of activities from the pituitary hormone. Thus, there is less binding to the lactogenic growth hormone receptors [49], so that its lactogenic activity is less [50].

Binding to the somatogenic receptors and GHBP is similar to that of the pituitary hormone. Most authors report an increase in IGF1 during pregnancy [51] and this increase appears to correlate well with the circulating concentrations of growth hormone variant. These changes may contribute to the coarsening of features which is very occasionally observed in pregnant women. The placental hormone also has similar effects on carbohydrate and lipid metabolism to normal growth hormone, but it is not known whether the variant contributes to the resistance to insulin found in pregnancy. Growth hormone does not appear to be important for lactation which occurs normally in growth hormone-deficient dwarfs.

Hypothalamo–pituitary–adrenal axis

Plasma cortisol concentrations increase in pregnancy [52,53], a rise which can be mimicked by injection of oestradiol into non-pregnant women. The elevated levels are due in part to oestrogen stimulation of the synthesis of transcortin which rises from 3.5 to 10 mg%. There is, however, a rise in free cortisol [54], which probably represents both an increase in metabolic clearance and increased adrenal production. Despite the elevated cortisol concentrations, late pregnant women do not become Cushingoid, reflecting reduced responsiveness to the hormone. Circadian variations in cortisol concentrations are maintained in the pregnant women [55,56] and responses to stressors such as surgery are still seen [57]. Furthermore, as in other situations, epidural anaesthetics reduce the cortisol response to labour and to caesarean section. This indicates that the maternal hypothalamo–pituitary axis continues to play an important role in the control of adrenal function.

There is, however, some evidence that the shape of the cortisol rhythm is altered in pregnancy [54]. In addition, dexamethasone fails to suppress urinary free-cortisol levels as it does in non-pregnant women [58]. Failure of dexamethasone inhibition is also observed in patients

with Cushing's syndrome. Another apparent inconsistency was the observation that plasma ACTH concentrations increase during pregnancy, whereas the elevated cortisol concentrations would normally be expected to suppress pituitary hormone release returning cortisol concentrations to normal. These observations could result from changes in the hypothalamic sensitivity to cortisol, but are also consistent with an ectopic source of ACTH, in this case the placenta. Rees *et al.* [58] demonstrated bio- and immunoactive ACTH in the placenta. ACTH, together with a number of other peptides including β-endorphin, is derived from a large precursor molecule pro-opiomelanocortin (POMC), and POMC-like mRNA has been identified in the placenta [59]. This placental POMC could also contribute to the observed increased circulating concentrations of β-endorphin.

A number of factors have been proposed to modify ACTH production by the placenta, including placental CRH. A substance effective in stimulating the release of ACTH from rat pituitary cells was extracted from human placentae by Shibasaki *et al.* [24]. The gene encoding preproCRH has now been shown to be expressed in the placenta [60], a large increase in preproCRH mRNA being seen late in pregnancy. Immunocytochemical studies indicate that the syncytiotrophoblast is the site of localization of immunoreactive CRH. Production of ACTH and CRH by the placenta is not suppressible *in vitro* with exogenous steroids; rather, CRH production seems to be stimulated [61,62]. Placental CRH is released into the circulation, circulating concentrations showing gradual increases in midpregnancy (Fig. 12.5) and increasing markedly towards term [63,64]. The concentrations achieved are of the order of 1 ng/ml compared to less than 10 pg/ml in the peripheral blood of men and non-pregnant women and 500 pg/ml in the hypothalamo-pituitary portal system. Such high concentrations of circulating CRH would be expected to exert a profound effect on the maternal pituitary. However, it has been demonstrated that most of the placental CRH circulates in association with a binding protein [18,19]. It has been suggested that the rapid transit time through the pituitary portal system is too rapid either for dis-

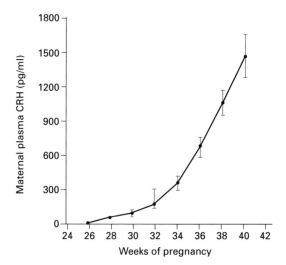

Fig. 12.5. Maternal plasma levels of immunoreactive CRH throughout pregnancy in the human. Values are given as means ± SEM (Redrawn from Campbell *et al.* [64]).

sociation of the CRH-binding protein complex or for the association of hypothalamic CRH with the binding protein [65]. However, the percentage of bound maternal CRH declines rapidly during the last 2 weeks of pregnancy [66], suggesting that CRH may have a role at term. The importance of the hypothalamo–pituitary–adrenal axis continues into lactation, cortisol being one of the hormones contributing to the process of continued milk secretion.

CRH is not the only hormone to influence ACTH secretion. The work of Gillies and Lowry [67] showed that vasopressin had a role and its importance in man has been demonstrated [68]. Vasopressin may have an important role to play in the control of pituitary ACTH during pregnancy. The response to peripherally administered CRH is reduced in human pregnancy, while work in primates suggests that vasopressin may be more effective during this period. It has been suggested, therefore, that placental CRH is responsible for the increased ACTH and cortisol concentrations observed in pregnancy, while other factors, especially vasopressin, contribute to acute stress induced changes in release from the pituitary [69].

Thyroid-stimulating hormone

There is a 15–20% increase in metabolic rate during pregnancy, largely due to the increasing metabolism of the placenta and fetus, and an increase in the size of the thyroid gland. This does not, however, appear to result from increasing concentrations of TSH and hence increased hypothalamic activity, despite the fall in free T_3. In the first trimester of pregnancy, there is a reduction in iodide absorption, probably as as result of increased renal filtration. This results in decreased plasma iodide and increased thyroid uptake of iodide from the blood. There is an increase in thyroid-stimulating activity as determined by bioassay, but this appears to be due to the high circulating concentrations of chorionic gonadotrophin possibly due to the common side chain with TSH. The thyroid-stimulating properties of this hormone may be sufficient to reduce plasma TSH concentrations and prevent the rise in TSH following thyrotrophin-releasing hormone administration [70,71]. At present it is not clear if there is a chorionic thyrotrophin, although thyrotrophin-releasing hormone has been extracted from the placenta. With regard to galactopoiesis, evidence from hypothyroid patients suggests that thyroid hormones do not play a significant role.

Gonadotrophins

The fall in the number of gonadotrophs during pregnancy is accompanied by a fall in the pituitary content and low basal plasma concentrations of LH and FSH. There is also a loss of the gonadotrophin response to GnRH administration [72]. The suppression of gonadotrophins during pregnancy is taken to be due to the high circulating concentrations of oestrogens and progesterone. However, there may be additional inhibitory effects from hCG which suppresses LH concentrations in postmenopausal women in the absence of changes in oestradiol [73] and from inhibin [74]. The elevated prolactin concentrations may also influence gonadotrophin release.

Circulating concentrations remain very low immediately after delivery and secretion of LH

366

and FSH remains suppressed during the early weeks of the puerperium. Stimulation with GnRH continues to give subnormal release of the gonadotrophins, although placental steroids decline rapidly over 2–3 days [75]. Over the ensuing weeks, the responsiveness gradually returns to normal. Plasma FSH remains low for up to 10 days [74], returning to the normal range within about 10–15 days postpartum. Luteinizing hormone is undetectable for up to 7 days postpartum [76] and if the mother does not breastfeed, pulstile LH secretion is re-established, whereas pulsatile release of LH is not seen in suckling mothers [77,78], and lactational amenorrhoea results. This spares the mother the additional stress of pregnancy while feeding an

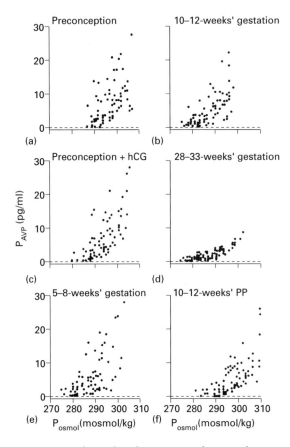

(a) Preconception
(b) 10–12-weeks' gestation
(c) Preconception + hCG
(d) 28–33-weeks' gestation
(e) 5–8-weeks' gestation
(f) 10–12-weeks' PP

P_{AVP} (pg/ml)

P_{osmol} (mosmol/kg)

Fig. 12.6. Relationship of P_{AVP} to P_{osmol} during a 2-hour hypertonic saline infusion in women at different stages of gestation and postpartum. The dashed line represents the lower of limit of detection of the assay. From Davison *et al.* [92] with permission.

infant. As shown in Fig. 12.7, suckling appears to suppress the normal pattern of pulsatile release of GnRH and hence LH, preventing normal growth of follicles [79]. Normal positive feedback of oestrogen is inhbited and the negative effects are enhanced [80].

The main factor involved is generally assumed to be prolactin, which suppresses not only the amount, but the frequency of pulsatile release of GnRH. Prolactin may also exert a direct effect on the gonadotrophs since GnRH-stimulated release from cultured pituitary cells is impaired in the presence of elevated prolactin concentrations, an effect reversed by bromocriptine [81]. Prolactin may also exert a direct effect on the ovary inhibiting ovarian oestrogen production. Much of the evidence for the central role of prolactin comes from animal studies and its importance in women has been questioned [82], the suggestion being that the reduced prolactin concentrations largely reflect a reduction in hypothalamic activity. The average time for ovulation in women who have lactated for at least 3 months is about 17 weeks and, if lactation is not prolonged, 70% of lactating women will have menstruated by about 36 weeks. By contrast, in non-lactating women the return of normal cyclic function and ovulation may be expected as soon as the second post-partum month, with ovulation occurring at an average of 9–10 weeks postpartum, so that by 12 weeks about 70% will have restored menses.

The posterior pituitary

Vasopressin

Many factors contribute to the increased fluid turnover in pregnancy, including increased fluid intake, increased metabolic rate and hyperventilation. Also, the extracellular fluid volume, including blood volume, increases and salt and water are retained. Plasma osmolality drops by about 10 mOsm/kg during pregnancy [83], mainly because of decreased concentration of sodium and its corresponding anions. However water balance is accurately regulated around the altered plasma volume and osmolality. For this to happen there must be a decrease in the osmotic threshold for drinking as well as for vasopressin secretion. That the hypothalamic osmoreceptors are effectively reset is demonstrated by the observation that on infusion of hypertonic saline the desire to drink occurs at a lower osmolality than postpartum [84]. Overall, there is also increased fluid intake, which appears to be due to primary polydipsia rather than increased urinary water loss [85]. Proof that any specific hormone is involved is lacking, but many hormones show increased effects during pregnancy, including angiotensin II which is a potent dipsogen [86].

While the changes in body fluid during pregnancy are more marked, changes are seen during the menstrual cycle of healthy women [87] and studies on the menstrual cycle provide additional insight to those in pregnancy. Control of vasopressin release is affected by the stage of the menstrual cycle [88] and it appears that this is due to the influence of gonadal steroids, since vasopressin concentrations fall on oophorectomy [89] and oestrogen replacement in postmenopausal women enhances vaso-

pressin release while progesterone is inhibitory [90]. This is consistent with the reported fall in the slope of the osmoregulatory line relating plasma vasopressin to osmolality in the luteal phase [91]. These authors also reported a fall in the osmotic threshold for vasopressin release and for severe thirst in the luteal phase. Davison *et al.* [92] found that during the third trimester of pregnancy women had measurable basal plasma vasopressin, despite the low osmolality, the values being similar to those 8–10 weeks postpartum. Concentrations could be normally suppressed with water loading and increased on hypertonic saline infusion, the osmotic threshold for release being decreased. There was also a decrease in the slope of the osmoregulatory line [93], which could be the result of altered osmoreceptor sensitivity and altered metabolic clearance. Clearance is unaltered early in pregnancy when the osmotic threshold is lowered, but increases some fourfold towards the end of pregnancy [94]. The presence of placental vasopressinase in the plasma, increased degradation in the

Fig. 12.7. Changes in plasma concentrations of LH and prolactin over a 24-hour period in a breast feeding woman at (a) 4 weeks postpartum and at (b) 16 weeks postpartum after the introduction of supplements in the same woman who remained amenorrhoeic until 22 weeks postpartum. ▼ indicates a suckling episode. From McNeilly [124] with permission of the authors and publishers.

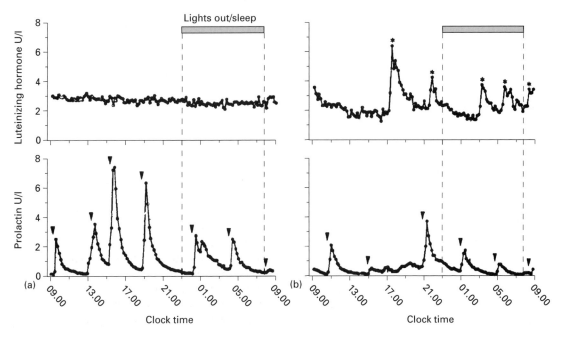

liver and kidney as well as degradation in the placenta could contribute to this increased clearance [94].

In addition to altered release of vasopressin during pregnancy, there may also be altered renal responsiveness [95]. The ability to excrete a water load depends on the stage of the pregnancy, Hytten and Klopper [96] reporting an increase in the second trimester with a marked reduction in the third trimester. Posture will contribute to the variations in the degree of urinary concentration [83,97]. The mobilization of fluid from the extremities during lateral reeumbency, for example, results in a number of changes including suppression of vasopressin release. There is, however, evidence that gonadal steroids affect the renal responsiveness to vasopressin during the oestrous cycle of the rat [98]. The kidney appears most responsive to vasopressin at times when the circulating concentrations of vasopressin are low [99,100], so that excessive changes in water loss are avoided. Preliminary studies in pregnant rats indicate that renal responsiveness to vasopressin may increase during pregnancy [101]. Studies on rats with congenital hypothalamic diabetes insipidus serve to confirm the postulated mechanisms underlying the increased water turnover in pregnancy. These animals too show a reduced osmolality during pregnancy and altered renal responsiveness to vasopressin [102]. Diabetes insipidus is a rare condition in the human and its occurrence in pregnancy is even more uncommon, with an incidence of 2–4/100 000 [103]. Pre-existing diabetes insipidus does not preclude pregnancy, although most patients require increased hormone replacement. Again this could be due to increased vasopressin clearance or relative renal resistance. The same factors could account for the transient diabetes experienced during pregnancy [104].

Oxytocin

Oxytocin is present in low circulating concentrations in the plasma of both men and women and shows a clear daily pattern of release with elevated concentrations during the night [105,106]. Hormone concentrations are also influenced by reproductive status with concentrations being elevated at the time of ovulation [107]. This is consistent with the observation that administration of oestrogen to postmenopausal women produces an increase in circulating oxytocin concentrations, which is unaffected by administration of a gestagen. When administered alone, however, medroxyprogesterone had a stimulatory effect [108]. Despite these observations on normally cycling women, oxytocin concentrations remain low during pregnancy and there is evidence from experimental animals that opioid-mediated mechanisms restrain oxytocin release during pregnancy [109]. Circadian rhythms of secretion are still observed [110] and it has been suggested that the pattern of hormone release may be important in the onset of parturition [111].

In contrast with studies of other mammalian species, circulating concentrations of oxytocin are not greatly elevated during parturition, an observation which was predicted on the basis of the infusion rates required to induce labour [112]. There is, however, a greatly enhanced uterine reponse to oxytocin concentrations with a dramatic upregulation of the oxytocin receptor. The very large increase in the number of oxytocin binding sites in all species studies led Soloff et al. [113] to propose that uterine oxytocin receptor up-regulation could be the trigger for parturition. Receptor regulation in the uterus depends on the oestrogen to progesterone ratio, with oestrogen up-regulating and progesterone down-regulating the binding sites. Hormone release is pulsatile and it has been observed that this produces a more effective stimulation of the uterus [114,115]. There is experimental evidence that dilation of the cervix is a stimulus for oxytocin secretion [116], so that a positive feedback loop could be established, which would help accelerate the process of delivery. This reflex is blocked by epidural anaesthesia in experimental animals [117], which has implications for management of labour in women. Oxytocin has been shown to be synthesized in a number of sites outside the hypothalamus including the human placenta, fetal membranes and decidua [118–120], but the significance of this observation in the context of parturition has yet to be established.

Oxytocin is also important for successful

lactation and, like prolactin, it is released in response to stimulation of the nipple. It acts on the myoepithelial cells which encircle the alveoli and ducts of the mammary gland, causing them to contract, thus reducing the size of the alveoli and widening the ducts [121]. This results in milk ejection. Oxytocin release is also influenced by psychological factors, so that stress may impair milk expression. Unlike the reflex release of prolactin, the milk ejection reflex can also be conditioned. Recently, interest has centred on central oxytocin release and studies on experimental animals indicate that the hormone produces a number of effects, including a role in the onset of maternal behaviour [122].

References

1 Saper C.B. (1990) Hypothalamus. In *The Human Nervous System*. Ed. G. Paxinos, p. 189. Academic Press, San Diego.

2 Harris G.W. (1972) Humours and hormones. *Journal of Endocrinology* **53**, ii–xxiii.

3 Theodosis D.T., Pierre K. & Poulain D.A. (1995) Adhesion molecules in the hypothalamo-neurohypophysial system: implications for structural plasticity. In *Neurohypophysis: Recent Progress in Vasopressin and Oxytocin Research*. Eds T. Saito, K. Kurokawa & S. Yoshida, p. 77. Elsvier, Amsterdam.

4 Doniach I. (1977) Histopathology of the anterior pituitary. *Clinics in Endocrinology and Metabolism* **6**, 3.

5 Rasmussen A.T. (1938) The proportions of the various subdivisions of the normal adult human hypophysis cerebri and the relative number of the different types of cells in the pars distalis with biometric evaluation of age and sex difference and special consideration of the basophilic invasion into the infundibular process. In *The Pituitary Gland*. Research Publications of the Association of Research on Nervous and Mental Disease **17**, p. 118. Williams and Wilkins, Baltimore.

6 Elster A.R., Sanders T.G., Vines F.S. & Chen M.Y. (1991) Size and shape of the pituitary gland during pregnancy and post partum: measurement with MR imaging. *Radiology* **181**, 531.

7 Goluboff L.G. & Ezrin C. (1969) Effect of pregnancy on the somatotroph and prolactin cell of the human adenohypophysis. *Journal of Clinical Endocrinology and Metabolism* **29**, 1533.

8 Dyson M. (1995) The endocrine system. In *Gray's Anatomy*, 38th edn, p. 1882. Churchill Livingstone, Edinburgh.

9 Stefaneau L., Kovacs K., Lloyd R.V., Scheithauer B.W., Young W.F., Sano T. & Jin L. (1992) Pituitary lactotrophs and mammotophs in pregnancy: a correlative in situ hybridisation and immunocytochemical study. *Virchows Archiv B Cell Pathology* **62**, 291.

10 De La Lastra M. & Llados C. (1977) Luteinising hormone content of the pituitary gland in pregnant and nonpregnant women. *Journal of Clinical Endocrinology and Metabolism* **44**, 921.

11 Scheithauer B.W., Sano T., Kovacs K.T., Young W.F., Ryan N. & Randall R.V. (1990) The pituitary gland in pregnancy: a clinicopathologic, immunohistochemical study of 69 cases. *Mayo Clinic Procedings* **65**, 461.

12 Hinshaw D.B., Hasso A.N., Thomson J.R. & Davison B.J. (1984) High resolution computed tomography of the posterior pituitary gland. *Neuroradiology* **26**, 299.

13 Tan S.L. & Jacobs H.S. (1986) Management of prolactinomas. *British Journal of Obststrics and Gynaecology* **93**, 1025.

14 Flerko B. (1980) The hypophysial portal circulation today. *Neuroendocrinology* **31**, 56.

15 Sheehan H.L. & Stanfield J.P. (1961) The pathogenesis of post partum necrosis of the anterior lobe of the pituitary gland. *Acta Endocrinlogica* **37**, 479.

16 Forsling M.L. & Grossman A. (1986) *Neuroendocrinology: A Clinical Text*, p. 47. Croom Helm, London.

17 Robinson I.C.A.F. (1991) Chronopharmacology of growth hormone and related peptides. *Advanced Drug Delivery Reviews* **6**, 57.

18 Orth D.N. & Mount C.D. (1987) Specific high affinity binding protein for corticotrophin-releasing hormone in normal human plasma. *Biochemical and Biophysical Research Communications* **143**, 411.

19 Linton E.A., Wolfe C.D.A., Behan D.P. & Lowry P.J. (1988) A specific carrier substance for human corticotrophin releasing factor in late gestational maternal plasma which could mask the ACTH-releasing activity. *Clinical Endocrinology* **28**, 315.

20 Robinson I.C.A.F., Carmignac D.F. & Fairhall K.M. (1993) Growth hormone (GH) receptors, GH binding protein and GH: an autoregulatory system? *Acta Paediatrica Suppl* **391**, 22.

21 Forsling M.L. (1976) *Antidiuretic Hormone*, p. 46. Eden Press, Montreal.

22 Forsling M.L. (1986) Regulation of oxytocin secretion. In *Current Topics in Neuroendocrinology. Vol 6. Neurobiology of Oxytocin*. Eds G. Ganten & D. Pfoff, p. 19. Springer Verlag, Berlin.

23 Webley G.E. & Hearn J.P. (1994) Embryo-maternal interactions during the establishment of pregnancy in primates. *Oxford Reviews in Reproductive Biology* **16**, 1.

24 Shibasaki T., Odagiri T., Shizume K. & Lin N. (1982) Corticotrophin releasing factor-like activity in human placental extracts. *Journal of Clinical Endocrinology and Metabolism* **55**, 384.

25 Gibbons J.M., Mituick M. & Chieffo V. (1975) In vitro biosynthesis of TSH and LH-releasing factors by human placenta. *American Journal of Obstetrics and Gynecology* **121**, 127.

26 Khodr G.S. & Siler-Khodr T.M. (1980) Placental luteinising hormone-releasing factor and its synthesis. *Science* **207**, 315.

27 Etzrodt H., Musch K., Schroder K.E. & Pfeffer E.F. (1980) Somatostatin-like activity in placenta, amniotic fluid and umbilical cord plasma. In *The Human*

370

Placenta. Eds A. Klopper, A. Genazzani & P.G. Croisignani, p. 277. Academic Press, London.

28 Watkins W.B. & Yen S.C.C. (1980) Somatostatin in cytotrophoblast of the immature human placenta: localisation by immunoperoxidase histochemistry. *Journal of Clinical Endocrinology and Metabolism* **50**, 969.

29 Jaffe R.B. (1991) Endocrine-metabolic alterations induced by pregnancy. In *Reproductive Endocrinology. Physiology, Pathophysiology and Clinical Management*, 3rd edn. Eds S.S.C.Yen & R.B. Jaffe, p. 183. Saunders, Philadelphia.

30 O'Leary P., Boyne P., Flett P., Beilby T. & James I. (1991) Longitudinal assessment of changes in reproductive homones during normal pregnancy. *Clinical Chemistry* **37**, 667.

31 Maurer R.A. (1982) Relationship between oestadiol, ergocryptine and thyroid hormone: effects on prolactin synthesis and prolactin messenger ribonucleic acid levels. *Endocrinology* **110**, 1515.

32 Rakoff J.S. & Yen S.C.C. (1978) Progesterone induced acute release of prolactin in oestrogen-primed ovariectomised women. *Journal of Clinical Endocrinology and Metabolism* **57**, 918.

33 Rigg L.A., Lein A. & Yen S.S.C. (1977) The pattern of increase in circulating prolactin levels during human gestation. *American Journal of Obstetrics and Gynaecology* **129**, 454–456.

34 Soares J., Faria T.N., Roby K.F. & Dob S. (1991) Pregnancy and the prolactin family of hormones; coordination of anterior pituitary, uterine and placental expression. *Endocrine Reviews* **12**, 402.

35 Mochizuki M., Morikawa H., Kawaguchi K. & Tojo S. (1976) Growth hormone, prolactin and chorionic somatomammotropin in normal and molar pregnancy. *Journal of Clinical Endocrinology and Metabolism* **43**, 614.

36 Boyer R.M., Finkelstein J.W., Kapen S. & Hellman L. (1975) Twenty four hour prolactin secretory patterns during pregnancy. *Journal of Clinical Endocrinology and Metabolism* **40**, 117.

37 Glasier A., McNeilly A.S. & Howie P.W. (1984) The prolactin response to suckling. *Clinical Endocrinology (Oxford)* **21**, 109.

38 Liu J.H. & Park K.H. (1988) Gonadotrophin and prolactin increases during the puerperium in non-lactating women. *Journal of Clinical Endocrinology and Metabolism* **66**, 839.

39 Robinson J.E. & Short R.V. (1977) Changes in breast sensitivity at puberty, during the menstrual cycle and at parturition. *British Medical Journal* **1**, 1188.

40 Masala A., Delitala G., Lo Dico G., Stoppelli I., Alagna S. & Devilla L. (1978) Inhibition of lactation and inhibition of prolactin release after mechanical breast stimulation in puerpural women given tamoxifen or placebo. *British Journal of Obstetrics and Gynaecology* **85**, 134.

41 Shu R.P.C. & Friesen H.G. (1980) Mechanism of action of prolactin in the control of mammary gland function. *Annual Reviews of Physiology* **42**, 83.

42 Posner B.I., Kelly P.A. & Friesen H.G. (1975) Prolactin receptors in rat liver: possible induction by prolactin. *Science* **188**, 57.

43 Franks S., Kiwi R. & Nabarro J.D.N. (1977) Pregnancy and lactation after pituitary surgery. *British Medical Journal* **1**, 882.

44 Ho K.Y., Elard W.S. & Blissard R.M. (1987) Effects of sex and age on the 24 h profile of growth hormone secretion in man: importance of endogenous estradiol concentrations. *Journal of Clinical Endocrinology and Metabolism* **64**, 51.

45 Tyson J.E., Rabinovittz D., Merimec J.J. & Friesen H. (1969) Response of plasma insulin and human growth homone to arginine in pregnant and post-partum females. *American Journal of Obstetrics and Gynecology* **103**, 313.

46 Mintz D.H., Stock R., Finster J.L. & Taylor A.L. (1965) The effect of normal and diabetic pregnancies on the growth hormone response to hypoglycaemia. *Metabolism* **17**, 54.

47 Frankenne F., Closset J., Gomez F., Scippo M.L., Smal J. & Hennen G. (1988) The physiology of growth hormones (GHs) in pregnant women and partial characterisation of the placental GH variant variant. *Journal of Clinical Endocrinology and Metabolism* **66**, 1171.

48 Eriksson L., Frankenne F., Eden S., Hennen G. & Schoultz B. (1989) Growth hormone 24-h serum profiles during pregnancy: lack of pulsatility for the secretion of the placental variant. *Journal of Clinical Endocrinology and Metabolism* **66**, 1171.

49 Ray J., Okamura H., Kelly P.A. Cooke N.E. & Liebhaber S.A. (1990) Human growth hormone variant demonstrates a receptor binding profile distinct from that of normal pituitary growth hormone. *Journal of Biological Chemistry* **265**, 7939.

50 MacLeod J.N., Worsley F., Ray, J., Friesen H.G., Liebhaber S.A. & Cooke N.E. (1991) Human growth hormone variant is a biologically active somatogen and lactogen *Endocrinology* **128**, 1298.

51 Hall K., Enberg G., Hellem E., Lindin G., Ottosson-Seeberger A., Sara V., Trygstad O. *et al.* (1984) Somatomedin levels in pregnancy: longitudinal study in healthy subjects and patients with growth hormone deficiency. *Journal of Clinical Endocrinology and Metabolism* **59**, 587.

52 Carr B.R., Parker C.R., Madden J.D., MacDonald P.C. & Porter J.D. (1981) Maternal plasma adrenocorticotrophin and cortisol relationships throughout human pregnancy. *American Journal of Obstetrics and Gynecology* **139**, 416.

53 Rees L.H. & Lowry P.J. (1978) ACTH and related peptides. In *Endocrine Function of the Human Adrenal Cortex.* Eds V.H.T. James, M. Serio, G. Guisli & L. Martinin, p. 33. Academic Press, London.

54 Nolten W.E. & Rueckert P.A. (1981) Elevated free cortisol index in pregnancy: possible regulatory mechanisms. *American Journal of Obstetrics and Gynecology* **139**, 492.

55 Patrick J., Challis J., Campbell K., Carmichael L., Natale R. & Richardson B. (1980) Circadian rhythms in maternal plasma cortisol and estriol concentrations at 30–31, 34–35 and 38–39 weeks gestational age. *American Journal of Obstetrics and Gynecology* **136**, 325.

56 Cousins L., Rigg L., Hollingsworth D., Meis P.,

Halberg F., Brink G. & Yen S.S. (1983) Qualitative and quantitative assessment of the circadian rhythm of cortisol in pregnancy. *American Journal of Obstetrics and Gynecology* **145**, 411.

57 Namba Y., Smith J.B., Fox G.S. & Challis J.G.R. (1980) Plasma cortisol concentrations during caesarian sections. *British Journal of Anaesthetics* **52**, 1027.

58 Rees L.H., Burke C.W., Chard T., Evans S.W. & Letchworth A.T. (1975) Possible placental origin of ACTH in normal human pregnancy. *Nature* **254**, 620.

59 Chen C.L., Chang C.-C., Kreiger D. & Bardin C.W. (1986) Expression and regulation of proopiomelanocortin-like gene in the ovary and placenta: comparison with the testis. *Endocrinology* **118**, 2382.

60 Frim D.M., Emanuel R.L., Robinson B.G., Smas C., Alder G.K. & Majzoub J.A. (1988) Characterisation and gestational regulation of corticotrophin-releasing hormone messenger RNA in human placenta. *Journal of Clinical Investignation* **82**, 287.

61 Robinson B.G., Emanuel R.L., Frim D.M. & Majzoub J.A. (1988) Glucocorticoid stimulates expression of corticotrophin-releasing hormone in human placenta. *Proceedings of the National Academy of Sciences of the USA* **85**, 5244.

62 Jones S.A., Brook A.N. & Challis J.G.R. (1989) Steroids modulate corticotrophin-releasing hormone production in human fetal membranes and placenta. *Jounral of and Metabolism* **70**, 1574.

63 Sasaki A., Liotta L.S., Luckey M.M., Margioris A.N., Suda T. & Kreiger D.T. (1984) Immunoreactive corticotrophin-releasing factor is present in human maternal plasma during the third trimester of pregnancy. *Journal of Clinical Endocrinology and Metabolism* **59**, 812.

64 Campbell E.A., Linton E.A., Wolfe C.D.A., Scraggs P.A., Jones M.T. & Lowry P.J. (1987) Plasma corticotrophin releasing hormone concentrations during pregnancy and parturition. *Journal of Clinical Endocrinology and Metabolism* **64**, 1054.

65 Linton E.A., Behan D.P., Saphier P.W. & Lowry P.J. (1990) Corticotrophin-releasing hormone (CRH)-binding protein: reduction in the adrenocorticotrophin-releasing activity of placental, but not hypothalamic CRH. *Journal of Clinical Endocrinology and Metabolism* **70**, 1574.

66 Linton E.A., Perkins A.V., Woods R.J., Eben F., Wolfe C.D.A., Behan D.P., Potter E. *et al.* (1993) Corticotrophin-releasing hormone-binding protein (CRH-B): plasma levels decreased during the third trimester of normal human prenancy. *Journal of Clinical Endocrinology and Metabolism* **76**, 265.

67 Gillies, G. & Lowry P. (1979) Corticotrophin releasing factor may be modulated by vasopressin. *Nature* **278**, 463.

68 Schulte H.M., Chrousos G.P., Gold, P.W., Booth J.D., Oldfield E.H., Cutler S.G.B. & Loriaux D.L. (1985) Continuous administration of synthetic ovine corticotrophin releasing factor in man. *Journal of Clinical Investigation* **75**, 1781.

69 Goland R.S., Wardlaw S.L., MacCarter G., Warren W.B. & Stark R.I. (1991) Adrenocorticotrophin and cortisol responses to vasopressin during pregnancy. *Journal of Clinical Endocrinology and Metabolism* **73**, 257.

70 Guillaume J., Schussler G.C. & Goldman J. (1985) Components of total serum thyroid concentrations during pregnancy: high free thyroxine and blunted thyrotrophin reponse to TSH-releasing hormone in the first trimester. *Journal of Clinical Endocrinology and Metabolism* **60**, 678.

71 Yoshimura M., Nishikawa M., Yoshikawi N., Horimoto M., Toyoda N.M., Sawaragi I. & Inada M. (1991) Mechanism of thyroid stimulation by human chrorionic gonaotrophin in sera of normal pregnant women. *Acta Endocrinoloigica* **124**, 173.

72 Rubinstein L.M., Parlow A.F. & Derzko Hershman J. (1978) Pituitary gonadotrophin response to LHRH in human pregnancy. *Obstetrics and Gynaecology* **52**, 172.

73 Miyake A., Tanizawa O., Aono T. & Kurachi K. (1997) Pituitary responses in LH secretion to LHRH in pregnancy. *Obstetrics and Gynaecology* **49**, 549.

74 Abe Y., Hasegawa Y., Miyamoto K., Yamaguchi M., Andoh A., Ibuki Y. & Igarashi M. (1990) High concentrations of plasma immunoreactive inhibin during normal pregnancy in women. *Journal of Clinical Endocrinology and Metabolism* **71**, 133.

75 Sheehan K.L. & Yen S.S.C. (1979) Activation of pituitary gonadotrophic function by an agonists of luteinisin releasing factor in the puerperium. *American Journal of Obstetrics and Gynecology* **135**, 755.

76 Kremer J.A., Borm G., Schellenkens L.A., Thomas C.M. & Rolland R. (1990) Pulsatile secretion of luteinising hormone and prolactin in lactating and non-lactating women and the response to naltrexone. *Journal of Clinical Endocrinology and Metabolism* **72**, 294.

77 Fox S.R. & Smith S.M. (1984) The suppression of pulsatile luteinising hormone secretion during lactation in the rat. *Endocrinology* **115**, 2045.

78 McNeilly A.S. (1984) Endocrine control of lactational infertility in women. In *Endocrinology Clinical Endocrinology and Metabolism*. Eds F. Labrie & L. Proulx, p. 803. Elsevier, New York.

79 Nunley W.C., Urban R.T., Evans W.S. & Veldhuis J.P. (1991) Preservation of pulsatile LH release during postpartum lactational amenorrhoea. *Journal of Clinical Endocrinology and Metabolism*, **30**, 629.

80 Baird D.T., McNeilly A.S., Sowers R.S. & Sharpe R.M. (1979) Failure of oestrogen-induced discharge of luteinising hormone in lactating women. *Journal of Clinical Endocrinology and Metabolism* **49**, 500.

81 Cheung C.Y. (1983) Prolactin suppresses LH secretion and pituitary responses to LHRH by a direct action at the pituitary. *Endocrinology* **113**, 632.

82 McNeilly A.S. (1988) Suckling and the control of gonadotrophin secretion. In *The Physiology of Reproduction*. Eds E. Knobil & J.D. Neil, p. 2323. Raven Press, New York.

83 Davison J.M., Valloton M.B. & Lindheimer M.D. (1981) Plasma osmolality and urinary concentration and dilution during and after pregnancy: evidence that lateral recumbancy inhibits maximal urinary concentrating ability. *British Journal of Obstetrics and Gynaecology* **88**, 472.

84 Davison J.M., Gilmore J., Durr J., Robertson G.L.

372

& Lindheimer M.D. (1984) Altered osmotic thresholds for vasopressin release and thirst in human pregnancy. *American Journal of Physiology* **246**, F105.

85 Olsson K. & Dahlborn K. (1985) Effects of asynthetic vasopressin analogue (desmopressin) in pregnant, lactating and anoestrous goats. *Acta Physiologica Scandinavica* **124**, 597.

86 Fitzsimons J.T. (1972) Thirst. *Physical Reviews* **52**, 468.

87 Greene R. & Dalton K. (1953) Premenstrual syndrome. *British Medical Journal* **1**, 1007.

88 Forsling M.L., Akerlund M. & Stromberg P. (1981) Variations in plasma concentrations of vasopressin during the menstrual cycle. *Journal of Endocrinology* **89**, 263.

89 Forsling M.L., Anderson C.H.M., Wheeler M.J. & Raju K.S. (1996) The effect of hormone replacement on neurohypophyseal hormone secretion in women. *Clinical Endocrinology* **44**, 39.

90 Forsling M.L., Stromberg P. & Akerlund M. (1982) Effect of ovarian steroids on vasopressin release. *Journal of Endocrinology* **95**, 147.

91 Spruce B.A., Baylis P.H., Burd J. & Watson M.J. (1985) Variations in osmoregulation of vasopressin during the human menstrual cycle. *Clinical Endocrinology* **22**, 37.

92 Davison J.M., Shills E.A., Philips P.R. & Lindheimer M.D. (1988) Serial evaluation of vasopressin release and thirst in human pregnancy: role of human chorionic gonadotrophin in the regulatory changes of gestation. *Jounal of Clinical Investigation* **81**, 798.

93 Lindheimer M.D., Barron W.M. & Davison J.M. (1988) Osmoregulaion of vasopressin release and thirst in pregnancy. In *Vasopressin: Integrative and Cellular Function*. Eds A.W. Cowley, J.-F. Liard & D.A. Ausiello, p. 265. Raven Press, New York.

94 Davison J.M., Sheills E.A., Philips P.R., Barron W.M. & Lindheimer M.D. (1993) Metabolic clearance of vasopressin and an analogue resistant to vasopressinase in human pregnancy. *American Journal of Physiology* **264**, F348.

95 Lindheimer M.D., Barron W.M. & Davison J.M. (1985) Water metabolism and vasopressin secretion in pregnancy. In *Vasopressin*. Ed. R.W. Schrier, p. 229. Raven Press, New York.

96 Hytten F.E. & Klopper A.I. (1963) Response to a water load in pregnancy. *Journal of Obstetrics and Gynaecology of the British Commonwealth* **70**, 402.

97 Theobald G.W. & Lundborg R.A. (1963) Changes in limb volume and in venous infusion pressures caused by pregnancy. *Journal of Obstetrics and Gynaecology of the British Commonwealth* **70**, 408.

98 Wang Y.-X., Crofton J.T., Liu H., Brooks D.P. & Share L. (1994) Effects of gonadectomy on sexually dimorphic antidiuretic action of vasopressin in conscious rats. *American Journal of Physiology* **267**, R536.

99 Forsling M.L. & Peysner K. (1988) Pituitary and plasma vasopressin concentrations and fluid balance throughout the oestrous cycle of the rat. *Journal of Endocrinology* **117**, 397.

100 Forsling M.L., Zhou Y. & Windle R.J. (1995) The natriuretic actions of vasopressin in the female rat: variations during the four days of the oestrous cycle. *Journal of Endocrinology* **148**, 457.

101 Hartley D., Stafford G., Zaman Z. & Forsling M.L. (1996) Does the renal responsiveness to vasopressin change during pregnancy and lactation in the rat? *British Journal of Pharmacology* **119**, 142.

102 Barron W.M., Durr J., Stamoutsos B.A. & Lindheimer M.D. (1985) Osmoregulation and vasopressin secretion during pregnancy in Brattleboro rats. *American Journal of Physiology* **248**, R29.

103 Hime M.C. & Richardson J.A. (1978) Diabetes insipidus and pregnancy: case report, incidence and review. *Obstetrics and Gynaecology Survey* **33**, 375.

104 Durr J.A. (1987) Diabetes insipidus in pregnancy. *American Journal of Kidney Disease* **9**, 276.

105 Landgraf H., Hacker R. & Buhl H. (1982) Plasma vasopressin and oxytocin changes in response to exercise and during the day-night cycle in man. *Endokrinologie* **8**, 281.

106 Forsling M.L. (1995) Daily rhythms of oxytocin secretion. *Advances in Experimental Medicine and Biology* **395**, 92.

107 Mitchell M.D., Haynes P.J., Anderson A.B.M. & Turnbull A.C. (1981) Plasma oxytocin concentrations during the menstrual cycle. *European Journal of Obstetrics, Gynaecology and Reproductive Biology* **12**, 195.

108 Bossmar T., Forsling M. & Akerlund M. (1995) Circulating oxytocin and vasopressin is influenced by ovarian steroid replacement in women. *Acta Obstetrica et Gynaecologica Sandinavica* **74**, 544.

109 Douglas A.J., Dye S., Leng G., Russell J.A. & Bicknell R.J. (1993) Endogenous opioid regulation of oxytocin secretion through pregnancy in the rat. *Journal of Neuoendocrinology* **5**, 307.

110 Honnebier M.B.O.M., Figuera J.P., Riviera J., Vale W. & Nathanielsz P.W. (1989) Studies on the role of oxytocin in late pregnancy in the pregnant rhesus monkey: plasma concentrations of oxytocin in the maternal circulation and throughout the 24 h day and the effect of the synthetic oxytocin analogue [–Mpa(CH$_3$)$_5$]$_1$, Me(Tyr^2, Orn^8) oxytocin on spontaneous nocturnal myometrial contractions. *Journal of Developmental Physiology* **12**, 225.

111 Fuchs A.R., Behrens O. & Liu H.C. (1992) Correlation of nocturnal increase in plasma oxytocin with a decrease in plasma estradiol/progesterone ratio in late pregnancy. *American Journal of Obstetrics and Gynecology* **169**, 159.

112 Theobald G.W., Robards M.F. & Suter P.E. (1969) Changes in myometrial sensitivity to oxytocin in man during the last six weeks of pregnancy. *Journal of Obstetrics and Gynaecology of the British Commonwealth* **76**, 385.

113 Soloff M.S., Alexandrova M. & Fernstrom M.J. (1979) Oxytocin receptors: triggers for parturition and lactation. *Science* **204**, 1313.

114 Cummisky K.C. & Dawood M.Y. (1990) Induction of labor with pulsatile oxytcoin. *American Journal of Obstetrics and Gynaecology* **163**, 1868.

115 Randolph G.W. & Fuchs A. (1989) Pulsatile administration enhances the effect and reduces the dose of oxytocin required for the induction of labour. *American Journal of Perinatology* **6**, 159.

116 Flint A.P.F., Forsling M.L., Mitchell M.D. & Turnbull A.C. (1975) Temporal relationship between changes in oxytocin and prostaglandin F levels in response to vaginal distension in the pregnant and puerpural ewe. *Journal of Reproduction and Fertility* **43**, 551.

117 Flint A.P.F., Forsling M.L. & Mitchell M.D. (1978) Blockade of the Ferguson reflex by lumbar epidural anaesthesia in the partuient sheep: effects on oxytocin secretion and uterine venous prostaglandin F levels. *Hormone and Metabolic Research* **10**, 545.

118 Chibbar R., Miller F.D. & Mitchell B.F. (1993) Synthesis of oxytocin in amnion, chorion and decidua may influence the timing of human parturition. *Journal of Clinical Investigation* **91**, 185.

119 Lefebvre D.L., Giaid A. & Zingg H.H. (1992) Expression of the oxytocin gene in rat placenta. *Endocrinology* **130**, 1185.

120 Lefebvre D.L., Giaid A., Bennet H., Lariviere R. & Zingg H.H. (1992) Oxytocin gene expression in rat uterus. *Science* **256**, 1553.

121 Linzell J.L. (1961) Recent advances in the physiology of the udder. *Veterinary Annals* **2**, 44.

122 De Wied D., Diamant M. & Fodor M. (1993) Central nervous system effects of the neurohypophysial hormones and related peptides. *Frontiers in Neuroendocrinology* **7**, 243.

123 Stanier M.W. & Forsling M.L. (1989) *Physiological Processes: An Introduction to Mammalian Physiology*, p. 310.

124 McNeilly A.S. (1993) Lactational amenorrhoea. *Endocrinology and Metabolism Clinics of North America* **22**, 59.

The Thyroid Gland

I.D. RAMSAY

The thyroid gland produces hormones which are important in the regulation of many aspects of cell metabolism, particularly heat and energy production. During pregnancy a picture of apparent physiological hyperthyroidism may develop because of the clinical features of emotional upset, heat intolerance, tachycardia, a hyperdynamic circulation and a goitre which may have a bruit over it. The basal metabolic rate (BMR) is elevated, as are the thyroid hormone concentrations in the blood. However, modern methods of investigation have demonstrated that thyroid function is basically normal during pregnancy, albeit disturbed by the pregnant state. The increase in the BMR can be accounted for by the metabolic contribution of the uterus and its contents and by the increased work of maternal heart and lungs [1] (Chapter 2).

The physiology of thyroid hormones

Iodine is essential for the manufacture of thyroid hormones, four atoms of it being present in every molecule of thyroxine (T_4) and three atoms in each molecule of tri-iodothyronine (T_3). Iodine in the diet is reduced to iodide and is absorbed by the wall of the small intestine. Iodide is avidly trapped by the thyroid gland under the influence of thyroid-stimulating hormone (TSH) produced by the pituitary gland. The iodide is oxidized in the thyroid gland and joined to tyrosyl groups to form iodotyrosines containing either one or two iodine atoms, called mono- and di-iodotyrosine, respectively, a conversion which takes place within thyroglobulin in the thyroid acinar cell. Linkage of the iodotyrosines then takes place. The junction of two molecules of di-iodotyrosine will form one molecule of thyroxine and that of one molecule of monoiodotyrosine with that of di-iodotyrosine will create one molecule of tri-iodothyronine. The thyroid gland seems preferentially to manufacture T_4 rather than T_3 in ordinary physiological situations [2]. The hormone–thyroglobulin complex is then stored within the lumen of the colloid follicle. Under the action of TSH, a small bud of thyroglobulin enters the thyroid acinar cell by a process of endocytosis and the thyroid hormones are released into the bloodstream. Any iodotyrosines present are deiodinated and the iodide is available for recycling (Fig. 13.1).

The thyroid hormones circulate in the blood largely bound to proteins. A specific protein, thyroxine-binding globulin (TBG), binds 85% of all the thyroxine, and another protein, thyroxine-binding pre-albumin (TBPA) binds most of the rest [3]. Albumin binds a very small fraction of T_4 and a minute amount (0.05%) exists as the free hormone. Tri-iodothyronine circulates in about one-sixtieth the concentration of T_4 but, because it is much less bound to the carrier proteins, its free fraction (0.5% of the total) assumes a relatively greater importance, being about one-

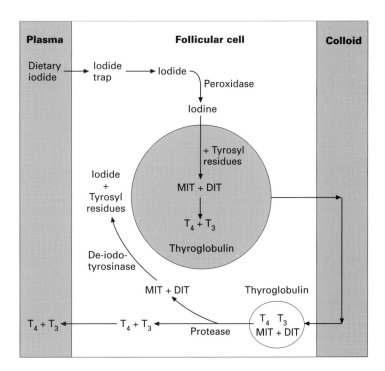

Fig. 13.1. The synthesis of thyroid hormones. MIT: mono-iodotyrosine; DIT: di-iodotyrosine; T_4: thyroxine; T_3: tri-iodothyronine.

seventh that of the concentration of free T_4. About 80% of the T_3 in the blood is derived from the monodeiodination of T_4 [4], and it is believed that T_3 is almost certainly the more important of the two hormones metabolically, T_4 probably acting mainly as a prohormone. This conversion of T_4 to T_3, in addition to the buffering of the hormones by protein binding, enables a steady state to prevail and prevents wild fluctuations in free hormone levels.

An additional way in which the amount of free T_3 may be regulated is the monodeiodination of T_4 to a relatively inert tri-iodothyronine called reverse T_3.

Control of thyroid hormone secretion

Although there may be some internal thyroidal regulatory mechanisms, the main control of thyroid hormone secretion is by the action of pituitary TSH. The secretion of TSH is in turn regulated by the negative feedback of the thyroid hormones on the anterior pituitary, raised levels suppressing secretion and reduced levels stimulating secretion (Fig. 13.2). In addition, a

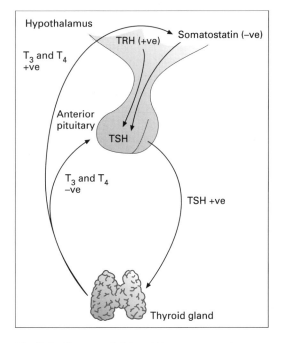

Fig. 13.2. The control of thyroid hormone secretion.

hypothalamic hormone, thyrotrophin-releasing hormone (TRH), passes down the neurohypophyseal portal system of veins to the anterior pituitary and modifies the way in which TSH responds to the negative feedback of thyroid hormones. For instance, if the concentration of thyroid hormones has been constantly low (as in a patient with borderline hypothyroidism), TRH will stimulate the anterior pituitary to synthesize and release TSH. The converse is true in thyrotoxicosis: TRH stimulation is ineffective and the thyrotrophs of the anterior pituitary do not make or release TSH [5]. Another hypothalamic hormone, somatostatin, has an inhibiting action on TSH secretion. It seems likely that raised levels of circulating thyroid hormones may stimulate the production of somatostatin (Fig. 13.2). In a normal person, other external factors such as intense environmental cold may stimulate TSH secretion, presumably via the hypothalamus. For a fuller review of thyroid physiology, see Braverman and Utiger [6].

The action of thyroid hormones

It is generally accepted that T_3 is the more important hormone metabolically. T_3 binds to cell membranes, nuclear receptors and mitochondria. Stimulation at the membrane level increases intracellular concentrations of substrates such as amino acids which can then, by nuclear transcription, be synthesized into proteins. Mitochondrial stimulation increases the capacity of the respiratory enzymes and the production of the high energy bonds of adenosine triphosphate [7]. Thyroid hormones are thus important in regulating the production of energy, in stimulating protein synthesis, in regulating carbohydrate and lipid metabolism, and in promoting growth in infancy and childhood. Normal levels of hormone in the first 2 years of life are absolutely essential for brain development; inadequate thyroid hormone production leads to cretinism.

Modification of thyroid physiology by pregnancy

During pregnancy there is a transfer of iodide and iodothyronines to the fetus [8], and, due to

the increased glomerular filtration rate, the renal clearance of iodide doubles, plasma inorganic iodide falls and thyroidal clearance of iodine rises to three times normal, enabling the absolute iodine uptake to remain within the normal range [9]. Radioactive iodine uptake is significantly elevated throughout pregnancy. The effects of stimulation by TSH and of suppression by T_3 on [132]I uptake are similar to those in non-pregnant subjects [10]. Radioactive iodine uptakes should not, of course, be routinely used in thyroid diagnosis because of radiation to the fetal thyroid.

It has been suggested [9] that relative iodine deficiency is responsible for the compensatory follicular hyperplasia in the thyroid [11] and the formation, at least according to the studies at Aberdeen, of a goitre in up to 70% of pregnant women [12]. Support for this comes from the fact that pregnant women in Iceland, who have a higher dietary iodine intake and higher plasma inorganic iodide levels than the Aberdeen women, do not have an increased prevalence of goitre compared with non-pregnant women [13]. Moreover, the clearance of iodine by the thyroid is not increased in the pregnant Icelandic women [13]. In the US, where a higher iodine content in the diet is provided by the general use of iodized salt, no significant difference in the prevalence of goitre [14,15] or in iodine balance was found between pregnant and non-pregnant women or between the antepartum and postpartum months in the pregnant patients [16], though there seems to be a small increase in thyroid volume, even in iodine-replete areas [17,18].

The actual stimulus for thyroid hyperplasia and increased thyroid clearance of iodide could be mediated by TSH. Although there have been reports of raised TSH levels during pregnancy [19–21], which other workers have been unable to confirm [22,23], the general consensus is that there is a rise in human chorionic gonadotrophin (hCG) during early pregnancy, accompanied by a fall in TSH within the normal range [17,24]. This is then followed by a rise in TSH during the last two trimesters of pregnancy. hCG is considered to stimulate the thyroid gland during early pregnancy [24–28]. hCG and TSH share a common α-subunit so hCG is capable of stimulating the TSH receptors. A normal rise of TSH in response to the injection of TRH has been found throughout pregnancy [21,23], apart from the first trimester [29] which is in keeping with this view. Certainly the amounts of hCG found in molar pregnancies can increase levels of T_3 and T_4 above normal [25,30–33]. Thyroid stimulation by a chorionic thyrotrophin is considered doubtful [34]. TRH activity has been found in placental tissue [35,36]. Any effect this had on thyroid function would have to be mediated by pituitary TSH.

Thyroxine-binding globulin

The increasing production of placental oestrogens during pregnancy induces a greater synthesis of TBG [37] by the liver. There is also a reduced clearance of TBG by the liver [38]. The concentration of TBG is doubled by the end of the first trimester [39,40] and it remains elevated throughout the rest of pregnancy. Because of the increased number of binding sites for thyroid hormones, the total amounts of both T_4 and T_3 are raised in the blood, the effect being greater on T_4 than on T_3, which is generally only raised in the last trimester [41–44]. Despite this, not all the binding sites are saturated and so older tests such as the T_3 resin uptake will give results which are in the hypothyroid range. However, the raised total and apparently hyperthyroid T_4, when combined with the hypothyroid T_3 resin uptakes, gives a free thyroxine index [45] which is usually within the normal range in pregnancy though some values may fall above the upper limit of normal [46].

The other less important thyroxine-binding protein, TBPA, actually decreases during pregnancy [39].

Free thyroid hormone concentrations

The general consensus of opinion is that free thyroxine concentrations, measured directly and not by calculation from total T_4 and T_3 resin uptake measurements, are normal in pregnancy [43,44,47,48], though some reports have suggested that they may decline as pregnancy progresses [17,42,49,50]. The differences may be explained by different techniques used for the measurement. The results using a commonly employed kit method (Amerlex) show a slight fall in free T_4 compared with the non-pregnant range by the second trimester and an even greater reduction by the third trimester [51]. Measurement of free T_4 in pregnancy is probably more accurate than the derived free thyroxine index [47] but where only that is available it provides an adequate guide to thyroid status, particularly when combined with highly sensitive TSH estimations (see below).

Free tri-iodothyronine concentrations are generally normal in pregnancy [42,43,48]. One study reported a 10% reduction in free T_3 but found a normal free T_3 index using a T_3 talc uptake to compensate for the increased amount of TBG concentration [44]. Recent experience with the Amerlex test shows a slight reduction in free T_3 levels in the second trimester, with a greater fall in the third trimester [51]. The amount of metabolically inactive reverse T_3 is slightly higher in maternal blood than in controls [52]; this is probably due to its increased binding to TBG.

Urinary excretion of thyroid hormones

There have been two reports of increased and one of normal excretion of unconjugated T_4 in pregnancy [41,42,48]. The urinary excretion of unconjugated T_3 was raised in one study [42] but not in two others [41,48], when renal T_3 clearances were also found to be normal [53]. The consensus of opinion is that net thyroxine turnover is unchanged in normal pregnancy [54].

Thyroid-stimulating hormone

The introduction of highly sensitive immunoradiometric (IRMA) assays for TSH [17,55] has added a new dimension to thyroid function testing in pregnancy. Elevated TSH levels indicate primary hypothyroidism and suppressed concentrations are found in thyrotoxicosis and in other thyroid diseases in which there may be autonomous thyroid function (multinodular goitre, adenoma).

Thyroid activity in labour

Total T_4 and T_3 have been shown to rise during labour though the free T_4 concentration remained stable [56,57]. It seems likely that an increase in plasma protein concentration, caused by a shift of fluid into the extravascular space, is responsible [56].

Thyroid activity in the puerperium

Following delivery, concentrations of TBG fall slowly back to normal during the next 6 weeks [39]. For this reason, the elevated total T_4 of pregnancy also declines to normal over the same period. Total T_3, being much less bound to TBG, shows an appreciable decline by 7 days postpartum [41], though not to normal levels.

The radioactive iodine uptake is still elevated at 1 week, but not at 6 weeks after delivery [9,10]. By 6 weeks, the renal clearance of iodine and the absolute iodine uptake by the thyroid have returned to normal, but the thyroid clearance rate does not reach control values until the 12 week postpartum [9].

Fetal thyroid hormones

The fetal thyroid and the pituitary–thyroid axis only become active at about the 12th week of gestation [58,59]. Before that time, the fetus is entirely dependent upon the mother for thyroid hormone [25,60]. During early pregnancy, even as early as 8 weeks, T_4, present in the coelomic fluid, may pass to the fetus via the yolk sac [61] and both T_4 and T_3 have been demonstrated in rat fetus before the onset of fetal thyroid function [62,63]. Placental T_4 accumulation remains high in the rat throughout pregnancy and it is possible that the increase in TBG is necessary to provide the transport of T_4 to the fetoplacental unit [64].

As the fetal thyroid hormone concentrations rise during the second and third trimester [58,59], there is an increased fetal need for iodide, which is transported across the placenta and is also provided by the monodeiodination of iodothyronines within the placenta [8].

At term, TSH and free T_4 are higher in the fetus than in the mother but free T_3 is less than half the maternal value [65,66]. The inactive hormone, reverse T_3, is present in high concentration in the umbilical cord, along with metabolically inactive sulphated iodothyronines [8]. It is thought that T_3 sulphate could act as a source of T_3 in fetal tissues which contain a sulphatase [8].

It has been shown that various tissues, including brain of rats and sheep, contain a type II deiodinase by the time of mid-gestation, allowing for the local conversion of the T_4 to T_3 [8]. This type II activity is increased in both normal fetuses and in fetuses with hypothyroidism and this would help to prevent impairment of brain development by converting the limited amount of maternal T_4 which has been transferred across the placenta into T_3 [8,67,68]. The amounts, however, seem to be insufficient to suppress the fetal hypothalamic–pituitary axis or to promote normal bone maturation [69].

Neonatal thyroid function

Childbirth, and the resultant cooling, induces in the full-term neonate a rise in TSH which peaks at about 70 mU/l 30 minutes after birth. The TSH then declines and reaches normal adult levels at 3–4 weeks of age [70,71]. Triiodothyronine and thyroxine levels become supranormal at 36–48 hours postpartum and decrease to adult values by 4 or 5 weeks [71].

Hyperthyroidism in pregnancy

Hyperthyroidism occurs in about 2.2 per 1000 pregnant white women and in 1.7 per 1000 pregnant black women [72]. In the majority, the cause of the hyperthyroidism is Graves' disease. In the days before therapy was available for this condition, the perinatal mortality was as high as 48% [73]. Even with treatment, there are slightly more stillbirths and neonatal deaths than in a normal population and the mean birthweight of white babies was found by Niswander and Gordon to be 363 g lower and of black babies 184 g lower than those born to normal women [72].

Since patients with untreated hyperthyroidism commonly are infertile, most women seen by obstetricians will already have been started on treatment before becoming pregnant. Hyperthyroidism, however, can start in pregnancy, particularly between the 10th and 15th week [74], and may sometimes be difficult to diagnose. Many of the features of pregnancy and hyperthyroidism are similar — emotional lability, heat intolerance, palpitations, palmar erythema and goitre — but failure to gain weight despite a good appetite, a rapid sleeping pulse and the presence of lid lag with or without exophthalmos or the presence of pretibial myxoedema, indicating the possibility of Graves' disease, should always suggest a diagnosis of hyperthyroidism. The total T_4 will usually be higher than the physiologically elevated T_4 of pregnancy and the T_3 resin uptake will not be as hypothyroid as it normally is in pregnancy. Indeed the T_3 resin uptake may be in the normal range, the reason being that, despite the large number of binding sites available on the increased amount of TBG in pregnancy, a greater proportion of them than normal are occupied by the excess T_4 produced by the overactive thyroid gland. The free thyroxine index, calculated from the product of the total T_4 and the T_4 resin uptake (expressed as a ratio) [75] will usually be clearly above the normal range. Nowadays direct measurements of free T_3 and free T_4, which are generally available, will show elevated levels in thyrotoxicosis and the new highly sensitive TSH estimations will demonstrate levels suppressed below the normal range. These TSH measurements have rendered the TRH test obsolete for the diagnosis of thyrotoxicosis.

It is important to remember that while Graves' disease may have gone into remission during pregnancy (and the treatment has been stopped), the disease is frequently exacerbated in the postpartum period, due to the reversal of the physiological immunosuppression of pregnancy [74,76–78].

Some patients with hyperemesis gravidarum may have thyrotoxicosis, which is usually transient and does not require medication with antithyroid drugs [79–81]. The mechanism may be through thyroidal stimulation by a form of hCG with higher thyrotrophic activity [82], though hyperemesis can also occur in Graves' disease during pregnancy.

Intrauterine and neonatal thyrotoxicosis

Although thyrotoxicosis in the fetus and newborn is regarded as rare, it has occurred in 10% of the babies born to patients seen by the author who have either a history of previous Graves' disease or Graves' disease during pregnancy [83]. Other authors quote prevalence rates of up to 20 or 25% [84–87]. The disease is caused by thyroid-stimulating immunoglobulins which pass across the placenta from the mother. The mothers often have marked exophthalmos, sometimes with pretibial myxoedema.

If possible, measurement of the maternal thyroid-stimulating antibodies should be carried out, as they can predict the development of fetal and neonatal thyrotoxicosis [88]. The older methods involved estimations of long-acting thyroid stimulator (LATS) and LATS protector [88], but newer methods such as the radioreceptor assay [89] show good correlations between the assay result and levels of T_3 and T_4 in affected fetuses [90]. In a mother who is not receiving antithyroid drugs during pregnancy, the fetus' uncontrolled hyperthyroidism will give rise to an abnormally high fetal heart rate of more than 160/per minute. It is now possible to obtain fetal blood by cordocentesis for thyroid hormone estimation in the initial diagnosis of fetal hyperthyroidism and for its subsequent management [91–93]. The babies of all mothers with thyroid disease, particularly those who have been hyperthyroid, should be observed by a skilled paediatrician.

Hypothyroidism in pregnancy

Hypothyroidism is commoner in pregnancy than hyperthyroidism; in one US study, it occurred in 9 per 1000 white women and 3 per 1000 black women [72]. The degree of hypothyroidism is usually fairly mild, since severe hypothyroidism leads to anovulation, mainly due to abnormal feedback of oestriol on the hypothalamus, and in some patients to hyperprolactinaemia, induced by hypothalamic release of TRH [94]. Mild hypothyroidism may remain unrecognized. It is important to diagnose hypothyroidism, since the abortion and stillbirth rates are double that of the general population [72,94]. One follow-up study of 7-year-old children of mothers with low thyroxine levels during pregnancy showed that their mean intelligence quotient was only 91 compared to that of 105 in children born of hypothyroid mothers who had received adequate hormone replacement during pregnancy [95]. However, a subsequent study found no evidence of physical or intellectual disability in children born to hypothyroid mothers [96].

The diagnosis may be suggested by excessive weight gain, cold intolerance, muscle aches and stiffness, a sleepy, puffy look to the face, a slow pulse, delayed relaxation of the ankle jerks and symptoms of carpal tunnel syndrome. The total T_4 will be inappropriately low for pregnancy but is frequently in the normal non-pregnant range because of the increased TBG. The T_3 resin uptake will be more hypothyroid than is normally seen in pregnancy and the calculated free thyroxine index will be low. Free T_4 levels are low. Total T_3 and free T_3 measurements are not useful diagnostically in hypothyroidism as they may be in the normal range. Because of the effect of low circulating thyroid hormone concentrations on the hypothalamic/pituitary feedback mechanism, the TSH will be high; this is the single most important diagnostic test for primary hypothyroidism. After treatment has been started, the dosage of thyroxine can be best monitored in pregnancy by ensuring that the free thyroxine index, or, preferably, free thyroxine concentrations are within the normal pregnancy range and that the TSH is also suppressed to within the normal range.

Postpartum thyroiditis

It is being recognized increasingly [97–100] that some women are predisposed to autoimmune thyroiditis and may, after delivery, develop a rise in thyroid antibody titre and biochemical evidence of thyroid dysfunction; this is due to the removal of the immunosuppressive effect of pregnancy [78,97,101–104]. Postpartum thyroiditis commonly begins with a transient episode of thyrotoxicosis, 1–3 months after parturition [105], due to autoimmune destruction of the gland, which remits after 2 or 3 months and the patient remains euthyroid [76,100]. However, about a third of these thyrotoxic patients pass into a hypothyroid phase, though the majority recover [76]. Some patients with postpartum thyroiditis, a quarter to a third of

the total, appear to start with hypothyroidism, again with eventual recovery of euthyroidism in the majority [76,100].

Twenty to twenty-five per cent of patients developing postpartum thyroiditis have a first-degree relative with autoimmune disease [106]. A titre of thyroid microsomal antibodies greater than 1/1600 during the first trimester of pregnancy increases the chances of postpartum thyroiditis [76,102,104,107]; indeed Hall et al. [100] found that 70% of those who had a positive family history of thyroid disease and positive thyroid antibodies at the first antenatal clinic visit developed the disease postpartum.

References

1 Hytten F.E. & Leitch J. (1971) The Physiology of Human Pregnancy, 2nd edn. Blackwell Scientific Publications, Oxford.
2 Singer P.A. & Nicoloff J.T. (1972) Estimation of the triiodothyronine secretion rate in euthyroid man. Journal of Clinical Endocrinology and Metabolism 35, 82.
3 Woeber K.A. & Ingbar S.H. (1968) The contribution of thyroxine-binding prealbumin to the binding of thyroxine in human serum, as assessed by immunoabsorption. Journal of Clinical Investigation 47, 1710.
4 Hesch R.-D. & Koehrle J. (1986) Intracellular pathways of iodothyronine metabolism. In Werner's The Thyroid: A Fundamental and Clinical Text. Eds S.H. Ingbar & L.E. Braverman, p. 154. J.B. Lippincott, Philadelphia.
5 Hall R., Evered D.C. & Tunbridge W.M.G. (1973) The role of TSH and TRH in thyroid disease. In 9th Symposium on Advanced Medicine. Ed. G. Walker, p. 15. Pitman Medical, London.
6 Braverman L.E. & Utiger R.D. (eds) (1991) Werner's The Thyroid: A Fundamental and Clinical Text, 6th edn. J.B. Lippincott, Philadelphia.
7 Ingbar S.H. (1985) The Thyroid Gland. In Williams' Textbook of Endocrinology, 7th edn. Eds J.D. Wilson & D.W. Foster, p. 682. W.B. Saunders, Philadelphia.
8 Burrow G.N., Fisher D.A. & Larsen P.R. (1994) Maternal and fetal thyroid function. New England Journal of Medicine 331, 1072.
9 Aboul-Khair S.A., Crooks J., Turnbull A.C. & Hytten F.E. (1964) The physiological changes in thyroid function during pregnancy. Clinical Science 27, 195.
10 Halnan K.E. (1958) The radioiodine uptake of the human thyroid in pregnancy. Clinical Science 17, 281.
11 Stoffer R.P., Koeneke I.A., Chesky V.E. & Hellwig C.A. (1957) The thyroid in pregnancy. American Journal of Obstetrics and Gynecology 74, 300.
12 Crooks J., Aboul-Khair S.A., Turnbull A.C. & Hytten F.E. (1964) The incidence of goitre during pregnancy. Lancet ii, 334.

13 Crooks H., Tulloch M.I., Turnbull A.C., Davidsson D., Skulason T. & Snaedal G. (1967) Comparative incidence of goitre in pregnancy in Iceland and Scotland. *Lancet* **ii**, 625.

14 Levy R.P., Newman D.M., Rejali L.S. & Barford D.A.G. (1980) The myth of goiter in pregnancy. *American Journal of Obstetrics and Gynecology* **137**, 701.

15 Long T.J., Felice M.E. & Hollingsworth D.R. (1985) Goiter in pregnant teenagers. *American Journal of Obstetrics and Gynecology* **152**, 670.

16 Dworkin H.J., Jacquez J.A. & Beierwaltes W.H. (1966) Relationship of iodine ingestion to iodine excretion in pregnancy. *Journal of Clinical Endocrinology and Metabolism* **26**, 1329.

17 Glinoer D., De Nayer P., Bourdoux P., Lemone M., Robyn C., Van Steirteghem A., Kinthaert J. *et al.* (1990) Regulation of maternal thyroid during pregnancy. *Journal of Clinical Endocrinology and Metabolism* **71**, 276.

18 Nelson M., Wickus G.G., Caplan R.H. & Beguin E.A. (1987) Thyroid gland size in pregnancy: an ultrasound and clinical study. *Journal of Reproductive Medicine* **32**, 888.

19 Lemarchand-Béraud T. & Vannotti A. (1969) Relationships between blood thyrotrophin level, protein bound iodine and free thyroxine concentration in man under normal physiological conditions. *Acta Endocrinologica (Kobenhavn)* **60**, 315.

20 Malkasian G.D. & Mayberry W.E. (1970) Serum total and free thyroxine and thyrotropin in normal and pregnant women, neonates and women receiving progestogens. *American Journal of Obstetrics and Gynecology* **108**, 1234.

21 Kannan V., Sinha M.K., Devi P.K. & Rastogi G.K. (1973) Plasma thyrotrophin and its response to thyrotropin releasing hormone in normal pregnancy. *Obstetrics and Gynecology* **42**, 547.

22 Odell W.D., Wilber J.F. & Utiger R.D. (1967) Studies of thyrotropin physiology by means of radioimmunoassay. *Recent Progress in Hormone Research* **23**, 47.

23 Kanazawa S., Nakamura A., Saida K. & Tojo S. (1976) Plancento-thyroidal relationship in normal pregnancy. *Acta Obstetrica et Gynaecologica Scandinavica* **55**, 201.

24 Ballabio M., Poshyachinda M. & Ekins R.P. (1991) Pregnancy-induced changes in thyroid function: role of human chorionic gonadotropin as putative regulator of maternal thyroid. *Journal of Clinical Endocrinology and Metabolism* **73**, 824.

25 Kenimer J.G., Hershman J.M. & Higgins H.P. (1975) The thyrotropin in hydatidiform moles is human chorionic gonadotropin. *Journal of Clinical Endocrinology and Metabolism* **40**, 482.

26 Pekonen F., Alfthan H., Stenman U.H. & Ylikorkala O. (1988) Human chorionic gonadotropin (hCG) and thyroid function in early pregnancy: circadian variation and evidence for intrinsic thyrotropic activity of hCG. *Journal of Clinical Endocrinology and Metabolism* **66**, 853.

27 Yoshikawa N., Nishikawa M., Horimoto M., Yoshimura M., Sawaragi S., Horikoshi Y., Sawaragi I. *et al.* (1989) Thyroid stimulating activity in sera of normal pregnant women. *Journal of Clinical Endocrinology and Metabolism* **69**, 891.

28 Kimura M., Amino N., Tamaki H., Mitsuda N., Miyai K. & Tanizawa O. (1990) Physiologic thyroid activation in normal early pregnancy is induced by circulating hCG. *Obstetrics and Gynecology* **75**, 775.

29 Guillaume J., Schussler G.C. & Goldman J. (1985) Components of the total serum thyroid hormone concentrations during pregnancy: high free thyroxine and blunted thyrotropin (TSH) response to TSH-releasing hormone in the first trimester. *Journal of Clinical Endocrinology and Metabolism* **60**, 678.

30 Nagataki S., Mizuno M., Sakamoto S., Irie M., Shizume K., Nakao K., Galton V.A. *et al.* (1976) Thyroid function in molar pregnancy. In *Thyroid Research*. Eds J. Robbins & L.E. Braverman, p. 535. Excerpta Medica, Amsterdam.

31 Uchimura H., Nagataki S., Tabuchi T., Mizuno M. & Ito K. (1976) The thyroid stimulating activity of highly purified preparations of human chorionic gonadotrophins. In *Thyroid Research*. Eds J. Robbins & L.E. Braverman, p. 37. Excerpta Medica, Amsterdam.

32 Pekary A.E., Jackson I.M., Goodwin T.M., Pang X.-P., Hein M.D. & Hershman J.M. (1993) Increased *in vitro* thyrotropic activity of partially sialated human chorionic gonadotropin extracted from hydatidiform moles of patients with hyperthyroidism. *Journal of Clinical Endocrinology and Metabolism* **76**, 70.

33 Tsuruta E., Tada H., Tamaki H., Kashiwa T., Asahi K., Takeoka K., Mitsuda N. *et al.* (1995) Pathogenic role of asiolo human chorionic gonadotropin in gestational thyrotoxicosis. *Journal of Clinical Endocrinology and Metabolism* **80**, 350.

34 Roti E., Gnudi A. & Braverman L.E. (1983) The placental transport, synthesis and metabolism of hormones and drugs which affect thyroid function. *Endocrine Reviews* **4**, 131.

35 Gibbons J.M., Mitnick M. & Chieffo V. (1975) In vitro biosynthesis of TSH- and LH-releasing factors by the human placenta. *American Journal of Obstetrics and Gynecology* **121**, 127.

36 Shambaugh G. III., Kubek M. & Wilber J.F. (1979) Thyrotropin-releasing hormone activity in the human placenta. *Journal of Clinical Endocrinology and Metabolism* **48**, 483.

37 Dowling J.T., Freinkel N. & Ingbar S.H. (1960) The effect of oestrogens upon the peripheral metabolism of thyroxine. *Journal of Clinical Investigation* **39**, 1119.

38 Ain K.B., Mori Y. & Refetoff S. (1987) Reduced clearance rate of thyroxine binding blobulin (TBG) with increased sialylation: a mechanism for estrogen-induced elevation of serum TBG concentration. *Journal of Clinical Endocrinology and Metabolism* **65**, 689.

39 Man E.B., Reid W.A., Hellegers A.E. & Jones W.S. (1969) Thyroid function in human pregnancy. III. Serum thyroxine binding prealbumin (TBPA) and thyroxine-binding globulin (TBG) of pregnant women aged 14 through 43 years. *American Journal of Obstetrics and Gynecology* **103**, 338.

40 Mulaisho C. & Utiger R.D. (1977) Serum thyroxine-binding globulin: determination by competitive

382

ligand-binding assay in thyroid disease and pregnancy. *Acta Endocrinologica (Kobenhavn)* **85**, 314.

41 Rastogi G.K., Sawhney R.C., Sinha M.K., Thomas Z. & Devi P.K. (1974) Serum and urinary levels of thyroid hormones in normal pregnancy. *Obstetrics and Gynecology* **44**, 176.

42 Finucane J.F., Griffiths R.S. & Black E.G. (1976) Altered patterns of thyroid hormones in serum and urine in pregnancy and during oral contraceptive therapy. *British Journal of Obstetrics and Gynaecology* **83**, 733.

43 Osathanondh R., Tulchinsky D. & Chopra I.J. (1976) Total and free thyroxine and triiodothyronine in normal and complicated pregnancy. *Journal of Clinical Endocrinology and Metabolism* **42**, 98.

44 Parslow M.E., Oddie T.H. & Fisher D.A. (1977) Evaluation of serum triiodothyronine and adjusted triiodothyronine (free triiodothyronine index) in pregnancy. *Clinical Chemistry* **23**, 490.

45 Clark F. & Horn D.B. (1965) Assessment of thyroid function by the combined use of the serum protein-bound iodine and resin uptake of ^{131}I-triiodothyronine. *Journal of Clinical Endocrinology and Metabolism* **25**, 39.

46 Goolden A.W.G., Gartside J.M. & Sanderson C. (1967) Thyroid status in pregnancy and in women taking oral contraceptives. *Lancet* **i**, 12.

47 Souma J.A., Niejadlik D.C., Cottrell S. & Rankel S. (1973) Comparison of thyroid function in each trimester of pregnancy with the use of triiodothyronine uptake, thyroxine iodine, free thyroxine, and free thyroxine index. *American Journal of Obstetrics and Gynecology* **116**, 905.

48 Shakespear R.A. & Burke C.W. (1976) Triiodothyronine and thyroxine in urine. I. Measurement and application. *Journal of Clinical Endocrinology and Metabolism* **42**, 494.

49 Ingbar S.H., Braverman L.E., Dawber N.A. & Lee G.Y. (1965) A new method for measuring the free thyroid hormone in human serum and an analysis of the factors that influence its concentration. *Journal of Clinical Investigation* **44**, 1679.

50 Thorson S.C., Wilkins G.E., Schaffrin M., Morrison R.T. & McIntosh H.W. (1972) Estimation of serum free thyroxine concentration by ultrafiltration. *Journal of Laboratory and Clinical Medicine* **80**, 145.

51 Parker J.H. (1985) Amerlex free triiodothyronine and free thyroxine levels in normal pregnancy. *British Journal of Obstetrics and Gynaecology* **92**, 1234.

52 Burman K.D., Read J., Dimond R.C., Strum D., Wright F.D., Patow W., Earl J.M. *et al.* (1976) Measurements of 3,3',5'-triiodothyronine (reverse T_3), 3,3'-1-diiodothyronine, T_3 and T_4 in human amniotic fluid and in cord and maternal serum. *Journal of Clinical Endocrinology and Metabolism* **43**, 1351.

53 Shakespear R.A. & Burke C.W. (1976) Triiodothyronine and thyroxine in urine. II. Renal handling, and effect of urinary protein. *Journal of Clinical Endocrinology and Metabolism* **42**, 504.

54 Dowling J.T., Appleton W.G. & Nicoloff J.T. (1967) Thyroxine turnover during human pregnancy. *Journal of Clinical Endocrinology and Metabolism* **27**, 1749.

55 Caldwell G., Kellett H.A. & Gow S.M. (1985) A new strategy for thyroid function testing. *Lancet* **i**, 1117.

56 Siersbaek-Nielsen K. & Morholm Hansen J. (1969) Variations in plasma thyroxine during labour and early puerperium. *Acta Endocrinologica (Kobenhavn)* **60**, 423.

57 Hotelling D.R. & Sherwood L.M. (1971) The effects of pregnancy on circulting triiodothyronine. *Journal of Clinical Endocrinology and Metabolism* **33**, 783.

58 Thorpe-Beeston J.G., Nicolaides K.H., Felton C.V., Butler J. & McGregor A.M. (1991) Maturation of the secretion of thyroid hormone and thyroid-stimulating hormone in the fetus. *New England Journal of Medicine* **324**, 532.

59 Ballabio M., Nicolini V., Jowett T., Ruiz de Elvira M.C., Ekins R.P. & Rodeck C.H. (1989) Maturation of thyroid function in normal human fetuses. *Clinical Endocrinology (Oxford)* **35**, 565.

60 Ekins R. (1985) Roles of serum thyroxine binding proteins and maternal thyroid hormones in fetal development. *Lancet* **i**, 1129.

61 Contempré B., Jauniaux E., Calvo R., Jurcovic D., Campbell S. & Morreale de Escobar G. (1993) Detection of thyroid hormones in human embryonic cavities during the first trimester of pregnancy. *Journal of Clinical Endocrinology and Metabolism* **77**, 1719.

62 Obregon M.J., Mallol J., Pastor R., Morreale de Escobar G. & Escobar del Rey F. (1984) L-thyronine and 3,5,3'-triiodothyronine in rat embryos before onset of fetal thyroid function. *Endocrinology* **114**, 305.

63 Woods R.J., Sinha A.K. & Ekins R.P. (1984) Uptake and metabolism of thyroid hormones by the rat fetus in early pregnancy. *Clinical Science* **67**, 359.

64 Ekins R.P., Sinha A.K., Pickard M.R., Evans I.M. & Al Yatama F. (1994) Transport of thyroid hormones to target tissues. *Acta Medica Austriaca* **21**, 26.

65 Robin N.I., Refetoff S., Gleason R.E. & Selenkow H.A. (1970) Thyroid hormone relationships between maternal and fetal circulations in human pregnancy at term: a study of patients with normal and abnormal thyroid function. *American Journal of Obstetrics and Gynecology* **108**, 1269.

66 Ramsay I., Kaur S. & Krassas G. (1983) Thyrotoxicosis in pregnancy: results of treatment by antithyroid drugs combined with T_4. *Clinical Endocrinology (Oxford)* **18**, 75.

67 Santini F., Cortelazzi D., Baggiani A.M., Marconi A.M., Beck-Peccoz P. & Chopra I.J. (1993) A study of the serum 3.5.3'-triiodothyronine sulphate concentration in normal and hypothroid fetuses at various gestational ages. *Journal of Clinical Endocrinology and Metabolism* **76**, 1583.

68 Vulsma T., Gons M.H. & de Vijlder J.J. (1989) Maternal-fetal transfer of thyroxine in congenital hypothyroidism due to a total organification deject or thyroid agenesis. *New England Journal of Medicine* **321**, 13.

69 Sack J., Kaiserman I. & Siebner R. (1993) Maternal-fetal T_4 transfer does not suffice to prevent the effects of in-utero hypothyroidism. *Hormone Research* **39**, 1.

70 Fisher D.A., Dussault J.H., Sack J. & Chopra I.J. (1977) Ontogenesis of hypothalamic-pituitary-

thyroid function and metabolism in man, sheep and rat. *Recent Progress in Hormone Research* **33**, 59.

71 Polk D.H. (1994) Diagnosis and management of altered fetal thyroid status. *Clinics in Perinatology* **21**, 647.

72 Niswander K.R. & Gordon M. (1972) *The Women and their Pregnancies*, p. 246. W.B. Saunders, Philadelphia.

73 Gardiner-Hill H. (1929) Pregnancy complicating simple goitre and Graves's disease. *Lancet* **i**, 120.

74 Amino N., Tanizawa O., Mori H., Iwatani Y., Yamada T., Kurachi K., Kumahara Y. *et al.* (1982) Aggravation of thyrotoxicosis in early pregnancy and after delivery in Graves' disease. *Journal of Clinical Endocrinology and Metabolism* **55**, 108.

75 Committee on Nomenclature of the American Thyroid Association (1976) Revised nomenclature for tests of thyroid hormones in serum. *Journal of Clinical Endocrinology and Metabolism* **42**, 595.

76 Amino N., Mori H., Iwatani Y., Tanizawa O., Kawashima M., Tsuge I., Ibaragi K. *et al.* (1982) High prevalence of transient *post partum* thyrotoxicosis and hypothyroidism. *New England Journal of Medicine* **306**, 849.

77 Hardisty C.A. & Munro D.S. (1983) Serum long acting thyroid protector in pregnancy complicated by Graves' disease. *British Medical Journal* **286**, 934.

78 Weetman A.P. & McGregor A.M. (1984) Autoimmune thyroid disease: developments in our understanding. *Endocrine Reviews* **5**, 309.

79 Dozeman R., Kaizer F.E., Cass O. & Pries J. (1983) Hyperthyroidism appearing as hyperemesis gravidarum. *Archives of Internal Medicine* **143**, 2202.

80 Jeffcoate W.J. & Bain C. (1985) Recurrent pregnancy-induced thyrotoxicosis presenting as hyperemesis gravidarum. *British Journal of Obstetrics and Gynaecology* **92**, 413.

81 Bober S.A., McGill A.L. & Tunbridge W.M.G. (1986) Thyroid function in hyperemesis gravidarum. *Acta Endocrinologica* **111**, 404.

82 Tsuruta E., Tada H., Tamaki H., Kashiwa T., Asahi K., Takeoka K., Mitsuda N. *et al.* (1995) Pathogenic role of asiolo human chorionic gonadotropin in gestational thyrotoxicosis. *Journal of Clinical Endocrinology and Metabolism* **80**, 350.

83 Ramsay I. (1991) Fetal and neonatal hyperthyroidism. *Contemporary Reviews in Obstetrics and Gynaecology* **3**, 74.

84 Tamaki H., Amino N., Takeoka K., Iwatani Y., Tachi J., Kimura M., Mitsuda N. *et al.* (1989) Prediction of later development of thyrotoxicosis or central hypothyroidism from the cord serum thyroid-stimulating hormone level in neonates born to mothers with Graves' disease. *Journal of Pediatrics* **115**, 318.

85 Mortimer R.H., Tyack S.A., Galligan J.P., Perry-Keene D.A. & Tan Y.M. (1990) Graves' disease in pregnancy: TSH receptor binding inhibiting immunoglobulins and maternal and neonatal thyroid function. *Clinical Endocrinology*, **32**, 141.

86 Matsuura N., Yamada Y., Nohara Y., Konishi J., Kasagi K., Endo K., Kojima H. *et al.* (1980) Familial neonatal transient hypothyroidism due to maternal

TSH-binding inhibitor immunoglobulins. *New England Journal of Medicine* **303**, 738.

87 Clavel S., Madec A.M., Bornet H., Deviller P., Stefanutti A. & Orgiazzi J. (1990) Anti-TSH receptor antibodies in pregnant patients with antoimmune thyroid disorders. *British Journal of Obstetrics and Gynaecology* **97**, 1003.

88 Dirmikis S.M. & Munro D.S. (1975) Placental transmission of thyroid stimulating immunoglobulins. *British Medical Journal* **ii**, 665.

89 Shewring G. & Smith B.R. (1982) An improved radioreceptor assay for TSH receptor antibodies. *Clinical Endocrinology* **17**, 409.

90 Mamotani N., Noh I., Oyanagi H., Ishikawa N. & Ito K. (1986) Antithyroid drug therapy for Graves' disease in pregnancy. *New England Journal Of Medicine* **315**, 24.

91 Porreco R.P. & Bloch C.A. (1990) Fetal blood sampling in the management of intrauterine thyrotoxicosis. *Obstetrics and Gynecology* **76**, 509.

92 Wenstrom K.D., Weiner C.P., Williamson R.A. & Grant S.S. (1990) Diagnosis of prenatal fetal hyperthyroidism using funipuncture. *Obstetrics and Gynecology* **76**, 513.

93 Hare J.Y. & Ludomirsky A. (1994) Cordocentesis; direct access to the fetal circulation for evaluating fetal wellbeing and thyroid function. *Current Opinion in Obstetrics and Gynaecology* **6**, 440.

94 Thomas R. & Reid R.L. (1987) Thyroid disease and reproductive dysfunction: a review. *Obstetrics and Gynecology* **70**, 789.

95 Man E.B. (1975) Maternal hypothyroxinaemia: development of 4 and 7 year old offspring. In *Perinatal Thyroid Physiology and Disease*. Eds D.A. Fisher and G.N. Burrow, p. 117. Raven Press, New York.

96 Montoro M., Collea J.V., Frasier S.D. & Mestman J.H. (1981) Successful outcome of pregnancy in women with hypothyroidism. *Annals of Internal Medicine* **94**, 31.

97 Amino N., Miyai K., Kuro R., Tanizawa O., Azukizawa M., Takai S., Tanaka F. *et al.* (1977) Transient post-partum hypothyroidism: fourteen cases with autoimmune thyroiditis. *Annals of Internal medicine* **87**, 155.

98 Ramsay I. (1986) *Post partum* thyroiditis: an underdiagnosed disease. *British Journal of Obstetrics and Gynaecology* **93**, 1121.

99 Nicolai T.F., Turney S.L. & Roberts R.C. (1987) *Post partum* lymphocytic thyroiditis. *Archives of Internal Medicine* **147**, 221.

100 Hall R., Fung H., Kologlu M., Collison K., Maro J., Parkes A.B., Harris B.B. *et al.* (1987) Thyroid disease and pregnancy. *Journal of Endocrinology* **112** (suppl).

101 Amino N., Kuro R., Tanizawa O., Tanaka F., Hayashi C., Kotani K., Kawashima M. *et al.* (1978) Changes of serum anti-thyroid antibodies during and after pregnancy in auto-immune thyroid diseases. *Clinical and Experimental Immunology* **31**, 30.

102 Amino N. & Miyai K. (1983) *Post-partum* autoimmune endocrine syndrome. In *Autoimmune Endocrine Disease*. Ed. T.F. Davies, p. 247. John Wiley and Sons, New York.

103 Zakarija M. & McKenzie J.M. (1983) Pregnancy-

384

associated changes in the thyroid-stimulating antibody of Graves' disease and the relationship to neonatal hyperthyroidism. *Journal to Clinical Endocrinology and Metabolism* **57**, 1036.

104 Amino N., Iwatani Y., Tamaki H., Mori H., Miyai K. & Tanizawa O. (1984) Mechanism of post partum thyroid disease. In *Endocrinology, Proceedings of the 7th International Congress of Endocrinology*, Quebec City, 1–7 July. Eds F. Labrie & L. Proulx, p. 461. Excerpta Medica, Amsterdam.

105 Ginsberg J. & Walfish P.G. (1977) Post-partum transient thyrotoxicosis with painless thyroiditis. *Lancet* **i**, 1125.

106 Farid N.R. & Bear J.C. (1983) Autoimmune disorders and the major histocompatability complex. In *Autoimmune Endocrine Disease*. Ed. T.F. Davies, p. 59. John Wiley and Sons, New York.

107 Jansson R., Bernander S., Karlsson A., Levin K. & Nilsson G. (1984) Autoimmune thyroid dysfunction in the *post partum* period. *Journal of Clinical Endocrinology and Metabolism* **58**, 681.

The Adrenal Gland

I.D. RAMSAY & RINA M. DAVISON

The adrenal cortex

The adrenal glands each weigh about 4 g and are situated at the upper pole of the kidneys. Each gland is composed of an outer cortex and an inner medulla. The cortex is divided into three recognizable zones:

1 The zone glomerulosa, a thin outer layer which is mainly responsible for aldosterone production.
2 The zona fasciculata, a wide zone of radiating strands, which produces cortisol.
3 The zona reticularis, a net-like structure adjacent to the medulla, which also manufactures cortisol as well as androgens and oestrogens.

The adrenal cortex, the ovaries and the placenta share the ability to synthesize steroid hormones from acetate or cholesterol. All the steroid-producing organs can make androgens and oestrogens, but only the adrenal cortex has the enzymes necessary for the manufacture of cortisol.

The basic structure of steroid hormones consists of three cyclohexane rings and one cyclopentane ring. The 17 carbon atoms of the rings are conventionally numbered as shown in Fig. 14.1. Oestrogens have an extra carbon atom (no. 18) attached at carbon atom 13 of the structure. When another carbon atom (no. 19) is added at the 10 position, the basic structure of the androgens is formed. Cortisol, like the other glucocorticoids, is a 21-carbon atom molecule with a two-carbon atom side chain (nos 20 and 21) attached at the 17 position on the ring. The synthesis of adrenal cortical hormones starts with acetate or cholesterol and proceeds via various steps catalysed by enzymes to the formation of glucocorticoids, mineralocorticoids, androgens and oestrogens [1] (Fig. 14.2).

Action of adrenal steroid hormones

Glucocorticoids promote the formation of glucose from protein (gluconeogensis), encourage glycogen deposition and increase fatty acid synthesis, as well as having an anti-insulin action. Glucocorticoids are also necessary for the excretion of water by the kidneys.

Mineralocorticoid activity is due largely to aldosterone, deoxycorticosterone having only one-twentieth of its potency. Aldosterone increases the reabsorption of sodium from the distal tubules of the kidney. The effect on increasing potassium excretion appears to be separate from the sodium retaining mechanism. Aldosterone also alters the distribution of sodium and potassium ions across cell membranes throughout the body.

Androgens, in the amounts produced by the normal adrenal, probably produce very little physiological effect apart from promoting secondary sexual hair growth.

Oestrogens are produced in such small quantities by the adrenal cortex that it is doubtful that they have any important physiological function during the reproductive years.

Circulation of hormones in the blood

Cortisol is 75% firmly, but reversibly, bound to a globulin called transcortin or corticosteroid-binding globulin (CBG) [2,3]. Another 15% is loosely bound to albumin and the remaining metabolically active 10% remains in the free form. Fifty to sixty per cent of aldosterone is bound to albumin, about 5–10% to CBG, and the remainder circulates in the free form [4].

Testosterone and oestradiol are bound to another globulin which is called sex hormone-binding globulin (SHBG) [5]. Oestrogens increase the amount of SHBG, whereas androgens decrease it. In a normal woman in the premenstrual phase, the relative preponderance of oestrogen secretion to that of androgens ensures that the free fraction of oestradiol is maintained at a much greater level than that of testosterone [6], since the binding constant for testosterone with SHBG is three times that of oestradiol [7].

Metabolism of hormones

The most important site of steroid hormone breakdown is the liver, where derivatives are linked to water-soluble glucuronides and sulphates and are excreted by the kidney. Urinary steroids can be measured by several methods and this may give rise to some confusion, because each method measures something different. Urinary 17-hydroxycorticosteroids (17-OHCS), measured by the Porter–Silber method, are derived from the glucocorticoids 11-deoxycortisol and cortisol. 17-Ketogenic steroids are steroids that can be converted into 17-ketosteroids by oxidation with sodium bismuthate, and they include pregnanetriol in addi-

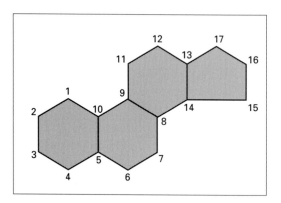

Fig. 14.1. The basic structure and numbering system of steroid hormones.

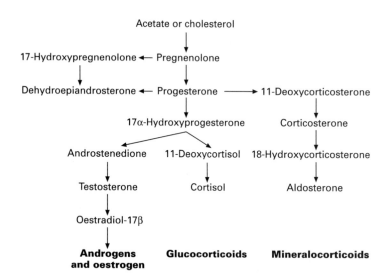

Fig. 14.2. The synthetic pathways of steroid hormones in the adrenal cortex.

tion to the glucocorticoids. The urinary free cortisol is related to the amount of unbound cortisol in blood and correlates well with the cortisol secretion rate. This technique has largely replaced methods for measuring 17-OHCS and 17-ketogenic steroids. Urinary 17-ketosteroids measured by the Zimmerman method mainly measure adrenal androgens such as dehydroepiandrosterone and androstenedione, but are a poor indicator of adrenal testosterone production. Aldosterone can also be measured in urine. The subject has been reviewed by Loraine and Bell [8]. Salivary cortisol has also proven a valid and reliable reflection of the unbound hormone in blood [9,10].

Control of adrenocortical hormones

The secretion of glucocorticoids is controlled by the secretion of adrenocorticotrophic hormone (ACTH) from the anterior pituitary gland. The production of ACTH is, in turn, governed by a substance called corticotrophin-releasing hormone (CRH), which is produced by the hypothalamus and which travels down the hypophysial portal system of veins to the anterior pituitary. The control of plasma cortisol is through a negative feedback of cortisol on the anterior pituitary and the hypothalamus. High levels of cortisol inhibit the CRH-induced secretion of ACTH by the pituitary, but also have an effect in diminishing the hypothalamic release of CRH. There is, in addition, a circadian rhythm of CRH production, so that levels of ACTH, and thus cortisol, are highest at about 8.00 a.m. and lowest at midnight. This rhythm can be over-ridden by stressful stimuli such as fear, pain and hypoglycaemia, all of which result in an increased secretion of cortisol. For a full review of this subject see Forsling and Grossman (Fig. 14.3) [11].

Although aldosterone production is stimulated to a certain extent by an acute rise in ACTH, its main means of control is via the renin–angiotensin system. Sodium loss, or a reduction in blood flow through the kidneys, leads to a release of renin from the juxtaglomerular apparatus. The renin hydrolyses renin substrate, produced by the liver, to form angiotensin I (A I). A I is then converted into

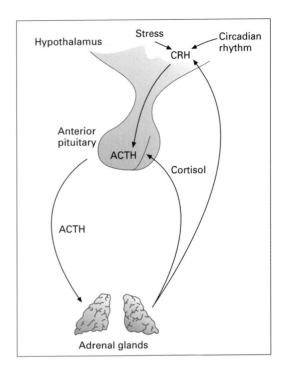

Fig. 14.3. The control of adrenocortical hormones.

angiotensin II (A II) which stimulates the adrenal to secrete aldosterone. Sodium retention, increase in blood volume or an increase in blood pressure leads to inhibition of renin release and a diminution of aldosterone secretion [12].

Cortical function in pregnancy

ACTH levels rise progressively in pregnancy, but within the normal range for non-pregnant subjects [13–15]. There is also a steady rise in total plasma cortisol [16–18] from 3 months of gestation until delivery [19]. Much of the increase in the plasma cortisol is due to its binding to CBG, the concentration of which rises steadily during pregnancy to twice normal values [3]. In addition to the increased amount of total plasma cortisol, the mean unbound cortisol is elevated in normal pregnancy with loss of diurnal variation — the midnight values being relatively higher, compared with controls, than the morning values [20,21]. There would thus appear to be a greater tissue exposure to unbound cortisol in late pregnancy [20]. Whether this could be responsible in part for such pseudo-Cushingoid features of pregnancy as striae gravidarum, impaired carbohydrate tolerance and hypertension remains controversial [22,23].

The increased amount of unbound cortisol in the plasma is reflected in an excretion of urinary free cortisol which more than doubles during the course of pregnancy [24]. The urinary free cortisols do not suppress normally with dexamethasone and, since ACTH is found in high concentration in the placenta, it is thought that the rise in plasma ACTH during pregnancy (see above) may be due to its production by the placenta and this may modulate pituitary–adrenal function in pregnancy [13–15,25–27].

The concentration of CRH in maternal plasma increases greatly during the last trimester of normal pregnancy, and is higher in women with pre-eclampsia [28,29].

Recently, a corticotrophin releasing factor (CRF) binding protein has been identified and cloned. It binds the circulating CRF, reducing its biological action during pregnancy, and may thus represent one of the major mechanisms used by target tissues to control CRF activity during pregnancy [30,31].

Amounts of 17-OHCS excreted in the urine actually decline in pregnancy due to a reduction in the amount of the tetrahydrometabolites of the glucocorticoids and the excretion of breakdown products which are not measured as 17-OHCS [32].

There is a slight rise in urinary 17-ketogenic steroids [33], but this probably is accounted for by metabolites of progesterone [34]. Cortisol secretion rates have been variously reported as increased [35] or reduced [36] in pregnancy. There is a prolonged half-life of cortisol in the blood [37].

Because of the considerable rise in SHBG [5], plasma testosterone rises during pregnancy and is highest at delivery [38,39]. However, unbound testosterone has been reported as normal [40], as is the testosterone production rate [41]. These facts are somewhat at variance with the finding of an increase in testosterone glucuronide in urine during late pregnancy [42].

There is a modest rise in 17-ketosteroid excretion [43], but the complexities of adrenal androgen metabolism in pregnancy have not been fully worked out. For instance, although urinary and plasma androsterone excretion has been shown to fall in late pregnancy [43,44] there is a rise in plasma 16β-hydroxydehydroepiandrosterone [45].

Renin and aldosterone

There is an oestrogen-induced increase [46] in plasma renin substrate during pregnancy. There may also be an increased sodium loss due to the raised glomerular filtration rate which is already present at the 12th week of gestation [47], the natriuretic effect of rising progesterone levels in the blood, and the fetal need of sodium. These factors lead to an increase in A II [48], and increased secretion, plasma concentration and excretion of aldosterone [49–56], and in fact the high level of aldosterone during pregnancy may play an important role in stabilizing blood pressure and maintaining the balance of water and electrolytes.

Plasma renin [57,58] and both plasma [52] and urinary aldosterone [50] are below normal in preeclampsia.

11-Deoxycorticosterone

The weaker mineralocorticosteroid 11-deoxycorticosterone (DOC) is of interest because it becomes elevated by the 8th week of gestation and in fact shows the greatest percentage increase of all adrenal steroids during pregnancy [59]. Since at 8 weeks neither cortisol nor corticosterone are significantly elevated, it is likely that something other than ACTH is responsible for the rise, particularly as DOC is not suppressible by dexamethasone at any stage of pregnancy [60,61]. It seems likely that the DOC is being produced by the fetoplacental unit [60].

DOC does not appear to change in response to alterations in salt balance during pregnancy [62], and plasma levels have been found to be unaltered [60] or decreased [63,64] in pre-eclampsia. However, before one can say that DOC has no part to play in the pathogenesis of pre-eclampsia, it would be necessary to compare free DOC levels with blood volume status in pre-eclampsia [65].

Cortical function in labour

There is an increased cortisol production rate [36,66], a rise in plasma cortisol, and an increase in the urinary excretion of 17-OHCS [16] during labour. These changes can all be attributed to a stress response.

Cortical function in the puerperium

Immediately after parturition there is a rise in the urinary excretion of 17-ketosteroids [33], which may be due to the stress of labour, because this excretion is normal by the next day. Plasma cortisol levels, raised during pregnancy and even more considerably elevated in labour, fall to normal within a week of parturition [19]. The raised plasma levels of testosterone and androstenedione decline to normal within a few days of delivery [38].

Fetal adrenocortical hormones

The fetal adrenal gland differs from that of the adult in that there is a relative deficiency of 3-β-dehydrogenase, the steroid-metabolizing enzyme directly involved in cortisol synthesis.

Fetal cortisol can arise from two alternative sources: transplacental passage of maternal cortisol, or synthesis from placental progesterone [67]. Recently, a significant correlation between fetal cortisol and progesterone was noted and it is likely that *in vivo*, placental progesterone is an important precursor of cortisol in the fetus [68]. There is a significant increase in plasma cortisol concentration with advancing gestational age, though lower than maternal levels, and it has been estimated that the contribution of maternal cortisol to fetal cortisol near term by placental passage, is between 25% and 50% [69].

Dehydroepiandrosterone sulphate (DHEAS) concentrations in the fetus decrease significantly with gestational age, and it has been postulated that the rising cortisol to DHEAS ratio may be a trigger for the initiation of labour [70].

Adrenal disorders in pregnancy

Addison's disease

Tiredness, nausea and vomiting, a tendency to hypoglycaemia and pigmentation may all be present in normal pregnancy, but if these symptoms are combined with weight loss, a diagnosis of Addison's disease should be considered. Following the decline in the prevalence of tuberculosis in this country, the most common cause of primary adrenal failure has become autoimmune adrenalitis. As 50% of patients with autoimmune adrenalitis have other endocrine disorders (D. Doniach, personal communication), the presence either in the patient or a close relative of other autoimmune diseases such as hypothyroidism, Hashimoto's thyroiditis, Graves' disease, pernicious anaemia or vitiligo should make one view the above symptoms in a pregnant woman with suspicion.

Measurement of the urea and electrolytes may suggest the diagnosis of adrenal failure. There may be hyponatraemia, hypochloraemia, hyperkalaemia, acidosis and a rise in blood urea. A basal plasma cortisol may be low but, on the other hand, can be in the normal range because of the increase in the binding protein CBG. The best test is to study the response of the plasma cortisol to the injection of tetracosactrin (Synacthen (Ciba)). In primary adrenal disease there will be no response.

The maintenance treatment of Addison's disease in the pregnant woman is 20 mg of hydrocortisone by mouth in the morning and 10 mg at night, together with a mineralocorticoid such as 9-α-fluorohydrocortisone, 0.1–0.2 mg daily. In severe adrenal failure or if the patient is vomiting, it is necessary to give the hydrocortisone parenterally and in adequate dosage—up to 100 mg 8 hourly is often required. If saline is being infused, there may not be any need to inject a mineralocorticoid such as deoxycorticosterone acetate since the cortisol has sufficient mineralocorticoid effect.

Acute adrenal failure

Acute adrenal failure sometimes occurs in pregnancy as a complication of pre-eclampsia or of shock following accidental or postpartum haemorrhage [71–73]. At necropsy, necrosis of adrenal cortical cells is found together with haemorrhage into the gland and thrombosis of the adrenal veins [74]. Another haemorrhagic type of adrenal failure, the Waterhouse–Friderichsen syndrome, may occur as a result of generalized septicaemia. Adrenal failure may also develop in women who have received treatment with steroids in the past year or two for such conditions as asthma and rheumatoid arthritis. The reason is that the feedback mechanism for the release of ACTH has not yet fully recovered from steroid suppression and is unable to respond appropriately to stress.

The patient may present clinically with profound coma and laboratory tests may only reveal severe hypoglycaemia which only responds to treatment with corticosteroids [75].

Acute adrenal failure may occur following parturition in a patient with previously undiagnosed Addison's disease, possibly due to increased stress and the possibility that the mother had been provided with some cortisol from the fetal adrenal during pregnancy [75]. Treatment is with 100 mg intravenous hydrocortisone hemisuccinate immediately and an infusion of 5% dextrose in 0.9% saline. Intramuscular hydrocortisone hemisuccinate 100 mg is then given after a short interval and repeated 8 hourly, or more often if indicated.

Steroid therapy in pregnancy

In women who are already receiving steroids when they become pregnant it is advisable to try and avoid the use of very high doses during the first trimester because this may give rise to an increased risk of congenital abnormalities [76]. ACTH therapy is best avoided in pregnancy since it may lead to an increased secretion of androgens by the maternal adrenal. In a female fetus, some degree of virilization of the external genitalia could take place.

Cushing's disease

Cushing's disease is rare, occurring in only 1.8 per million of the population each year [74]. Since amenorrhoea and anovulation are usually present, Cushing's disease is rarely associated with pregnancy [77]. Just over half of the reported cases have been due to an adrenal adenoma or carcinoma, which form a minority in the non-pregnant state, pituitary dependent disease being the commonest cause; the reason for this is uncertain [77–80].

Cushing's disease has the clinical features of weight gain, hypertension, glycosuria and abdominal striae. All of these can also be found in pregnancy, but the presence of a rounded moon face, a buffalo hump on the shoulders, hirsuitism, acne and a proximal myopathy should suggest Cushing's disease.

The biochemical diagnosis may be difficult. Both in normal pregnancy and in Cushing's disease there is a rise in plasma cortisol [16,17,18], loss of diurnal variation of plasma cortisol [20,21], and an increase in urinary free cortisol [24], 17-ketogenic [18] steroids and 17-ketosteroids [43]. Even plasma ACTH levels may not be of great help. In patients with adrenal adenoma or carcinoma, the plasma ACTH concentrations should be very low, but a confusing factor could be the production of ACTH by the placenta [13,14]. For these reasons pregnant patients with suspected Cushing's disease are best referred to an endocrinologist, experienced in adrenal disorders, for investigation.

The fetal loss rate in untreated Cushing's disease is 26% and of the live births nearly half are premature [78]. Once the diagnosis has been made, localization studies can be carried out on the pituitary by magnetic resonance imaging (MRI) and on the adrenal by ultrasonography (US) or MRI.

If no tumour is shown on MRI scanning of the pituitary, the diagnosis may be made by the procedure of bilateral inferior petrosal sinus corticotrophin sampling before and after CRH stimulation; this can be performed safely during pregnancy [81].

If the pituitary gland investigations are normal and an adrenal tumour is suspected, adrenal computerized tomography (CT) may be justifiable if US or MRI has been unhelpful. Experience with treatment of Cushing's syndrome in pregnancy has been limited to 16 cases out of 67. Bilateral or unilateral adrenalectomy in 11 cases has been followed by birth at term in 7, premature birth in 3 and a still birth at 20 weeks [78–80,82].

Medical treatment with metyrapone has been used successfully in a few limited cases but there is a risk of hypertension [78,83], and a marked rise in deoxycorticosterone [61].

Congenital adrenal hyperplasia

Congenital adrenal hyperplasia occurs in 1 in 5000 to 1 in 10000 births, of which 90% are due to a deficiency of the enzyme 21-hydroxylase. Undiagnosed females presenting in adult life tend to be infertile and hirsute, but girls treated in childhood and adolescence have a fertility rate of 64% [64], although this is substantially less with the salt-losing form [84–86]. The major problem in those who go to term is that of cephalopelvic disproportion [84]. The patient's normal dose of steroid drugs should be continued throughout pregnancy.

Primary hyperaldosteronism

Primary hyperaldosteronism (Conn's syndrome) is rare during pregnancy [87–89]. It may present as hypertension or be accompanied by other symptoms of aldosterone excess, such as polyuria, polydipsia, tetany, muscle weakness and periodic paralysis [90]. Plasma aldosterone is higher than normally seen in pregnancy and renin is suppressed [87,91]. Conservative management with hypotensive drugs and potassium supplements may allow the patient to go to term, after which a definitive surgical procedure can be carried out [87].

The adrenal medulla

The adrenal medulla secretes the catecholamines adrenaline and noradrenaline. Secretion occurs in response to stimuli transmitted from the hypothalamus down the preganglionic sympathetic neurones to the adrenal medulla. The hypothalamus responds to various stimuli such as fear, cold and hypoglycaemia.

The catecholamines exert their action by stimulating two different types of receptor in the body which have been designated alpha and beta. α-Receptors are in the main excitatory, though, in the gut, stimulation of α-receptors causes inhibition. On the whole β-receptors are inhibitory. Noradrenaline is principally a stimulator of α-receptors, whereas adrenaline can stimulate both types of receptor.

The net effect of noradrenaline is to increase peripheral resistance in the circulation, leading to a rise in blood pressure. This causes a reflex bradycardia. Adrenaline stimulates sweating, pilo-erection, dilatation of the pupils, tachycardia and the breakdown of liver glycogen. It relaxes the smooth muscle of arterioles (particularly in muscle), bronchioles, intestines, bladder and uterus.

Medullary function in pregnancy

Plasma levels of adrenaline and noradrenaline are the same in pregnancy as in the non-pregnant state [92]. There is a rise in both hormones during labour. Adrenaline concentrations return to normal within 3–21 minutes of delivery, though noradrenaline remains high during this period and may even rise. The changes during delivery can be attributed to stress. Possibly the rise in noradrenaline following delivery is related to changes in plasma volume.

There is no evidence that catecholamines contribute to pregnancy-induced hypertension. Plasma adrenaline remains unchanged, while noradrenaline levels fall, but rise to normal following childbirth and the restoration of the blood pressure [93,94]. However, in pre-eclampsia, raised plasma free adrenaline has been correlated with the increase in blood pressure, suggesting that a rise in sympathetic tone may be an aetiological factor [95], although it is possible that the raised adrenaline levels could be related to stress of pre-eclampsia or the muscular activity associated with convulsions in eclampsia [95,96].

Phaeochromocytoma during pregnancy

This catecholamine secreting tumour is estimated to occur in 1 in 50000 term pregnancies, but is more often than not misdiagnosed in pregnancy as pre-eclampsia or essential hypertension [97]. Studies show a 58% maternal and 56%

fetal mortality rate in undiagnosed phaeochromocytoma in pregnancy. However, this has vastly reduced in the last 5 years to about 17% and 15% respectively [98,99]. The following constellation of symptoms should always raise the question of phaeochromocytoma: paroxysmal or sustained hypertension, paroxysmal or postural hypotension, sweating, palpitations and tachycardia, anxiety, nausea and vomiting. Suspicion should be stronger if there is a family history of phaeochromocytoma, hyperparathyroidism, neurofibromatosis or medullary carcinoma of the thyroid. The diagnosis is best made by measurement of resting, supine plasma adrenaline and noradrenaline; this is more reliable than urinary catecholamine metabolites and vanillylmandelic acid [100]. Since methyldopa may raise levels of urinary vanillylmandelic acid, patients should be investigated after being taken off medication for 1 week [100–101]. Another approach has been to measure catecholamines in platelets, since the half-life in platelets is much longer than that in plasma [102].

As soon as the diagnosis has been made, treatment should be carried out. After the α-adrenoreceptor blocking agent phenoxybenzamine has controlled the blood pressure, the β-adrenoreceptor blocking drug propranolol may be used to control the heart rate and any arrhythmias. However, since phenoxybenzamine has possible teratogenic effects, labetalol can be substituted during the first 16 weeks of gestation [103]. α-Adrenoreceptor blockade has been successful in reducing both maternal and fetal mortality by over 60% [104]. Prazosin has recently been suggested as an alternative to phenoxybenzamine [105], as it acts presynaptically to inhibit the release of noradrenaline and hence decreases the risk of associated tachycardia. Localization studies can be safely carried out by US or by MRI [106] which is preferred to CT, as it eliminates the risk of radiation exposure to the mother and fetus. Following localization, the tumour can be removed surgically. If the fetus is of a viable age, caesarean section should be performed at the same time [107], though medical treatment alone has been used successfully to control the phaeochromocytoma until such time as the fetus was mature enough for a section to be carried out [108–110]. Spontaneous labour and vaginal delivery should be avoided as they may lead to a sudden rise in catecholamines [101,107,108].

References

1 Temple T.E. & Liddle G.W. (1970) Inhibitors of adrenal steroid biosynthesis. *Annual Review of Pharmacology* **10**, 199.
2 Daughaday W.H. (1958) Binding of corticosteroids by plasma proteins. III. The binding of corticosteroid and related hormones by human plasma and plasma fractions as measured by equilibrium dialysis. *Journal of Clinical Investigation* **37**, 511.
3 Doe R.P., Fernandez R. & Seal U.S. (1964) Measurement of corticosteroid-binding globulin in man. *Journal of Clinical Endocrinology and Metabolism* **24**, 1029.
4 Burke C.W. (1973) *The Adrenal Cortex in Practical Medicine*, p. 16. Gray-Mills, London.
5 Anderson D.C. (1974) Sex-hormone-binding globulin. *Clinical Endocrinology* **3**, 69.
6 Burke C.W. & Anderson D.C. (1972) Sex-hormone-binding globulin is an oestrogen amplifier. *Nature* **240**, 38.
7 Brooks R.V. (1975) Androgens. In The Testis. Eds W.R. Butt & D.R. London. *Clinics in Endocrinology and Metabolism* **4**, 503.
8 Loraine J.A. & Bell E.T. (1976) *Hormone Assays and Their Clinical Application.* Churchill Livingstone, Edinburgh.
9 Dorn L.N. & Susannan E.J. (1993) Serum and saliva cortisol relations in adolescents during pregnancy and the early post partum period. *Biological Psychiatry* **34**, 226.
10 Kirschbaum C. & Hellhammer D.H. (1994) Salivary cortisol in psychoneuroendocrine research: recent developments and applications. *Psychoneuroendocrinology* **19**, 313.
11 Forsling M.L. & Grossman A. (1986) *Neuroendocrinology: A Clinical Text.* Croom Helm, London.
12 Beevers D.G., Brown J.J., Cuesta V., Davies D.L., Fraser R., Lebel M., Lever A.F., Morton I.I., Oelkers W., Robertson J.I.S., Schalekamp M.A. & Tree M. (1975) Inter-relationships between plasma angiotensin 11, arterial pressure, aldosterone and exchangeable sodium in normotensive and hypertensive man. *Journal of Steroid Biochemistry* **6**, 779.
13 Genazzani A.R., Fraioli F., Hurlimann I., Fioretti P. & Felber J.P. (1975) Immunoreactive ACTH and cortisol plasma levels during pregnancy. Detection and partial purification of corticotrophin-like placental hormone: the human chorionic corticotrophin (hCG). *Clinical Endocrinology* **4**, 1.
14 Rees, L.H., Burke C.W., Chard T., Evans S.W. & Letchworth A.T. (1975) Possible placental origin of ACTH in normal human pregnancy. *Nature* **254**, 620.
15 Carr B.R., Parker C.R., Madden J.D., MacDonald P.C. & Porter J.C. (1981) Maternal plasma adrenocorticotrophin and cortisol relationships throughout

human pregnancy. *American Journal of Obstetrics and Gynecology* **139**, 416.

16 Assali N.S., Garst J.B. & Voskian J. (1955) Blood levels of 17-hydroxycorticosteroids in normal and toxemic pregnancies. *Journal of Laboratory and Clinical Medicine* **46**, 385.

17 Gottfried I., Goldberg S. & Lewenthal H. (1965) Rapid screening test for adrenal cortical function. *Lancet* **i**, 607.

18 Goldberg S., Lewenthal H., Gottfried I. & Ben-Aderet N. (1966) Free 11-hydroxycorticosteroids in plasma in normal pregnancies and in cases of fetal death and missed abortion. *American Journal of Obstetrics and Gynecology* **95**, 892.

19 Bayliss R.I.S., Browne J.C.McC., Round B.P. & Steinbeck A.W. (1955) Plasma-17-hydroxycorticosteroids in pregnancy. *Lancet* **i**, 62.

20 Burke C.W. & Roulet F. (1970) Increased exposure of tissues to cortisol in late pregnancy. *British Medical Journal* **i**, 657.

21 Galvao-Teles A. & Burke C.W. (1973) Cortisol levels in toxaemic and normal pregnancy. *Lancet* **i**, 737.

22 Browne F.J. (1958) Aetiology of pre-eclamptic toxaemia and eclampsia: fact and theory. *Lancet* **i**, 115.

23 Sophian J. (1958) Actiology of pre-eclamptic toxaemia and eclampsia. *Lancet* **i**, 434.

24 Murphy B.E.P. (1968) Clinical evaluation of urinary cortisol determinations by competitive protein-binding radioassay. *Journal of Clinical Endocrinology and Metabolism* **28**, 343.

25 Waddel B.J. & Burton P.J. (1993) Release of bioactive ACTH by perfused human placenta at early and late gestation. *Journal of Endocrinology* **136**, 345.

26 Goland R.S., Jozak S. & Conwell I. (1994) Placental corticotrophin-releasing hormone and the hypercortisolism of pregnancy. *American Journal of Obstetrics and Gynecology* **171**, 1287.

27 Goland R.S., Conwell I.M., Warren W.B. & Wardlaw S.L. (1992) Placental corticotrophin releasing hormone and pituitary adrenal function during pregnancy. *Neuroendocrinology* **56**, 742.

28 Laatikainen T., Virtanen T., Kaaja R., Salminen K. & Lappalainen T. (1991) Corticotrophin-releasing hormone in maternal and cord plasma in preesclampsia. *European Journal of Obstetrics, Gynecology and Reproductive Biology* **39**, 19.

29 Ransanen I., Salminen K. & Lappalainen T. (1990) Response of plasma immunoreactive beta-endorphin and corticotrophin to isometric exerise in uncomplicated pregnancy and in pregnancy induced hypertension. *European Journal of Obstetrics, Gynecology and Reproductive Biology* **35**, 119.

30 Lowry P.J. (1993) Corticotrophin releasing factor and its binding protein in human plasma. *Ciba Foundation Symposium* **172**, 108.

31 Petralgia F., Potter E., Cameron V.A., Sutton S., Behan D.P., Woods R.J., Sawchenks P.E. *et al.* (1993) Corticotrophin releasing factor binding protein is produced by human placenta and intrauterine tissues. *Journal of Clinical Endocrinology and Metabolism* **77**, 919.

32 Layne D.S., Meyer C.J., Vaishwanar P.S. & Pincus G. (1962) The secretion and metabolism of cortisol and aldosterone in normal and steroid treated women.

Journal of Clinical Endocrinology and Metabolism **22**, 107.

33 Appleby J.I. & Norymberski J.K. (1957) The urinary excretion of 17-hydroxycorticosteroids in human pregnancy. *Journal of Endocrinology* **15**, 310.

34 Beck P., Eaton C.J., Young I.S. & Kupperman H.S. (1968) Metyrapone response in pregnancy. *American Journal of Obstetrics and Gynecology* **100**, 327.

35 Cope C.L. & Black E. (1959) The hydrocortisone production in late pregnancy. *Journal of Obstetrics and Gynaecology of the British Empire* **66**, 404.

36 Migeon C.J., Kenny F.M. & Taylor F.H. (1968) Cortisol production rate. VIII. Pregnancy. *Journal of Clinical Endocrinology and Metabolism* **28**, 661.

37 Christy N.P., Wallace E.Z., Gordon W.E.L. & Jailer I.W. (1959) On the rate of hydrocortisone clearance from plasma in pregnant women and in patients with Laennec's cirrhosis. *Journal of Clinical Investigation* **38**, 299.

38 Mizuno M., Labotsky J., Lloyd C.W., Kobayashi T. & Murasawa Y. (1968) Plasma androstenedione and testosterone during pregnancy and in the newborn. *Journal of Clinical Endocrinology and Metabolism* **28**, 1133.

39 Tyler J.P.P., Newton J.R. & Collins W.P. (1975) Variations in the concentration of testosterone in peripheral venous plasma from healthy women. *Acta Endocrinologica (Kobenhavn)* **80**, 542.

40 Rivarola M.A., Forest M.G. & Migeon C.J. (1968) Testosterone, androstenedione and dehydroepiandrosterone in plasma during pregnancy and at delivery: concentration and protein binding. *Journal of Clinical Endocrinology and Metabolism* **28**, 34.

41 Gandy H.M. (1977) Androgens. In *Endocrinology of Pregnancy*. Eds F. Fuchs & A. Klopper, p. 123. Harper and Row, Hagerstown, Md.

42 Ismail A.A.A., Harkness R.A. & Loraine J.A. (1967) Observations on urinary testosterone excretion during the menstrual cycle and in pregnancy. Abstract. *Acta Endocrinologica (Kobenhavn)* (Suppl. 119), 50.

43 Birke G., Gemzell C.A., Plantin L.O. & Robbe H. (1958) Plasma levels of 17-hydroxycorticosteroids and urinary excretion pattern of keto-steroids in normal pregnancy. *Acta Endocrinologica (Kobenhavn)* **27**, 389.

44 Hankin M.E. & Cox R.I. (1969) Peripheral plasma 11-deoxy-17-oxosteroids: alterations during pregnancy. *Australian and New Zealand Journal of Obstetrics and Gynaecology* **9**, 105.

45 Sekihara H., Sennett J.A., Liddle G.W., McKenna T.J. & Yarbo L.R. (1976) Plasma 16β-hydroxydehydroepiandrosterone in normal and pathological conditions in man. *Journal of Clinical Endocrinology and Metabolism* **43**, 1078.

46 Skinner S.L., Lumbers E.R. & Symonds E.M. (1969) Alterations by oral contraceptives of normal menstrual changes in plasma renin activity, concentration and substrate. *Clinical Science* **36**, 67.

47 Sims E.A.H. & Krantz K.E. (1958) Serial studies of renal function during pregnancy and the puerperium in normal women. *Journal of Clinical Investigation* **37**, 1764.

48 Dlisterdieck G. & McElwee G. (1971) Estimation of

394

angiotensin II concentration in human plasma by radioimmunoassay: some applications to physiological and clinical states. *European Journal of Clinical Investigation* **2**, 32.

49 Venning E.H. & Dyrenfurth I. (1956) Aldosterone excretion in pregnancy. *Journal of Clinical Endocrinology and Metabolism* **16**, 426.

50 Rinsler M.G. & Rigby B. (1957) Function of aldosterone in the metabolism of sodium and water in pregnancy. *British Medical Journal* **ii**, 966.

51 Weir R.J., Paintin D.B., Robertson I.I.S., Tree M., Fraser R. & Young J. (1970) Renin, angiotensin and aldosterone relationships in normal pregnancy. *Proceedings of the Royal Society of Medicine* **63**, 1101.

52 Weir R.J., Paintin D.B., Brown J.J., Fraser R., Lever A.F., Robertson J.I.S. & Young J. (1971) A serial study in pregnancy of the plasma concentration of renin, corticosteroids, electrolytes and proteins and of haematocrit and plasma volume. *Journal of Obstetrics and Gynaecology of the British Commonwealth* **78**, 590.

53 Smeaton T.C., Andersen G.J. & Fulton I.S. (1977) Study of aldosterone levels in plasma during pregnancy. *Journal of Clinical Endocrinology and Metabolism* **44**, 1.

54 Alhenc-Gelas F., Tache A. & Saint-Andre J.P. (1986) In *Advances in Nephrology*, vol. 15, p. 25. Eds J.P. Grunfeld, M.H. Maxwell, J.F. Bach, J. Crosnier & J.L. Funck-Brentano. Year Book Medical Publishers, Chicago.

55 Dal L.T. (1993) Relation between somatostatin, atrial natriuretic peptide beta-endorphin, aldosterone and pregnancy induced hypertension. *Chinese Journal of Obstetrics and Gynaecology* **303**, 718.

56 Tsai Y.L., Wu S.J., Chen Y.M. & Hsie H. (1993) Changes in renin activity, aldosterone level and electrolytes in pregnancy induced hypertension. *Journal of the Formosan Medical Association* **92**, 514.

57 Brown J.J., Davies D.L., Doak P.B., Lever A.F., Robertson J.I.S. & Trust P. (1965) Plasma-renin concentration in hypertensive disease of pregnancy. *Lancet* **ii**, 1219.

58 Brown J.J., Davies D.L., Doak P.B., Lever A.F., Robertson J.I.S. & Trust P. (1966) Plasma-renin concentration in the hypertensive disease of pregnancy. *Journal of Obstetrics and Gynaecology of the British Commonwealth* **73**, 410.

59 Wintour E.M., Coghlan J.P., Oddie C.J., Scoggins B.A. & Walters W.A.W. (1978) A sequential study of adrenocorticosteroid level in human pregnancy. *Clinical and Experimental Pharmacology and Physiology* **5**, 399.

60 Brown R.D., Strott C.A. & Liddle G.W. (1972) Plasma deoxycorticosterone in normal and abnormal human pregnancy. *Journal of Clinical Endocrinology and Metabolism* **35**, 736.

61 Nolten W.E., Lindheimer M.D., Oparil S. & Ehrlich E.N. (1978) Desoxycorticosterone in normal pregnancy. I. Sequential studies of the secretory patterns of desoxycorticosterone, aldosterone and cortisol. *American Journal of Obstetrics and Gynecology* **132**, 414.

62 Ehrlich E.N., Nolten W.E., Oparil S. & Lindheimer M.D. (1976) Mineralocorticoids in normal pregnancy. In *Hypertension in Pregnancy*. Eds M.D. Lindheimer, A.I. Katz & F.P. Zuspan, p. 189. John Wiley, New York.

63 Weir R.J., Fraser R., Morton J.J., Tree M. & Wilson A. (1973) Angiotensin, aldosterone and DOC in hypertensive disease of pregnancy. *Scottish Medical Journal* **18**, 64.

64 Weir R.J., Doig A., Fraser R., Morton J.J., Parboosingh J., Robertson J.I.S. & Wilson A. (1976) Studies of the renin-angiotensin-aldosterone system, cortisol, DOC and ADH in normal and hypertensive pregnancy. In *Hypertension in Pregnancy*. Eds M.D. Lindheimer, A.J. Katz & F.P. Zuspan, p. 251. John Wiley, New York.

65 Lindheimer M.D., Katz A.I., Nolten W.E., Oparil S. & Ehrlich E.N. (1977) Sodium and mineralocorticoids in normal and abnormal pregnancy. In *Advances in Nephrology*, vol. 7. Eds J. Hamburger, J. Crosnier, J.P. Grunfeld & M.H. Maxwell, p. 33. Year Book Medical Publishers, Chicago.

66 Fajardo M.C., Florido J. & Villaverde C. (1994) Plasma levels of beta-endorphin & ACTH during labor and immediate puerperium. *European Journal of Obstetrics, Gynaecology and Reproductive Biology* **55**, 10.

67 Solomons C.L., Bird C.E., Ling W., Iwamiya M. & Young P.C.M. (1967) Formation and metabolism of steroids in the fetus and placenta. *Recent Progess in Hormone Research* **23**, 297.

68 Donaldson A., Nicholini V., Symes E., Rodeck C. & Tannirandorn Y. (1991) Fetal adreno-cortical steroids and precursors. *Clincial Endocrinology* **35**, 447.

69 Beitens I.Z., Bayard F., Ances I.G., Kowarski A. & Migeon C. (1973) The metabolic clearance rate, blood production, interconversion, and transplacental passage of cortisol and cortisone in pregnancy near term. *Paediatric Research* **7**, 509.

70 Svec F. (1990) Antiglucocorticoid activity of dehydroepiandrosterone. *Clinical Research* **38**, 28.

71 Shearman R.P. (1957) Acute adrenocortical insufficiency in obstetrics and gynaecology. *Journal of Obstetrics and Gynaecology of the British Empire* **64**, 14.

72 Yarnell R.W., D'Atton M.E. & Steinbock V.S. (1994) Pregnancy complicated by pre-eclampsia and adrenal insufficiency. *Anesthesia and Analgesia* **78**, 176.

73 Guivarch-Leveque A., Vovan J.M., Le Bervet J.Y., Broux P.L. & Giraud J.R. (1993) Acute adrenal gland decompensation in the immediate post partum. *Journal of Gynecology, Obstetrics and Reproductive Biology (Paris)* **22**, 879.

74 Nabarro J. & Brook C. (1975) Diseases of the adrenal cortex. *Medicine* **8**, 351.

75 Drucker D., Shumak S. & Angel A. (1984) Schmidt's syndrome presenting with intrauterine growth retardation and post partum Addisonian crisis. *American Journal of Obstetrics and Gynecology* **149**, 229.

76 Popert A.J. (1962) Pregnancy and adrenocortical hormones: some aspects of their interaction in rheumatic diseases. *British Medical Journal* **i**, 967.

77 Kreines K. & DeVaux W.D. (1971) Neonatal adrenal insufficiency associated with maternal Cushing's syndrome. *Pediatrics* **47**, 516.

78 Gormley M.J.J., Hadden D.R., Kennedy T.L., Montgomery D.A.D., Murnaghan G.A. & Sheridan B.

(1982) Cushing's syndrome in pregnancy; treatment with metyrapone. *Clinical Endocrinology* **16**, 283.

79 Sheeler L.R. (1994) Cushing's syndrome and pregnancy. *Endocrinology and Metabolism Clinics of North America* **23**, 619.

80 Aron D.C., Schnall A.M., Sheelar L.R. (1990) Cushing's syndrome and pregnancy. *American Journal of Obstetrics and Gynecology* **162**, 244.

81 Pinnett M.G., Pan Y.Q., Oppenheim D., Pinnette S.G. & Blackstone J. (1994) Bilateral inferior petrosal sinus corticotropin sampling with corticotropin releasing hormone stimulation in a pregnant patient with Cushing's syndrome. *American Journal of Obstetrics and Gynecology* **171**, 563.

82 Kiplani A., Buckshee K. & Ammini A.C. (1993) Cushing's syndrome complicating pregnancy. *Australian and New Zealand Journal of Obstetrics and Gynecology* **33**, 428.

83 Close C.F., Mann M.C., Watts J.F. & Taylor K.G. (1993) ACTH independent Cushing's syndrome in pregnancy with spontaneous resolution after delivery; control of the hypercortisolism with metapyrone. *Clinical Endocrinology (Oxford)* **39**, 375.

84 Klingensmith G.J., Garcia S.C., Jones H.W., Migeon C.J. & Blizzard R.M. (1977) Glucocorticoid treatment of girls with congenital adrenal hyperplasia: effects on height, sexual maturation, and fertility. *Journal of Pediatrics* **90**, 996.

85 Mulaikal R.M., Migeon C.J., Rock J.A. (1987) Fertility rates in female patients with CAH due to 21-hydroxylase deficiency. *New England Journal of Medicine* **316**, 178.

86 Feldman S., Billaud L., Thalaard J.C. & Raux-Demay M.C. (1992) Fertility in women with late onset adrenal hyperplasia due to 21-hydroxylase deficiency. *Journal of Clinical Endocrinology and Metabolism* **74**, 635.

87 Hammond T.G., Buchanan J.D., Scoggins B.A., Thatcher R. & Whitworth J.A. (1982) Primary hyperaldosteronism in pregnancy. *Australian and New Zealand Journal of Medicine* **12**, 537.

88 Casper F., Seufert R., Riedmiller H. & Baver H. (1990) Primary adosteronism in pregnancy. *Gynaecological Research* **30**, 16.

89 Neerof M.G., Shlossman P.A., Poll D.S., Ludonirsky A. & Weiner S. (1991) Idiopathic aldosteronism in pregnancy. *Obstetrics and Gynecology* **78**, 489.

90 Crane M.G., Andes J.P., Harris J.J. & Slate W.G. (1964) Primary aldosteronism in pregnancy. *Obstetrics and Gynecology* **23**, 200.

91 Gordon R.D., Fishman L.M. & Liddle G.W. (1967) Plasma renin activity and aldosterone secretion in a pregnant woman with primary aldosteronism. *Journal of Clinical Endocrinology and Metabolism* **27**, 385.

92 Lederman R.P., McCann D.S. & Work B. (1977) Endogenous plasma epinephrins and norepinephrins in last-trimester pregnancy and labour. *American Journal of Obstetrics and Gynecology* **129**, 5.

93 Rubin P.C., Butters L., McCabe R. & Reid J.L. (1986) Plasma catecholamines in pregnancy induced hypertension. *Clinical Science* **71**, 111.

94 Tinkanen H., Roarus M. & Metsa-Ketela T. (1993) Catecholamine concentration in venous plasma and cerebrospinal fluid in normal and complicated pregnancy. *Gynecologic and Obstetrics Investigation* **35**, 7.

95 Øian P., Kjeldsen S.E., Eide I. & Norman N. (1985) Adrenaline and pre-eclampsia. *Acta Medica Scandinavica* (Suppl. **693**), 29.

96 Moodley J., McFadyen M.L., Dilray A. & Ranjiah S. (1991) Plasma noradrenaline and adrenaline levels in eclampsia. *South African Medical Journal* **80**, 191.

97 Harper M.A., Murnahan G.A., Kennedy L., Hadden D.R. & Atkinson A.B. (1989) Phaeochromocytoma in pregnancy. *British Journal of Obstetrics and Gynaecology* **96**, 594.

98 Hart J.J. (1990) Phaeochromocytoma. *American Family Physician* **42**, 163.

99 Potts J.M. & Larrimer J. (1994) Pheochromocytoma in a pregnant patient. *Journal of Family Practice* **38**, 290.

100 Bravo E.L., Tarazi R.C., Gifford R.W. & Stewart B.H. (1979) Circulating and urinary catecholamines in pheochromocytoma: diagnostic and pathophysiologic implications. *New England Journal of Medicine* **301**, 682.

101 Griffen J.B., Norman P., Douvas S., Martin I.N. & Morrison J.C. (1984) Pheochromocytoma in pregnancy: diagnosis and collaborative management. *Southern Medical Journal* **77**, 1325.

102 Plouin P.F., Chatellier G., Tougest M.A., Duclos J.M., Pagny J.Y., Comol P. & Menarch J. (1988) Recent developments in phaeochromocytoma diagnosis and imaging. *Advances in Nephrology* **17**, 275.

103 Oliver M.D., Brownjohn A.M. & Vinall P.S. (1990) Medical management of phaeochromocytoma in pregnancy. *Australian and New Zealand Journal of Obstetrics and Gynaecology* **30**, 263.

104 Stenstrom G. & Swolin K. (1985) Pheochromocytoma in pregnancy: experience of treatment with phenoxybenzamine in three patients. *Acta Obstetrica et Gynaecologica Scandinavica* **64**, 357.

105 Venuto R., Burstein P. & Schneider R. (1984) Pheochromocytoma: antepartum diagnosis and management with tumour resection in the puerium. *American Journal of Obstetrics and Gynecology* **150**, 431.

106 Greenberg M., Moawad A.H., Wieties B.M., Goldberg L.I., Kaplan E.I., Greenberg B. & Lindheimer M.D. (1986) Extraadrenal pheochromocytoma: detection during pregnancy using MR imaging. *Radiology* **161**, 475.

107 Pinaud M., Souron R., Le Neel J.C., Lopes P., Murat A. & L'Hoste F. (1985) Bilateral phaeochromocytoma in pregnancy: anaesthetic management of combined caesarian section and tumour removal. *European Journal of Anaesthiology* **2**, 395.

108 Schenker J.G. & Granat M. (1982) Phaeochromocytoma and pregnancy: an updated appraisal. *Australian and New Zealand Journal of Obstetrics & Gynecology* **22**, 1.

109 Griffith M.I., Felts J.H., James F.M., Meyers R.T., Shealy G.M. & Woodruff L.F. (1974) Successful control of pheochromocytoma in pregnancy. *Journal of the American Medical Association* **229**, 437.

110 Lyons C.W. & Colmorgen G.H.C. (1988) Medical management of phaeochromocytoma in pregnancy. *Obstetrics and Gynecology* **72**, 450.

The Ovary

DIANA HAMILTON-FAIRLEY
& M.R. JOHNSON

Introduction

The exact role of the ovary during pregnancy is difficult to define for so many of its steroid and peptide products are produced by the placenta. The most prominent of the steroids are oestrogen and progesterone while the peptides include activin and inhibin, relaxin and the binding protein follistatin. Relaxin is the only peptide whose origin remains principally ovarian throughout pregnancy and it is also the only one that does not seem to play an important role in folliculogenesis. Since our knowledge of the role that relaxin plays during pregnancy and parturition has increased considerably over the last few years, a significant part of this chapter is dedicated to this peptide.

The concept that there is no ovarian contribution to the coordinated endocrine events of pregnancy is difficult to accept but equally difficult to confirm since the design of suitable in-vivo human experiments is fraught with ethical problems. The placenta has its own hypothalamic–pituitary axis acting as an endocrine feedback system between the fetus and the mother. Whether this system has any effect on ovarian function or whether ovarian steroids play any part in the regulation of the fetomaternal hypothalamic–pituitary axis is not known. This chapter will, therefore, not dwell on this area but look further back at the functioning of the ovary in the development of the oocyte, at conception, on luteal function and the maintenance of early pregnancy. We will examine the role of the hypothalamic–pituitary axis on folliculogensis and pregnancy and the role of ovarian peptides in the maintenance of pregnancy and parturition.

The ovarian cycle

The role of follicle-stimulating hormone and luteinizing hormone

Ensuring the growth and maturation of the oocyte is the most important function of the ovary. A few days before the onset of menstrual bleeding, a decrease in the production of 17β-oestradiol (E2) and progesterone leads to a positive feedback on the hypothalamus and pituitary gland so that concentrations of gonadotrophin-releasing hormone (GnRH) from the hypothalamus and follicle-stimulating hormone (FSH) from the pituitary both rise (Fig. 15.1). They are released in a pulsatile fashion — each pulse occurring approximately every 90 minutes. A small increase in luteinizing hormone (LH) concentrations is also found. The role of LH is to increase the production of androstenedione and testosterone from the thecal cells — a monolayer of cells surrounding the antral follicles which contain the immature oocyte. FSH acts upon the enzyme aromatase within the inner monolayer of granulosa cells converting androstenedione and testosterone to E2 (the two-cell theory of steroidogenesis, Fig. 15.2 [1–4]). This is associated with the production of an E2-rich fluid (liquor folliculi) which

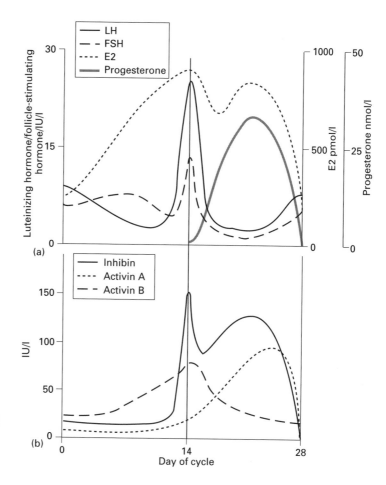

Fig. 15.1. Intra-ovarian regulation of principal metabolic pathways by endocrine, paracrine and autocrine factors.

causes the follicles to enlarge as cystic structures within the ovary.

The majority of the follicles which begin this growth process fail to enlarge beyond 8 mm in diameter and become atretic. The precise mechanism for the selection of a single dominant follicle is not well understood but there is evidence to suggest that the follicle that becomes dominant (at about 10–12 mm in diameter) develops LH receptors on the surface of the granulosa cells while the follicles that become atretic do not develop these receptors [5]. The increasing concentration of E2 has a positive feedback on FSH production and a negative feedback on LH concentrations until the E2 concentration reaches levels of 600–1200 pmol/l at a follicular diameter of 18–22 mm in diameter. This leads to a positive feedback on the pituitary and a several-fold increase in LH and FSH concentra-tions. The role of the rise in FSH concentrations in the process of ovulation is not well under-stood. In contrast, the role of LH has been shown to halt follicular growth, the granulosa cells become luteinized and start to produce proges-terone as well as E2 (Fig. 15.1). The oocyte undergoes the completion of the meiotic meta-phase I with an unequal division of the oocyte cytoplasm leading to the development of the first polar body. Meiosis is again frozen and will only be finally completed at the time of concep-tion with the extrusion of the second polar body. Thirty-six hours following the LH surge, the oocyte is released from the ovary into the peri-toneal cavity to be picked up by the fimbriae of the fallopian tube.

There is increasing evidence that LH plays an important role in oocyte maturation. Its pres-ence in excessive concentrations during the

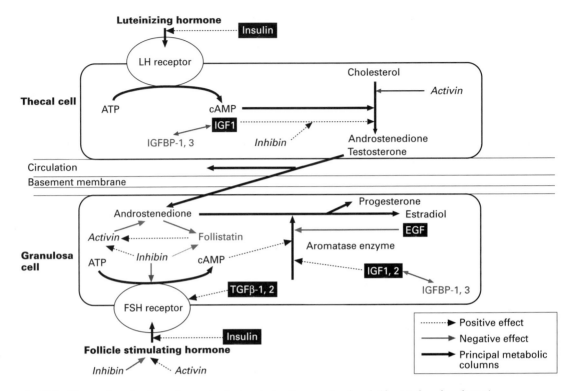

Fig. 15.2. Changes in endocrine and paracrine factors during the menstrual cycle (day 14, day of ovulation).

early to midfollicular phases of the menstrual cycle has been found to be associated with an increased risk of early pregnancy loss [6,7]. Since LH receptors seem to develop when the follicle reaches 10–12 mm in diameter, it has been suggested that the premature presence of LH may accelerate oocyte maturation to the detriment of oocyte quality. This has been borne out by the finding in in-vitro fertilization that oocyte quality and fertilization rates are adversely affected by the presence of endogenous LH levels prior to the follicles achieving a mature diameter of 18–20 mm. As a result, down-regulation of the pituitary using GnRH analogues has become routine practice in superovulation induction for in-vitro fertilization with improved fertilization and implantation rates.

The gonadotrophins undoubtedly play a vital role in follicular growth but it has been known now for many years that intrafollicular and intraovarian factors also play a vital part in the regulation of the ovarian cycle both in the maturation of the oocyte and the maintenance of the corpus luteum.

Paracrine factors in the control of ovarian function

Insulin-like growth factors 1 and 2 and their binding proteins

The insulin-like growth factors (IGFs) are a family of homologous, low molecular weight, single-chain polypeptide growth factors containing three intrachain disulphide bonds which promote cellular mitosis and differentiation in a number of systems. They are very similar to proinsulin in their structure and function with each having the ability to bind to the other's receptors although with varying degrees of specificity. In-situ hybridization histochemistry has shown that the granulosa cells of developing follicles are the principal site of IGF1 expression *in vivo* [8]. mRNA transcripts have been found in preantral and antral follicles but not in the corpus luteum or atretic follicles. Using solution hybridization ribonuclease protection assay, the granulosa cells from immature hypophysectomized rats were found to be the only site of IGF1 production while IGF2 was solely produced in the thecal-interstitial cells. In the human, however, IGF2 mRNA transcripts were found in granulosa-luteal cells and were regulated by trophic hormones in a similar fashion to the transcripts of the cholesterol side-chain cleavage P_{450} enzyme [9]. This suggests that IGF1 and IGF2 play different roles within the ovary and may act as co-ordinators of activity between the two cell layers according to the two-cell hypothesis of ovarian steroidogenesis (Fig. 15.2).

The IGFs are found bound to a family of insulin-like growth factor binding proteins (IGFBPs) in serum, amniotic fluid and media from several cultured cell types. Six IGFBPs, numbered 1–6, have been identified in humans, of which IGFBP-3 is the principal protein found in serum where it circulates as a 150 kDa complex. IGFBP-1 is the main binding protein found in amniotic fluid and has a molecular weight of 25 kDa. IGFBP-2 has been found in the rat and human central nervous system and neonatal serum with a molecular weight of 35 kDa. The other IGFBPs, 4, 5 and 6, have been found in several tissues, including media from culture breast carcinoma cells, fibroblasts and osteoblasts [10].

In-vitro experiments in the rat, pig and human have all shown that granulosa cells produce both IGF1, IGF2 and several of the IGFBPs in varying quantities [10]. Zhou and Bondy [11] have shown, however, that in the human IGF2 but not IGF1 is found in the mature human granulosa cells, particularly in antral and atretic follicles. IGF1 has been shown to enhance FSH stimulated granulosa cell E2 and progesterone production in addition to thecal testosterone production [12]. IGF2 seems to produce a similar effect only in the presence of insulin [13].

The actions of these growth factors may be modulated by the concentrations of the IGF-binding proteins and a distinctive intraovarian pattern of IGFBP2-5 mRNA has been isolated from follicular fluid in pigs [12] while mRNAs for IGFBP-2, -3, -4 and -5 are reported in rat ovary [14–18] and IGFBP-1, -2, -3 and -4 [19–21] in human luteinizing granulosa cells. IGFBP-1 has been localized to these cells and corpora lutea using immunohistochemistry where the synthesis of IGFBP-1 regulated by adenylate cyclase

and protein kinase C pathways occurs. FSH and IGF1 inhibit IGFBP-1 synthesis. Although IGFBP-1 was not detected in follicular fluid during the follicular phase, mRNA expression was found in the granulosa cells of dominant follicles. IGFBP-2 is also synthesized by luteinizing granulosa cells and inhibited by human chorionic gonadotrophin (hCG) and other cyclic AMP stimulators. IGFBP-3 mRNA expression has been described in thecal cells of all types of follicle but is also found in the granulosa cells of dominant follicles while IGFBP-2, 4, 5 gene expression was confined mostly to the granulosa cells of atretic follicles [22]. IGFBP-3 and -2 were found to inhibit DNA synthesis and FSH-stimulated steroid production by cultured rat preovulatory granulosa cells.

Follicular growth is associated with a decrease in intrafollicular IGFBP concentrations while an increase in IGFBP concentrations has been found in atretic folliculuses [12], implying that the IGFs are essential for follicular growth, maturation and ovulation. A recent study compared the granulosa cell production of IGF1 and IGF2 and IGFBPs from different sized follicles from women with normal ovaries and those with polycystic ovaries. The production of IGF1, IGF2 and the IGFBPs from the granulosa cells of antral follicles was similar in the two groups. In contrast, the granulosa cells from the larger follicles obtained from normal ovaries showed an increase in IGF2 and IGFBP-1 and -3 and a decrease in the levels of IGFBP-2. The granulosa cells from large follicles obtained from women with polycystic ovaries produced similar concentrations of IGF1 and IGF2 and IGFBP-1 and -3 to those found in antral follicles which may reflect the failure of these follicles to mature [13]. It is known that women with polycystic ovaries, particularly those who are obese or hyperinsulinaemic, are more likely to be anovulatory and suffer miscarriages [23–25]. It is, therefore, possible that an abnormality in the paracrine regulation of oocyte development may lead to the failure of follicular growth or the release of immature or prematurely matured oocytes and thus play a role in the pathogenesis of anovulation and early pregnancy loss. It is impossible to comment on the role of ovarian IGFs and their binding proteins during pregnancy because they are found in such large quantities in the decidua, placenta and amniotic fluid, but the ovarian contribution probably plays little or no part in the maintenance of pregnancy.

Interleukin-1, epidermal growth factor and the transforming growth factors

Interleukin-1 (IL-1) is a polypeptide cytokine which is predominantly produced by activated macrophages. Its precise role in intraovarian regulation is not well understood but evidence demonstrating intraovarian production and the presence of receptors and ligands within the ovary is now well documented [26]. IL-1 is not produced exclusively by macrophages and there is evidence in the mouse that the granulosa cell may be actively involved in the secretion of various IL-1 components, namely IL-1α and IL-1β [27]. The production of IL-1 has been shown to be hormone dependent and it seems to be able to enhance a wide variety of activities associated with ovulation, including an increase in prostaglandin, collagenase, nitric oxide, aerobic glycolysis and hyaluronic acid production with variable effects on steroidogenesis [26]; for example, both IL-1α and IL-1β amplified the production of 20α-dihydroprogesterone by luteal cells, with IL-1β having a greater effect than IL-1α. The activities of IL-1β are all essential components in the maturation of the oocyte and finally in ovulation [27,28]. This has led to the speculation that IL-1β may play a central role in the intraovarian regulation of these events and the finding of an increase in IL-1 midcycle supports this concept [29]. The role of other members of the interleukin family is unknown, although IL-6 has been shown to be produced by rat granulosa cells and may play a role in their differentiation and growth [30].

Epidermal growth factor (EGF) is a single chain of 53 amino acids with three internal intrasulphide bonds. In-situ hybridization has shown that EGF is produced by most tissues, including granulosa cells [31]. EGF has been shown to inhibit FSH-stimulated E2 production by human granulosa cells in vitro [32] and their proliferation and differentiation. In sheep, it has been shown to inhibit inhibin secretion in addition to E2 and to enhance progesterone secretion

[33]. Its role in vivo has not been established but it would be logical for there to be an intraovarian inhibitor during the follicular phase in order to help in the selection of the dominant follicle.

The transforming growth factors TGFα and TGFβ1 have been detected in thecal interstitial cells. TGFα, a 50 amino acid polypeptide, is not only structurally similar to EGF but also binds to the same receptor with a similar potency. It has been localized to the thecal cell layer [33] and found to suppress granulosa cell differentiation, leading to the possibility that it acts as another paracrine factor in the relationship between the thecal and granulosa cell layers. TGFα has been found to play a role in the paracrine regulation of cell differentiation in many different cell types, e.g. the development of fetal ovaries [34] and in surface and epithelial ovarian carcinoma [35].

TGFβ, a homodimer related to inhibin which has two identical 112-amino acid chains, has been localized by histochemical techniques to rat granulosa, thecal and luteal cells [36,37]. In contrast to EGF, TGFβ1 and TGFβ2 seem to act as counter-regulators by increasing FSH receptor messenger RNA concentrations [38,39], thus acting as regulators of granulosa cell proliferation and differentiation. The ways in which all these factors interrelate in oocyte development is not yet fully understood but they are all important pieces in the fine tuning of perfect oocyte development.

The role of inhibin, activin and follistatin

Inhibin and activin are dimeric proteins. Inhibin is a heterodimer, with an α- and a β-subunit, while activin is a homodimer of the β-subunit. There is a single form of the α-subunit, but two forms of the β-subunit which are designated A and B. Thus, inhibin may be either inhibin A or inhibin B, and activin may be activin-A, activin-B or activin-AB, depending on the type of the β subunit (Fig. 15.3). Both activin and inhibin are a part of a structurally related family which includes TGFβ and Müllerian duct inhibitory factor (MIF). The actions of inhibin appear to be limited to the reproductive axis, while those of activin affect not only other endocrine systems, but also cell growth and differentiation. Only the reproductive effects of each hormone will be considered.

Inhibin

Circulating inhibin is derived from the ovary during the menstrual cycle and probably for the early part of pregnancy [40–42], thereafter the placenta is likely to become the predominant source [43]. Inhibin circulates bound to α-2 macroglobulin, which does not inhibit bio-

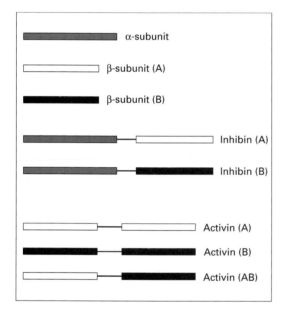

Fig. 15.3. Activin and inhibin subunits and molecules.

activity, but which may interfere with measurement [44]. Follistatin, the predominant inhibin-binding protein in follicular fluid, appears not to bind inhibin significantly in the circulation, and its effect on inhibin bioactivity is uncertain [44]. During the early and middle follicular phase, the serum levels of inhibin remain unchanged, but rise in the late follicular phase to a peak which coincides with the midcycle gonadotrophin surge; thereafter, following an initial decline, they rise, only to decline again prior to the onset of menstruation [45–47] (Fig. 15.4). If pregnancy occurs, inhibin levels rise until the 8th week of pregnancy, then decline until the 16th week and remain unchanged until the beginning of the third trimester, when they rise again to a peak at around 36 weeks [43,45]. Inhibin levels decline with age, possibly because of a reduction in the number of oocytes available; this reduction is inverse to the rise in FSH found during the premenopausal period.

During the menstrual cycle, inhibin mRNA synthesis may be assessed with oligonucleotide probes directed to the α-subunit and the β-subunits, and the site of peptide synthesis by immunohistochemistry with specific antibodies. In the human, such studies suggest that inhibin is synthesized in the granulosa cells of the small antral follicles and the corpus luteum (Table 15.1) [41]. Secretion by the developing follicle appears to be regulated by FSH [48] perhaps in a protein kinase A (PKA)-dependent manner [49]. During the luteal phase, inhibin is secreted

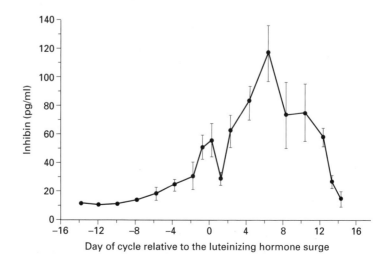

Fig. 15.4. The circulating levels of inhibin (SD) dimer during the menstrual cycle. (Adapted from Muttukrushna *et al.* [47].)

Table 15.1. Factors increasing the synthesis of activin and inhibin in ovary. (No factors have been identified which reduce the ovarian synthesis of either peptide.)

Peptide	Site or cells	Factor
Inhibin (unspecified)	Antral follicle granulosa cells	FSH
	Corpus luteum	LH
Activin (unspecified)	Granulosa cells	FSH, LH, GnRH, follistatin, inhibin

Table 15.2. The action of activin and inhibin in the pituitary.

Peptide	Site or cells	Action
Inhibin-A	Pituitary cells *in vitro*	Increases β–B subunit synthesis
Inhibin (unspecified)	Pituitary	Reduces circulating levels of FSH
		Reduces pituitary expression of FSH-β subunit mRNA
		No effect on GnRH-stimulated FSH release
		Reduces GnRH receptor expression
Activin-A	Pituitary cells *in vitro*	Increases follistatin release
		Reduces β–B subunit synthesis
Activin (unspecified)	Gonadotrophs *in vitro*	Increased FSH synthesis and secretion and FSH-β mRNA expression
	Somatotrophs *in vitro*	Reduced GH synthesis and secretion
	Lactotrophs *in vitro*	Reduced prolactin synthesis and secretion
	Corticotrophs *in vitro*	Reduced ACTH synthesis and secretion
	Pituitary *in vivo*	Stabilizes FSH mRNA
		Promotes GnRH receptor expression
		Augments GnRH-stimulated LH release

ACTH: adrenocorticotrophic hormone; GH: growth hormone.

by the corpus luteum, and is LH dependent [50–52] (Table 15.2). The mechanisms regulating pituitary synthesis of inhibin and activin are not known.

Strong negative correlations have been demonstrated between the circulating levels of inhibin and FSH, supporting the hypothesis that inhibin has an endocrine role in the modulation of FSH secretion [52–54]. However, similar negative correlations exist between oestrogen and FSH during the menstrual cycle; moreover, it is probably oestrogen, and not inhibin, that is responsible for the suppressed levels of FSH during pregnancy and the puerperium prior to the resumption of the normal cycle [54].

Peripheral administration of inhibin reduced circulating levels of FSH in both rats and primates, and FSH-β mRNA levels in the rat pituitary [55]. However, inhibin does not affect GnRH-stimulated FSH release, nor does inhibin appear to alter either the basal or stimulated production of the LH-β subunit [56,57]. While not affecting GnRH stimulated FSH release directly, inhibin reduces the expression of the GnRH receptor [58]. In addition to its effects on circulating FSH levels, during oestrus in the rat, inhibin attenuates the progesterone surge, while in metoestrus, it has no effect on FSH, but increases E2 levels while reducing those of progesterone [59].

Contrast studies in which inhibin has been immunoneutralized have failed to show any increase in the circulating levels of FSH in either the follicular or the luteal phases of the Macaque monkey, suggesting that inhibin may have a limited endocrine role in the regulation of FSH in primates [60,61]. These studies, like the early assay, relied on antibodies directed against the α-subunit, and may have served only to bind free α-subunit and not to neutralize inhibin. However, if inhibin-immunoneutralizing antibodies are added to pituitary cell cultures, basal FSH secretion is increased. This suggests that the inhibin produced locally in the pituitary acts in a paracrine manner to inhibit FSH secretion [62]. In a further twist to the activin–inhibin interaction, the addition of inhibin-A to pituitary cultures not only inhibits FSH release, but also promotes the synthesis of the β-form of the B-subunit of activin and inhibin, i.e. increases activin-B synthesis (Table 15.2) [62].

The production of inhibin by the antral follicle granulosa cells suggests that it may have paracrine effects. These have been investigated, but virtually exclusively *in vitro*; thus, these studies only suggest possible in-vivo effects. Inhibin has no effect on IGF1 induced testosterone secretion by human thecal cells obtained from antral follicles, but the addition of LH to the IGF1 pretreated cells results in an increase in androstenedione, dihydroepiadrostenedione, testosterone and progesterone secretion, which, with the exception of progesterone synthesis, is then enhanced by the addition of inhibin [63,64]. Overall, such data suggest that granulosa cell-derived inhibin may act on the adjacent thecal cell layer to promote the supply of androgens to be aromatized to oestrogens, but inhibin has little if any effect on progesterone synthesis in the human. Inhibin has been reported to reduce FSH-stimulated production of oestrogen by granulosa cells [65] (Table 15.3).

The free α-subunit may have actions in its own right, as it has been shown to bind to FSH and GnRH receptors [66,67]. However, the functional significance of the free α-subunit remains at present uncertain.

Activin

Activin is a homodimer of the β-subunit of inhibin with a molecular weight of 28 kDa. Given that there are two forms of the β-subunit, activin may exist as A-A, B-B or A-B (Fig. 15.3). Activin has a range of effects; these include the stimulation of FSH secretion, induction of erythrodifferentiation, and potentiation of gonadotrophin receptor expression on ovarian cells. Only those effects which relate to the female reproductive system will be considered.

Despite the fact that human follicular fluid contains all three types of the activin molecule, the evidence suggests that during the menstrual cycle either none of them are present in the peripheral circulation [68], or that the levels remain unchanged [46]. Like inhibin, circulating activin is bound predominantly to α-2 macroglobulin and, to a lesser extent, follistatin; the reverse is true in follicular fluid [43]. While follistatin inhibits activin bioactivity, α-2 macroglobulin does not [44].

In primates, activin synthesis has been identified in the preovulatory follicle of the Macaque ovary. In-situ hybridization identified moderate amounts of the α-subunit and of both forms of the β-subunit mRNA, while in the corpus luteum only a small amount of both forms of the β-subunit were found [41]. In preantral follicles and prior to ovulation, there are high levels of the B-form of the β-subunit. Pos-

Table 15.3. The action of activin and inhibin in the human ovary.

Peptide	Site or cells	Action
Inhibin (unspecified)	Human thecal cells, pretreated with IGF1 and stimulated with LH	Increases synthesis of androstenedione, dihydroepiandrostenedione, testosterone
	Human granulosa cells, stimulated by FSH	Reduced FSH-stimulated oestradiol release
Activin-A	Granulosa cells	Reduces basal and hCG-stimulated synthesis of P450-scc and P450-c17
Activin (unspecified)	Oocyte	Stimulates resumption of meiosis
	Thecal cells	Inhibits androgen production
	Granulosa cells	Inhibits progesterone production
	Luteal cells	Inhibits hCG-induced progesterone production, inhibits basal and FSH-induced aromatase production

tovulation, high levels of the α-subunit and of the A-form of the β-subunit mRNA were detected [41]. In the human ovary, the granulosa cells may make activin at all stages of development, but also synthesize follistatin which may modulate the effects of activin. The thecal cells appear to synthesize activin only in the dominant follicle [41]. Human granulosa cells cultured *in vitro* from freshly removed ovaries express α- and β-A and, to a lesser extent, β-B. These data suggest that in early pregnancy the corpus luteum produces inhibin-A and activin-A [69]. The primate and human pituitary may also synthesize activin [70,71], although its function within the pituitary is not known.

Ovarian synthesis of activin in the rat and human appears to be controlled by FSH, LH and GnRH, the first two via cyclic adenosine morophosphate (cAMP) and the last via protein kinase C (PKC) (Table 15.2) [49,71]. In addition, activin synthesis is enhanced by follistatin and inhibin (Table 15.2) [62].

In the pituitary, activin, like inhibin, is co-secreted with the gonadotrophins [72], and acts on the gonadotrophs to enhance FSH synthesis and secretion. However, it also inhibits the synthesis and secretion of growth hormone (GH) by the somatotrophs, adrenocorticotrophic hormone (ACTH) by the corticotrophs, and prolactin by the lactotrophs (Table 15.2) [56,62,73,74]. Indeed, the pituitary contains three activin receptor types—I, II and IIB—which have been localized to cell lines representing all of the above cell types with the exception of the lactotrophs [62]. Little evidence exists as to regulation of their expression, but the expression of the type II receptor mRNA is regulated by a non-steroidal factor which is not inhibin and which acts independently of GnRH [75].

Although activin is present in human follicular fluid, it is probably inhibited by follistatin [76]. The addition of activin to granulosa cells inhibited progesterone production in a cAMP-dependent mechanism [77]. This effect was inhibited by follistatin, but not α_2-macroglobulin [78]. In cultured human thecal cells activin inhibited androgen production [63] and in dispersed luteal cells both basal and hCG-induced progesterone production was inhibited [79,80]. Mitogenesis in luteinizing granulosa cells was

promoted [80] but basal and FSH-stimulated aromatase activity was inhibited [79]. Activin-A reduced the basal and hCG-stimulated increase in the mRNA levels of two key enzymes in steroid hormone synthesis, cholesterol side chain cleavage (P450 scc) and 17α-hydroxylase (P450c17) (Table 15.3) [72].

In amphibians, it has been shown that activin may play a role in embryogenesis, and in gene knockout studies it seems that maternal activin is essential for normal embryonic development [82]. The effects of activin on the developing embryo are probably modulated by follistatin as its mRNA has been shown to be expressed in the developing embryo [83].

Follistatin

Follistatin was originally described in 1987 [41], because of its ability to inhibit FSH secretion [84,85]. It occurs in several forms with a molecular weight of between 31 and 39 kDa. It is a single chain peptide synthesized in the ovary, placenta, fetal membranes, decidua and pituitary [41,86,87]. It binds both activin and inhibin through their common β-subunit, but two molecules of follistatin are required to inhibit activin's bioactivity completely [88]. It appears that follistatin has no inherent activity of its own, and its effects are limited to the inhibition of activin bioactivity [89]. It is uncertain whether it affects inhibin bioactivity.

It is synthesized in the rat and human ovary in an FSH-dependent manner [41]. It is synthesized in the somatotrophs of the rat pituitary [86], its synthesis and secretion is enhanced by activin, but reduced by inhibin and testosterone [87]. In the circulation it binds both activin and inhibin, but it is relatively less important as a carrier protein than α-2 macroglobulin [44].

The renin–angiotensin system

Over the last few years evidence has been presented of a renin–angiotensin system which is specific to the ovary [90]. The principal active peptide of this system is angiotensin II (A II), which is converted from the decapeptide angiotensin I, which in its turn is cleaved from angiotensinogen by renin—an aspartyl protease.

High levels of A II are found in preovulatory follicles and the whole activity of the system has been shown to vary during the cycle reaching a peak midcycle. The role of A II is not clear but it may be involved in oocyte maturation and possibly in ovulation itself. The pathogenesis of the rather bizarre ovarian hyperstimulation syndrome which can follow the development of multiple dominant follicles during assisted conception cycles remains obscure. The syndrome occurs early in the luteal phase and is prolonged by pregnancy. It includes the development of massive ovarian enlargement, ascites, hypercoagulability and haemoconcentration resulting in a profound metabolic disturbance and fluid imbalance which may have serious consequences for the patient including death. The renin–angiotensin system has been implicated in its development because of the well-known effects of the renal renin–angiotensin system on electrolyte and fluid homeostasis.

Other postulated functions of A II include a role in the formation of the corpus luteum, growth of new blood vessels, which is an important part of folliculogenesis, and the maintenance of the corpus luteum and the regulation of progesterone production by luteal cells. How this system fits into the paracrine control of ovarian function of pregnancy requires a great deal of further research.

Progesterone production

Following the midcycle LH surge and the release of the oocyte, the granulosa cells become luteinized and start to produce progesterone in addition to E2. The levels of progesterone continue to rise into the midluteal phase (Fig. 15.1). The function of the corpus luteum is known to be critical for the maintenance of early pregnancy since its removal before 6–7 weeks of pregnancy leads to miscarriage [91]. There has been a longstanding debate on the existence of a luteal phase defect (LPD) as a cause of subfertility and miscarriage. The prevalence of LPD in subfertility has been reported to vary between 3.5 and 20% and in recurrent miscarriage 23 and 60% [92]. The cause of LPD is multifactorial and its diagnosis is often difficult to establish. An endometrial biopsy showing 3 or more days' discrepancy from the expected finding for the day of the cycle seems to have become accepted as the diagnostic gold standard, although the day of the LH surge is not usually identified accurately [93]. Many clinicians, therefore, do not believe in this condition or do not believe that the prevalence is as high as some of the studies indicate, since the diagnostic criteria are not strictly defined. Another study has suggested that most women have one or two imperfect cycles each year but do not suffer from subfertility or miscarriage [R. Fleming and I. Coutts, personal communication], leading to the conclusion that LPD may be an underdiagnosed and overtreated reproductive endocrine disorder [92].

Clinical manifestations of LPD include a short luteal phase causing intermenstrual bleeding, premenstrual spotting and polymenorrhoea. It has therefore been proposed that luteal phase support with progesterone or hCG may improve the outcome of treatment for anovulation or recurrent pregnancy loss. A review paper which examined four papers on the effect of exogenous progesterone administration on the outcome of pregnancy has shown that only one of the four studies was randomized and demonstrated an improved pregnancy outcome, but this was a very small study (44 patients) which did not take into account the natural regression to the mean of pregnancy loss. The other studies were retrospective and two of them used several different treatment patterns and showed no difference for women treated with progestagens who conceived spontaneously. There is therefore insufficient evidence to support the use of progestagens for luteal phase support as a treatment for subfertility or recurrent pregnancy loss [94]. One study subdivided the women with recurrent miscarriage into those with a regular cycle and those with oligomenorrhoea and found that hCG support in early pregnancy led to an improved pregnancy outcome in those with oligomenorrhoea but did not affect the outcome in women with a regular cycle [95].

The demise of the corpus luteum appears to be controlled by both ovarian (oxytocin) and uterine factors ($PGF_{2\alpha}$) in sheep [96]. The uterus plays a dominant role in smaller mammals such as the guinea pig but in the sheep involution is secondary to an interaction between the two. In primates there is indirect evidence that a similar mechanism exists but the ovarian role appears to be dominant and the uterus has little function in this regard. In the sheep there is no reduction in the ovarian or uterine production and accumulation of $PGF_{2\alpha}$ nor in the number of receptors or binding capacity of $PGF_{2\alpha}$ in the corpus luteum. The other principal group of prostaglandins PGE_1 and PGE_2 seem to be blood-borne antiluteolysins that counteract the effects on the corpus luteum of $PGF_{2\alpha}$. The early embryo suppresses the response of the corpus luteum to $PGF_{2\alpha}$ by a number of mechanisms; the first is by the secretion of omega interferon which inhibits the production of $PGF_{2\alpha}$ by the uterus, the second by an increase in the production of PGE_1 and PGE_2, and this may protect the placental secretion of progesterone from $PGF_{2\alpha}$ and prevent the demise of the corpus luteum. Whether any of these mechanisms are relevant in the human is unknown.

The role of the ovary in pregnancy

Maintenance of corpus luteum function

Trophoblast-derived hCG rescues the corpus luteum, preventing the normal progression to atresia and maintaining corpus luteum synthesis of progesterone and E2. It is synthesized and secreted by the preimplantation embryo as early as 7 days postfertilization in vitro [97], and there is an abundance of hCG receptors on the corpus luteum at the appropriate time during the luteal phase [98]. Several studies during early pregnancy have failed to find any relationship between the circulating immunoreactive or bioactive levels of hCG and the levels of progesterone or E2 [99–101], suggesting that either they are not related or that the relationship is more complicated and involves either the rate of rise of hCG or its receptor occupancy. In-vitro experiments investigating the regulation of hCG production during the first trimester suggest that E2 [102] and insulin [103] may inhibit trophoblastic production of hCG while GnRH and interleukin-1 have been shown to stimulate hCG production [104].

However, following superovulation and in-vitro fertilization (IVF), circulating levels of both progesterone and E2 decline despite the presence of increasing levels of hCG, and there is no relationship between them [105]. This suggests that either another factor is involved in the modulation of steroid synthesis by the corpus luteum [101,106,107], or that the function of the corpus luteum is preprogrammed. Thus, the embryo may either synthesize a factor itself, or induce the synthesis of a factor in either the trophoblast or endometrium, which is superimposed upon, or supersedes the luteotrophic effect of hCG [99–101,106,107]. Indeed, that this putative modulator of corpus luteum function is derived from or regulated by the embryo is suggested by the presence of a direct relationship between the circulating levels of hCG and both progesterone and E2 in anembryonic pregnancies [108]. Thus, the embryo itself — either directly or indirectly — becomes the prime determinant of steroid synthesis by the corpus luteum. Evidence from a study of heterotopic pregnancy suggests that the developing embryo supersedes hCG and controls the corpus luteum function itself. The embryo may achieve this by regulating the synthesis of a factor produced by the endometrium in response to implantation [106]. This factor has been reported to reduce the expression of hCG receptors in the corpus luteum as has been reported previously [109], or it may antagonize hCG activity.

Thus, while it is established that in early pregnancy, hCG, synthesized by the developing trophoblast, acts on the corpus luteum, preventing atresia and maintaining steroid synthesis, it is possible that another factor supersedes this effect of hCG, or that the corpus luteum in terms of steroid synthesis is preprogrammed to decline.

The luteoplacental shift

Csapo and Pulkkinen, in a series of studies, demonstrated that the corpus luteum is redundant after 6–7 weeks' gestation [91]. However, corpus luteum dysfunction is thought to be one of the many causes of early pregnancy loss through reduced levels of progesterone. The luteoplacental shift is when the predominant source of circulating levels of oestrogen and progesterone shifts from being the corpus luteum to being the placenta. Its timing by the measurement of steroid levels alone is complicated by the ever-increasing placental contribution to the circulating pool. Even 17-hydroxyprogesterone, once held to be the product of the corpus luteum alone [110,111], has now been shown to be synthesized in considerable amounts and released by the developing placenta [112]. As implied above, placental steroid synthesis must be capable of supporting a pregnancy from between 6 and 7 weeks [91], but the exact time of the luteoplacental shift has been difficult to define, and probably varies between pregnancies. Certainly, the placenta seems to become the dominant source of E2 earlier than it does for progesterone in IVF pregnancies [113]. Moreover, the timing of the luteoplacental shift is likely to be of critical importance only when the life of the corpus luteum is reduced or placental development impaired.

Relaxin

Relaxin was discovered in 1926, and in 1930 it was identified as a water-soluble fraction of porcine ovaries which relaxed the guinea pig symphysis pubis. It has a molecular weight of 6000 kDa and is a member of the insulin-IGF-nerve growth factor family. It is formed of two chains, with two inter-chain and one intra-chain disulphide bond. Two relaxin genes exist in the human, both on chromosome 9 [114]. Controversy exists as to whether both genes or only human relaxin-2 is expressed. Like insulin, it is synthesized as a pre-pro-hormone, and is cleaved to the active moiety with the production of a C-peptide (Fig. 15.5). It is present in the peripheral circulation unbound in the last days of the menstrual cycle prior to the onset of menstruation, and throughout pregnancy.

During the menstrual cycle, relaxin is present in the peripheral circulation within 6–8 days of the LH surge and is undetectable by the onset of menstruation (Fig. 15.6) [113]. It is likely that peripheral relaxin is derived exclusively from the corpus luteum during the normal cycle, since higher concentrations of relaxin are found in the venous blood draining the ovary bearing the corpus luteum compared with no detectable levels of relaxin in either the contralateral ovarian vein or in the peripheral blood [115]. In addition, relaxin mRNA has been localized in the corpus luteum from the midluteal phase

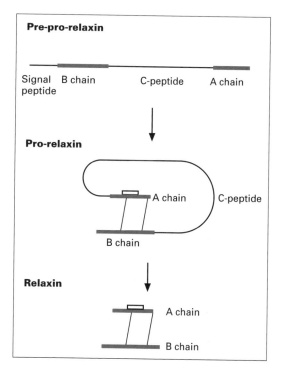

Fig. 15.5. The synthetic pathway of relaxin.

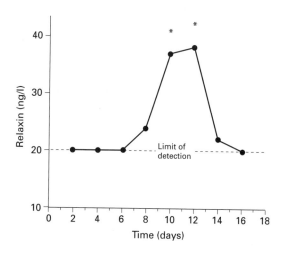

Fig. 15.6. The geometric means of the plasma levels of relaxin during the luteal phase of the menstrual cycle in 9 normal volunteers. The asterisk (*) indicates a significant elevation over baseline ($P < 0.05$). From Johnson *et al.* [113].

and pregnancy [116], coinciding with its detection in peripheral plasma [113]. With conception and implantation, plasma levels of relaxin rise rapidly and peak towards the end of the first trimester, thereafter they decline and remain

408

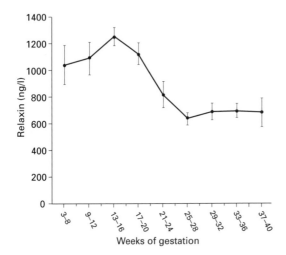

Fig. 15.7. The means of the plasma levels of relaxin (SEM) at 4-week intervals between 5 and 40 weeks of gestation.

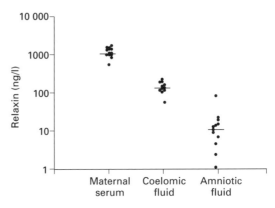

Fig. 15.8. The log concentration of relaxin in maternal serum, coelomic fluid and amniotic fluid in 15 normal pregnancies between 8 and 11 weeks' gestation. The horizontal bar represents the median value. From Johnson et al. [121].

unchanged for the remainder of pregnancy (Fig. 15.7) [117].

During pregnancy, the exclusive source of circulating relaxin is the corpus luteum, since although relaxin mRNA has been isolated from the placenta [118], placental relaxin does not appear to contribute to the circulating pool [119]. The distribution of relaxin between maternal and fetal compartments has been studied previously although in only a few subjects. This study suggested that at term relaxin is not present in cord blood, but may be present in amniotic fluid in low concentrations [120] (1 of 10 samples). In a larger study, relaxin was not detected in any samples of fetal plasma obtained between 19 weeks' gestation and term, but relaxin was detected in samples of amniotic fluid obtained from 10 weeks' gestation to term [121] and in samples of coelomic fluid obtained between 7 and 12 weeks' gestation (Fig. 15.8) [121]. Thus, relaxin may be available to the developing embryo and fetus from as early as 7 weeks' gestation, either by absorption from the coelomic fluid or by trandermal diffusion across the non-keratinized fetal skin. Indeed, as the fetal heart rate (FHR) is related to maternal levels of relaxin [122], it does appear that maternal relaxin is available to the developing conceptus, and may be able to influence fetal development.

Relaxin immunoreactivity has been localized

to the chorionic cytotrophoblast, syncytiotrophoblast, the cells of the placental base plate and decidua (M.R. Johnson, personal data, and [118]). The recent identification of relaxin mRNA in the syncytiotrophoblasts of the placenta has confirmed the site of relaxin synthesis. Relaxin mRNA was not detected prior to 19 weeks' gestation [123]; this precludes the placenta as a source of amniotic fluid relaxin and increases the likelihood that it is derived by simple diffusion from the maternal circulation. The association between the increase in relaxin mRNA expression and the onset of labour suggests that placental relaxin may be involved in this process, possibly acting locally to modulate the synthetic activity of the decidua and fetal membranes.

During the menstrual cycle, corpus luteum synthesis of relaxin is regulated either directly or indirectly by LH. hCG administered on alternate days from early in the luteal phase seems to have no effect on relaxin synthesis, but when the onset of administration is later in the luteal phase, relaxin synthesis is increased [124]. In addition, when hCG is used as a luteal phase support, circulating relaxin levels are increased in early pregnancy above those of the control group [125]. Furthermore, the addition of hCG to granulosa cells *in vitro* enhanced relaxin synthesis [126]. As these early studies suggested, the circulating levels of gonadotrophins during the luteal phase are shown to affect corpus luteum function during pregnancy [127,128]. Relaxin synthesis by the corpus luteum is, therefore, programmed within the first few weeks of pregnancy [128]. Thus, while in the pig corpus luteum function appears to be determined during the cycle of conception [129] and in the rat it is regulated by conceptus number [130], in the human corpus luteum function during pregnancy is determined both in the cycle of conception and during early pregnancy.

Factors other than hCG may modulate the circulating levels of relaxin during pregnancy, as suggested by the increase in serum levels of relaxin following the administration of PGE_1 for induction of a therapeutic abortion [131]. At term, the administration of $PGF_{2\alpha}$ or oxytocin for the induction of labour did not alter serum relaxin levels [132]. The relationship between relaxin and the prostaglandins has been examined using cultured discs of amniotic membranes *in vitro*. These were obtained either following prelabour elective caesarean section at term (CS group) or normal vaginal delivery (NVD group) were cultured *in vitro*. Following the addition of relaxin to the cultures, the production of PGE was reduced in the CS group and increased in the NVD group although the increase was only statistically significant in those in whom the onset of labour was associated with intact membranes [133]. Thus, before labour, relaxin inhibits the release of prostaglandins from the fetal membranes, and prostaglandins increase the circulating levels of relaxin. During labour, however, relaxin increases prostaglandin production from the fetal membranes and prostaglandins have no effect on relaxin levels. Any relationship between relaxin and oxytocin in the human is not yet clear, but in the rat, it is possible that relaxin enhances the oxytocin synthesis and/or release [134].

Little is known about the importance of relaxin during the menstrual cycle or early pregnancy. Work in primate suggests that it may promote the growth of the endometrium, myometrium and cervix [135]. In addition, in-vitro relaxin is able to enhance the endometrial production of pro-renin, aromatase, prolactin and IGFBP-1 [136–139]. However, there is no evidence to support an essential role for relaxin

during early pregnancy in the human, as ovum donation pregnancies may be established and maintained in its absence [119]. Relaxin does not appear to influence the outcome of these pregnancies adversely since birth weight, the incidence of miscarriage, preterm labour and pre-eclampsia are all similar to the normal population [140]. In a single case report, however, the second stage of labour was prolonged and delivery was with forceps [141].

Despite the fact that relaxin has been identified as one of the most potent inotrophic and chronotrophic agents in the isolated rat atrial preparation known to man [141], there is no evidence of any relationship between maternal heart rate and maternal plasma relaxin levels [122]. However, maternal relaxin levels proved to be related independently to FHR, as did hCG [122]. A strong relationship between β-hCG subunit levels and the FHR had been reported previously [143]. While hCG itself has no recognized effects on the heart, it is known to regulate relaxin synthesis; thus, the relationship between hCG and FHR may be indirect, mediated through maternal relaxin levels.

Recently, a negative relationship has been identified between the levels of plasma relaxin and uterine blood flow, suggesting that relaxin and E2 may act in opposition to regulate uterine blood flow [144]. Taken with the evidence that relaxin promotes endometrial growth [135], and stimulates the secretory function of the endometrium [136–138,144], it is possible that relaxin has a role in the regulation of placental development.

Relaxin levels have been reported to be elevated [143,144], similar [145] and reduced [146] during pregnancies which end in preterm labour. The most obvious mechanism by which an association between preterm labour and relaxin levels may exist is through the ability of relaxin to inhibit myometrial contractility. Thus, it would be expected that prior to the onset of preterm labour, relaxin levels would be reduced. However, since relaxin also promotes cervical ripening, and such an effect may be expected to induce labour, it might be argued that preterm labour is an effect of elevated levels of relaxin. In addition, relaxin is associated with lower uterine blood flow [143], which may impair placental development, which in turn is associated with preterm labour and reduced birth weight [147], again supporting the notion that elevated levels of relaxin during early pregnancy could be associated with preterm labour and low birth weight. Relaxin may have any number of conflicting effects in relation to the time of onset of labour; however, the mean levels of relaxin during labour at term were found to be higher in labours of spontaneous onset than in those of induced onset, again supporting the hypothesis that relaxin promotes the onset of labour (M.R. Johnson, personal data). No associations have been reported between antenatal levels of relaxin and any other complications of pregnancy.

During labour, low relaxin levels were associated with reduced rates of cervical dilatation in multiparous women and in labours of induced onset, and with lower average uterine activity integrals in nulliparous women and in labours of spontaneous onset (M.R. Johnson, personal data). These data suggest that endogenous relaxin is active *in vivo*, despite conflicting reports from in-vivo and in-vitro studies [148–151], and that during labour in the human endogenous relaxin acts to inhibit myometrial contractility and reduce cervical resistance. Thus, relaxin acts in the same manner in the human, rat and pig, promoting cervical compliance and inhibiting myometrial contractility. These actions implicate relaxin in the regulation of the rate of progress of labour and ultimately in determining its outcome.

In summary, the role of relaxin during the menstrual cycle and pregnancy is unclear. However, relationships have been demonstrated between maternal relaxin levels and FHR, uterine blood flow, the onset of labour and the progression of labour. These suggest that endogenous relaxin may affect fetal and placental development, as well as promoting the onset of labour. During labour itself, relaxin appears to modulate cervical resistance and myometrial contractility.

The uteroplacental circulation

Following conception, the immediate outcome of pregnancy is determined by the processes of implantation and subsequently by the development of the placenta. Given a viable embryo, the outcome of these processes is probably determined by the endometrium. The factors involved in the regulation of the endometrial response to implantation are uncertain, but recently uterine blood flow has been suggested to affect the chances of implantation following embryo transfer [152], and this is probably mediated through an effect on endometrial receptivity.

In the human, pregnancy-induced changes in the uterine circulation have been related closely to trophoblast infiltration of the placental bed and the concomitant erosion of the spiral arteries. However, in some animals such as horses, pigs and all ruminants, placental bed infiltration and erosion of the spiral arteries does not occur, yet the conceptus is adequately supplied with maternal blood [153]. This suggests that the process of trophoblast invasion is not strictly necessary for the development of the placenta. Furthermore, evidence from ectopic pregnancies and miscarriages suggests that trophoblast invasion of the placental bed is not necessary for the occurrence of the changes in the uterine circulation of early pregnancy [154–156]. Thus, other factors, probably derived from the maternal circulation, are likely to be responsible for the pregnancy-induced changes in the uterine circulation. Indeed, an inverse relationship has been reported between E2 levels and the resistance index and pulsatility index of the uterine artery [157]. Such an effect is consistent with the suggested effects of oestrogens on the general vasculature. More recent data suggest that relaxin is also an important factor in the determination of the uterine artery resistance index and pulsatility index, such that higher levels of relaxin have been associated with an increase in these indices [141]. Thus, in early pregnancy, parameters of uterine blood flow are associated with the circulating levels of maternal hormones. These data support the assertion that the changes in uterine blood flow which occur in early pregnancy may be determined by alterations in maternal endocrinology and are not secondary to trophoblast invasion of the decidua. Clearly, in midpregnancy, the importance of trophoblast invasion is critical to the maintenance of adequate uteroplacental perfusion. The factors which regulate this have yet to be defined.

Summary

The role of the ovary in pregnancy is principally one of ensuring good oocyte development, maturation and release followed by adequate progesterone and relaxin production by the corpus luteum. The regulation of these functions is controlled by the hypothalamic–pituitary axis and several intraovarian paracrine regulators which inter-relate in order to maximize perfect conditions for conception and implantation. Relaxin is the only peptide which is produced exclusively by the ovary during pregnancy and it seems to play a role in placental and embryonic development including the regulation of the FHR. Its functions continue throughout pregnancy, culminating in an apparently vital role in labour.

References

1 Hillier S.G., Reichert L.E. & van Hall E.V. (1981) Control of preovulatory follicular oestrogen biosynthesis in the human ovary. *Journal of Clinical Endocrinology and Metabolism* **49**, 851.

2 McNatty K.P., Makris A., Osathanondh R. & Ryan K. (1980) Thecal tissue from ovarian follicles in vitro. *Steroids* **36**, 53.

3 Tsang B.K., Armstrong D.T., & Whitfield J.F. (1980) Steroid biosynthesis by isolated human ovarian follicular cells in vitro. *Journal of Clinical Endocrinology and Metabolism* **51**, 1407.

4 McNatty K.P., Makris A., DeGrazia C., Osathanondh R. & Ryan K. (1980) Steroidogenesis by recombined follicular cells from the human ovary in vitro. *Journal of Clinical Endocrinology and Metabolism* **51**, 1286.

5 Yamoto M., Shima K. & Nakano R. (1992) Gonadotrophin receptors in human ovarian follicles and corpora lutea throughout the menstrual cycle. *Hormone Research* **37**(Suppl. 1), 5.

6 Regan L., Owen E. & Jacobs H.S. (1990) Hypersecretion of LH, infertility and spontaneous abortion. *Lancet* **ii**, 1141.

7 Watson H., Kiddy D.S., Hamilton-Fairley D., Scanlon M.J., Barnard C., Collins W.P., Bonney R.C. *et al.* (1993) Hypersecretion of luteinising hormone and ovarian steroids in women with recurrent early miscarriage. *Human Reproduction* **8**, 829.

8 Oliver J.E., Aitman T.J., Powell J.F., Wilson C.A. & Clayton R.N. (1989) Insulin-like growth factor-1 gene expression in rat ovary is confined to the granulosa cells of developing follicles. *Endocrinology* **127**, 3249.

9 Voutilainen R. & Miller W.L. (1987) Coordinate trophic hormone regulation of mRNAs for insulin like growth factor-II and the cholesterol side chain cleavage P450 ssc, in human steroidogenic tissues. *Proceedings of the National Academy of Science USA* **84**, 1590.

10 Giudice L.C. (1992) Insulin like growth factors and ovarian follicular development. *Endocrine Reviews* **13**, 641.

11 Zhou J. & Bondy C. (1993) Anatomy of the human ovarian insulin-like growth factor system. *Biology of Reproduction* **48**, 467.

12 Mason H.D., Margara R., Winston R.M.L., Seppälä M., Koistinen R. & Franks S. (1993) IGF-1 (Insulin like growth factor-1) inhibits production of IGF binding protein-1 while stimulating estradiol secretion in granulosa cells from normal and polycystic human ovaries. *Journal of Clinical Endocrinology and Metabolism* **76**, 1275.

13 Mason H.D., Willis D.S., Holly J.M. & Franks S. (1994) Insulin preincubation enhances insulin like growth factor-2 action on steroidogenesis in human granulosa cells. *Journal of Clinical Endocrinology and Metabolism* **78**, 1265.

14 Nakatani A., Shimasaki S., Erickson G.F. & Ling N. (1991) Tissue specific expression of four insulin like growth factor binding proteins (1,2,3,4) in the rat ovary. *Endocrinology* **129**, 1521.

15 Riciarelli E., Hernandez E.R., Hurwitz A., Schwander J. & Adashi E.Y. (1991) The ovarian expression of the anti-gonadotropic insulin like growth factor binding protein-2 is theca-interstitial cell selective: evidence for hormonal regulation. *Endocrinology* **129**, 2266.

16 Riciarelli E., Hernandez E.R., Tedeschi C., Botera L.F., Kokia E., Rohan R.M., Rosenfeld R.G. *et al.* (1992) Rat ovarian insulin like growth factor binding protein-3: a growth hormone-dependent theca-interstitial cell-derived antigonadotrophin. *Endocrinology* **130**, 3092.

17 Erickson G.F., Nakatani A., Ling N. & Shamasaki S. (1992) Cyclic changes in insulin like growth factor binding protein-4 (IGFBP-4) mRNA in the rat ovary. *Endocrinology* **130**, 625.

18 Erickson G.F., Nakatani A., Ling N. & Shamasaki S. (1992) Localisation of insulin like growth factor binding protein-5 (IGFBP-5) mRNA in rat ovaries during the estrous cycle. *Endocrinology* **130**, 1867.

19 Koistinen R., Suikkari A.-M., Tiitinen A., Kontula K. & Seppala M. (1990) Human granulosa cells contain insulin like growth factor binding protein (IGFBP-1) mRNA. *Clinical Endocrinology* **32**, 635.

20 Giudice L.C., Milki A.M., Milkowski D.A. & El Danasouri I. (1991) Human granulosa contain messenger ribonucleic acids encoding insulin like growth factor binding proteins (IGFBPs) and secrete IGFBPs in culture. *Fertility and Sterility* **56**, 475.

21 Giudice L.C., Dsupin B.A., Irwin J.C. & Eckert R.L. (1992) Identification of insulin like growth factor binding proteins in human oviduct. *Fertility and Sterility* **57**, 475.

22 El-Roeiy A., Roberts V.J., Shimassaki S., Ling N. & Yen S.S.C. (1992) Localisation, expression of insulin like growth factor binding proteins (IGFBPs) 1–6 in normal, polycystic (PCO) human ovaries. *Proceedings of the 48th Annual Meeting of the American Fertility Society* pS9 (Abstract 0-020).

23 Kiddy D.S., Sharp P.S., White D.M., Scanlon M.F., Mason H.D., Bray C.S., Polson D.W. *et al.* (1990) Differences in clinical and endocrine features between obese and non-obese subjects with polycystic ovary

412

syndrome: an analysis of 263 consecutive cases. *Clinical Endocrinology* **32**, 213.

24 Sharp P.S., Kiddy D.S., Reed M.J., Anyaoku V., Johnston D.G. & Franks S. (1991) Correlation of plasma insulin and insulin like growth factor-1 with indices of androgen transport and metabolism in women with polycystic ovary syndrome. *Clinical Endocrinology* **35**, 253.

25 Hamilton-Fairley D., Kiddy D., Watson H., Paterson C. & Franks S. (1992) Association of moderate obesity with a poor pregnancy outcome in women with polycystic ovary syndrome treated with low dose gonadotrophin. *British Journal of Obstetrics and Gynaecology* **99**, 128.

26 Hurwitz A., Loukides J., Ricciarelli E., Botero L., Katz E., McAllister J.M., Garcia J.E. *et al.* (1992) The human intraovarian interleukin-1 (IL-1) system: highly compartmentalised and hormonally dependent regulation of the genes encoding IL-1, its receptor, and its receptor antagonist. *Journal of Clinical Investigation* **89**, 1746.

27 Simon C., Frances A., Piquette G. & Polan M.L. (1994) Immunohistochemical localisation of the interleukin-1 system in the mouse ovary during follicular growth, ovulation and luteinisation. *Biology of Reproduction* **50**, 449.

28 Brannstrom M., Wang L. & Norman R.J. (1993) Ovulatory effect of interleukin-1β on the perfused rat ovary. *Endocrinology* **132**, 399.

29 Takehara Y., Dharmaraajan A.M., Kaufman G. & Wallach E.E. (1994) Effect of interleukin-1β on ovulation in the in-vitro perfused rabbit kidney. *Endocrinology* **134**, 1788.

30 Polan M.L., Loukides J.A. & Honig J. (1994) Interleukin-1 in human ovarian cells and in peripheral blood monocytes increases during the luteal phase: evidence for a midcycle surge in the human. *American Journal of Obstetrics and Gynecology* **170**, 1000.

31 Goroscope W.C. & Spangelo B.L. (1993) Interleukin 6 production by rat granulosa cells in vitro: effect of cytokines, follicle stimulating hormone and cyclic 3′,5′-adenosine monophosphate. *Biology of Reproduction* **50**, 38.

32 Mason H.D., Margara R., Winston R.M.L., Beard R.W., Reed M.J. & Franks S. (1990) Inhibition of oestradiol production by epidermal growth factor in human granulosa cells of normal and polycystic ovaries. *Clinical Endocrinology* **33**, 511.

33 Murray J.F., Downing J.A., Evans G., Findlay J.K. & Scaramuzzi R.J. (1993) Epidermal growth factor acts directly on the sheep ovary in vivo to inhibit 17-β oestradiol and inhibin secretion and enhance progesterone secretion. *Journal of Endocrinology* **137**, 253.

34 Osathanondh R. & Villa-Komaroff L. (1993) Expression of messenger ribonucleic acid for epidermal growth factor receptor and its ligands, epidermal growth factor and transforming growth factor-α, in human first- and second trimester fetal ovary and uterus. *American Journal of Obstetrics and Gynecology* **168**, 1569.

35 Jindal S.K., Snoey D.M., Lobb D.K. & Dorrington J.H. (1994) Transforming growth factor localisation and role in surface epithelium of normal ovaries and in

ovarian carcinoma cells. *Gynaecological Oncology* **53**, 17.

36 Schmid P., Cox D., van der Putten H., McMaster G.K. & Bilbe G. (1994) Expression of THF-β and TGF-β type II receptor mRNA in mouse folliculogenesis: stored maternal TGF-β2 message in oocytes. *Biochemical and Biophysical Research Communication* **201**, 649.

37 Bendell J.J. & Dorrington J. (1988) Rat theca-interstitial cells secrete a tranforming growth factor-β-like factor that promotes growth and differentiation in rat granulosa cells. *Endocrinology* **123**, 941.

38 Flanders K.C., Thompson N.L. & Cissel D.S. (1989) Transforming growth factor-β1: histochemical localisation with antibodies to different epitopes. *Journal of Cell Biology* **108**, 653.

39 Dunkel L., Tilly J.L., Shikone T., Nishimori K. & Hsueh A.J.W. (1994) Follicle stimulating hormone receptor expression in the rat ovary: increases during prepubertal development and regulation by the opposing actions of transforming growth factor β and α. *Biology of Reproduction* **50**, 940.

40 Illingworth P.J., Reddi K., Smith K.B. & Baird D.T. (1991) The source of inhibin secretion during the human menstrual cycle. *Journal of Clinical Endocrinology and Metabolism* **73**, 667.

41 Roberts V.J., Barth S., el-Roeiy A. & Yen S.S. (1993) Expression of inhibin/activin subunits and follistatin messenger ribonucleic acids and proteins in ovarian follicles and the corpus luteum during the human menstrual cycle. *Journal of Clinical Endocrinology and Metabolism* **77**, 1402.

42 Fraser H.M., Lunn S.F., Cowen G.M. & Saunders P.T. (1993) Localisation of inhibin/activin subunit mRNAs during the luteal phase in the primate ovary. *Journal of Molecular Endocrinology* **10**, 245.

43 Muttukrishna S., George L., Fowler P.A., Groome N.P. & Knight P.G. (1995) Measurement of serum concentrations of inhibin-A (alpha-beta A dimer) during human pregnancy. *Clinical Endocrinology* **42**, 391.

44 Krummen L.A., Woodruff T.K., DeGuzman G., Cox E.T., Baly D., Mann E., Garg S. *et al.* (1993) Identification and characterisation of binding proteins for inhibin and activin in human serum and follicular fluids. *Endocrinology* **132**, 431.

45 Lambert-Messerlian G.M., Hall J.E., Sluss P.M., Taylor A.E., Martin K.A., Groome N.P., Crowley W.F. Jr *et al.* (1994) Relatively low levels of dimeric inhibin circulate in men and women with polycystic ovarian syndrome using a specific two-site enzyme-linked immunosorbent assay. *Journal of Clinical Endocrinology and Metabolism* **79**, 45.

46 Demura R., Suzuki T., Tajima S., Mitsuhashi S., Odagiri E., Demura H. & Ling N. (1993) Human plasma free activin and inhibin levels during the menstrual cycle. *Journal of Clinical Endocrinology and Metabolism* **76**, 1080.

47 Muttukrishna S., Fowler P.A., Groome N.P., Mitchell G.G., Robertson W.R. & Knight P.G. (1994) Serum concentrations of dimeric human inhibin during the spontaneous human menrual cycle and after treatment with exogenous gonadotrophins. *Human Reproduction* **9**, 1634.

48 Fraser H.M., Smith K.B., Reddi K. & Lunn S.F. (1990) Inhibin secretion after treatment with an LHRH agonist and subsequent ovarian hyperstimulation induced by FSH in the macaque (Macaca arctoides). *Journal of Reproduction and Fertility* **89**, 441.

49 Miyanaga K., Erickson G.F., DePaolo L.V., Ling V. & Shimasaki S. (1993) Differential control of activin, inhibin and follistatin proetins in cultured rat granulosa cells. *Biochemical and Biophysical Research Communications* **15**, 253.

50 Smith K.B. & Fraser H.M. (1991) Control of progesterone and inhibin secretion during the luteal phase in the macaque. *Journal of Endocrinology* **128**, 107.

51 McLachlan R.I., Cohen N.L., Vale W.W., Rivier J.E., Burger H.G., Bremner W.J. & Soules M.R. (1989) The importance of luteinising hormone in the control of inhibin and progesterone secretion by the human corpus luteum. *Journal of Clinical Endocrinology and Metabolism* **68**, 1078.

52 Roseff S.J., Bangah M.L., Kettel M., Vale W., Rivier J., Burger H.G. & Yen S.S.C. (1989) Dynamic changes in the circulating inhibin levels during the luteal–follicular transition of the human menstrual cycle. *Journal of Clinical Endocrinology and Metabolism* **69**, 1033.

53 Hall J.E., Schoenfeld D.A., Martin, K.A. & Crowley, W.F. Jr (1991) Hypothalamic gonadotrophin-releasing hormone secretion and follicle stimulating hormone dynamics during the luteal-follicular transition. *Journal of Clinical Endocrinology and Metabolism* **73**, 667.

54 Le Nestor E., Marraoui J., Lahlou N., Roger M., de Ziegler D. & Bouchard P. (1993) Role of estradiol in the rise in follicle stimulating hormone levels during the luteal–follicular transition. *Journal of Clinical Endocrinology and Metabolism* **77**, 439.

55 Burger H.G., Hee J.P., Mamers P., Bangah M., Zissimos M. & McCloud P.I. (1994) Serum inhibin during lactation: relation to the gonadotrophins and gonadal steroids. *Clinical Endocrinology* **41**, 771.

56 Carroll R.S., Kowash P.M., Lofgren J.A., Schwall R.H. & Chin W.W. (1991) In vivo regulation of FSH synthesis by inhibin and activin. *Endocrinology* **129**, 3299.

57 Weiss J., Crowley W.F. Jr, Halvorson L.M. & Jameson J.L. (1993) Perifusion of rat pituitary cells with gonadotropin-releasing hormone, activin and inhibin reveals distinct effects on gonadotropin gene expression and secretion. *Endocrinology* **132**, 2307.

58 Braden T.D. & Conn P.M. (1992) Activin A stimulates the synthesis of gonadotrophin-releasing hormone receptors. *Endocrinology* **130**, 2101.

59 Woodruff T.K., Krummen L., Lyon R.J., Stocks D.L. & Mather J.P. (1993) Recombinant human inhibin-A and recombinant human activin-A regulate pituitary and ovarian function in the adult female rat. *Endocrinology* **132**, 2332.

60 Fraser H.M., Smith K.B., Lunn S.F., Cowen G.M., Morris K. & McNeilly A.S. (1992) Immunoneutralisation and immunocytochemical localisation of inhibin alpha subunit during the mid-luteal phase in the stump tail macaque. *Journal of Endocrinology* **133**, 341.

61 Fraser H.M., Tsonis C.G., Lunn S.F. & Saunders P.T.

(1993) Paper presented to the annual meeting of the Society for the Study of Fertility, Cambridge.

62 Bilezikjian L.M., Corrigan A.Z. & Vale W.W. (1994) Activin-B, inhibin-B and follistatin as autocrine/paracrine factors of the rat anterior pituitary. In *Frontiers of Endocrinology 3. Inhibin and Inhibin Related Proteins.* Eds H.G. Burger, J.K. Findlay, D.M. Robertson, D.M. de Kretser & F. Petraglia, p. 81. Ares-Serono Symposia, Rome.

63 Hillier S.G., Yong E.L., Illingworth P.J., Baird L., Schwall R.H. & Mason A.J. (1991) Effect of recombinant activin on androgen synthesis in cultured human thecal cells. *Journal of Clinical Endocrinology and Metabolism* **72**, 1206.

64 Sugino H., Nakamura T., Hasegawa Y., Miyamoto K., Abe Y., Igarashi M., Eto Y. *et al.* (1988) Erythroid differentiation factor can modulate follicular granulosa cell functions. *Biochemical and Biophysical Research Communication* **153**, 281.

65 Hillier S.G., Yong E.L., Illingworth P.J., Baird D.T., Schwall R.H. & Mason A.J. (1991) Effect of recombinant inhibin on androgen synthesis in cultured human thecal cells. *Molecular and Cellular Endocrinology* **75**, R1.

66 Schneyer A., Sluss P., Whitcomb R., Martin K., Sprengel R. & Crowley W. (1991) Precursors of a-inhibin modulate follicle stimulating hormone receptor binding and biological activity. *Endocrinology* **129**, 1987.

67 Woodruff T.K., Krummen L., Baly D., Wong W.L., Garg S., Sadick M., Davis G. *et al.* (1994) Inhibin and activin measured in human serum. In *Frontiers of Endocrinology 3. Inhibin and Inhibin Related Proteins.* Eds H.G. Burger, J.K. Findlay, D.M. Robertson, D.M. de Kretser & F. Petraglia, p. 55. Ares-Serono Symposia, Rome.

68 Eramaa M., Heikinheimo K., Tuuri T., Hilden K. & Ritvos O. (1993) Inhibin and activin subunit mRNA expression in human granulosa-luteal cells. *Molecular and Cellular Endocrinology* **92**, R15.

69 Attardi B., Marshall G.R., Zorub D.S., Winters S.J., Miklos J. & Plant T.M. (1992) Effects of orchidectomy on gonadotropin and inhibin subunit messenger ribonucleic acid in the pituitary of the rhesus monkey (Macaca mulatta). *Endocrinology* **130**, 1238.

70 Alexander J.M., Swearingen B., Tindall G.T. & Klibanski A. (1995) Human pituitary adenomas express endogenous inhibin subunit and follistatin messenger ribonucleic acids. *Journal of Clinical Endocrinology and Metabolism* **80**, 147.

71 Rabinovici J., Spener S.J., Doldi N. & Jaffe R.B. (1994) Localisations and action of activin in the human ovary and adrenal gland. In *Frontiers of Endocrinology 3. Inhibin and Inhibin Related Proteins.* Eds H.G. Burger, J.K. Findlay, D.M. Robertson, D.M. de Kretser & F. Petraglia, p. 191. Ares-Serono Symposia, Rome.

72 Roberts V.J., Peto C.A., Vale W. & Sawchenko P.E. (1992) Inhibin/activin subunits are co-stored with LH and FSH in secretory granules in the rat anterior pituitary gland. *Neuroendocrinology* **56**, 214.

73 Li R., Phillips D.M. & Mather J.P. (1995) Activin promotes ovarian follicle development in vitro. *Endocrinology* **136**, 849.

414

74 Fraser H.M., Lunn S.F., Whielaw P.F. & Hillier S.G. (1995) Induced luteal regression: differential effects on follicular and luteal inhibin/activin subunit mRNAs in the marmoset monkey. *Journal of Endocrinology* **144**, 201.

75 Dalkin A.C., Gilrain J.T. & Marshall J.C. (1994) Ovarian regulation of pituitary inhibin subunit and activin receptor type II gene expression: evidence for a nonsteroidal inhibitory substance. *Endocrinology* **135**, 944.

76 Sadatsuki M., Tsutsumi O., Sakai R., Eto Y., Hayashi N. & Taketani Y. (1993) Presence and possible function of activin-like substance in human follicular fluid. *Human Reproduction* **8**, 1392.

77 Li W., Yuen B.H. & Leung P.C. (1992) Inhibition of progestin accumulation by activin-A in human granulosa cells. *Journal of Clinical Endocrinology and Metabolism* **75**, 285.

78 Cataldo N.A., Rabinovici J., Fujimoto V.Y. & Jaffe R.B. (1994) Follistatin antagonizes the effects of activin-A on steroidogenesis in human luteinizing granulosa cells. *Journal of Clinical Endocrinology and Metabolism* **79**, 272.

79 Rabinovici J., Spencer S.J., Doldi N., Goldsmith P.C., Schwall R. & Jaffe R.B. (1992) Activin-A as an intraovarian modulator: actions, localisation, and regulation of the intact dimer in human ovarian cells. *Journal of Clinical Investigation* **89**, 1528.

80 Di Simone N., Lanzone A., Petraglia F., Ronsisvalle E., Caruso A. & Mancuso S. (1994) Effect of activin-A on progesterone synthesis in human luteal cells. *Fertility and Sterility* **62**, 1157.

81 Fraser H.M., Lunn S.F., Cowen G.M. & Saunders P.T., Rabinovici J., Spencer S.J. & Jaffe R.B. (1990) Recombinant human activin-A promotes proliferation of human luteinised pre-ovulatory granulosa cells in vitro. *Journal of Clinical Endocrinology and Metabolism* **71**, 1396.

82 Vassalli A., Matzuk M.M., Gardner H.A., Lee K.F. & Jaenisch R. (1994) Activin/inhibin beta A subunit gene disruption leads to defects in eyelid development and female reproduction. *Genes and Development* **15**, 414.

83 Huylebroek D., Verschueren K. & De Waele P. (1994) Activins: multipotent regulators of cellular function, differentiation and development. In *Frontiers of Endocrinology 3. Inhibin and Inhibin Related Proteins.* Eds H.G. Burger, J.K. Findlay, D.M. Robertson, D.M. de Kretser & F. Petraglia, p. 271. Ares-Serono Symposia, Rome.

84 Xiao S., Farnworth P.G. & Findlay J.K. (1992) Interaction between activin and follicle stimulating hormone-suppressing protein/follistatin in the regulation of basal inhibin production by cultured rat granulosa cells. *Endocrinology* **131**, 2365.

85 Ueno N., Ling N., Ying S.-Y., Esch F., Shimasaki S. & Guillemin R. (1987) Isolation and partial purification of follistatin: a single chain Mr 35 000 monomeric protein that inhibits the release of follicle stimulating hormone. *Proceedings of the National Academy of Science USA* **84**, 8282.

86 De Kretser D.M., Foulds L.M., Hancock M. & Robertson D.M. (1994) Partial characterisation of inhibin, activin and follistatin in the term human placenta. *Journal of Clinical Endocrinology and Metabolism* **79**, 502.

87 Petraglia F., Gallinelli A., Grande A., Florio P., Amram A., Ferrari S., Genazzani A.R. *et al.* (1994) Local production and action of follistatin in human placenta. *Journal of Clinical Endocrinology and Metabolism* **78**, 205.

88 Sugino H., Sugino K. & Nakamura T. (1994) The activin-binding protein. In *Frontiers of Endocrinology 3. Inhibin and Inhibin Related Proteins.* Eds H.G. Burger, J.K. Findlay, D.M. Robertson, D.M. de Kretser & F. Petraglia, p. 69. Ares-Serono Symposia, Rome.

89 DePaolo L.V., Mercado M., Guo Y. & Ling N. (1993) Increased follistatin (activin-binding protein) gene expression in rat anterior pituitary tissue after ovariectomy may be mediated by pituitary activin. *Endocrinology* **132**, 2221.

90 Lightman A., Palumbo A., de Cherney A.H. & Naftolin F. (1989) The ovarian renin–angiotensin system. *Seminars in Reproductive Endocrinology* **7**, 79.

91 Csapo A.I. & Pulkkinen M. (1978) Indispensibility of the human corpus luteum in the maintenance of early pregnancy luteectomy evidence. *Obstetrical and Gynecological Survey* **33**, 69.

92 Soules M. (1987) Luteal phase defect: an underdiagnosed and overtreated reproductive endocrine disorder. *Clinics in North American Obstetrics and Gynaecology* **41**, 856.

93 McNeely M. & Soules M. (1988) The diagnosis of luteal phase defect: a critical review. *Fertility and Sterility* **50**, 1.

94 Karamadian L.M. & Grimes D.A. (1992) Luteal phase deficiency: effect of treatment on pregnancy rates. *American Journal of Obstetrics and Gynecology* **167**, 1391.

95 Quenby S. & Farquharson R.G. (1994) Human chorionic gonadotrophin supplementation in recurrent pregnancy loss: a controlled trial. *Fertility and Sterility* **62**, 708.

96 Weems C.W., Vincent D.L. & Weems Y.S. (1992) Role of prostaglandins (PG) F2alpha,E1,E2, adenosine, oestradiol 17 beta, histone-H2A and progesterone of conceptus, uterine and ovarian origin during early pregnancy in the ewe. *Reproduction, Fertility and Development* **4**, 289.

97 Dokras A., Sargent I.L., Ross C., Gardener R.L. & Barlow D.H. (1991) The human blastocyst: morphology and human chorionic gonadotrophin secretion in vitro. *Human Reproduction* **6**, 1143.

98 Rajaniemi J.J., Ronnberg L., Kauppila A., Ylostalo P., Jalkanen M., Saastamoinen J., Selander K. *et al.* (1981) Luteinizing hormone receptors in human ovarian follicles and corpora lutea during the menstrual cycle and pregnancy. *Journal of Clinical Endocrinology and Metabolism* **108**, 307.

99 Hubinont C.J., Thomas C. & Schwers J.F. (1987) Luteal function in ectopic pregancy. *American Journal of Obstetrics and Gynecology* **156**, 669.

100 Kratzer P.G. & Taylor R.N. (1990) Corpus luteum function in early pregnancies is primarily determined by the rate of change of human chorionic

gonadotropin levels. *American Journal of Obstetrics and Gynecology* **163**, 1497.

101 Norman R.J., Buck R.H., Kemp M.A. & Joubert S.M. (1988) Impaired corpus luteum function in ectopic pregnancy cannot be explained by altered human chorionic gonadotropin. *Journal of Clinical Endocrinology and Metabolism* **66**, 1166.

102 Sharma S.C., Purohit P. & Rao A.J. (1993) Role of oestradiol-17 beta in the regulation of synthesis and secretion of human chorionic gonadotrophin by first trimester human placenta. *Journal of Molecular Endocrinology* **11**, 91.

103 Barnea E.R., Neubrun D. & Shurtz-Swirski R. (1993) Effect of insulin on human chorionic gonadotrophin secretion by placental explants. *Human Reproduction* **8**, 858.

104 Steele G.L., Currie W.D., Leung E.H., Yuen B.H. & Leung P.C. (1992) Rapid stimulation of human chorionic gonadotropin secretion by interleukin-1 beta from perifused first trimester trophoblast. *Journal of Clinical Endocrinology and Metabolism* **75**, 783.

105 Johnson M.R., Riddle A.F., Grudzinskas J.G., Sharma V., Campbell S., Collins W.P., Lightman S.L. *et al.* (1993) Endocrinology of IVF pregnancies during the first trimester. *Human Reproduction* **8**, 316.

106 Johnson M.R., Bolton V.N., Riddle A.F., Sharma V., Nicolaides K.H., Grudzinskas J.G. & Collins W.P. (1993) Interactions between the embryo and corpus luteum. *Human Reproduction* **8**, 1496.

107 Lower A.M., Yovich J.L., Hancock C. & Grudzinskas J.G. (1993) Is luteal function maintained by factors other than chorionic gonadotrophin in early pregnancy? *Human Reproduction* **8**, 645.

108 Johnson M.R., Riddle A.F., Sharma V., Collins W.P., Nicolaides K.H. & Grudzinskas J.G. (1993) Placental and ovarian hormones in anembryonic pregnancy. *Human Reproduction* **8**, 112.

109 Khan-Dawood F.S. & Dawood M.Y., (1991) Human corpus luteum: chorionic gonadotropin receptors during ectopic pregnancy. *Fertility and Sterility* **57**(Suppl. q-183).

110 Tulchinsky D. & Hobel C.J. (1974) Plasma human chorionic gonadotropin, estrone, estradiol, estriol, progesterone and 17a-hydroxyprogesterone in human pregnancy. *American Journal of Obstetrics and Gynecology* **117**, 884.

111 Yoshimi T., Strott C.A., Marshall J.R. & Lipsett M.B. (1969) Corpus luteum function in early pregnancy. *Journal of Clinical Endocrinology and Metabolism* **29**, 225.

112 Nowroozi K., Check J.H., O'Shaughnessy A. & Shapse D. (1991) Measurement of 17-hydroxyprogesterone levels during the first trimester of donor oocyte pregnancies. *Human Reproduction* (Abstracts of the 7th Annual Meeting of ESHRE), P27.

113 Johnson M.R., Carter G., Grint C. & Lightman S.L. (1993) Relaxin in the menstrual cycle. *Acta Endocrinologica* **129**, 121.

114 Crawford R.J., Hudson P., Shine J., Niall H.D., Eddy R.L. & Shows T.B. (1984) Two human relaxin genes are on chromosome 9. *EMBO Journal* **3**, 2341.

115 Khan-Dawood F.S., Goldsmith L.T., Weiss G. & Dawood M.Y. (1989) Human corpus luteum secretion

of relaxin, oxytocin, and progesterone. *Journal of Clinical Endocrinology and Metabolism* **68**, 627.

116 Ivell R., Hunt N., Khan-Dawood F. & Dawood M.Y. (1989) Expression of the human relaxin gene in the corpus luteum of the menstrual cycle and in the prostate. *Molecular and Cellular Endocrinology* **66**, 251.

117 Bell R.J., Eddie L.W., Lester A.R., Wood E.C., Johnston P.D. & Niall H.D. (1987) Relaxin in human pregnancy serum measured with an homologous radioimmunoassay. *Obstetrics and Gynecology* **69**, 585.

118 Sakbun V., Koay E.S. & Bryant-Greenwood G.D. (1987) Immunocytochemical localization of prolactin and relaxin c-peptide in human decidua and placenta. *Journal of Clinical Endocrinology and Metabolism* **65**, 339.

119 Johnson M.R., Abdalla H., Allman A.C.J., Wren M.E., Kirkland A. & Lightman S.L. (1991) Relaxin levels in ovum donation pregnancies. *Fertility and Sterility* **56**, 59.

120 Weiss G., O'Byrne E.M., Hochman J., Steinetz B.G., Goldsmith L. & Flitcraft J.G. (1978) Distribution of relaxin in women during pregnancy. *Obstetrics and Gynecology* **52**, 569.

121 Johnson M.R., Jauniaux E., Jurkovic D., Campbell S. & Nicolaides K.H. (1994) The levels of relaxin in embryonic fluids and maternal serum and during the first trimester of normal pregnancies. *Human Reproduction* **9**, 1561.

122 Sakbun V., Ali S.M., Greenwood F.C. & Bryant-Greenwood G.D. (1990) Human relaxin in the amnion, chorion, decidua parietalis, basal plate, and placental trophoblast by immunocytochemistry and northern analysis. *Journal of Clinical Endocrinology and Metabolism* **70**, 508.

123 Quagliarello J., Goldsmith L., Steinetz B., Lustig D.S. & Weiss G. (1980) Induction of relaxin secretion in non-pregnant women by human chorionic gonadotropin. *Journal of Clinical Endocrinology and Metabolism* **51**, 74.

124 Johnson M.R., Okokon E., Collins W.P., Sharma V. & Lightman S.L. (1991) The effect of human chorionic gonadotropin and pregnancy on the circulating levels of relaxin. *Journal of Clinical Endocrinology and Metabolism* **72**, 1042.

125 Gagliardi C.L., Goldsmith L.T., Saketos M., Weiss G. & Schmidt C.L. (1992) Human chorionic gonadotropin stimulation of relaxin secretion by luteinized human granulosa cells. *Fertility and Sterility* **58**, 314.

126 Johnson M.R., Abbas A.A., Irvine R., Norman-Taylor J.Q., Grudzinskas J.G., Collins W.P. & Nicolaides K.H. (1994) The regulation of corpus luteum function. *Human Reproduction* **9**, 41.

127 Anderson L.L., Adair V., Stromer M.H. & McDonald W.G. (1983) Relaxin production and release after hysterectomy in the pig. *Endocrinology* **113**, 677.

128 Golos T.G. & Sherwood O.D. (1982) Control of corpus luteum function during the second half of pregnancy in the rat: a direct relationship between conceptus number and both serum and ovarian relaxin levels. *Endocrinology* **111**, 872.

129 Seki K., Uesato T. & Kato K. (1987) Serum relaxin concentrations in women following the administra-

416

tion of 16,16-dimethyl-trans-delta 2-PGE1 methyl ester during early pregnancy. *Prostaglandins* **33**, 739.

130 Hochman J., Weiss G., Steinetz B.G. & O'Byrne E.M. (1978) Serum relaxin concentrations in prostaglandin- and oxytocin-induced labor in women. *American Journal of Obstetrics and Gynecology* **130**, 473.

131 Lopez-Bernal A., Bryant-Greenwood G.D., Hansell D.J., Hicks B.R., Greenwood F.C. & Turnbull A.C. (1987) Effect of relaxin on prostaglandin E production by human amnion: changes in relation to the onset of labour. *British Journal of Obstetrics and Gynaecology* **94**, 1045.

132 Jones S.A. & Summerlee A.J. (1986) Effects of porcine relaxin on the length of gestation and duration of parturition in the rat. *Journal of Endocrinology* **109**, 85.

133 Hisaw F.L. & Hisaw F.L. (1964) Effect of relaxin on the uterus of monkeys (macaca mulatta) with observations on the cervix and symphysis pubis. *American Journal of Obstetrics and Gynecology* **89**, 141.

134 Tseng L., Mazella J. & Chen G.A. (1987) Effect of relaxin on aromatase activity in human endometrial stromal cells. *Endocrinology* **120**, 2220.

135 Huang C.J., Stromer M.H. & Anderson L.L. (1991) Abrupt shifts in relaxin and progesterone secretion by aging luteal cells: luteotropic response in hysterectomized and pregnant pigs. *Endocrinology* **128**, 165.

136 Poisner A.M., Thrailkill K., Poisner R. & Handwerger S. (1990) Relaxin stimulates the synthesis and release of prorenin from human decidual cells: evidence for autocrine/paracrine regulation. *Journal of Clinical Endocrinology and Metabolism* **70**, 1765.

137 Zhu H.H., Huang J.R., Mazella J., Rosenberg M. & Tseng L. (1990) Differential effects of progestin and relaxin on the synthesis and secretion of immunoreactive prolactin in long term culture of human endometrial stromal cells. *Journal of Clinical Endocrinology and Metabolism* **71**, 889.

138 Brooks A.A., Johnson M.R., Steer P.J. & Abdalla H.I. (1995) Birth weight: nature or nurture? *Early Human Development* **42**, 29.

139 Eddie L.W., Cameron I.T., Leeton J.F., Healy D.L. & Renou P. (1990) Ovarian relaxin is not essential for dilatation of cervix (Letter). *Lancet* **336**, 243.

140 Kakouris H., Eddie L.W. & Summers R.J. (1992) Cardiac effects of relaxin in rats. *Lancet* **339**, 1076.

141 Rotsztejn D., Rana N. & Dmowski W.P. (1993) Correlation between fetal heart rate, crown-rump length, and β-human chorionic gonadotrophin levels during the first trimester of well timed conceptions resulting from infertility treatment. *Fertility and Sterility* **59**, 1169.

142 Jauniaux E., Johnson M.R., Ramsay B., Jurkovic D., Meuris S. & Campbell S. (1994) The role of relaxin in the development of the uteroplacental circulation in early pregnancy. *Obstetrics and Gynecology* **84**, 338.

143 Petersen L.K., Skajaa K. & Uldbjerg N. (1992) Serum relaxin as a potential marker for preterm labour. *British Journal of Obstetrics and Gynaecology* **99**, 292.

144 Weiss G., Goldsmith L.T., Sachdev R., Von Hagen S. & Lederer K. (1993) Elevated first-trimester serum relaxin concentrations in pregnant women following ovarian stimulation predict prematurity risk and preterm delivery. *Obstetrics and Gynecology* **82**, 821.

145 Bell R.J., Eddie L.W., Lester A.R., Wood E.C., Johnston P.D. & Niall H.D. (1988) Antenatal serum levels of relaxin in patients having preterm labour. *British Journal of Obstetrics and Gynaecology* **95**, 1264.

146 Szlachter B.N., Quagliarello J., Jewelewicz R., Osathanondh R., Spellacy W.N. & Weiss G. (1982) Relaxin in normal and pathogenic pregnancies. *Obstetrics and Gynecology* **59**, 167.

147 Johnson M.R., Riddle A.F., Grudzinskas J.G., Sharma V., Collins W.P., Lightman S.L. & Nicolaides K.H. (1993) Reduced circulating placental protein levels during the first trimester are associated with preterm labour and low birth weight. *Human Reproduction* **8**, 1942.

148 Szlachter N., O'Byrne E., Goldsmith L., Steinetz B.G. & Weiss G. (1980) Myometrial inhibiting activity of relaxin-containing extracts of human corpora lutea of pregnancy. *American Journal of Obstetrics and Gynecology* **136**, 584.

149 MacLennan A.H., Green R.C., Grant P. & Nicolson R. (1986) Ripening of the human cervix and induction of labor with intracervical purified porcine relaxin. *Obstetrics and Gynecology* **68**, 598.

150 MacLennan A.H. & Grant P. (1991) Human relaxin: in vitro response of human and pig myometrium. *Journal of Reproductive Medicine* **36**, 630.

151 Bell R.J. (1994) Two randomized, double-blind, placebo-controlled studies of vaginal recombinant human relaxin for cervical ripening prior to the induction of labour. In *Progress in Relaxin Research.* Eds A. MacLennan & G. Tregear. World Scientific Publishing, Singapore.

152 Steer C.V., Campbell S., Tan S.L., Crayford T., Mills C., Mason B. & Collins W.P. (1991) The use of transvaginal color flow imaging after in vitro fertilisation to identify optimum uterine conditions before embryo transfer. *Fertility and Sterility* **57**, 372.

153 Burton G.J. (1992) Human and animal models: limitations and comparisons. In *The First Twelve Weeks of Gestation.* Eds E. Barnea, J. Hustin & E. Jauniaux, p. 469. Springer Verlag, Heidelberg.

154 Jurkovic D., Jauniaux E. & Campbell, S. (1992) Doppler ultrasound investigations of pelvic circulation during the menstrual cycle and early pregnancy. In *The First Twelve Weeks of Gestation*, Eds E. Barnea, J. Hustin & E. Jauniaux, p. 78. Springer-Verlag, Heidelberg.

155 Kurjak A., Zalud I., Salighagic A., Crvenkovic G. & Matijevic R. (1991) Transvaginal color Doppler in the assessment of abnormal early pregnancy. *Journal of Perinatal Medicine* **19**, 155.

156 Arduini D., Rizzo G. & Romanini C. (1991) Doppler ultrasonography in early pregnancy does not predict adverse pregnancy outcome. *Ultrasound in Obstetrics and Gynecology* **1**, 180.

157 Jauniaux E., Jurkovic D., Delonge-Desnoek J. & Meuris S. (1992) Influence of human chorionic gonadotrophin, oestradiol, and progesterone on uteroplacental and corpus luteum blood flow in normal early pregnancy. *Human Reproduction* **7**, 1467.

The Placenta

Placental Metabolism

T. CHARD

From the time of implantation onwards, the human placenta secretes large quantities of hormonal and non-hormonal compounds. Some of these are structural proteins, enzymes, metabolic intermediates etc., which are a normal component of cells throughout the body and thus are not in any way specific to the placenta. Such non-specific compounds include growth factors [1], proto-oncogenes [2], tumour suppressor genes (p53) [3], hormone receptors, pro-renin and active renin [4], and the enzymes involved in steroid synthesis and inter-conversion; the latter do not differ from those in other steroid-producing tissues [5]. In addition, the placenta contains low concentrations of adrenocorticotrophic hormone (ACTH)-related peptides and hypothalamic-releasing hormones which are virtually identical to their hypothalamic–pituitary counterparts [6–9], together with releasing hormone receptors [10], transcription factors [11] and significant concentrations of interferon alpha and other cytokines [12,13].

Some of the materials produced by the placenta are secreted into the mother, most notably a range of specific proteins, and large quantities of steroid hormones. The secreted proteins include a series of products which are usually described as specific to this organ; the characteristics and properties of the most familiar of these placental proteins are listed in Table 16.1. The major steroids are oestriol and progesterone. The function of these materials is poorly understood even though, for example, protein synthesis by the trophoblast accounts for 12–16% of the amino acids transferred from mother to fetus [14]. Furthermore, none of these materials is entirely specific; i.e. occurring only in the placenta and not in any other site. All these steroids are secreted by the normal ovary. Many of the classical proteins of the human placenta can be found in relatively high concentrations in seminal plasma in men [15] and in ovarian follicular fluid in women [16,17]. Small amounts of human chorionic gonadotrophin (hCG) can be found in many normal tissues [18,19], and some is secreted by the pituitary gland, especially in women after the menopause [20,21].

Site of synthesis of placental products

The principal source of all the products discussed in this chapter is the trophoblast layer of the placenta, although in the case of steroids, preformed steroid precursors are derived from

Table 16.1. Some properties of the placental proteins. Note that the functions are always proposed. There is no clear evidence for the reality of most of these functions except in experimental situations. Immunosuppressive properties have not been listed: these have been postulated for all of the placental proteins but never proven [175]. The table does not include placental proteins which are now known to be produced by maternal tissues (endometrium) (placental protein 12 [PP12; now identified as insulin-like growth factor binding protein-1 (IGFBP-1)]; placental protein 14 [PP14, also known as glycodelin]).

Name and synonyms	Chromosomal origin	Molecular weight (kDa)	Proposed functions
Human chorionic gonadotrophin (hCG)			
None	α-subunit is coded by a single gene on 6q.21.1–q23	α-subunit 14.5	Stimulates the corpus luteum to produce progesterone and oestrogens in early pregnancy
	β-subunit is coded by a family of seven genes on 19q.13.32	β-subunit 22.2	Thyrotrophic activity Stimulates testosterone production by fetal testis
Human placental lactogen (hPL)			
Human chorionic somatomammotrophin (hCS) (and others)	Gene has two subunits (A and B) on 17q22–q24	21–23	Lactotrophic activity Metabolic activity (on mother and fetus) including anti-insulin effects Erythropoietic activity
Human placental growth hormone (hPGH)			
None	hGH-V or hGH-2 gene on 17q22–q24	22–23	Closely related to both pituitary growth hormone and placental lactogen but with greater somatotrophic activity than the latter
Schwangerschaftsprotein-1 (SP1)			
Trophoblast-specific β1 globulin Pregnancy-associated placental protein-C (PAPP-C) Pregnancy-specific β1 glycoprotein (psβ1G) Trophoblast-specific β-glycoprotein (TSG)	19q13.1	90–110	Unknown
Placental protein 5 (PP5)			
None	Unknown	36.6–42	Protease inhibition Analogue of antithrombin III
Placental alkaline phosphatase (PLAP)			
Heat-stable alkaline phosphatase	2q37	130	IgG-Fc receptor
Cystine aminopeptidase (CAP)			
Oxytocinase	Unknown	300	Protection of uterus against effects of oxytocin
Pregnancy-associated plasma protein-A (PAPP-A)			
None	9q33.1	800	Protease inhibitor (including elastase)

the mother and especially from the fetus. From about 12 weeks of pregnancy onwards, the trophoblast is in direct contact with the general maternal circulation via the intervillous space, whereas it is separated from fetal blood by a basement membrane and the vascular endothelium of the fetal capillaries. This explains why placental proteins are found in high levels in the mother but relatively low levels in the fetus; steroids, by contrast, are found at equivalent or higher concentrations in the fetus. Prior to 12 weeks, the situation is more complex. At this earlier stage there is little or no circulation of blood in what will later become the intervillous space [22–24]. Furthermore, there is a large area of extraplacental trophoblast (the chorionic membrane) which lies between the extra-embryonic coelom and the maternal decidua (Fig. 16.1); this area of the trophoblast, which seems to be inactive later in pregnancy, could be an important source of proteins such as hCG in the first few weeks of pregnancy [25].

The trophoblast of the chorionic villi includes an outer layer of syncytiotrophoblast and an inner layer of cytotrophoblast (Fig. 16.2). The latter consists of isolated cells which are prominent in the early placenta but become very

sparse towards term. The source of most of the products discussed here is believed to be the syncytiotrophoblast, though some have suggested that the placental releasing hormones, together with inhibin and relaxin, are secreted by the cytotrophoblast. Furthermore, the cytotrophoblast could be a source of molecules such as hCG and human placental lactogen (hPL) before 6 weeks' gestation [26]. The evidence for the tissue origin of placental products is largely based on immunohistochemistry. This technique sometimes yields ambivalent results, so that reports in the literature include identification of virtually all placental products in every cell and tissue type within the placenta. Thus the view that the origin is always the syncytiotrophoblast represents the most commonly held view but is not necessarily definitive. Some of the doubts arise from the difficulty of identifying a given cell type within an organ as complex as the placenta. For example, cells may be described as decidual (i.e. of maternal origin) when in fact they are part of the extensive but often wrongly identified extravillous trophoblast [27]. Similar problems can arise with other experimental systems (in-vitro culture) in which separation of fetal and maternal tissues is

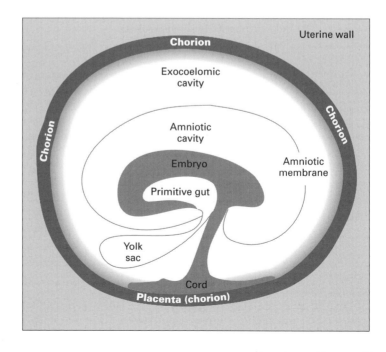

Fig. 16.1. Diagram to demonstrate the major structures present in an 8-week pregnancy. Note that the chorion (trophoblast) is the main source of placental proteins, and that at this stage of pregnancy the extraplacental chorion may be a major source of placental products secreted into the mother.

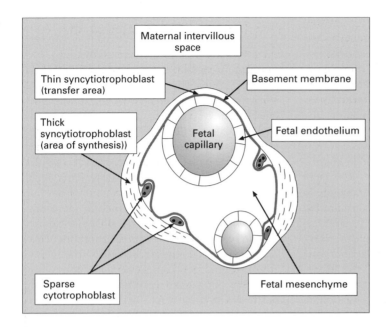

Fig. 16.2. A cross-section of a chorionic villus in a mature placenta.

required. There are also pitfalls for the unwary histochemist. The trophoblast has specific receptors for proteins such as ferritin and the immunoglobulins; these receptors have the ability to bind immunological reagents non-specifically.

The earliest stage at which the trophoblast begins active secretion has been the subject of several studies. Most agree that hCG and steroid secretion by human embryos in tissue culture occurs around 7 days after fertilization [28–30].

Mechanisms of synthesis

Within the trophoblast itself, the mechanisms of synthesis and secretion are similar to mechanisms in other tissues and steroid-producing glands [5]. However, there is a unique biosynthetic pathway for the production of oestriol (reviewed by Kuss [31]). The placenta derives cholesterol from low-density lipoproteins in the maternal circulation and removes the sidechain to form the 21-carbon steroid pregnenolone. The fetal adrenal converts this to the C19 androgen, dehydroepiandrosterone, which in turn is 16-hydroxylated and conjugated to sulphate in the fetal liver. This compound is taken up by the placenta, where the sulphate is removed [32] and ring A is aromatized to form

oestriol [33,34]. Thus, secretion of oestriol into the mother reflects the activity of both fetus and placenta, and this remarkable piece of physiology led to the classic endocrine concept of the fetoplacental unit [35].

The trophoblast is remarkable for the uniqueness, range and quantity of materials produced. What features of this tissue might be associated with this extraordinary phenomenon?

The trophoblast is a syncytium

The only tissues other than the trophoblast which may exist as a syncytium (i.e. multiple nuclei within one cell) are inflammatory giant cells and some tumour cells. The analogy with tumour cells might well be relevant, because a wide range of tumours of non-trophoblastic origin can sometimes secrete hCG [36,37]. However, the invasive cells of the trophoblast are the cytotrophoblast or extravillous trophoblast. Unlike the villous syncytiotrophoblast, these cells do not characteristically secrete placental products.

The trophoblast is a transfer tissue

From a functional point of view, the trophoblast might be described as analogous to the surface epithelia of other organs responsible for transfer such as the lung, kidney and gut. However, these do not secrete placental proteins or steroids. Furthermore, the analogy is tenuous because with these organs the transfer is between the bloodstream and the outside of the body rather than between two circulations.

The trophoblast is a male organ

Evidence from studies on mouse gametes and embryos has suggested the intriguing hypothesis that the maternal genome is necessary for the development of the embryo while the presence of the paternal pronucleus is associated with development of the trophoblast [38]. Thus, the paternal haploid set might be imprinted on the trophoblast and determine which set of genes becomes active. It is notable but perhaps overspeculative to point out that the only other major site of placental protein synthesis is the male reproductive tract [15].

The trophoblast is directly exposed to the maternal bloodstream (the surface release hypothesis)

All cells in the body contain the same genome and thus have the potential to secrete placental products. What is actually secreted might be determined by the anatomical location of a given cell. The unique feature of villous trophoblast cells is that the cell membrane is directly adjacent to the bloodstream in the intervillous space, while most other secretory cells in the body are separated from the circulation by a layer of blood vessel endothelium and its basement membrane. This anatomical relationship could also explain why placental proteins are secreted almost exclusively into the mother. Attractive though this surface-release hypothesis is in late pregnancy, there are a number of pieces of countervailing evidence. Especially notable is the fact that intervillous blood flow does not begin until after 12 weeks of pregnancy; prior to that time the intervillous space contains an acellular fluid [22,23]. However, Meuris and colleagues [39] have suggested that the peak of hCG corresponds to the earliest time at which intervillous bloodflow can be observed by Doppler ultrasound.

Distribution of placental products

The levels of placental proteins in the fluids surrounding the early fetus are shown in Table 16.2.

In the circulation, the highest concentrations of placental proteins are found in maternal blood and the lowest in fetal blood; levels in amniotic fluid are intermediate [40]. This is consistent with the fact that the fetal microcirculation restricts transfer of large molecules [41]. By contrast, the levels of steroids are usually higher in the fetal compartment (10-fold higher in the case of oestriol and progesterone).

The circulating concentration in the mother is the result of a balance between plasma volume, metabolic removal and the rate of input from the placenta. The pattern of increase of some of the placental proteins shown in Table 16.1 is illustrated in Fig. 16.3. With most proteins, and the steroid progesterone, there is a slow rise during the first trimester, then a more rapid rise during the midtrimester and early third trimester, followed by a plateau towards term. This sigmoid curve is very similar to that of the weight of the placenta itself. Exceptions to this pattern are those of hCG, which shows a rapid early rise to reach a peak at 8–10 weeks [25,30], and oestriol and pregnancy-associated plasma protein-A (PAPP-A), which show a steady increase throughout pregnancy with no plateau towards term [42].

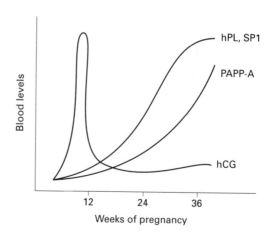

Fig. 16.3. The pattern of circulating levels of some placental proteins throughout pregnancy.

Table 16.2. Median values of placental products in amniotic fluid, extra-embryonic coelomic fluid and maternal serum at 8–12 weeks' gestation. Modified from Zhou *et al.* [176] and Iles *et al.* [177].

Protein	Amniotic fluid	Extra-embryonic coelomic fluid	Maternal serum	Reference
hCG (IU/ml)	1.7	245.0	157.0	[60]
Total β-subunit of hCG (IU/ml)	6.73	410.0	410.0	[60]
Free β-subunit of hCG (µg/ml)	0.262	17.3	0.3	[60]
hCG (IU/ml)	1.0	120.0	81.0	[178]
hPL (ng/ml)	30.0	80.0	210.0	[179]
PAPP-A (mIU/ml)	<10.0	26.0	1220.0	[177]

Metabolism of placental products

The main sites of metabolism of the placental proteins are the liver and kidneys, and some are excreted in the urine. The urine concentrations relative to those in blood vary greatly between the different proteins: with hPL, the urinary levels are one-tenth or less of those in the circulation; with hCG, the levels are almost identical in the two fluids. In urine, most of the hCG is in the form of the metabolic fragment known as β-core. This is derived from the β-subunit. It lacks sequences of amino acids at both the N- and C-terminus; cleavage of a loop between residues 45 and 57 yields a two-chain structure held together by disulphide bonds [43]. One aspect of metabolism which is of practical clinical importance is the time-to-time variations of levels in maternal blood or urine. Of the observed variation, some is due to the method of measurement (estimation by immunoassay typically has a coefficient of variation of 5–10%). True biological variation has to be added to this technical distribution range. Despite claims that the plasma concentration of placental proteins may follow a set pattern or rhythm within a 24-hour period, these have never been confirmed. There is, however, random time-to-time fluctuation which ranges between 5 and 15% for all materials studied [44–47]. Such a random fluctuation is frequently interpreted as pulsatile release, though the phenomenon could equally be due to changes in clearance or metabolism. Similarly, and contrary to widely held views, there is no diurnal rhythm of urine hCG levels; the hormone is not more concentrated in an early morning specimen [48].

Table 16.3. The half-lives of various placental proteins, as measured following delivery of the placenta.

Product	Half-life
hPL	15–20 minutes
hCG	5–10 hours
SP1	20–30 hours
PAPP-A	4.2 days
PP5	30 minutes

The placental steroids are also metabolized in the liver and kidneys and a small proportion are excreted unchanged. The bulk of progesterone is converted to 20α-hydroxyprogesterone [49] and eventually metabolized to pregnanediol and excreted in the urine as pregnanediol glucuronide [50]. The bulk of oestriol is excreted as the sulphate and glucuronide conjugates [5].

The half-lives of some placental proteins are listed in Table 16.3. In all cases, the half-life has two or more components: an initial fast decline as the product clears from the circulation, and a more extended phase as the product leaves the extravascular compartments. The literature on half-lives is often confusing because of a failure to identify which phase is involved. The half-lives of the steroid hormones are typically 20–30 minutes, but the situation is rendered complex by such factors as the formation of metabolites and recirculation.

Function of placental products

The most important function of the placenta is

transport of nutrients, gases and waste products between the fetus and the mother. What then is the function of the placental products? It is generally presumed that naturally occurring biological materials exist for a purpose. In the case of the specific products of the placenta, this purpose would be the adjustment of the physiology of the mother to yield the environment best suited to the survival of the child. In this respect, it is notable that the postulated functions of the placental proteins are confined almost exclusively to the mother. For example, despite the somatotrophic activity of hPL, there is little evidence that it has a direct role in fetal growth [51], though some have suggested that fetal tissues are more susceptible to the stimulatory effect of hPL and hCG [52]. The possibility that placental hCG stimulates testosterone output by the fetal testis in midtrimester is attractive but unproven [53–55].

Even in the mother, many of the proposed functions of placental products are speculative rather than definitive. Amongst the protein products, the sole exception appears to be hCG: there is little doubt that this is the major luteotrophic signal from an early pregnancy. The corpus luteum contains luteinizing hormone (LH)/hCG receptors [56]. Progesterone production by granulosa-luteal cells can be stimulated by very small amounts of hCG, though there appears to be no direct relationship between the circulating levels of progesterone and hCG in early pregnancy [57]. It is notable that no pregnancy has ever been described in which hCG is absent. Another possible exception is PAPP-A; absence of this molecule is associated with the Cornelia de Lange syndrome in the fetus [58]. But, even here, the pregnancy itself is normal.

It is widely believed that only the intact heterodimer of hCG has biological activity. However, a single chain protein which contains both α- and β-subunits has biological activity [59]. Similarly, there is growing evidence that the isolated subunits can have biological activity. Thus, the α-subunit, which is present in very high concentrations, especially in the coelomic fluid (Table 2 of Ref. 60) can stimulate prolactin secretion by the endometrium [61]. The β-subunit may act as a growth factor [62].

Of the placental steroids, it is widely accepted that progesterone plays an important role in the maintenance of pregnancy, ensuring that the uterus does not contract as a result of the presence of the expanding conceptus. Up to the 8th week of pregnancy, removal of the corpus luteum results in abortion [63]. In the human, the best recent experimental evidence for this hypothesis is the fact that pregnancy can be terminated by administration of the progesterone-receptor antagonist, mifepristone [64]. In vitro, however, progesterone may stimulate human myometrial contractility [65].

Evidence for an important functional role of oestriol is less cogent. It has been proposed that changing steroid levels, with a decrease in progesterone and an increase in oestrogens, play an important part in the onset of labour [66–70]. There is no doubt that this occurs in animals, but the evidence in humans is thin and disputed [71–73]. Furthermore, progesterone levels in the myometrium are constant throughout pregnancy and there is no excess adjacent to the placenta [74].

It has been suggested that most of the functions of the trophoblast products are entirely autocrine: that their primary function is to monitor the environment of the placenta, a 'placental radar' and, thereby, to ensure homogeneity of the all-important transfer functions [75]. This view of the lack of endocrine function of placental proteins is supported by some experiments of nature: rare pregnancies in which a specific product is almost totally deficient. Deficiencies of placental sulphatase (leading to very low levels of oestriol) [50], hPL [76] and SP1 [77] have been described. With occasional exceptions [78], pregnancies in which these defects are present are usually entirely normal in every other respect, making it difficult to suggest that placental products serve an essential biological role.

There is also evidence for paracrine function of placental hormones: for example, hCG may stimulate secretion of prorenin by the placenta [79], formation of gap junctions in the trophoblast [80], and inhibit oxytocin-induced contractions of the myometrium [81]. Receptors for hCG are present in the fetal membranes [82].

Control mechanisms of placental products

The mechanisms which control the production of placental proteins are as enigmatic as the functions. Even when a mechanism has been proposed (for example, the control of hPL release by maternal lipids and carbohydrates), the evidence is disputed and subject to alternative explanations [83]. The only situation in which a significant and unambiguous short-term change in maternal levels of placental products has been shown is the dramatic rise in placental protein 5 levels that follows intravenous injection of small doses of heparin [84]. There are no other examples of changes of this speed and magnitude.

Many authors have speculated that there might exist, within the placenta itself, a control system for hCG comparable to that of the hypothalamic–pituitary gonadal axis. All of the relevant factors are present (releasing hormones, releasing hormone receptors, gonadotrophins, steroids) and all are in the closest possible proximity. However, firm evidence for this hypothesis is limited to a large number of virtually identical in-vitro studies, the findings of which can easily be criticized:

1 some of the tissue culture studies use very high levels of active agents that do not reflect the in-vivo situation;

2 in most studies, only a single target product was measured and it is not possible to judge the specificity of the effect;

3 while some studies suggest that there could be interactions at the intracellular level (e.g. between GnRH and hCG), there is no evidence that such interactions play any significant role in the time-to-time variation of hCG levels in blood;

4 there is little or no effect of GnRH levels on hCG in vivo [85–87];

5 the placenta of some species (e.g. the rabbit) may contain high levels of GnRH but does not secrete chorionic gonadotrophin [88];

6 inadvertent administration of GnRH-agonists during early pregnancy does not affect the outcome of the pregnancy [89]. Similarly, the suggestion that hCG secretion may be influenced by progesterone [90] is not supported by studies using progesterone antagonists in vivo [91].

Other and less specific factors might also influence placental hormone secretion. For example, co-incubation of trophoblast with endometrium leads to a reduction in the secretion of hCG and hPL [92].

There is also a lack of information on mechanisms which control placental steroid secretion. No experimental manipulation in vivo (other than disruption of the pregnancy) can alter progesterone levels. Oestriol levels can be influenced by alteration in precursor steroid supply from the fetal adrenal: low levels are found in anencephaly and fetal adrenal hypoplasia, or if fetal adrenal function is inhibited by administration of corticosteroids [93]. However, none of these situations reflect on the time-to-time control of oestriol levels in a normal pregnancy.

The absence of classical control mechanisms constitutes an argument for the surface release hypothesis. According to this, the potential for placental synthesis would be directly related to the total mass of the trophoblast; the rate of release (and secondarily of synthesis) would be a function of the concentration of the substance in maternal blood in the intervillous space; and the latter would, in turn, depend on the rate of blood flow in the intervillous space [94]. This is conceptually very similar to the proposal that pituitary hormone release is partly controlled by mass action direct feedback [95]. Specific evidence showing the dependence of placental synthesis on uteroplacental bloodflow is available from studies of the conversion of maternal dehydroepiandrosterone sulphate into oestradiol [96–98]. Further evidence is provided by the observation that the placenta possesses hCG receptors [99–102] and that addition of hCG can inhibit the release of hCG by placental tissues in vitro [103] — equivalent to short-short loop or mass-action feedback. The surface release hypothesis may well apply in mid- to late pregnancy. It is compatible with the fact that no investigation has clearly demonstrated a diurnal rhythm of placental proteins [45,47]. The surface release hypothesis might account for the peak of hCG in early pregnancy, since this peak is coincident with the establishment of intervillous bloodflow [39]. As already noted, other anatomical features may explain this phenomenon, in particular the activity of the extraplacental chorion before this comes into contact with fetal tissues.

The absence of control mechanisms for 'specific' products does not necessarily apply to all materials in this tissue. The cytochrome enzyme complex P-450, for example, is responsible for detoxification of drugs and carcinogens and is increased in the placentas of smokers when compared to those of non-smokers [104].

Miscellaneous factors that may affect levels of placental products in the maternal circulation include:

1 Smoking. Levels of hCG are lower in smokers than in non-smokers [105–107]. There is no specific effect of smoking on maternal hPL levels though, as expected, growth-retarded babies of smokers have low levels [108].

2 Race. Asian mothers have high hPL levels [109]. Median hCG levels are higher in blacks than in whites [110–112], though some have not been able to confirm this observation [113,114]. Bogart [113] was able to show a 9.8% difference after correction for maternal weight, and also showed that levels in orientals were 16% higher than those in white women.

3 Prostaglandins. Both extra- and intra-amniotic injections of prostaglandins decrease maternal hPL levels, probably by a direct effect on hPL synthesis [115].

4 Fetal sex. From approximately 18 weeks the maternal levels of hCG, hPL and Schwangerschaftsprotein 1 (SP1) may be higher in association with a female fetus [116,117] but there is no variation at earlier stages [118].

5 Maternal weight. There is an inverse relationship between maternal weight and circulating hCG levels [106,113,119].

6 Maternal haemoglobin. There is an inverse correlation between hCG and hPL levels and maternal haemoglobin concentration at 10 weeks of pregnancy [120].

Receptors in the placenta

As a generalization, whenever a specific receptor has been sought in the placenta, it has been found. Examples include receptors for hormones [99,121–126], releasing hormones [127], growth factors [128–133], cytokines [134–136] and many other biologically active compounds.

Though the existence of a receptor clearly indicates that ligand binding can occur, the functional significance of this is often enigmatic. Thus, the doubts about the function of specific placental products (see above) must extend equally to the association of these products with receptors in the tissue of origin. One possibility already noted [75] is that the receptor plays an autocrine role in the control of production of its specific ligand. This has been clearly demonstrated in the case of hCG [99].

Circulating binding proteins in the placenta

Placental extracts typically contain large quantities of the circulating binding proteins — for example, those for steroid hormones, thyronines and peptides. However, the bulk of this material can be attributed to the maternal blood which often constitutes a substantial part of a placental extract. There is little or no evidence for specific synthesis of such proteins by the placenta. The increase in circulating levels which is characteristic of pregnancy can almost always be attributed to an increase in maternal synthesis in response to placental steroids.

Some clinical applications of measurement of placental products

Early diagnosis of pregnancy

The early diagnosis of pregnancy usually depends on the detection of hCG in maternal urine or blood. Chorionic gonadotrophin first appears in maternal serum and urine shortly after the time of implantation [30]. The possibility of earlier detection by measurement of an early pregnancy factor has not been substantiated [137]. Once hCG appears, the levels increase with a linear-log relationship [138]. Given the ubiquitous nature of hCG at low concentrations (<15 IU/l), in clinical practice a single estimation of hCG should only be considered to be definitive if it is greater than 15 IU/l or if a lower level of hCG is seen to increase twofold at an interval of 3 days. If hCG has been administered therapeutically, estimations should be delayed until clearance of the exogenous hCG has occurred, i.e. a delay of up to 14 days. Other placental proteins associated with pregnancy, such as hPL and PAPP-A, are not candidates for early detection, since the rise in concentration in maternal blood cannot be easily identified until after 6 weeks of amenorrhoea.

Early pregnancy failure (biochemical pregnancies)

For a woman who wishes to become pregnant, the chance of producing a viable offspring in any one ovarian cycle is approximately 25%. Many estimates have been made of the frequency of very early pregnancy failure, several based on studies of the transient appearance of hCG during a potentially fertile cycle. These are known as biochemical pregnancies because this constitutes the sole evidence of a pregnancy. Estimates of the incidence of these biochemical pregnancies vary from 8 to 55% [139].

Threatened and spontaneous miscarriage

Levels of placental proteins [140–142] and progesterone [143] in the mother have been used to predict the outcome in women with vaginal bleeding in early pregnancy [140,141]. As a general rule, concentrations of placental products are reduced in association with threatened miscarriage in which the outcome is fetal loss, but normal in cases in which the pregnancy proceeds. For clinical prediction, measurement of these compounds may be unnecessary if fetal life can be demonstrated by ultrasound [144], though low levels of placental products (such as hCG, or SP1) have been shown *prior* to fetal demise [145]. It has been suggested by some that levels of PAPP-A are good predictors of fetal outcome in cases in which fetal heart action has been demonstrated but which spontaneously abort [17]. A deviation from the normal rise in blood levels of hCG is suggestive of failed pregnancy even before ultrasound can provide useful information [146]. It has been claimed that a single hCG determination at 14–16 days after embryo or gamete transfer is highly predictive of pregnancy outcome [147].

Anembryonic pregnancy

Blood levels of hCG have been shown to be low at 4 weeks' gestation in women who subsequently are shown to have blighted ovum; mean levels of maternal PAPP-A, oestradiol and progesterone fall some 3 weeks later [148].

Ectopic pregnancy

The main value of biochemical tests in this condition, and in particular the measurement of hCG, is to alert the clinician to the possibility of a pregnancy-related disorder in a woman presenting with lower abdominal pain, and to exclude this if a negative result (i.e. <25 IU/l) is obtained [149,150]. Stabile and her colleagues [151] reported a sensitivity of 100% for detection using hCG in conjunction with ultrasound. For detection of pregnancy, a simple non-quantitative method (e.g. a dipstick [152]) is appropriate. Quantitative estimates of hCG have been used to distinguish between an extra-uterine and an intrauterine pregnancy. Kadar and colleagues originally described a discriminatory hCG zone. The concept of this is that in normal pregnancies there is a concentration of hCG below which a gestation sac can never be seen by ultrasound, a level above which it can always be seen, and an intervening zone in which it can be seen in some women but not in others. If serum hCG is greater than 6500 IU/ml (>3000 IU/ml in a more recent study [153]), and a gestation sac cannot be seen, then an ectopic pregnancy is very likely [154–156]. Similar findings have been reported with SP1 and PAPP-A (secretion of PAPP-A being more severely compromised) [157,158] and progesterone [143,159–161]. Not surprisingly, combinations of markers have better predictive efficiency than single markers [162,163]. Some authors have expressed scepticism about the value of hCG and other analytes in distinguishing between different types of early pregnancy complications [164]. It has been suggested that women who are at high risk of an ectopic pregnancy should be routinely screened by hCG assays [165]. This group might include pregnancies by in-vitro fertilization.

Screening for Down's syndrome

One of the most striking clinical applications of measurement of placental proteins is in screening for Down's syndrome and other chromosomal abnormalities in early pregnancy [166]. In the presence of a Down's syndrome fetus there are complex changes in the levels of fetoplacental products in the maternal circulation. These include a general reduction in products of the fetus (alphafetoprotein, oestriol) and increased or occasionally decreased levels of placental proteins. The underlying mechanism of these changes is not understood. There are two main theories:

1 That the Down's syndrome pregnancy is immature relative to a normal pregnancy (this would explain the low levels of fetal products and the increased levels of hCG, but not the increased levels of other placental proteins).

2 That there is fetoplacental imbalance with a general decrease in fetal products and an increase in placental products (but this does not account for the greatly reduced levels of PAPP-A in the late first trimester).

In addition, there are two theories to explain the particular case of the increase in hCG:

1 In a Down's pregnancy there may be persistence of the extra-embryonic coelom. The chorion lining of this structure may be the principal source of the first trimester peak of hCG [25].

2 There is a mechanistic link via interferon-α (IFN-α). Thus, it is known that, under experimental conditions, IFN-α can influence hCG secretion [167]. Furthermore, the receptor for IFN-α lies on chromosome 21 and, in theory, the levels of this receptor might be increased in Down's syndrome.

Chorionic villus sampling

It is well recognized that maternal serum alphafetoprotein levels can show a substantial rise following invasive procedures in early pregnancy, notably amniocentesis [168], chorionic villus sampling (CVS) [169] and surgical [170] or medical termination [171]. This is almost certainly the result of fetomaternal haemorrhage. There is no significant change in proteins and hormones of placental origin following CVS [169].

Fetal well-being in late pregnancy

The levels of placental products, including most proteins and steroids, are reduced in cases of placental insufficiency in late pregnancy. This includes a number of complications, often of mixed aetiology, such as perinatal death, perinatal asphyxia and intrauterine growth retardation. Until the mid-1980s, measurement of placental products, especially hPL and oestriol, were widely used to identify the fetus at risk of these complications [172,173]. However, as with most tests of fetal well-being, there was a high incidence of false-positives and false-negatives, and in the past 10 years these tests have been almost entirely replaced by biophysical procedures, ultrasound imaging, antenatal cardiotocography and Doppler blood flow studies [174].

Conclusions

Pregnancy is associated with the secretion of an extraordinarily wide range of placental products into the mother. Measurement of some of these products in maternal blood has proved to be of considerable clinical value. Yet the biological role of many of these materials remains entirely enigmatic.

References

1 Ohlsson R. (1989) Growth factors, protooncogenes and human placental development. *Cell Differentiation and Development* **28**, 1.

2 Johnson P.M., Lyden T.W. & Mwenda J.M. (1990) Endogenous retroviral expression in the human placenta. *American Journal of Reproductive Immunology* **23**, 115.

3 Marzusch K., Ruck P., Horny H.-P., Dietl J. & Kaiserling E. (1995) Expression of the p53 tumour suppressor gene in human placenta: an immunohistochemical study. *Placenta* **16**, 101.

4 Downing G.J., Poisner A.M. & Barnea E.R. (1995) First-trimester villous placenta has high prorenin and active renin concentrations. *American Journal of Obstetrics and Gynecology* **172**, 864.

5 Albrecht E.D. & Pepe G.J. (1990) Placental steroid hormone biosynthesis in primate pregnancy. *Endocrine Reviews* **11**, 124.

430

6 Lee J.N., Seppala M. & Chard T. (1981) Characterization of placental luteinizing hormone releasing factor-like material. *Acta Endocrinologica* **96**, 394.

7 Baird A., Wehrenberg W.B., Bohlen P. & Ling N. (1985) Immunoreactive and biologically active growth hormone-releasing factor in the rat placenta. *Endocrinology* **117**, 1598.

8 Riley S.C. & Challis J.R.G. (1991) Corticotrophin-releasing hormone production by the placenta and fetal membranes. *Placenta* **12**, 105.

9 Challis J.R.G., Matthews S.G., Van Meir C. & Ramirez M.M. (1995) The placental corticotrophin-releasing hormone-adrenocorticotrophin axis. *Placenta* **16**, 481.

10 Bramley T.A., McPhie C.A. & Menzies G.S. (1992) Human placental gonadotrophin-releasing hormone (GnRH) binding sites. I. Characterization, properties and ligand specificity. *Placenta* **13**, 555.

11 Bamberger A.M., Bamberger C.M., Pu L.P., Puy L.A., Loh Y.P. & Asa S.L. (1995) Expression of pit-1 messenger ribonucleic acid and protein in the human placenta. *Journal of Clinical Endocrinology and Metabolism* **80**, 2021.

12 Chard T. (1989) Interferon in pregnancy. *Journal of Developmental Physiology* **11**, 271.

13 Chard T. (1995) Cytokines in implantation. *Human Reproduction Update* **1**, 385.

14 Carroll M.J. & Young M. (1983) The relationship between placental protein synthesis and transfer of amino acids. *Biochemistry Journal* **210**, 99.

15 Salem H.T., Menabawey M., Seppala M., Shaaban M.M. & Chard T. (1984) Human seminal plasma contains a wide range of trophoblast specific proteins. *Placenta* **5**, 413.

16 Westergaard J.G., Sinosich M.J. & Grudzinskas J.G. (1985) Pregnancy associated plasma protein A (PAPP-A) in preovulatory, nonovulatory, and atretic human ovarian follicles during the natural cycle. *Annals of the New York Academy of Science* **442**, 205.

17 Westergaard J.G., Teisner B., Sinosich M.J., Madsen L.T. & Grudzinskas J.G. (1985) Does ultrasound examination render biochemical tests obsolete in the prediction of early pregnancy failure? *British Journal of Obstetrics and Gynaecology* **92**, 77.

18 Braunstein G.D., Kamdar V., Rasor J., Swaminathan N. & Wade M.E. (1991) Widespread distribution of chorionic gonadotrophin-like substance in normal tissues. *Journal of Clinical Endocrinology and Metabolism* **49**, 917.

19 Yoshimoto Y., Wolfsen A.R., Hirose F. & Odell W.D. (1979) Human chorionic gonadotropin-like material: presence in normal human tissues. *American Journal of Obstetrics and Gynecology* **134**, 729.

20 Armstrong E.G., Ehrlich P.H., Birken S., Schlatterer J.P., Siris E., Hembree W.C. & Canfield R.E. (1984) Use of a highly sensitive and specific immunoradiometric assay for detection of human chorionic gonadotropin in urine of normal, nonpregnant and pregnant individuals. *Journal of Clinical Endocrinology and Metabolism* **59**, 867.

21 Huang S.C., Chen R.J., Hsieh C.Y., Wei P.Y. & Ouyang P.C. (1984) The secretion of human chorionic gonadotrophin-like substance in women employing contraceptive measures. *Journal of Clinical Endocrinology and Metabolism* **58**, 646.

22 Hustin J. & Schaaps J.P. (1987) Echographic and anatomic studies of the maternotrophoblastic border during the first trimester of pregnancy. *American Journal of Obstetrics and Gynecology* **157**, 162.

23 Jauniaux E., Jurkovic D., Campbell S. & Hustin J. (1992) Doppler ultrasonographic features of the developing placental circulation: correlation with anatomic findings. *American Journal of Obstetrics and Gynecology* **166**, 585.

24 Jauniaux E., Jurkovic D. & Campbell S. (1995) In vivo investigation of the placental circulations by Doppler echography. *Placenta* **16**, 323.

25 Chard T., Iles R. & Wathen N. (1995) Why is there a peak of human chorionic gonadotrophin (hCG) in early pregnancy? *Human Reproduction* **10**, 1837.

26 Maruo T., Ladines-Llave C.A., Matsuo H., Manato A.S. & Mochizuki M. (1992) A novel change in cytologic localization of human chorionic gonadotropin and human placental lactogen in first-trimester placenta in the course of gestation. *American Journal of Obstetrics and Gynecology* **167**, 217.

27 Panigel M. (1986) Anatomy and morphology. *Clinical Obstetrics and Gynaecology* **13**, 421.

28 Fishel S.B., Edwards R.G. & Evans C.J. (1984) Human chorionic gonadotropin secreted by preimplantation embryos cultured in vitro. *Science* **233**, 816.

29 Gunn L.K., Homa S.T., Searle M.J. & Chard T. (1994) Lack of evidence for the production of interferon-alpha-like species by the cultured human embryo. *Human Reproduction* **9**, 1522.

30 Chard T. (1992) Pregnancy tests: a review. *Human Reproduction* **7**, 701.

31 Kuss E. (1994) The fetoplacental unit of primates. *Experimental Clinical Endocrinology* **102**, 135.

32 French A.P. & Warren J.C. (1966) Sulfatase activity in the human placenta. *Steroids* **8**, 79.

33 Klausner D.A. & Ryan K.J. (1964) Estriol secretion by the human term placenta. *Journal of Clinical Endocrinology and Metabolism* **24**, 101.

34 Siiteri P.K. & MacDonald P.C. (1966) Placental estrogen biosynthesis during human pregnancy. *Journal of Clinical Endocrinology* **26**, 751.

35 Diczfalusy E. (1962) Endocrinology of the fetus. *Acta Obstetrica et Gynecologica Scandinavica* **41**, 45.

36 Braunstein G.D. (1983) hCG expression in trophoblastic and nontrophoblastic tumors. In *Oncodevelopmental Markers: Biologic, Diagnostic, and Monitoring Aspects*. Ed. W.H. Fishman, p. 351. Academic Press, New York.

37 Iles R.K. & Chard T. (1991) Human chorionic gonadotrophin expression by bladder cancers: biology and clinical potential. *Journal of Urology* **145**, 453.

38 Szulman A.E. (1988) Trophoblastic disease: clinical pathology of hydatidiform moles. *Obstetric and Gynecology Clinics of North America* **15**, 443.

39 Meuris S., Nagy A.M., Delogne-Desnoeck J., Jurkovic D. & Jauniaux E. (1995) Temporal relationship between the human chorionic gonadotrophin peak and the establishment of intervillous blood flow in early pregnancy. *Human Reproduction* **10**, 947.

40 Grudzinskas J.G., Evans D.G., Gordon Y.B., Jeffrey D. & Chard T. (1978) Pregnancy specific beta-1-glycoprotein in fetal and maternal compartments. *Obstetrics and Gynecology* **52**, 43.

41 Firth J.A. & Leach L. (1996) Not trophoblast alone: a review of the contribution to the fetal microvasculature to transplacental exchange. *Placenta* **17**, 89.

42 Stabile I., Grudzinskas J.G. & Chard T. (1988) Clinical applications of pregnancy protein estimations with particular reference to pregnancy-associated plasma protein A (PAPP-A). *Obstetric and Gynecological Survey* **43**, 73.

43 Lee C.L., Iles R.K., Shepherd J.H., Hudson C.N. & Chard T. (1991) The purification and development of a radioimmunoassay for beta-core fragment of human chorionic gonadotrophin in urine: applications as a marker of gynaecological cancer in premenopausal and postmenopausal women. *Journal of Endocrinology* **130**, 481.

44 Grudzinskas J.G., Obiekwe B.C. & Frumar A.M. (1979) Circulating levels of pregnancy specific beta-1-glycoprotein in late pregnancy, nyctohemeral and day-to-day variation and variation during labour. *British Journal of Obstetrics and Gynaecology* **86**, 973.

45 Houghton D.J., Newnham J.P., Lo K., Rice A. & Chard T. (1982) Circadian variation of circulating levels of four placental proteins. *British Journal Obstetrics and Gynaecology*. **89**, 831.

46 Houghton D.J., Perry L., Newnham J.P. & Chard T. (1983) Nyctohemeral variation in the level of 'unconjugated' oestriol in maternal serum. *Journal of Obstetrics and Gynaecology* **3**, 221.

47 Rose N.C., Canick J.A., Knight G.J., Pulkkinen A., Tumber M.B., Mennuti M.T. & Palomaki G.E. (1994) Second-trimester diurnal variation of maternal serum alpha-fetoprotein, human chorionic gonadotropin, and unconjugated oestriol: is it present and does it affect the prediction of a patient's risk for fetal Down syndrome? *Prenatal Diagnosis* **14**, 947.

48 Kent A., Kitau M.J. & Chard T. (1991) Absence of diurnal variation in urinary chorionic gonadotrophin excretion at 8–13 weeks gestation. *British Journal of Obstetrics and Gynaecology* **98**, 1180.

49 Brian-Little A. & Billiar R.B. (1983) Progestagens. In *Endocrinology of Pregnancy*. Eds A.R. Fuchs & A. Klopper p. 92. Harper & Row, Philadelphia.

50 Taylor N.F. (1982) Placental sulphatase deficiency. *Journal of Inherited Metabolic Disease* **5**, 164.

51 Houghton D.J., Shackleton P., Obiekwe B.C. & Chard T. (1984) Relationship of maternal and fetal levels of human placental lactogen to weight and sex of the fetus. *Placenta* **5**, 455.

52 Hill D.J., Crace C.G. & Milner R.D.G. (1985) Incorporation of 3H thymidine by isolated fetal myoblasts and fibroblasts in response to human placental lactogen (hPL): possible mediation of hPL action by release of immunoreactice SM-C. *Journal of Cell Physiology* **125**, 337.

53 Abramovich R., Baker T.D. & Neal P. (1974) Effect of human chorionic gonadotrophin on testosterone secretion by the foetal human testis in organ culture. *Journal of Endocrinology* **60**, 179.

54 Molsberry J.L., Carr B.R., Mendelson C.R. & Simpson I.R. (1982) Human chorionic gonadotrophin binding to human fetal tests as a function of gestational age. *Journal of clinical Endocrinology and Metabolism* **55**, 791.

55 Word R.A., George F.W., Wilson J.D. & Carr B.R. (1989) Testosterone synthesis and adenylate cyclase activity in the early human fetal testis appear to be independent of human chorionic gonadotropin control. *Journal of Clinical Endocrinology and Metabolism* **69**, 204.

56 Nakamo R., Yamato M. & Nishimori K. (1995) Possibler existence of luteinizing hormone/chorionic gonadotropin receptors in human corpora lutea during early pregnancy. *Early Pregnancy: Biology and Medicine* **1**, 37.

57 Johnson M.R., Ridler A.F., Irvine R., Sharma V., Collins W.P., Nicolaides K.H. & Grudzinskas J.G. (1993) Corpus luteum failure in ectopic pregnancy. *Human Reproduction* **8**, 1491.

58 Westergaard J.G., Chemnitz J., Teisner B., Poulsen H.K., Ipsen L., Beck B. & Grudzinskas J.G. (1983) Pregnancy-associated plasma protein-A: a possible marker in the classification and prenatal diagnosis of Cornelia de Lange syndrome. *Prenatal Diagnosis* **3**, 225.

59 Sugahara T., Pixley M.R., Minami S., Perlas E., Ben-Menahem D., Huseh A.J.W. & Boime I. (1995) Biosynthesis of a biologically active single peptide chain containing the human common α and chorionic gonadotropin β subunits in tandem. *Proceedings of the National Academy of Science USA* **92**, 2041.

60 Iles R.K., Wathen N.C., Campbell D.J. & Chard T. (1992) Human chorionic gonadotrophin and subunit composition of maternal serum and coelomic and amniotic fluids in the first trimester of pregnancy. *Journal of Endocrinology* **135**, 563.

61 Blithe D.L., Richards R.G. & Skarulis M.C. (1991) Free alpha molecules from pregnancy stimulate secretion of prolactin from human decidual cells: a novel function for free alpha in pregnancy. *Endocrinology* **129**, 2257.

62 Gillott D.J., Iles R.K. & Chard T. (1966) The effects of beta-human chorionic gonadotrophin on the in vitro growth of bladder cancer cell lines. *British Journal of Cancer* **73**, 323.

63 Csapo A., Pulkkinen M.O. & Wiest W.G. (1973) Effects of luteectomy and progesterone replacement therapy in early pregnant patients. *American Journal of Obstetrics and Gynecology* **115**, 759.

64 Howell R.J.S., Olajide F., Teisner B., Grudzinskas J.G. & Chard T. (1989) Circulating levels of placental protein 14 and progesterone following Mifepristone (RU38486) and Gemeprost for termination of first trimester pregnancy. *Fertility and Sterility* **52**, 66.

65 Fu X., Rezapour M., Lofgren M., Ulmsten U. & Backstrom T. (1993) Unexpected stimulatory effect of progesterone human myometrial contractile activity in vitro. *Obstetrics and Gynecology* **82**, 23.

66 Darne J., McCarrigle H.H.G. & Lachelin G.C.L. (1987) Saliva oestriol, oestradiol, oestrone and progesterone levels in pregnancy: spontaneous labour at term is preceded by a rise in the saliva oestriol: progesterone ratio. *British Journal of Obstetrics and Gynaecology* **94**, 227.

67 Darne J., McGarrigle H.H.G. & Lachelin G.C.L. (1987) Increased saliva oestriol to progesterone ratio before idiopathic preterm delivery: a possible predictor for preterm labour? *British Medical Journal* **294**, 270

68 Csapo A.I., Knobil E., van der Molen H.J. &

432

Wiest W.G. (1971) Peripheral plasma progesterone levels during human pregnancy and labor. *American Journal of Obstetrics and Gynecology* **110**, 630.

69 Turnbull A.C., Flint A.P.F., Jeremy J.Y., Patten P.T., Keirse M.J.N.C. & Anderson A.B.M. (1974) Significant fall in progesterone and rise in oestradiol levels in human peripheral plasma before onset of labour. *Lancet* **i**, 101.

70 Raja R.L.T., Anderson A.B.M. & Turnbull A.C. (1974) Endocrine changes in premature labour. *British Medical Journal* **ii**, 67.

71 Lewis P.R., Galvin P.M. & Short R.V. (1987) Salivary oestriol and progesterone concentrations in women during late pregnancy, parturition and puerperium. *Journal of Endocrinology* **115**, 177.

72 Chew P.C.T. & Ratnam S.S. (1976) Serial plasma progesterone levels at the approach of labour. *Journal of Endocrinology* **69**, 163.

73 Chew P.C.T. & Ratnam S.S. (1976) Serial levels of plasma oestradiol-17β at the approach of labour. *Journal of Endocrinology* **71**, 267.

74 Batra S. & Bengtsson L.P. (1978) 17β-estradiol and progesterone concentrations in myometrium of pregnancy and their relationship to concentrations in peripheral plasma. *Journal of Endocrinology* **46**, 622.

75 Chard T. (1993) Placental radar. *Journal of Endocrinology* **138**, 177.

76 Simon P., Decoster C., Brocas H., Schwers J. & Vassart G. (1986) Absence of human chorionic somatomammotropin during pregnancy associated with two types of gene deletion. *Human Genetics* **74**, 235.

77 Grudzinskas J.G., Gordon Y.B., Davies B., Humphreys J., Brudenell M. & Chard T. (1979) Circulating levels of pregnancy specific beta-1-glycoprotein in pregnancies complicated by diabetes mellitus. *British Journal of Obstetrics and Gynaecology* **86**, 978.

78 Rich D.E.E. & Johansen K.A. (1993) Placental sulfatase deficiency and congenital ichthyosis with intrauterine fetal death: case report. *American Journal of Obstetrics and gynecology* **168**, 570.

79 Downing G.J., Maulik D. & Poinser A.M. (1996) Human chorionic gonadotropin stimulates placental prorenin secretion: evidence for autocrine/paracrine regulation. *Journal of Clinical Endocrinology and Metabolism* **81**, 1027.

80 Cronier L., Bastide B., Herve J.C., Beleze J. & Malassine A. (1994) Gap junctional communication during human trophoblast differentiation: influence of human chorionic gonadotrophin. *Endocrinology* **135**, 402.

81 Eta E., Ambrus G. & Rao Ch.V. (1994) Direct regulation of human myometrial contractions by human chorionic gonadotrophin. *Journal of Clinical Endocrinology and Metabolism* **79**, 1582.

82 Toth P., Li X., Lei Z.M. & Rao Ch.V. (1996) Expression of human chorionic gonadotropin (hCG)/luteinizing hormone receptors and regulation of the cyclooxygenase-1 gene by exogenous hCg in human fetal membranes. *Journal of Clinical Endocrinology and Metabolism* **81**, 1283.

83 Pavlou C., Chard T., Landon J. & Letchworth A.T. (1973) Circulating levels of human placental lactogen in late pregnancy: the effects of glucose loading, smoking and exercise. *European Journal of Obstetrics, Gynecology and Reproductive Biology* **3**, 45.

84 Menabawey M., Silman R.E., Rice A. & Chard T. (1985) Dramatic increase of placental protein 5 levels following injection of small doses of heparin. *British Journal of Obstetrics and Gynaecology* **92**, 207.

85 Kim S.J., Nam Koong S.E., Lee J.W., Jung J.K., Kang B.C. & Park J.S. (1987) Response of human chorionic gonadotrophin to luteinising hormone-releasing hormone stimulation in the culture media of normal human placenta, choriocarcinoma cell lines and in the serum of patients with gestational trophoblastic disease. *Placenta* **8**, 257.

86 Perez Lopez L.R., Robert J. & Teigeiro J. (1984) Prl, TSH, FSH, beta-hCG and oestriol response to repetitive (triple) LRH/TRH administration in the third trimester of human pregnancy. *Acta Endocrinologica (Copenhagen)* **106**, 400.

87 Iwashita M., Kudo Y., Shinozaki Y. & Takeda Y. (1993) Gonadotropin-releasing hormone increases serum human chorionic gonadotropin in pregnant women. *Endocrinology Journal* **40**, 539.

88 Bergh P.A., Anderson T.L. & Hofmann G.E. (1991) Immunohistochemical localization of gonadotropin releasing hormone during implantation in the New Zealand white rabbit. *American Journal of Obstetrics and Gynecology* **164**, 1127.

89 Chang S.Y. & Soong Y.K. (1995) Unexpected pregnancies exposed to leuprolide acetate administered after the mid-luteal phase for ovarian stimulation. *Human Reproduction* **10**, 204.

90 Szilagyi A., Benz R. & Rossmanith W.G. (1993) Human chorionic gonadotropin secretion from the early human placenta; in vitro regulation by progesterone and its antagonist. *Gynecological Endocrinology* **7**, 241.

91 Olajide F., Howell R.J.S., Wass J.A.H., Holly J.M.P., Bohn H., Grudzinskas J.G., Chapman M.G. *et al.* (1989) Circulating levels of placental protein 12 and chorionic gonadotrophin following RU38486 and Gemeprost for termination of first trimester pregnancy. *Human Reproduction* **4**, 337.

92 Katsuragawa H., Kanzaki H., Inoue T., Hirano T., Narukawa S., Watanabe H. & Mori T. (1995) Endometrial stromal cell decidualization inhibits human chorionic gonadotrophin and human placental lactogen secretion by co-cultured trophoblasts. *Human Reproduction* **10**, 3028.

93 Simmer H.H., Frankland M. & Greipel M. (1975) On the regulation of fetal and maternal 16α-hydroxydehydroepiandrosterone and its sulfate by cortisol and ACTH in human pregnancy at term. *American Journal of Obstetrics and Gynecology* **121**, 646.

94 Chard T. (1986) Placental synthesis. In *Clinics in Obstetrics and Gynaecology: The Human Placenta*. T. Chard, p. 447. WB Saunders Company, London.

95 Kastin A.J., Arimura A. & Schally A.V. (1971) Mass action-type direct feedback control of pituitary release. *Nature* **231**, 29.

96 Everett, R.B. Porter, J.C., MacDonald, P.C. & Gant,

N.F. (1980) Relationship of maternal plasma dehydroandrosterone sulfate through placental estradiol formation. *American Journal of Obstetrics and Gynecology* **136**. 435.

97 Fritz M.A., Stanczyk F.Z. & Novy M.J. (1985) Relationship of uteroplacental blood flow to the placental clearance of maternal dehydroepiandrosterone through estradiol formation in the pregnant baboon. *Journal of Clinical Endocrinology and Metabolism* **61**, 1023.

98 Senner J.W., Stanczyk F.Z., Fritz M.A. & Novy M.J. (1985) Relationship of uteroplacental blood flow to placental clearance of maternal plasma C-19 steroids: evaluation of mathematical models. *American Journal of Obstetrics and Gynaecology* **153**, 573.

99 Reshef E., Lei Z.M., Rao C.V., Pridham D.D., Chegini N. & Luborsky J.L. (1990) The presence of gonadotropin receptors in nonpregnant human uterus, human placenta, fetal membranes and decidua. *Journal of Clinical Endocrinology and Metabolism* **70**, 421.

100 Lei Z.M. & Rao C.V. (1992) Gonadotropin receptors in human fetoplacental unit: implications for hCG as an intracrine, paracrine and endocrine regulator of human fetoplacental function. In *Trophoblast Research: Placental Signals: Autocrine and Paracrine Control of Pregnancy*, 6th edn. Ed. L. Cedard & A. Firth, p. 213. University of Rochester Press, Rochester, N.Y.

101 Shi Q.J., Lei Z.M., Rao C.V. & Lin J. (1993) Novel role of human chorionic gonadotropin in differentiation of human cytotrophoblasts. *Endocrinology* **132**, 1387.

102 Iwashita M., Evans M.I. & Catt K.J. (1986) Characterization of a gonadotropin-releasing hormone receptor site in term placenta and chorionic villi. *Journal of Clinical Endocrinology and Metabolism* **62**, 127.

103 Licht P., Cao H., Lei Z.M., Rao C.V. & Merz W.E. (1993) Novel self-regulation of human chorionic gonadotropin biosynthesis in term pregnancy human placenta. *Endocrinology* **133**, 3014.

104 Song E.J., Gelboin H.V. & Park S.S. (1985) Monoclonal antibody-directed radioimmunoassay detects cytochrome P-450 in human placenta and lymphocytes. *Science* **228**, 490.

105 Bernstein L., Pike M.C., Lobo R.A., Depue R.H., Ross R.K. & Henderson B.E. (1989) Cigarette smoking in pregnancy results in marked decrease in maternal hCG and oestradiol levels. *British Journal of Obstetrics and Gynaecology* **96**, 92.

106 Bartels I., Hoppe-Sievert B., Bockel B., Herold S. & Caesar J. (1993) Adjustment formulae for maternal serum alpha-fetoprotein, human chorionic gonadotropin, and unconjugated oestriol to maternal weight and smoking. *Prenatal Diagnosis* **13**, 123.

107 Cuckle H.S., Wald N.J., Densem P., Knight G.J., Haddow J.E., Palomaki G.E. & Canick J.A. (1990) The effect of smoking in pregnancy on maternal serum alpha-fetoprotein, unconjugated oestriol, human chorionic gonadotrophin, progesterone and dehydroepiandrosterone sulphate levels. *British Journal of Obstetrics and Gynaecology* **97**, 272.

108 Lee J.N., Grudzinskas J.G. & Chard T. (1980) Circulating human placental lactogen (HPL) levels in relation to smoking during pregnancy. *Journal of Obstetrics and Gynaecology* **1**, 87.

109 Bissenden J.G., Scott P.H., Hallum J., Mansfield H.N. & Scott P. (1981) Racial variations in tests of fetoplacental function. *British Journal of Obstetrics and Gynaecology* **88**, 109.

110 Simpson J.L., Elias S., Morgan C.D., Shulman L., Umstot E. & Anderson R.N. (1990) Second trimester maternal serum human chorionic gonadotrophin and unconjugated oestriol levels in blacks and whites. *Lancet* **335**, 1459.

111 Muller F. & Boue A. (1990) A single chorionic gonadotropin assay for maternal screening for Down's syndrome. *Prenatal Diagnosis* **10**, 389.

112 Kulch P., Keener S., Matsumoto M. & Crandall B.F. (1993) Racial differences in maternal serum human chorionic gonadotropin and unconjugated oestriol levels. *Prenatal Diagnosis* **13**, 191.

113 Bogart M.H., Jones O.W., Felder R.A., Best R.G., Bradley L., Butts W., Crandall B. *et al.* (1991) Prospective evaluation of maternal serum human chorionic gonadotropin levels in 3428 pregnancies. *American Journal of Obstetrics and Gynecology* **165**, 663.

114 Petrocik E., Wassman E.R. & Kelly J.C. (1989) Prenatal screening for Down syndrome with maternal serum human chorionic gonadotropin levels. *American Journal of Obstetrics and Gynecology* **161**, 1168.

115 Ylikorkala O. & Pennanen S. (1973) Human placental lactogen (hPL) levels in maternal serum during abortion induced by intra- and extra amniotic injection of prostaglandin F2-alpha. *Journal of Obstetrics and Gynaecology of the British Commonwealth* **80**, 927.

116 Obiekwe B.C. & Chard T. (1983) Placental proteins in late pregnancy: relation to fetal sex. *Journal of Obstetrics and Gynaecology* **3**, 163.

117 Leporrier N., Herrou M. & Leymarie P. (1992) Shift of the fetal sex ratio in hCG selected pregnancies at risk for Down syndrome. *Prenatal Diagnosis* **12**, 703.

118 Muller F., Aegertier P. & Boue A.(1993) Prospective maternal serum human chorionic gonadotropin screening for the risk of fetal chromosome anomalies and of subsequent fetal and neonatal deaths. *Prenatal Diagnosis* **13**, 29.

119 Suchy S.F. & Yeager M.T. (1990) Down syndrome screening in women under 35 with maternal serum hCG. *Obstetrics and Gynecology* **76**, 20.

120 Wheeler T., Sollero C., Alderman S., Landen J., Anthony F. & Osmond C. (1994) Relation between maternal haemoglobin and placental hormone concentrations in early pregnancy. *Lancet* **343**, 511.

121 Maaskant R.A., Bogic L.V., Gilger S., Kelly P.A. & Bryant-Greenwood G.D. (1996) The human prolactin receptor in the fetal membranes, decidua, and placenta. *Journal of Clinical Endocrinology and Metabolism* **81**, 396.

122 Shinozaki H., Minegishi T., Nakamura K., Tano M., Miyamoto K. & Ibuki Y. (1995) Type II and type IIB activin receptors in human placenta. *Life Science* **56**, 1699.

123 Knock G.A., Sullivan M.H., McCarthy A., Elder M.G., Polak J.M. & Wharton J. (1994) Angiotensin II (AT1) vascular binding sites in human placentae from normal-term, preeclamptic and growth retarded

434

pregnancies. *Journal of Pharmacology and Experimental Therapy* **271**, 1007.

124 Lafond J., Simoneau L., Savard R. & Lajeunesse D. (1994) Calcitonin receptor in human placental syncytiotrophoblast brush border and basal plasma membranes (published erratum appears in *Molecular Cell Endocrinology* **103**, 171). *Molecular and Cellular Endocrinology* **99**, 285.

125 Kingdom J.C., McQueen J., Ryan G., Connell J.M. & Whittle M.J. (1994) Fetal vascular atrial natriuretic peptide receptors in human placenta: alteration in intrauterine growth retardation and preeclampsia. *American Journal of Obstetrics and Gynaecology* **170**, 142.

126 Horie K., Takakura K., Imai K., Liao S. & Mori T. (1992) Immunohistochemical localization of androgen receptor in the human endometrium, decidua, placenta and pathological conditions of the endometrium. *Human Reproduction* **7**, 1461.

127 Clifton V.L., Owens P.C., Robinson P.J. & Smith R. (1995) Identification and characterization of a corticotrophin-releasing hormone receptor in human placenta. *European Journal of Endocrinology* **133**, 591.

128 Cooper J.C., Sharkey A.M., McLaren J., Charnock-Jones D.S. & Smith S.K. (1995) Localization of vascular endothelial growth factor and its receptor, flt, in human placenta and decidua by immunohistochemistry. *Journal of Reproduction and Fertility* **105**, 205.

129 Evain-Brion D. & Alsat E. (1994) Epidermal growth factor receptor and human fetoplacental development [Review]. *Journal of Pediatric Endocrinology* **7**, 295.

130 Kojima K., Kanzaki H., Iwai M., Hatayama H., Fujimoto M., Narukawa S., Higuchi T. *et al.* (1995) Expression of leukaemia inhibitory factor (LIF) receptor in human placenta: a possible role for LIF in the growth and differentiation of trophoblasts. *Human Reproduction* **10**, 1907.

131 Saito S., Fukunaga R., Ichijo M. & Nagata S. (1994) Expression of granulocyte colony-stimulating factor and its receptor at the fetomaternal interface in murine and human pregnancy. *Growth Factors* **10**, 135.

132 Jokhi P.P., Chumbley G., King A., Gardner L. & Loke Y.W. (1993) Expression of the colony stimulating facto-1 receptor (c-fms product) by cells at the human uteroplacental interface. *Laboratory Investigations* **68**, 308.

133 Holmgren L., Claesson-Welsh L, Heldin C.H. & Ohlsson R. (1992) The expression of PDGF alpha- and beta-receptors in subpopulations of PDGF-producing cells implicates autocrine stimulatory loops in the control of proliferation in cytotrophoblasts that have invaded the maternal endometrium. *Growth Factors* **6**, 219.

134 Baergen R., Benirschke K. & Ulich T.R. (1994) Cytokine expression in the placenta. The role of interleukin 1 and interleukin 1 receptor antagonist expression in chorioamnionitis and parturition. *Archives of Pathology and Laboratory Medicine* **118**, 52.

135 Paulesu L., Romagnoli R., Cintorino M., Ricci M.G. & Garotta G. (1994) First trimester human trophoblast expresses both interferon-gamma and interferon-gamma-receptor. *Journal of Reproductive Immunology* **27**, 37.

136 Yelavarthi K.K. & Hunt J.S. (1993) Analysis of p60 and p80 tumor necrosis factor-alpha receptor messenger RNA and protein in human placentas *American Journal of Pathology* **143**, 1131.

137 Chard T. & Grudzinskas J.G. (1987) Early pregnancy factor. *Biological Research in Pregnancy* **8**, 53.

138 Kadar N., Bohrer M., Kemman E. & Shelden R. (1993) A prospective randomized study of the chorionic gonadotropin-time relationship in early gestation: clinical implications. *Fertility and Sterility* **60**, 409.

139 Chard T. (1991) Frequency of implantation and early pregnancy loss in natural cycles. *Baillière's Clinical Obstetrics and Gynaecology* **5**, 179.

140 Niven P.A.R., Chard T. & Landon J. (1972) Placental lactogen levels as a guide to the outcome of threatened abortion. *British Medical Journal* **3**, 799.

141 Salem H.T., Ghaneimah S.A., Shaaban M.M. & Chard T. (1984) Prognostic value of biochemical tests in the assessment of fetal outcome in threatened abortion. *British Journal of Obstetrics and Gynaecology* **91**, 382.

142 Pedersen J.F., Ruge S. & Sorensen S. (1995) Depressed serum levels of human placental lactogen in first trimester vaginal bleeding. *Obstetrica Gynecologica Scandinavica* **74**, 27.

143 Al-Sebai M.A.H., Kingsland C.R., Diver M., Hipkin L. & McFadyen I.R. (1995) The role of a single progesterone measurement in the diagnosis of early pregnancy failure and the prognosis of fetal viability. *British Journal of Obstetrics and Gynaecology* **102**, 364–369.

144 Stabile I., Grudzinskas J.G. & Campbell S. (1987) Ultrasonic assessment of complications during first trimester pregnancy. *Lancet* **ii**, 1237.

145 Johnson M.R., Riddle A.F., Grudzinskas J.G., Sharma V., Collins W.P. & Nicolaides K.H. (1993) The role of trophoblast dysfunction in the aetiology of miscarriage. *British Journal of Obstetrics and Gynaecology*, **100**, 353.

146 Check J.H. & Lurie D. (1992) Analysis of serum human chorionic gonadotrophin levels in normal, singleton, mutiple and abnormal pregnancies. *Human Reproduction* **7**, 1176.

147 Heiner S.J., Kerin J.F., Schmidt L.L. & Wu T.C.J. (1992) Can a single, early quantitative human chorionic gonadotropin measurement in an in vitro fertilization-gamete intrafallopian transfer program predict pregnancy outcome. *Fertility and Sterility* **58**, 373.

148 Yovich J.L., McColin J.C., Wilcox D.L., Grudzinskas J.G. & Bolton A.E. (1986) The prognostic value of beta hCG, PAPP-A, oestradiol and progesterone in early human pregnancies and the effect of medroxy progesterone acetate. *Australian and New Zealand Journal of Obstetrics and Gynacology* **26**, 59.

149 Jouppila P., Seppala M. & Chard T. (1980) Pregnancy specific beta-1 glycoprotein in complications of early pregnancy. *Lancet* **i**, 667.

150 Seppala M., Ranta T., Tontti K., Stenman U.H. & Chard T. (1980) Use of a rapid hCG-beta subunit

radioimmunoassay in acute gynaecological emergencies. *Lancet* **i**, 165.

151 Stabile I., Campbell S. & Grudzinskas J.G. (1988) Can ultrasound reliably diagnose ectopic pregnancy? *British Journal of Obstetrics and Gynaecology* **95**, 1247.

152 Norman R.J., Lowings C. & Chard T. (1985) Dipstick method for human chorionic gonadotropin suitable for emergency use on whole blood and other fluids *Lancet* **7**, 19.

153 Kadar N., Bohrer M., Kemman E. & Shelden R. (1994) The discriminatory human chorionic gonadotropin zone for endovaginal sonography: a prospective, randomized study. *Fertility and Sterility* **61**, 1016.

154 Kadar N. (1983) Ectopic pregnancy. In *Progress in Obstetrics and Gynaecology*. Ed. J. Studd, p. 305. Churchill Livingstone, Edinburgh.

155 Rottem S. & Timor-Tritsch I.E. (1988) *Transvaginal Ultrasonography*. p. 125. Heinemann Medical Books, London.

156 Keith S.C., London S.N., Weitzman G.A., O'Brien T.J. & Miller M.M. (1993) Serial transvaginal ultrasound scans and beta-human chorionic gonadotropin levels in early singleton and multiple pregnancies. *Fertility and Sterility* **59**, 1007.

157 Chemnitz J., Tornehave D., Teisner B., Poulsen H.K. & Westergaard J.G. (1994) The localisation of pregnancy proteins (hPL, SP1 and PAPP-A) in intra- and extrauterine pregnancies. *Placenta* **489**, 494.

158 Sinosich M.J. (1985) Biological role of pregnancy-associated plasma protein A in human reproduction. In *Proteins of the Placenta*. Eds P. Bischof & A. Klopper, p. 184. Karger, Basel.

159 Stern J.J., Voss F. & Coulam C.B. (1993) Early diagnosis of ectopic pregnancy using receiver-operator characteristic curves of serum progesterone concentrations. *Human Reproduction* **8**, 775.

160 Stovall T.G., Ling F.W., Carson S.A. & Buster J.E. (1992) Serum progesterone and uterine curettage in differential diagnosis of ectopic pregnancy. *Fertility Digest* **57**, 456.

161 Stovall T.G., Ling F.W., Cope B.J. & Buster J.E. (1989) Preventing ruptured ectopic pregnancy with a single serum progesterone. *American Journal of Obstetrics and Gynecology* **160**, 1425.

162 Grosskinsky C.M., Hage M.L., Tyrey L., Christakos A.C. & Hughes C.L. (1993) hCG, progesterone, alphafetoprotein, and estradiol in the identification of ectopic pregnancy. *Obstetrics and Gynecology* **81**, 705.

163 Stovall T.G., Ling F.W., Andersen R.N. & Buster J.E. (1992) Improved sensitivity and specificity of a single measurement of serum progesterone over serial quantitative beta-human chorionic gonadotrophin in screening for ectopic pregnancy. *Human Reproduction* **7**, 723.

164 Ledger W.L., Sweeting V.M. & Chatterjee S. (1994) Rapid diagnosis of early ectopic pregnancy in an emergency gynaecology service: are measurements of progestereone, intact and free beta human chorionic gonadotrophin helpful? *Human Reproduction* **9**, 157.

165 Cacciatore B., Stenman U.H. & Ylostalo P. (1994) Early screening for ectopic pregnancy in high-risk symptom-free women. *Lancet* **343**, 517.

166 Chard T. & Macintosh M. (1995) Screening for Downs syndrome. *Current Medical Litcraturc: Obstetrics and Gynaecology* **1**, 3.

167 Iles R.K. & Chard T. (1989) Enhancement of ectopic beta-human chorionic gonadotrophin expression by interferon. *Journal of Endocrinology* **123**, 501.

168 Chard T., Kitau M.J., Ledward R., Coltart T., Embury S. & Seller M.J. (1975) Elevated levels of maternal plasma alphafetoprotein after amniocentesis. *British Journal of Obstetrics and Gynaecology* **83**, 33.

169 Knott P.D., Chan B., Ward R.H.T., Chard T., Grudzinskas J.G., Petrou M. & Model B. (1988) Changes in circulating alphafetoprotein and human chorionic gonadotrophin following chorionic villus sampling. *European Journal of Obstetrics, Gynecology and Reproductive Biology* **27**, 277.

170 Naik K., Kitau M., Setchell M.E. & Chard T. (1988) The incidence of fetomaternal haemorrhage following elective termination of first-trimester pregnancy. *European Journal of Obstetrics, Gynecology and Reproductive Biology* **27**, 355.

171 Chard T., Olajide F. & Kitau M. (1990) Changes in circulating alphafetoprotein following administration of mifepristone in first trimester pregnancy. *British Journal of Obstetrical and Gynaecology* **97**, 1030.

172 Beischer N., Brown J., Parkinson P. & Walstab J. (1991) Urinary oestriol assay for monitoring fetoplacental function. *Australian and New Zealand Journal of Obstetrics and Gynaecology* **31**, 1.

173 Chard T. & Klopper A. (1982) *Placental Function Tests*. Springer-Verlag, Berlin.

174 Chard T. (1987) What is happening to placental function tests? *Annals of Clinical Biochemistry* **24**, 435.

175 Chard T. & Grudzinskas J.G. (1992) Placental proteins and steroids and the immune relationship between mother and fetus. In *Immunological Obstetrics*. Eds C.B. Coulam, W. Page Faulk & J.A. Mclntyre, p. 282. W.W. Norton & Company, New York.

176 Zhou A.M., Tewari P.C., Bluestein B.I., Caldwell G.W. & Larsen F.L. (1993) Multiple forms of prostate-specific antigen in serum: differences in immuno-recognition by monoclonal and polyclonal assays. *Clinical Chemistry* **39**, 2483.

177 Iles R.K., Wathen N.C., Sharma K.B., Campbell J., Grudzinskas J.G. & Chard T. (1994) Pregnancy-associated plasma protein A levels in maternal serum, extraembryonic coelomic and amniotic fluids in the first trimester. *Placenta* **15**, 693.

178 Jauniaux E., Gulbis B., Jurkovic D., Schaaps J.P., Campbell S. & Meuris S. (1993) Protein and steroid levels in embryonic cavities in early human pregnancy. *Human Reproduction* **8**, 782.

179 Wathen N.C., Cass P.L., Campbell D.J., Kitau M.J. & Chard T. (1992) Levels of placental protein 14, human placental lactogen and unconjugated oestriol in extraembryonic coelomic fluid. *Placenta* **13**, 195.

PART 6

The Fetus

Conception to Implantation

G. COTICCHIO & S. FISHEL

Embryogenesis begins during oogenesis. E.B. WILSON, 1925

Follicular and oocyte growth

Throughout the historical ages, the ability of the oocyte to support the formation of a new organism has stimulated the interest of philosophers and scientists. Both classical embryology studies and recent findings suggest that successful fertilization and development of the embryo depend on the accomplishment of processes occurring in both the nuclear and cytoplasmic components of the oocyte during oogenesis. This has direct implications for assisted reproduction technology. Current methods for assessing oocyte quality in routine in-vitro fertilization (IVF) are poorly informative, yet this factor largely affects the ability of the embryo to develop and implant.

During fetal life, primordial germ cells are first distinguishable in the yolk sac by alkaline phosphatase staining [1]. These cells migrate through the dorsal mesentery of the hindgut, reach the genital ridges and invade the indifferent gonads after the 26th day post-fertilization in humans [2]. Here, germ cells, commonly referred to as oogonia, lose their motility and undergo rapid proliferation. When the proliferative phase is completed, oogonia are transformed into oocytes. This change is followed by entry into the meiotic prophase. Chromosomes, consisting of two sister chromatids, condense at leptotene, establish synapses with their homologues at zygotene, undergo recombination at pachytene, but prematurely arrest in the diplotene stage, before the first meiotic division takes place [3]. The oocyte nucleus, known as the germinal vesicle, does not undergo further development until ovulation, remaining arrested at this stage of meiosis, also referred to as the dictyate stage, for up to forty or more years. In humans, entry into meiosis is not a synchronized event for all oogonia. Although in a proportion of germ cells meiosis can start as soon as the second month of gestation, some oogonia do not enter meiosis until the 7th month of gestation [4]. Entry into meiosis is accompanied by extensive attrition. The number of oocytes is approximately 7 millions at the 5th month of gestation, but there are no more than 1 million germ cells in the infant at birth [5]. The reason for such a massive phenomenon of cell death is not known. However, since this event is temporally associated with chromosome recombination at pachytene [6], it has been speculated that this could reflect the need to eliminate oocytes characterized by gross meiotic anomalies.

Entry into meiosis is followed by the formation of the primordial follicle. Somatic cells, probably derived, at least in some mammals, from the mesonephric tissue [7], are induced

440 to differentiate into granulosa cells, forming a flattened monolayer around the oocyte. The oocyte is the causal element for this process of differentiation, as pathological or experimental oocyte loss prevents the determination of the somatic component of the primordial follicle.

At birth, the pool of primordial follicles represents a non-renewable source of non-growing germ cells and its accidental loss invariably leads to a permanent state of infertility. This pool rests in the ovarian cortex and progressively decreases with age [8], with only a few follicles remaining in the ovaries of post-menopausal women. Atresia, a process of programmed follicular cell death, plays a significant role in the depletion of the non-growing follicles [9]. Initiation of follicular growth is the other factor involved in the reduction of the pool of primordial follicles. The departure of the primordial follicle from the non-growing pool may occur at any time from fetal life throughout infancy, puberty and reproductive life. It is not clear what triggers follicle growth at this early stage. Although gonadotrophins may exert a priming action during fetal life [10], they appear not to be involved in promoting the early stages of follicle growth. Vice versa, local growth-regulating factors are thought to play a major role in this process [11]. Growth is accompanied by migration through the ovarian tissue [12]. Primordial follicles, which are situated in the ovarian cortex, progressively move towards the medullary region, as they start to grow. Formation of the antrum reverses this movement, forcing follicles towards the surface of the organ. However, the large majority of developing follicles are destined to degenerate at some stage of the growth phase (Fig. 17.1). In fact, only a minute fraction, approximately 0.05% in humans, of the original number of primordial follicles achieves ovulation.

Follicle development is essential for oocyte function. The oocyte resting in the primordial follicle is incompetent to complete meiosis, achieve fertilization and support the development of the embryo. The non-growing oocyte is only apparently 'quiescent', showing the measurable synthetic activity required to repair and replace cellular components over a prolonged period of time. In order to achieve full com-

Fig. 17.1. Schematic illustration of follicular growth and selection. The relative size of the various types of follicles is not drawn to scale and their number does not reflect the corresponding proportion in the entire follicle population. Despite the fact that growing follicles are continuously recruited from the primordial pool, only a very small proportion of them achieve ovulation during reproductive life. The follicles which are not destined to ovulate undergo degeneration (atresia) at some stage of their growth, including the primordial phase.

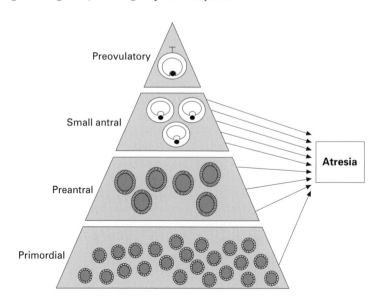

petence, the oocyte has to undergo increase in mass, complete nuclear maturation and promote a series of cytoplasmic changes which are believed to be fundamental for supporting early development, despite being only partially understood.

The human primordial oocyte measures about 35 μm. Over a period of several months [13], the human oocyte volume undergoes a fourfold expansion, reaching the final size of 120 μm shortly after antrum formation. This expansion parallels the rate of accumulation of proteins and RNAs. Mammalian embryos rely on maternal support for their growth. Therefore they are not expected to accumulate yolk in their cytoplasm, as opposed to species whose development occurs in the external environment. Nevertheless, it is not entirely clear yet if mammalian oocytes build up a small reserve of non-informational material needed by the early embryo.

During oocyte growth, the germinal vesicle also increases in size, although the overall nucleus to cytoplasm ratio progressively decreases. In the human oocyte, chromatin is not entirely dispersed at any stage of growth and individual chromosomal threads are still visible. Chromosomes are locally decondensed to form lateral loops, where RNA transcription actively occurs [14]. Numerous nucleoli are also formed in order to synthesize large amounts of rRNA.

In small oocytes, cytoplasmic organelles are mainly confined in the perinuclear region. Onset of growth coincides with their migration towards the oocyte surface [15,16]. Small vesicles form from the dissociation of the Golgi apparatus, to assist the release of glycoproteins into the extracellular environment. With some delay after the initiation of growth, cortical granules are also generated. In the mature egg, they migrate to a position close to the plasmalemma and the release of their contents, following sperm-mediated activation, is essential to prevent polyspermic fertilization. Mitochondria also undergo significant changes during oocyte growth. They increase in size, acquire an oval or round shape, and their internal cristae transform into columnar structures. The maternal mitochondrial complement is vital to the embryo, as very little contribution, if any, comes from the spermatozoon [17]. Both rough and smooth endoplasmic reticula (ER) are distinguishable in the growing oocyte, although they are not particularly conspicuous.

The beginning of the growth phase coincides with the activation of the synthesis of rRNA, tRNA and other small RNAs. These RNAs accumulate until meiotic resumption, when their levels start to decrease [18]. Poly(A)+ RNA, which directs protein synthesis, is also accumulated and accounts for about 8% of the total RNA contents of the mature egg. It is worth noting that, although maternal transcripts in the mammalian embryo play a less crucial role compared to other species, such as *Xenopus laevis*, nevertheless, during maturation and at least the first cell cycle of the fertilized egg, protein synthesis entirely relies on stored RNA [19].

Large amounts of proteins are also produced in the developing oocyte to provide components essential to the increase in its cell mass. To this end, cytoskeletal proteins. RNA-binding proteins, zona pellucida proteins (see below), membrane-bound proteins and housekeeping enzymes are synthesized. Some of these enzymes may persist after fertilization until the 4–8-cell stage [20]. So, in mammals, proteins are also stored in the growing oocyte and used at a later stage by the early embryo.

Zona pellucida

In the human, the zona pellucida is an extracellular vestment measuring approximately 15 μm in thickness, progressively laid down during oogenesis as soon the resting oocytes start the growth phase, apparently without contribution from adjacent granulosa cells [21]. It shows a fibrillogranular structure, permeable to enzymes, immunoglobulins and small viruses. The surface arrangement is different on the inner and outer surfaces. Cytoplasmic channels pass from the attendant corona radiata cells through the zona pellucida, interacting with the oocyte in the form of gap junctions, and the retraction of these processes prior to fertilization has been suggested to leave channels for the passage of spermatozoa [22]. The properties of the zona pellucida vary at different stages, and increases in porosity before fertilization presumably facilitate sperm penetration. After fertilization, the zona pellucida is covered with oviductal glycosaminoglycans. Also at this time, the properties of the zona pellucida change, becoming less soluble to proteases, low pH or the disruption of covalent and non-covalent bonds. The zona pellucida is antigenic and immunization can prevent follicular growth, ovulation, and fertilization in several species. Sperm–egg interactions can be inhibited by antibodies raised against zona pellucida proteins [23]. In humans, anti-zona antibodies are thought to be involved in some cases of infertility.

At the molecular level, the zona pellucida is made up of three major extensively glycosylated proteins, ZP1 (200 kDa), ZP2 (120 kDa) and ZP3 (83 kDa), possessing both N-linked and O-linked oligosaccharide side chains connected to the polypeptide structure through asparagine and serine/threonine residues, respectively [24]. These proteins form a porous mesh in which polymers of ZP2-ZP3 are interconnected by heterodimers of ZP1. ZP3 is responsible for species-specific egg sperm recognition and induction of the acrosome reaction through a specific O-linked oligosaccharide [25,26]. ZP2 plays a distinct role, by binding acrosome-reacted sperm and assisting their penetration through the zona [27].

The molecular genetics of human ZP3 [28] and ZP2 [29] has been researched in detail. In particular, ZP3 is a 424 residues protein characterized by many serine and threonine subunits, potentially available for O-linked glycosylation. Zona pellucida proteins are not related to other extracellular matrix components and are highly conserved among mammalian species. ZP3 expression is specifically regulated during oocyte development. In fact, the number of ZP3 transcripts is progressively increased during the growth phase, is partially reduced when the oocyte reaches full size, and is dramatically decreased to non significant levels at fertilization [24].

Control of meiosis

Meiosis fulfils two fundamental functions: it creates new combinations of genes by reshuffling the maternal and paternal genomes and generates haploid gametes required for sexual reproduction. For unknown reasons, in the mammalian female, meiosis is initiated several years before eggs achieve full maturation. As described above, this process is arrested in the diplotene stage, before the segregation of homologue chromosomes. This early arrest probably meets the need of having a diploid set of chromosomes during oocyte growth, in order to ensure the expression of both maternal and paternal alleles during this crucial phase.

The meiotic cycle is designed on the scheme of the mitotic cycle. In somatic cells, the cell cycle is divided into distinct phases. During the mitotic phase, or M phase, nuclear division occurs and the cell is separated into two daughter cells. In the interval between two consecutive mitoses, cells undergo growth during the G_1 and G_2 phases and replicate their nuclear DNA during the S phase. A biochemical device, the cell cycle control system, promotes the accomplishment of the various phases and coordinates them in a fixed order according to the sequence $M \rightarrow G_1 \rightarrow S \rightarrow G_2 \rightarrow M$, to ensure that cells double their mass before undergoing division and the number of chromosomes is not altered throughout repeated cycles of division. This control system acts at specific checkpoints, where it can prevent the triggering of the following phase, if essential events of the preceding phase have not been completed. Figure 17.2 shows the three major checkpoints [30]:

1 Start, at the end of the G_1 phase, the system checks that the cell has undergone a sufficient rate of growth before undertaking DNA replication.

2 Entry, at the end of the G_2 phase, the system does not promote mitosis unless all DNA is replicated and the cell has undergone further growth.

3 Exit, during the M phase, chromosome segregation and cell division are prevented if chromosomes are not correctly aligned on the mitotic spindle.

The cell cycle control system has been shown to be essentially the same in organisms as different as human and yeast, although minor differences may exist. The whole system is based on the activity of protein kinases and relative regulatory components [31]. Some of these proteins are highly conserved and many of them are

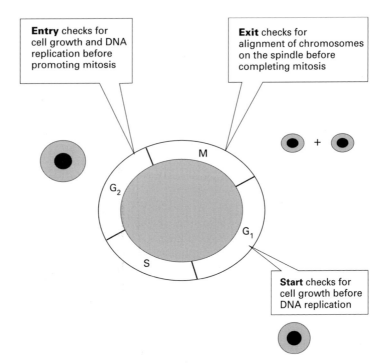

Entry checks for cell growth and DNA replication before promoting mitosis

Exit checks for alignment of chromosomes on the spindle before completing mitosis

Start checks for cell growth before DNA replication

Fig. 17.2. Schematic representation of the cell division cycle. Newly formed cells increase their mass during the G_1 and G_2 phases, duplicate their DNA during the S phase and undergo cell division during the M phase. In this cyclical process, the **start**, **entry** and **exit** checkpoints are strategically positioned to ensure that the various phases take place provided that appropriate conditions exist.

encoded by proto-oncogenes. Two families of proteins play a fundamental role in the control system. One is a group of cyclin-dependent protein kinases (Cdk) which promote downstream events of the various phases of the cycle by phosphorylating specific proteins on serine and threonine residues. The other one is a group of regulatory proteins, cyclins, which bind to Cdk thereby promoting the kinase activity of these enzymes. Alteration of the levels of these proteins is a major mechanism by which the control of the cell cycle is achieved at specific checkpoints. In fact, fluctuating levels of cyclins lead to periodic formation of active Cdk-cyclin complexes in order to determine the pace of the various events occurring throughout the cycle. Other important components of the cell cycle control system are a series of protein kinases and phosphatases which phosphorylate and dephosphorylate specific sites on Cdk and cyclin, thereby regulating the activity of these components irrespective of their levels.

The components that control meiosis are fundamentally the same as those of the mitotic cycle, although their regulation is probably dif-ferent, as meiosis gives rise to the generation of a haploid cell. In meiosis, the first division is immediately followed by the second division, without intervening cell growth and DNA synthesis, according to the sequence M(mitotic) $\rightarrow$ $G_1 \rightarrow S \rightarrow G_2 \rightarrow$ 1st meiotic division $\rightarrow$ 2nd meiotic division. This chain of events is controlled at two principal checkpoints, the diplotene stage (corresponding to the G_2 phase of the mitotic cycle) in immature oocytes and the metaphase of the 2nd meiotic division (MII) in fully mature oocytes. Under physiological conditions, the signals that trigger the resumption of meiosis at these checkpoints are the luteinizing hormone (LH) surge at ovulation [32] and sperm penetration at fertilization, respectively. Resumption at the checkpoint between G_2 and the metaphase of the 1st meiotic division (MI) is triggered by activation of a specific type of Cdk/cyclin complex, referred to as M-phase promoting factor, or MPF, derived from the association of the Cdk p34[cdc2] with the cyclin B type [33]. This activity gradually increases during the G_2/MI transition, peaks at MI, decreases during the intervening period between MI and MII

444

when the oocyte extrudes the first polar body and again reaches high levels in MII-arrested oocytes (Fig. 17.3) [34]. At this stage, sperm penetration causes a calcium-mediated drop of MPF activity [35] which induces extrusion of the second polar body and completion of meiosis.

Non-growing oocytes are arrested in the meiotic prophase and are intrinsically incompetent to resume meiosis. In contrast, irrespective of the LH-mediated signal, fully grown oocytes can resume meiosis and progress to MII when released from antral follicles and cultured *in vitro* [36,37]. It follows that, at some stage of their growth, oocytes acquire the ability to progress through the cycle. In the mouse, it has been shown that this ability is gradually developed, as oocytes which are not quite fully grown can achieve resumption at the first checkpoint, undergoing germinal vesicle breakdown, but prematurely arrest at MI [38]. The inability of incompetent oocytes to resume meiosis is probably due to inadequate levels of components of the cell cycle control mechanism. In the mouse, although in growing and fully grown oocytes the

levels of cyclin B are the same, the levels of the other MPF component, p34cdc2, are lower in the smaller oocytes [39]. An abrupt increase in p34cdc2 levels at the time of the acquisition of the ability to progress to MI suggests that inadequate MPF activity is responsible for the incompetence of small oocytes. It has also been speculated that partially competent oocytes are incapable of promoting a drop in MPF activity in order to progress beyond MI. Persistent high levels of MPF have been shown to occur in the meiotic block of LT/Sv mice, in which most oocytes are arrested at MI even when they are fully grown [40].

As already described, until ovulation, the follicular environment exerts an inhibitory effect on the ability of fully grown oocytes to resume meiosis and progress to MII. Several lines of evidence suggest that, at least in rodents, high levels of cyclic adenosine 3′,5′-monophosphate (cAMP) are directly involved in maintaining the meiotic block at diplotene, as soon as the oocyte develops meiotic competence [41]. It is not known how this effect is achieved, but it is

Fig. 17.3. Changes in p34cdc2 kinase activity during maturation and fertilization. By a cascade of events which is not fully understood, the LH surge at midcycle triggers an increase in p34cdc2 activity and consequent breakdown of the germinal vesicle. Further changes in the same activity drive the oocyte to the metaphase of meiosis II. Until sperm penetration, high p34cdc2 kinase activity arrests the oocyte at this stage, preventing premature completion of meiosis and parthenogenetic development.

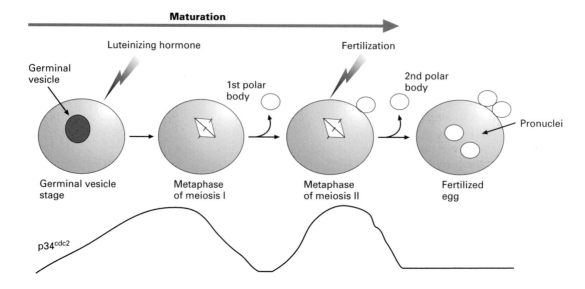

suspected that cAMP promotes a cascade of events which prevent MPF activation. cAMP has also been suggested to prevent meiotic resumption in human oocytes [42]. In mice, a drop in cAMP levels occurs during germinal vesicle breakdown, but it is not clear if this is the principal cause for meiotic resumption. Oscillations in intracellular calcium are thought be the principal signal which directly determines MPF activation and reinitiation of the meiotic cycle [43]. This view is supported by the fact that that calcium is a universal regulator of the cell cycle [30]. Furthermore, calcium has been shown to promote meiotic resumption in various non-mammalian species and calcium changes have been observed during germinal vesicle breakdown in the mouse [44]. Calcium also plays a key role in the reinitiation of the meiotic cycle at MII during fertilization [45]. Significantly, the role of calcium is consistent with LH action. In fact, it is known that binding of this hormone to its receptor on granulosa cells can give rise to increase in intracellular calcium [46]. As granulosa cells, cumulus cells and the oocyte form a functional syncytium due to the presence of gap junctions, it has been suggested that LH-induced calcium changes in the granulosa cells may be conveyed to the oocyte, thereby triggering meiotic resumption [47]. Further experiments also suggest that calcium is required to progress past MI [48].

Oocyte maturation

Fully grown oocytes from large antral follicles respond to LH or administration of human chorionic gonadotrophin (hCG) with the resumption of the meiotic cycle. Approximately 22–24 hours after the onset of maturation, the human oocyte undergoes germinal vesicle breakdown. Prior to this, local foci of chromatin condense and the pairs of bivalent chromosomes retract from the nuclear envelope. Transcription ceases. The chromosomes further condense and thicken, and kinetochores, large multiprotein complexes localized in the centromeric regions, appear associated with microtubules during the formation of the meiotic spindle. The meiotic spindle migrates to the periphery of the oocyte, regulated probably by actin microfilaments and microtubules [49]. By approximately 32 hours after the onset of maturation, the oocytes are in metaphase I. This phase lasts for a few hours, proceeding to anaphase I and telophase I. By approximately 36 hours, the first polar body is extruded from the oocyte as it develops to metaphase II.

Maturation of the nuclear component of the oocyte is delayed until immediately prior to fertilization. Perhaps the explanation of this program lies in the fact that the correct alignment of chromosomes on the meiotic spindle in the mature oocyte is a quite unstable condition. Therefore, achieving nuclear maturation and arrest at MII immediately before fertilization may be interpreted as a safeguard mechanism designed to minimize the risk of aneuploidy, i.e. the occurrence of an extra or missing chromosome, due to instability of the spindle and consequent chromosome dispersion.

A number of pathological conditions are related to anomalies of nuclear maturation. In contrast with other species, humans present a very high frequency of aneuploidy. This genetic condition is the most frequent cause of mental retardation and pregnancy loss, accounting for 8% of all pregnancies [50]. With the exception of sex chromosomes, aneuploidy is principally due to non-disjunction of bivalents occurring during the first meiotic division of maternal meiosis (Fig. 17.4) [51]. Less frequently, aneuploid gametes may arise for errors occurring during the maternal second meiotic division or paternal meiosis.

Interestingly, non-disjunction at MI or MII and abnormal rate of recombination between homologue chromosomes are strongly associated with maternal age [52,53]. Recombination is completed before birth, so it is unlikely to be responsible for age-related meiotic errors. Two different hypotheses can be proposed to explain these observations: (a) increased maternal age leads to augmented ovulation of oocytes resulting from abnormal recombination [54]; (b) compared to oocytes from young individuals, ageing oocytes are more prone to undergo meiotic errors during the segregation of chromosomes with abnormal recombination [55]. Although conclusive data are not available, the latter hypothesis appears more likely. In fact, there are

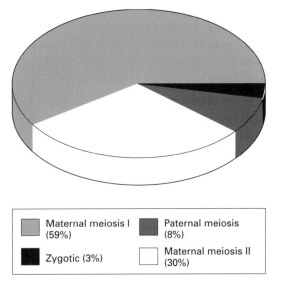

Maternal meiosis I (59%)

Paternal meiosis (8%)

Zygotic (3%)

Maternal meiosis II (30%)

Fig. 17.4. Incidence of the various causes of aneuploidy in the human conceptus. Anomalies in chromosome segregation in the developing embryo are infrequent. Vice versa, errors occurring during maternal meiosis, especially during meiosis I, are the most important cause for the generation of this condition. Anomalies in paternal meiosis play a secondary role. It is thought that, in older women, ageing oocytes are more likely to undergo meiotic errors during the segregation of chromosomes with abnormal recombination as a consequence of decreased function of cellular components, such as mitochondria.

no convincing data suggesting a mechanism by which primordial oocytes are selectively induced to initiate the growth phase depending on their status. Vice versa, it is plausible that oocyte function, including chromosome segregation, can be compromised as result of ageing [56].

Various agents can cause disruption of meiosis, some of which include various cryopreservatives, acid Tyrode's solution and environmental factors such as alcohol abuse, drugs used in chemotherapy and smoking [57].

The same signal which triggers nuclear maturation also induces a series of poorly understood cytoplasmic changes (cytoplasmic maturation) which are essential to successful fertilization and development. *In vivo* as well as *in vitro*, a significant proportion of oocytes which have undergone full nuclear maturation are unable to

fertilize or develop successfully, irrespective of sperm function. This poses the fundamental question as to why meiotically mature oocytes possess different developmental ability. Contrary to many invertebrates and other vertebrates, it is not yet possible to obtain clear biochemical evidence of oocyte cytoplasmic factors, typically proteins or mRNA, involved in the development of the early mammalian embryo. Consequently, in the absence of morphological or biochemical markers, it is not known which are the optimal conditions to achieve cytoplasmic competence in the 'mature' oocyte. Not surprisingly, determination of oocyte quality is reckoned to be probably the most difficult task in human IVF [58]. Nevertheless, although the essential nature of cytoplasmic maturation is far from being clear, evidence accumulated in recent years has started to give new insights into this process.

At fertilization, the ability of the oocyte to respond to the penetration of the spermatozoon with a series of intracellular calcium transients is an essential requisite for prevention of polyspermic fertilization, completion of meiosis, formation of pronuclei and, possibly, determination of postfertilization events [45]. During oogenesis, calcium-releasing mechanisms have been recently proven to undergo modification. In particular, in the mouse, the sensitivity of these mechanisms progressively increases during maturation, reaching the maximum just before the time of fertilization [59]. At this stage, in fact, oocytes respond to the spermatozoon with transients which are larger, longer and with different spatial organization compared to those detected in fully grown immature oocytes. The cellular basis of this process is not known, although the ER which is a major store of intracellular calcium, is suspected to be involved. During maturation, this organelle undergoes extensive redistribution involving dispersal throughout the oocyte cortex [60]. Receptors responsive to the signals which induce release of intracellular calcium are also redistributed on the membrane of the organelle, and this could modify the ability of the ER to release its calcium stores. Using thimerosal, an artificial calcium-releasing agent, it has been recently shown that human oocytes develop the ability to generate calcium changes during maturation [61].

Studies carried out in the mouse and pig [62,63] have shown that, during maturation, the increasing ability to decondense the sperm nucleus parallels the accumulation of glutathione. This thiol is thought to be an important factor required for processing sperm chromatin. This hypothesis is supported by the finding that artificial inhibition of glutathione synthesis prevents the decondensation of sperm chromatin [62]. However, this function is likely to depend also on other factors still unknown.

Size appears to be uninformative in the assessment of the degree of maturation of the oocyte. In the mouse, oocytes from both large and small antral follicles can mature in vitro, fertilize and develop to the two-cell stage with similar frequency. However, the rate of blastocyst formation in oocytes from small follicles is much smaller than that of the other group [64]. As oocytes from both groups have the same size, qualitative differences must exist. Since the embryonic genome is activated approximately at the two-cell stage in the mouse [19], immature oocytes are likely to be restricted in their developmental potential for the inability to activate the embryonic genome.

During maturation, selective modification, translation and degradation of specific mRNA have been proven to occur, as in the case of the tissue plasminogen activator (tPA) mRNA [65]. This suggests that selective control of mRNA utilization is a potential mechanism by which the oocyte can modulate its function during maturation.

The mature ovulated oocyte

The fully mature oocyte is a unique cell. The most evident characteristic is its size, measuring about 120 μm in diameter. Evenly distributed on the entire surface, the plasmalemma presents a dense array of microvilli containing bundles of actin ramifying into the cortical cytoskeleton below. In some cases the zona pellucida may appear particularly thick. It has been suggested that this can impede hatching of the blastocyst [66], but conclusive evidence is not available in this respect.

The oocyte is surrounded by a cloud of cumulus cells dispersed in a matrix of hyaluronic acid produced during maturation. The mature oocyte is thought to continue to interact with cumulus cells. But at this stage, there is no direct communication through gap junctions between the two types of cells, as the LH surge causes retraction of the cytoplasmic processes departing from the cumulus cells more closely associated to the oocyte. So germ and somatic cells probably interact through diffusible factors [67].

The cortical region of the oocyte contains several thousands of cortical granules derived from the centrifugal migration of vesicles associated with the Golgi apparatus. In primates and domestic species, the cortical region also presents a homogeneous layer of polymerized actin [68] which may contribute to the incorporation of the sperm head. In these species, oocytes also show significant similarities with reference to the microtubular organization, which essentially consists of the meiotic spindle [69,70]. This structure is located in the cortex, slightly tapered at the poles and radially oriented. The human meiotic spindle is particularly sensitive to suboptimal temperatures which are known to cause irreparable damage [71]. This clearly poses practical problems in the manipulation of oocytes for clinical IVF and all possible measures must be taken to minimize temperature-mediated damage. Oocytes aged in vitro are also prone to cytoskeletal dysfunction. In humans, cytoplasmic microtubular structures are not visible. So, the mature oocyte lacks an endogenous microtubule organizing centre which is essential for pronuclear formation and cell division. At fertilization, the sperm contributes to the cytoskeletal structure with its own microtubule organizing centre [72]. The fact that the mouse oocyte is characterized by a cytoskeletal structure with quite different characteristics indicates that this species is not necessarily an appropriate model for the study of the human oocyte.

Maternal mitochondria are a fundamental resource for the zygote. Paternal contribution, if any, is negligible. In the mouse, it has been recently found that paternal mitochondria are selectively eliminated during the very early phases of development [73]. Mitochondria are believed to be involved in the process of ageing. Over a prolonged period of time, in ageing tissue, mitochondria accumulate deleterious changes in their DNA, resulting from the action of reactive oxygen species and the absence of the protective function of chromosomal proteins. This damage obviously contributes to reduce the efficiency of cellular functions. Oocytes from older women are known to be affected by deletions in a proportion of their mitochondrial DNA population, which may contribute to the reduced fertility of these individuals.

A clearer understanding of the genetics, cell biology and cytoskeletal activity of the human oocyte is urgently required. Normal oocyte maturation *in vitro* is a goal worthy of every scientific effort because of the clinical imperative. There is now the potential to use immature oocytes from women undergoing follicular stimulation for conception *in vitro*—in, for example, polycystic ovarian disease — in whom *in vivo* oocyte maturation is either difficult or impossible. Furthermore, the generation of healthy mature oocytes from primordial follicles would aid those women undergoing cryopreservation of their ovarian tissue prior to treatment for cancer. However, it is clear from the above discussion that oocyte maturation is a complex process and the exquisitely balanced regulatory systems must be maintained to prevent a high incidence of chromosomal and other anomalies arising in the mature oocyte. In the near future, in-vitro oocyte maturation from small antral follicles is a realistic possibility for routine therapy; the generation of mature oocytes by growing follicles *in vitro*, however, is a much more difficult objective to achieve.

Male germ cells

The generation of the mature male gamete during spermatogenesis occurs on a different timescale from oogenesis. Unlike in the female, where oogonia divide during fetal life, in the male spermatogonia do not show signs of mitotic activity during prenatal and prepubertal life. At puberty spermatogonia begin actively to divide giving rise to three different cell types, A (A0, A1, A2, A3, A4), intermediate and B [74]. This mitotic phase is atypical, as in many cases the resulting cells are not physically independent units, being connected by cytoplasmic bridges.

Primary spermatocytes are formed from the development of type B spermatogonia. These cells activate the programme of meiotic division, duplicating their chromosomes and undergoing the long meiotic prophase during which new assortments of genes are generated. During the first meiotic division, the two components of each pair of bivalent chromosomes are segregated into two distinct daughter cells, the secondary spermatocytes. Each of these cells rapidly undergoes the second meiotic division, producing two haploid spermatids.

Although spermatids are genetically mature, i.e. haploid, they need to undergo dramatic changes in their structure and function to produce a highly specialized cell, the spermatozoon, capable of migrating through the female genital tract and fusing with the ovulated egg. This process of terminal differentiation is referred to as *spermiogenesis* [75], and in humans it occurs over a period of about 3 weeks. This transformation consists mainly in the condensation of the nuclear chromatin, development of the cisternae of the Golgi apparatus into the acrosomal vesicle, migration of the pair of centrioles to the pole opposite to the acrosome, formation of the tail axoneme, duplication of mitochondria, and their organization into a helical structure in the midpiece region. More than half of the cytoplasm of the spermatid is shed during this process, giving rise to the highly compacted cellular organization of the spermatozoon.

RNA and protein synthesis essentially occur during the diploid phase of spermatogenesis. Although the question remains controversial, it has been suggested that specific genes may be expressed at some point of the haploid phase [76]. In this respect it is interesting to note that haploid cells, including spermatids, present intercellular bridges through which specific mRNA can be conveyed.

Testicular sperm are not fully mature gametes. In the epididymis they undergo extensive cell surface modifications, consisting in spatial rearrangement and post-transitional modifications of pre-existing components, as well as addition of new macromolecules derived from the epididymal epithelium [77]. These changes are essential to develop motility. However, ability to fertilize is fully achieved only after further modifications occurring in the female tract. The genetic material may also be modified at post-testicular stages. In the mouse, it has been recently shown that specific genes are epigenetically modified through methylation [78], although the significance of this phenomenon is not fully understood.

Transport and preparation of the fertilizing spermatozoon

It is now well established that the transport of sperm through the female reproductive tract is predominantly independent of their inherent motility. Factors such as sperm concentration and linear velocity may be more relevant for the penetration through the oocyte–cumulus complex and, probably, the cervical mucus. However, within a few hours of coitus, only a few hundred spermatozoa reach an ampulla and these may be a highly selective population with a greater facility to penetrate the oocytes, as evidenced from animal studies [79].

During transit through the reproductive tract, sperm gain the capacity to fertilize the oocyte through a process referred to as capacitation. This is poorly understood but it is clear that it can take place outside the female reproductive tract as sperm removed from seminal plasma and washed into simple culture medium can undergo capacitation. Current research indicates that sterols may be removed in conjunction with various other changes in the lipid bilayer [80,81] and cholesterol may be removed and mannose receptors may migrate to the acrosomal and post acrosomal surface [82].

Many of the spermatozoa undergoing capacitation display a hyperactive form of movement and an increased lateral head displacement. Capacitation is a prerequisite to the acrosome reaction. During capacitation or the initiation of the acrosome reaction, spermatozoa change from oxidative to glycolytic metabolism; intra-cellular calcium levels increase, as does cAMP, in response to enhanced activity of adenylate cyclase. Biological induction of the acrosome reaction may require the activity of protein kinases A and C and guanosine triphosphate (GTP)-binding proteins, or G-proteins [83]. Purified zona pellucida receptor ZP3 triggers a high incidence of acrosome reaction in a given population of spermatozoa, similar to that produced by a calcium ionophore [84,85].

Morphologically, the start of the acrosome reaction is observed as interspersed areas of fusion between the outer acrosomal and plasma membranes, thereby releasing the content of the acrosome vesicle, which includes various enzymes, proteases and hydrolyses. This calcium-dependent process is linked to the activation of spermatozoa calmodulin [86] with a role for the angiotensin-converting enzyme.

It is still debated whether capacitation is required for spermatozoa to pass through the cumulus oophorus, although the contents of the acrosome may be required to depolymerize the hyaluronidate matrix, but it is believed that hyperactive motility generates a boring-type action to drive the acrosome-reacted spermatozoon through the zona pellucida. Hence, the fertilizing spermatozoon probably undergoes its acrosome reaction once bound to the zona pellucida, and especially the glycoprotein ZP3. Although other physiological agents, such as progesterone and follicular fluid, can induce the acrosome reaction, probably the most potent biological stimulant is ZP3 [84,85].

Second messenger systems such as calcium, pH, cAMP, calcium-dependent phospholipase, G-proteins and altered cyclic nucleotide metabolism are all implicated in the regulation of the acrosome reaction and hyperactivation [87].

Sperm binding and gamete fusion

The binding of a spermatozoon to the zona pellucida takes places in two phases, an initial weak binding followed by a firmer, permanent attachment [86]. Although sperm–egg fusion *per se* can occur across species, as in the case of the hamster egg penetration assay, sperm–zona binding, in contrast, is highly species-specific.

Even in those species in which cross-binding can occur — for example, rhesus monkey, squirrel monkey, rabbit, mouse, hamster and human — actual cross-fertilization will only arise once the zona pellucida is removed. Recognition of the glycoprotein components of the zona pellucida, principally ZP3, by receptors situated on the sperm surface accounts for the specificity of sperm–egg interaction.

In particular, ZP3 serine/threonine O-linked oligosaccharide chains are presumed to confer species specificity to sperm–zona binding [25]. It has been suggested that these side chains are specifically recognized by a complementary receptor, the enzyme β-1,4 galactosyltransferase, found on mouse spermatozoa [88]. Other sperm plasma membrane proteins may contribute to determine species-specific interaction. sp56, detected in mice [89], has a high affinity for ZP3. This protein is a homomultimeric peripheral membrane protein which binds to the zona of unfertilized oocytes, but not fertilized zygotes. sp56 appears also to be present only in acrosome-intact spermatozoa, but not in acrosome-reacted spermatozoa. The molecular biology of sp56 indicates that it is a member of a superfamily of protein receptors. It is, however, apparently absent in human sperm, and the lack of sperm–egg recognition between human and mouse might be due to the presence or absence of this class of proteins [90].

In addition to its involvement in species-specific recognition, ZP3 is also thought to be responsible in the regulation of sperm function. ZP3 synthesized from cDNA, and recombinant human ZP3 are extremely effective in inducing the acrosome reaction [83].

After the acrosome reaction, the spermatozoa are purported to be released from their binding to ZP3, and interact with ZP2 through acrosin, a trypsin-like protease, for establishing a secondary tight binding to the zona. This interaction probably occurs via a carbohydrate-binding domain located at the N-terminus of the sperm protein. PH20, a sperm antigen characterized in guinea pigs [91], is also suspected to be involved in the interaction with ZP2.

Penetration through the zona pellucida is a combination of lysis of the zona by zona lysins released from the acrosomal cap and also at the perforatorium, in combination with an enhanced kinetic motility (hyperactivation) providing the necessary thrust. Both thrust and enzymatic activity are required [83].

As the spermatozoa enter the perivitelline space, they come in contact with the plasma membrane of the oocyte (oolemma). As the sperm head comes in contact with the microvilli on the oolemma, the sperm tail is still beating outside the zona pellucida before being eventually drawn into the oocyte.

The post-acrosomal region of the acrosome-reacted spermatozoon is the point of fusion with the oolemma. At this stage the sperm plasma membrane is incorporated within the oolemma and the sperm tail becomes immotile. After fusion between the sperm head and the vitelline membrane microvilli, the latter retract and draw the spermatozoon into the ooplasm via subcortical layers of actin and myosin filaments. The adhesion peptides integrin, present on egg membranes, and disintegrin, present on sperm membranes, may be primarily involved in the sperm–egg fusion [92].

Oocyte activation

The trigger for fertilization

At fertilization, the sperm contributes to the formation of the zygote with its genomic complement and, in some species, the centriole. It is also responsible for delivering the message that triggers egg development. The series of changes which accompany fertilization is referred to as oocyte activation. These changes consist of cortical granule exocytosis, decondensation of the sperm head, completion of maternal meiosis and extrusion of the second polar body and pronuclei formation. The latter two events are the most conventional criteria to assess activation in routine IVF.

In many organisms, fusion of the sperm with the egg causes an immediate change in the potential of the oocyte membrane [93]. In mammals, this response does not have obvious function and it is not clear whether it is involved in generating a fast block to polyspermy, which is known to occur in other species.

The fundamental signal triggered by the

sperm for oocyte activation is a change in intracellular calcium levels [94]. In mammalian species, this change consists of repetitive oscillations, unlike in invertebrate eggs where only a monotonic variation occurs. In the human egg, these oscillations appear to have a duration of about 120 seconds, a frequency of 10–35 min and can last for several hours [95]. There is no doubt as to the importance of this event, since treatment of mouse eggs with an intracellular calcium chelator abolishes calcium oscillations and inhibits cortical granule exocytosis and reinitiation of the cell cycle [45]. The immediate source for the generation of calcium changes appears to be an intracellular store, probably the endoplasmic reticulum [94]. The initial calcium release induced by the sperm is presumed to trigger further calcium release by a mechanism of calcium-induced calcium release (CICR) similar to that described in muscle [96]. This poses the question of how the sperm can initially transmit its activating signal to the internal store. Various theories have been formulated in this respect [97]. It has been suggested that molecules on the sperm plasma membrane may exert a hormone-like action by binding to complementary receptors on the oocyte plasmalemma coupled to G-proteins. This would lead to stimulation of a phospholipase C and consequent generation of inositol $(1,4,5)$-triphosphate $(InsP_3)$, which induces release of calcium, and diacylglycerol, which activates protein kinase C. Different experiments support this theory; nevertheless, the existence of the most important components, an agonist on the sperm and a receptor on the egg, has not been demonstrated.

The sperm oscillin hypothesis appears to be supported by more convincing evidence. Several experiments have shown that hamster and boar sperm contain a soluble cytosolic factor that, when injected in eggs, induces calcium oscillations which mimic those triggered at fertilization [98]. In the hamster, this factor has recently been identified as an oligomeric protein with a subunit of M_r 33K whose sequence shows similarity with a prokaryote hexose phosphate isomerase [99]. However, the precise mechanism of action of this protein has not been elucidated. These two theories may not necessarily be

mutually exclusive, since it cannot be ruled out that parallel pathways may concur to produce the same effect.

Block to polyspermy

An important function of calcium changes associated with sperm–egg interaction is the prevention of polyspermic fertilization. In mammals, this is fundamentally achieved through modification of the zona pellucida (zona reaction). Other studies, specially those using subzonal insemination [100], have also suggested that a secondary block to polyspermy may occur at the level of the oocyte plasmalemma, possibly following sperm-induced depolarization.

Zona reaction is caused as the cortical granules — estimated in mammalian eggs to be in excess of 4000 lying just beneath the vitelline surface—fuse with the oolemma [101] as a result of sperm-induced intracellular calcium change. The cortical granules are lysosomal-like vesicles and, upon fusion with the oolemma, release proteases, peroxidases and glycosidases into the perivitelline space, causing a change in the binding properties and texture of the zona pellucida, often described as zona hardening. The zona hardening has been described as a transformation of ZP3 to ZA3f via modifications in O-linked oligosaccharides by the cortical granule glycosidases. This results in the loss of the ability of ZP3 to bind sperm and induce the acrosome reaction [26]. Hence, ZP3f utilized from fertilized oocytes are a poor model for studying sperm–zona interaction and induction of the acrosome reaction. These data, mainly for mice, are supported in part by the confirmed modification of at least one human zona protein during sperm–egg fusion [102]. ZP2 is also transformed into ZP2f after proteolysis, thus preventing further tight binding of sperm and penetration through the zona [103].

Reinitiation of the cell cycle

Sperm-induced calcium changes are thought to affect MPF function, thereby promoting reinitiation of the cell cycle. Continuing high levels of MPF ensure that the mature oocytes are arrested

452 at metaphase II until sperm penetration occurs. The kinase activity of MPF is responsible, directly or indirectly, for the maintenance of this arrest. Direct MPF targets are lamin proteins, which contribute to the structure of the nuclear envelope, histone H1, a chromatin component, and microtubule-associated proteins. In mature oocytes, persistent action of MPF on these targets prevents, respectively, reformation of the oocyte nucleus, maintenance of metaphase chromosomes in a highly condensed state and formation of the meiotic spindle. Indirect effects of MPF are probably derived from cascades of phosphorylations.

High levels of MPF are ensured by the action of a cytostatic factor (CSF) [104], whose essential

Fig. 17.5. Hypothetical model for cyclin degradation and MPF (p34cdc2-cyclin complex) inactivation at fertilization. In the mature oocyte the action of cytostatic factor (not shown in the figure) is thought to prevent cyclin destruction, ensuring high MPF levels. At fertilization, sperm-induced calcium oscillations are believed to activate calmodulin-dependent protein kinase II. This, in turn, promotes loss of cytostatic factor activity and cyclin modification (ubiquitination) required for its degradation through activated proteolytic activity (proteasome). Loss of p34cdc2 kinase activity determines cellular events necessary for the progression of the cell cycle, such as chromosome decondensation, pronuclear formation and disassembly of the meiotic spindle. From Whitaker [159] with permission.

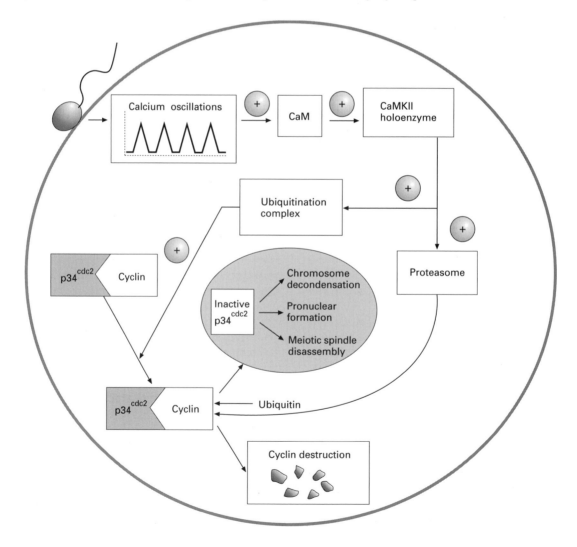

component is the product of the *c-mos* proto-oncogene. CSF action protects cyclin against proteolytic degradation, thereby preventing MPF inactivation. Calcium changes at fertilization move this delicate equilibrium (Fig. 17.5). Release of intracellular calcium is thought to activate calmodulin-dependent protein kinase II, which in its turn promotes proteolytic degradation of CSF and cyclin B [35]. However, since cyclin B is degraded before CSF destruction [105], it is likely that inhibition of CSF activity precedes its proteolytic inactivation.

Following MPF inactivation, the egg will resume meiosis proceeding from metaphase II to anaphase II, telophase II and extrusion of the second polar body. Sometimes, unfertilized eggs may appear to have two polar bodies, as a result of the fragmentation of the first polar body. After extrusion of the second polar body, abnormal activation may lead to re-formation of a metaphase-like configuration, referred to as MIII [106].

Pronuclear formation

Within the ooplasm, the sperm head enlarges as its chromatin decondenses involving reduced glutathione. The sperm head has been observed to decondense within a few hours after penetration, following disintegration of the sperm nuclear envelope. At this stage the spermatozoon DNA is encased by protamines, which are subsequently replaced by histones synthesized by the oocyte [107].

Although the male pronucleus is sometimes formed first, from about 12 hours post insemination *in vitro* the beginnings of both the male and female pronuclei can be seen in the ooplasm. The sperm midpiece and tail can also be observed close to the male pronucleus, as these have been incorporated with the fertilizing spermatozoon.

In normal conditions, both gametes contribute a haploid chromosome set. But various anomalies can arise at this stage. Morphologically observed 3 pronucleate eggs can be a result of dispermy; these can result in diandric triploids or diandric diploids — which can progress to the hydatidiform mole. The first or second polar body can be retained within the oocyte resulting in digynic triploids, having two maternal and one paternal chromosome sets. Further extrusion of a pronucleus can arise resulting in normal diploidy — as with the diandric triploids which lose a male pronucleus — or digyny. Triploids can also arise when eggs are fertilized by a diploid spermatozoon.

The pronucleus stage is estimated to last for up to 24 hours after insemination. During this period the pronuclei duplicate their DNA, enlarge to a terminal size and, although formed in different parts of the ooplasm, migrate to apposition, with their nucleoli aligned along the area of contact. The chromosomes condense into prophase of the first cleavage division and the pronuclei break down, initiating syngamy [108]. The mitotic spindle then forms on the metaphase plate and divides at anaphase progressing through the phases of mitosis.

In mature oocytes of human and ruminant species, centrioles are not detectable. At fertilization, sperm contributes to the mitotic apparatus with its own centrioles which direct the apposition of the pronuclei, duplicate and migrate to opposite poles of the juxtaposed pronuclei.

Genomic imprinting

The contribution of both the maternal and paternal genomes is essential to the constitution of the zygote, as it has been found that they do not play equivalent roles during development in the formation of the embryo and extraembryonic structures. In humans, diandric diploids fail to give rise to a proper embryo, producing only a peculiar embryonic tumour formed from a population of placenta-like cells [109]. Likewise, parthenogenetic activation of mouse eggs, whose diploidy is derived from duplication of maternal chromosomes or suppression of polar body formation, are not able to develop properly, generating an embryo largely deficient in the extraembryonic structures [110]. Interestingly, it has been recently shown that chimaeric parthenogenetic ↔ normal human embryos can result in viable offspring [111].

The development of parthenogenetic and androgenetic embryos shows that, although maternal and paternal chromosomes encode equivalent genetic information (with exception of the Y-specific genes) they retain some memory or imprint of the gametic origin and behave differently according to whether they are inherited from the mother or from the father. In the humans, the loss of the chromosomal region 15q11-13 results in distinct syndromes depending on whether the paternal or the maternal region is lost. Failure to inherit the paternal region causes the Prader–Willi syndrome, characterized by retarded motor development, hypotonia and feeding difficulty. Conversely, loss of the maternal region causes the Angelman syndrome, producing diverse symptoms such as ataxia, seizure and hyperactivity. These findings are consistent with the hypothesis that only one allele, either paternal or maternal, of certain genes is expressed during development. In fact in the mouse embryo, only the paternal allele of the *Igf-2* gene is expressed [112]. Conversely, the gene encoding the receptor of this factor, *Igf-2r*, is expressed only when inherited from the mother [113].

There is evidence that, at least in some cases, imprinting results from a gamete-specific pattern of DNA methylation. This epigenetic modification affects, either positively or negatively, gene transcription, leading to the expression of only one allele of imprinted genes during development. Transgenic experiments have shown that imprinting is a reversible condition. This allows that the epigenetic information of imprinted genes is erased by extensive hypomethylation during primordial germ cell formation and, subsequently, re-established during meiosis, through *ex novo* methylation, according to the sex of the developing embryo.

However, DNA methylation may not be the only type of DNA modification involved in genomic imprinting. In fact, conversion between alternative forms of chromatin structure may provide an additional mechanism by which epigenetic information is cyclically introduced and erased for the differential expression of imprinted genes.

Recent concerns have arisen with the potential use of human spermatids for conception *in vitro* via intra-cytoplasmic sperm injection technology. In fact, it is not entirely clear if epigenetic changes in the DNA constitution and cytoplasmic events which may occur during spermiogenesis may be important for the gener-ation of a healthy offspring. Gamete cell cycle phenomena, the role of the sperm centriole, and genomic imprinting have all been discussed [114].

Cleavage and the pre-implantation embryo

Following syngamy and completion of the first mitotic division, the zygote undergoes cleavage into two equal size cells. In the second cleavage division, which takes place independently for each blastomere, the plane of division is at right angles to the parental blastomere. This procedure continues with successive cleavage divisions resulting in an increasing number of smaller size cells, each dividing at an independent rate. This results in the pre-implantation embryo increasing its cell number without increasing its mass, i.e. cleavage rather than growth, and with perfectly healthy embryos often having an odd number of blastomeres. Indeed, perfectly normal human births have arisen from embryos at the five or more cell stage with blastomeres representing three different stages (viz: a two-cell-sized blastomere, four-cell-sized blastomere and eight-cell-sized blastomere) [115]. Cleavage is regulated by both epigenetic and genetic determining factors. Cleavage divisions are timed from the moment of sperm entry and activation of the oocyte by an inbuilt genetic 'clock' and unidentified regulatory cytoplasmic factors [116].

During the early cleavage stage, each blastomere is said to be totipotent, i.e. capable of generating all the cell types of the adult organism, as evidenced by individual blastomeres of two-cell mouse embryos developing into identical twins. Estimates to the limits of this totipotence have been the eight cell in both sheep and rabbits, and from cryopreserved human embryos with degenerating blastomeres. This potential has been described in the human up to the eight-cell stage [117].

It is during this cleavage period that the first stages of differentiation occur. The first crucial event occurs at the late eight-cell stage, when loosely connected blastomeres become compacted together, giving rise to a spherical arrangement. Extensive modifications of the blastomeres determine a process of radial self-polarization:

1 The nuclei move toward the basal inner portion of the blastomeres;

2 At the apical pole endocytic vesicles accumulate;

3 Microvilli are organized at the areas of cell surface where adjacent blastomeres are in contact;

4 At the basal lateral sides gap junctions and tight junctions are formed.

E-cadherin is thought to play role in compaction. At the two-cell stage this protein is uniformly distributed on the membrane of the blastomeres, but during compaction the E-cadherin molecules migrate to the areas where blastomeres are in contact [118]. In addition, antibodies to E-cadherin prevent compaction from taking place. There is evidence that intercellular contact may act by inducing a local signalling system which involves the activation of intracellular messengers and, ultimately, the downstream events resulting in compaction. In fact, chemical stimulation of the protein kinase C or diacylglycerol pathways cause the four-cell mouse embryo to undergo premature compaction [119]. The overall result of these events is that the blastomeres reinforce their intercellular contacts and the inner portion of the embryo is sealed off from the surrounding environment.

A proportion of the following cleavage planes are parallel to the outer surface, yielding one or two small inner apolar cells, while the remaining radial cleavages produce larger outer polar cells. Most of the descendants of the outer cells form the trophectoderm which does not contribute to the constitution of the embryo proper, generating the embryonic portion of the placenta. Conversely, the inner cells of the 16-cell stage (and a small proportion of trophectoderm cells of the 32-cell stage) yield the inner cell mass (ICM) which is responsible for the development of the embryo [120]. Studies comparing the biochemical make-up of internal and external blastomeres have also shown that these two groups of cells are characterized by diverse patterns of gene expression, since they synthesize distinct pools of proteins. By the 64-cell expanded blastocyst stage, the ICM and the tro-phectoderm are irreversibly determined in their developmental pathway, neither of them contributing to the cell population of the other group [121]. It seems that positional information, inside position as opposed to outside position, is the causal factor that establishes whether a blastomere of the morula stage will give rise to the trophoectoderm or the ICM. The causative mechanism is still unclear. Internal and external cells differ in the nature of the surrounding environment as well as in the arrangement of intercellular junctions. This may be responsible for the initial diversification occurring at the 16-cell stage. Various experiments support this view. In the mouse, individual totipotent 4-cell embryo blastomeres, when fused to a four- to 16-cell embryo, produce cells localized in the yolk sac or in the postimplantation embryo, depending on whether they have been placed outside the recipient morula or have been surrounded by other blastomeres [122]. The most accepted explanation of this phenomenon is that the position itself produces this initial pattern of differential specification. However, although it is very unlikely, it has not been definitively ruled out that external blastomeres inherit a cytoplasmic determinant localized radially at the periphery of the embryo. Obviously this hypothesis assumes that this determinant is very labile, as isolated blastomeres do not show any restriction of their potency.

Ultrastructurally, the early cleavage stage blastomeres have different characteristics compared to the later cleavage stages and fully formed somatic cells. For example, the mitochondria in the early-stage blastomeres differentiate by elongation and the development of more cristae and become opposed to the endoplasmic reticulum. Lysosomes which display arylsulphatase activity eventually differentiate into secondary lysosomes with the typical morphology; the Golgi complex is modified to autophagic vacuoles necessary for removing damaged tissue and other cell components. Blebbing of the outer sheet of nuclear membranes has been recorded in the human embryo until the eight-cell stage, and this system has been purported to be responsible for transporting nucleolar materials to the cytoplasm as nucleoli and nucleolar rRNA synthesis become active at the eight-cell stage [123].

Communication between blastomeres occurs through gap junctions resembling immature desmosomes, spindle midbodies and microvilli within the intercellular spaces up to approximately the four-cell stage. Thereafter the cytoplasmic organelles differentiate with the formation of complete desmosomes and tight junctions [124]. The injection of dyes into blastomeres indicates they act as a syncytial network.

During the initial cleavage stages, genetic information appears to have a maternal origin. As we have already noted, the growing oocyte accumulates the various types of RNA during the growth phase. But a decrease in this store begins at meiotic resumption, continuing during the first divisions. In the mouse, at the two-cell stage, most of the stored rRNA has been degraded and the great majority of poly(A)+ RNA, which is the fraction readily available for translation, has disappeared [18]. It has also been shown that, after fertilization, new species of poly(A)+ RNA appear in the absence of transcription, by the processing of primary transcripts. Indeed, selective mechanisms of recruitment of specific RNAs into the poly(A)+ pool are thought to be a fundamental requirement during early development in a large variety of species. So, the very early stage of development critically depends on inherited information stored in the mature oocyte. But the zygotic genome must soon be activated. This occurs at the two-cell stage in the mouse [19], whereas the rabbit embryo begins transcriptional activity only at the eight- to 16-cell stage. In the human zygote, conspicuous transcription starts at the four- to eight-cell stage [125], although some genes may be expressed before the second mitotic division. In mice and rabbits, transcription activation is temporally associated with changes in chromatin structure, derived by acetylation of histone H4 [126]. The large subunit of RNA polymerase II also undergoes changes which are presumed to affect its function, since at fertilization it is phosphorylated on its C-terminal domain and translocated into the pronuclei, while further phosphorylation occurs at the time of gene transcription [127].

Transitions in chromatin structure and RNA polymerase II function represent general mechanisms of regulation. Additional levels of control must also exist for modulating the expression of individual genes. GAL-4, *rig* and *oct-3* are examples of regulatory factors which are thought to be involved in the transcription of determined set of genes, such as those involved in housekeeping functions and establishment of totipotency.

Differences may exist between embryos of different sex. It has been suggested that male embryos grow more rapidly than female embryos due to the transcription from the sex-determining genes *Sry* and *Zfy* as shown in mouse studies [128].

As preimplantation development proceeds, the embryonic genome becomes more active, expressing both maternal and paternal characteristics. Following blastocyst differentiation and expansion, hCG begins to be secreted [129,130].

Gene regulation may occur at the level of whole chromosomes. In the early cleavage stages, between approximately the four- to eight-cell and the morula stages, each of the two X-chromosomes in female embryos is active. The paternal copy of the X-chromosome is preferentially inactivated in trophectodermal cells, in the extraembryonic ectoderm and proximal endoderm. However, in cell lines destined for fetal tissues, the maternal and paternal X-chromosomes are inactivated randomly. X-inactivation is irreversible, except in rare instances, such as in oogonia.

The genetic control of pattern formation in the development of mammals is still poorly understood. Nevertheless, new evidence is beginning to show that the development of highly evolved species probably shares amazing similarities with that of lower organisms, despite fundamental differences in the layout of the body plan. In the *Drosophila* embryo, the identity of segmental units is defined by the segment-specific expression of a complex (*HOM-C*) of homeotic genes whose products are characterized by a conserved domain, known as homeodomain. In mammals, *Hox* genes also encode for proteins containing the homeodomain. Remarkably, *Hox* genes are expressed and appear to determine the identity of segmental units, such as the hindbrain, somites and axial skeleton [131]. In addition, like *Drosophila*, the order of the *Hox* genes along the chromosome is collinear with their pattern of expression along the embryonic axis. If differentiation mechanisms are conserved among species throughout early development, it could be speculated that, in mammals, determination of the cell fate during early cleavage may be directed by genes operating and already found in lower biological systems.

The human embryo reaches the midpoint of the two-cell stage approximately 32–34 hours after insemination *in vitro*, the four-cell stage at approximately 50 hours, the eight-cell stage at approximately 65 hours, the morula stage at approximately 95 hours and the blastocyst, in excess of 100 cells, at approximately 110 hours. The earliest time for blastocyst hatching is during the 6th day after fertilization. There is some debate as to whether the cleavage rate seen *in vitro* is slower than that *in situ* within the female reproductive tract. Growth and differentiation are, however, at a constant rate and abnormal developmental times for cleavage arrest signify abnormal growth probably related to chromosomal anomalies; embryos grown *in vitro*, however, may be subjected to suboptimal conditions, including undue light, high oxygen concentrations or variations in pH, temperature, isotonicity, or toxins, including trace elements and heavy metals, in the culture medium. It has been suggested that the four- to eight-cell stage is sensitive to extraneous fluctuations as this is the time of the onset of embryonic genome transcription. The cleaving embryo is sensitive to growth factors and cytokines released in the autocrine loop from adjacent embryonic cells (or the mother). Numerous growth factors, such as insulin and insulin-like growth factors (IGFs), epidermal growth factor (EGF), platelet-derived growth factor, transforming growth factor-β (TGF-β), colony-stimulating factor-1, have been shown to be present in human embryos, and having effects on their development *in vitro* [132,133].

At blastulation, the inner cell mass, present at one pole of the embryo, is enclosed by a single-cell layer of trophectoderm cells, and the whole is encased in the zona pellucida. DNA-specific fluorochromes can distinguish the two cell types permitting analysis of these distinct cells at this stage. Partial apoptosis occurs, as in most blastocysts a certain number of inner cell mass and trophectoderm cells have degenerated [134]. The purpose of this putative programmed cell death is unclear. The formation of the blastocoelic cavity occurs during a rise in intracellular calcium concentration and the establishment of electrical polarity between the apical–basal regions of the cells. Blastocoelic fluid probably arises as a result of the action of the transmembrane enzyme, Na^+/K^+ ATPase, which uses ATP to pump Na^+ into intracellular spaces followed by uptake of water. This mechanism has been illustrated in the rabbit blastocyst [135] as morulae exposed to ouabain will show impaired blastocoelic formation.

The blastocoelic fluid contains newly synthesized proteins from both types of cells of the blastocyst (some of which are not secreted into culture medium), nutrients and various factors influencing growth and metabolism of the embryo, particularly the inner cell mass cells. The trophectoderm is linked to the cells of the inner cell mass by desmosomes, gap junctions and tight junctions and there is no basal lamina between the two tissues. Trophectoderm, when fully differentiated, resembles epithelial-like tissue using epithelium-like transport of ions and water to generate the blastocoelic cavity. Approaching the time of differentiation of the blastocysts, large molecules such as laminin are secreted, and type IV collagen is found on the mural trophectoderm (that opposing the inner cell mass), and fibronectin on the surface of the inner cell mass cells. These substances may be involved in cell migration and proliferation, while other high molecular weight glycoproteins may be involved in cell to cell adhesion between the trophoblast and the endometrium.

The blastocyst before implantation

The blastocyst must be free of its zona pellucida before attachment to the endometrium and subsequent implantation. *In vitro*, this occurs by a process of hatching approximately 7 days after conception. Morphologically, the zona pellucida

458 thins and the blastocyst fully expands. By reduction and expansion of the blastocoelic fluid, the blastocyst undergoes a series of contraction and expansion movements and this, coupled with a small digested hole in the zona pellucida, causes the trophectoderm to 'squeeze' through, forming a characteristic trophectoderm bleb.

In mice, the zona pellucida is digested by trypsin synthesized in focal regions of the trophectoderm, but *in vivo* the zona pellucida is not removed before implantation and it is assumed that uterine zona lysins completely digest the zona pellucida. There is no evidence of this in the human, whereas there is evidence for the production of trypsin over the whole surface of the trophectoderm. The hatching of the human embryo *in vitro* (Fig. 17.6) occurs through a very small digested hole in the zona pellucida on approximately day 7 after insemination. The proportion of hatching has been reported as low as 20–30%, which probably reflects, in part, suboptimal in-vitro culture conditions in addition to defects in the chromosome/genetic make-up of the embryo *per se*.

During culture *in vitro*, the zona pellucida may become hardened as a result of cortical granule release, or the presence of oximes and free radicals from other cellular components (e.g. cumulus cells, corona cells, spermatozoa, etc.). This hardened zona pellucida may impair hatching, although the incidence of this condition, and whether or not it is a problem *in vivo*, has yet to be proven. There exist uncontrolled reports that, in some patients (those with thick zona pellucidae, high follicle-stimulating hormone in the peripheral system, women over the age of 40 and/or those with repeated failure of implantation) there may be an improved chance of implantation if the assisted hatching procedure is applied [136]. This procedure is usually performed using a microneedle filled with an acid solution gently to digest a portion of the zona pellucida, equivalent to 20–30 μm, although some prefer the use of an erbium-yttrium-aluminium laser.

Once the human embryo has hatched, actual growth, i.e. increase in mass as distinct from *cleavage* during the preimplantation period, commences. The inner-cell mass differentiates into the embryonic disc which will give rise to hypoblast and epiblast, and occupies a polar position as a concave mass surrounded by the trophectoderm. During the preimplantation period, the human blastocyst prepares for implantation with distinct morphological and biochemical activities. Trophoblast cells contain microvilli and the embryos have characteristically large cytotrophoblastic nuclei, intracellular junctions between trophoblastic cells have been established and the differentiating endoderm synthesizes significant amounts of glycogen. Biochemically, studies have detected the secretion of hCG from the blastocyst stage [129], although the quantity of secretion can be affected by the ability of the blastocyst to hatch [130]. It has been computed [128] that the production of 16 000 mIU by the 10th day and 160 000 mIU of hCG by the 14th day is necessary for survival *in vivo*. There is also some evidence for the release of LH-RH by the human blastocyst, which is similar to that of the rhesus monkey [137].

The post-hatching period is coincident with preparations for implantation which include the expression of heparin sulphate proteoglycan, integrin E8 receptor αS17 βS11, IGF-R and EGF-R receptors, amongst others, on the trophectoderm cells. The inner-cell mass produces fibronectin and its binding molecule in addition to both polar and mural trophoblast tissue.

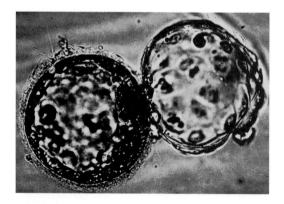

Fig. 17.6. Blastocyst almost completely hatched out of the zona pellucida. Some spermatozoa are still attached to the zona.

There is evidence that this binds to uterine fibronectin [138]. In mice, leukemia inhibitory factor (LIF) is required for implantation and mRNA for the LIF receptor has been identified on human blastocysts [139].

Embryo–maternal communication

Communication between the embryo and mother, sometimes termed maternal recognition of pregnancy, is considered an essential prerequisite for successful implantation. A plethora of substances transmitted in each direction have been identified, many of which are assumed to be acting as signals. Postulated roles for many of these substances are thought to involve immuno-suppressive action, regulation of prostaglandin, interferon and superoxide production, as well as regulation of uterine vasculature permeability.

The most widely studied embryonic signal is hCG, which is essential for the maintenance of corpus luteum function. The rate of hCG secretion is a discriminator of embryonic health [140,141]. Retarded secretion of hCG could be a result of a reduced trophoblast cell number, inhibited growth rate of the blastocyst, ectopic implantation, corpus luteum insufficiency, failure or inadequate penetration of the cytotrophoblasts into the decidua, or an inadequate villous structure.

The release of hCG by the trophoblast appears to be regulated by trophoblastic LH-RH which, in turn, may be controlled by EGF, TGF, activin and inhibin. The rate of increase of hCG can be used to identify ectopic implantation in 50% of cases, and in 25% of cases those patients who have a poorly developing embryo or a missed abortion [142].

hCG is luteotrophic and binds to ovarian receptors rescuing the deteriorating corpora lutea, resulting in an elevation of peripheral progesterone concentration. hCG also binds to the embryonic trophoblast and appears to affect the differentiation of syncytiotrophoblast from cytoblasts after implantation.

Another widely studied embryonic signal is the embryo-derived platelet activating factor (EDPAF, or PAF) which arises within 48 hours after fertilization [143]. Suggested functions for PAF include increasing vascular permeability, inducing thrombocytopenia, regulating the prostaglandin synthetase system, activation of uterine and systemic platelets, and influencing the vasodilatation and oedema of the decidua. Endometrium receptors for EDPAF are linked to calcium ion transport systems and phospholipase C. Early pregnancy factor (EPF) has also been the subject of debate for a number of years. Attempts to extract EPF from preimplantation embryos have been made by many workers, and it has been implicated as having an immunosuppressive role at implantation [144]. It has also been suggested to affect the production of prostaglandins and superoxides, and it has been implicated in the inhibition of IgG expression in mononuclear and other cells. Other substances implicated in signalling to the mother at the peri-implantation period include the following various steroids, proteins and metabolites:

- Inhibin (detected in Marmoset monkey embryos);
- TGF-β and IGF2;
- hCG;
- PAF (or EDPAF: also produced by the endometrium);
- Embryonic proteases;
- Oestrogen and progesterone;
- Interferon;
- Embryo-derived histamine-releasing substances;
- Plasma protein C;
- Prostaglandins;
- Embryo-derived β-inhibin.

Uterine preparation for implantation

There is much discussion in humans as to the timing of the window of implantation. The uterus becomes sensitive to implantation for a defined period, which varies between species. The primary events leading to implantation are apposition of the embryo and uterus, adhesion and penetration by the embryo. During the early luteal phase, and in preparation for implantation, the uterus undergoes considerable biochemical, physiological and cellular changes.

After ovulation, the uterine glands become tortuous, spiral arteries form, and the endometrium thickens and becomes oedematous as implantation approaches. Pinopods, microvilli and apical protrusions are present approximately 6 days after ovulation (20th day of the natural cycle) and remain for approximately 3 days. The disappearance of these pinopods by the 8th day after ovulation has been implicated as the endpoint for the period of implantation which occurs during the presence of the pinopods. These pinopods absorb molecules and fluid from the lumen, reducing the potential cavity and increasing apposition between the endometrium and embryo. At this time, biochemical changes occur on the surface of the epithelial cells, providing an overall electronegative charge as a result of the appearance of sugar residues and colloidal iron. Binding sites for lectins differentiate, and these have been shown to be deficient in women with primary infertility [145]. Major changes also occur in the glandular epithelium which accumulate giant mitochondria and glycogen particles and are responsible for the secretion of mucopolysaccharides and proteinaceous and lipid components into the intracellular spaces [146].

The regulation of uterine activity is controlled by steroids, with oestradiol affecting the development during the proliferative phase. During the secretory phase, however, progesterone regulates the type of secretory phase changes, and progesterone receptors are present in stroma, decidual and myometrial cells, in addition to smooth muscle, glandular epithelium and endothelium to varying degrees [147]. It is the action of progesterone that stimulates stromal oedema, increasing vascularity and overall secretory activity of the uterus. Its action is probably fundamental in priming the decidua for implantation [148]. Pinopods will not form in the absence of progesterone. Progesterone has been implicated in the following activities:

- Increases blood volume;
- Stimulates endometrial cellular secretion;
- Acts as an immunosuppressant;
- Stimulates prolactin synthesis;
- Inhibits phospholipase C;
- Affects oestrogen receptor distribution;
- Activates 17-OH dehydrogenase;

- Activates pinopod formation;
- Promotes fibronectin synthesis;
- Stimulates decidual cells.

Several prostaglandins are produced by the uterus including $F_{2\alpha}$ and PGE_2, synthesis of which is regulated by the luteal steroids. In numerous animal species, but not apparently humans, PGF_2 acts as a luteolysin, and as such it has been implicated as a cause of dysmenorrhoea. It is present in the epithelium or the oviductal mucosa in endometriotic patients. Prostaglandins have also been implicated in the regulation of decidual function.

A host of other substances have been implicated in uterine regulation, including growth factors, cytokines and adhesion molecules, and many of these have been reviewed previously [149–151]. Ligands or specific receptors for cytokines and adhesion molecules have been detected on blastocysts, but the precise nature of the interaction between these substances and the respective endometrial/embryonic tissues remains to be elucidated. Many proteins are actively secreted by the uterus [152], with specific proteins being released from the various tissue types in the endometrium at different phases during the cycle. For example, a 24 kDa heat-shock protein is at maximal secretion during the luteal phase during pinopod formation and has been associated with pinpointing the implantation-receptive endometrium [153].

For implantation to occur, decidualization is a necessary prerequisite, and this arises as a result of embryonic signalling or as activated macrophages release local factors such as tumour necrosis factor [154]. Decidualization involves modification of the stroma and decidua which change in vascular permeability. The decidua has cells which generally increase in size and become polyploid as a result of genomic endoreduplication. These support the invading blastocyst during implantation by producing a matrix of proteins and adhesive molecules, particularly laminin. Other substances produced by stromal and decidual cells are fibronectin, entactin, desmin, vimentin, collagen types I–V, heparin and proteoglycans [155]. Decidual stroma is endocrinologically active producing prolactin, which is postulated to be a luteotrophin, and it can synthesize the formation of cholesterol from β-lipoprotein and albumin.

The blastocyst produces enzymes, particularly proteases, which may aid penetration of the human epithelial basement membrane. In mice the pentasaccharide lacto-N-fucopentose-1 has been postulated as an essential component for implantation. It is expressed on mouse uterine epithelia with the corresponding receptor carried on the trophectoderm [156]. The embryo releases collagenase which may degrade endometrial collagen, and embryonic prostaglandins may enhance uterine permeability. Subsequent to adhesion, the embryo must penetrate between the epithelial cells of the competent uterus, presumably using its enzymes, to obtain contact with the uterine stroma. The blastocyst invades the stroma, perhaps by preferential attachment of the trophoblast to fibronectin [157], but major histocompatibility antigens are not expressed in response to the trophoblast cells. A comprehensive review of the differentiation of syncytiotrophoblasts and cytotrophoblast and the formation of chorionic villi is discussed elsewhere.

During the process of implantation, the blastocyst is developing at an incredible rate, allocating specific cells to various lineages, with differentiation of the primitive endoderm into the visceral yolk sac endoderm and parietal endoderm, and the inner cell mass giving rise to the epiblast which forms the floor of the amniotic cavity. During this period of gastrulation and tissue formation, there is extensive gene regulation and control, also involving a considerable amount of embryonic cell death or controlled apoptosis. A detailed review of organogenesis is published elsewhere [158].

Acknowledgments The authors wish to acknowledge the considerable help and support of Rosie Metcalf, Helen McDermott, Susan Corner and Sarah Gee in the preparation of this manuscript.

References

1 Ginsburg M., Snow M.H.L. & McLaren A. (1990) Primordial germ cells in the mouse embryo during gastrulation. *Development* **110**, 521.

2 Witschi E. (1948) Migration of the germ cells of human embryos from the yolk sac to the primitive gonadal folds. *Contributions to Embryology of the Canegie Institution of Washington* **32**, 67.

3 Baker T.G. & Frauchi L.L. (1967) The fine structure of oogoina and oocytes in human ovaries. *Journal of Cell Science* **2**, 213.

4 Peters H. (1976) Intrauterine gonadal development. *Fertility and Sterility* **27**, 493.

5 Baker T.G. (1963) A quantitative and cytological study of germ cells in human ovaries. *Proceedings of the Royal Society of Britain* **158**, 417.

6 Speed R.M. (1988) The possible role of meiotic pairing anomalies in the atresia of human fetal oocytes. *Human Genetics* **78**, 260.

7 Byskov A.G. (1975) The role of the rete ovarii in meiosis and follicle formation in the cat, mink and ferret. *Journal of Reproduction and Fertility* **45**, 201.

8 Faddy M.J., Gosden R.G., Gougeon A., Richardson S.J. & Nelson J.F. (1992) Accelerated disappearance of ovarian follicles in mid-life: implications for forecasting menopause. *Human Reproduction* **7**, 1342.

9 Gougeon A., Ecochard R. & Thalabard J.C. (1994) Age-related changes of the population of human ovarian follicles: increase in the disappearance rate of non-growing and early growing follicles: in aging women. *Biology of Reproduction* **50**, 653.

10 Baker T.G. & Scrimgeour J.B. (1980) Development of the gonad in the normal and anencephalic human fetuses. *Journal of Reproduction and Fertility* **60**, 193.

11 Packer A., Hsu Y.C., Besmer P. & Bachvarova R.F. (1994) The ligand of the *c-kit* receptor promotes oocyte growth. *Developmental Biology* **161**, 194.

12 Gosden R.G. (1985) The causes and consequences of ovarian ageing. In *Biology of Menopause*. Ed. R.G. Gosden, p. 188. Academic Press, London.

13 Gougeon A. (1986) Dynamics of follicular growth in the human: a model from preliminary results. *Human Reproduction* **1**, 81.

14 Davidson E.H. (1986) *Gene Activity in Early Development*, 3rd edn. p. 328. Academic Press, Orlando.

15 Szollosi D. (1972) Changes of some cell organelles during oogenesis in mammals. In *Oogenesis*. Eds J.D. Biggers & A.W. Schuetz, p. 47. University Park Press, Baltimore, Md.

16 Wassarman P.M. & Josefowicz W.J. (1978) Oocyte development in the mouse: an ultrastructural comparison of oocytes isolated at various stages of growth and meiotic competence. *Journal of Morphology* **156**, 209.

17 Gyllensten U., Wharton D., Josefsson A. & Wilson A.C. (1991) Paternal inheritance of mitochondrial DNA in mice. *Nature* **352**, 255.

18 Piko L. & Klegg K.B. (1982) Quantitative changes in total RNA, total poly(A), and ribosomes in early mouse embryos. *Developmental Biology* **89**, 362.

19 Clegg K.B. & Piko L. (1983) Quantitative aspects of RNA synthesis and polyadenylation in 1-cell and 2-cell mouse embryos. *Journal of Embryology and Experimental Morphology* **74**, 169.

462

20 West J.D., Flockhart J.H., Angell R.R., Hillier S.G., Thatcher S.S., Glasier A.F., Rodger M.W. *et al.* (1989) Glucose phosphate isomerase activity in mouse and human eggs and pre-embryos. *Human Reproduction* **4**, 82.

21 Zamboni L. & Upadhyay S. (1983) Germ cell differentiation in mouse adrenal glands. *Journal of Experimental Zoology* **228**, 173.

22 Familiari G., Nottola S.A., Macchiarelli G., Micara G., Aragona C. & Motta P.M. (1992) Human zona pellucida during in vitro fertilization: an ultrastructural study using saponin, ruthenium red, and osmium-thiocarbohydrazide. *Molecular Reproduction and Development* **32**, 51.

23 Koyama K., Hasegawa A., Inoue M. & Isojima S. (1991) Blocking of human sperm–zona interaction by monoclonal antibodies to a glycoprotein family (ZP4) of porcine zona pellucida. *Biology of Reproduction* **45**, 727.

24 Wassarman P.M. (1988) Zona pellucida glycoproteins. *Annual Review of Biochemistry* **57**, 415.

25 Florman H.M. & Wassarman P.M. (1985) O-linked oligosaccharides of mouse egg ZP3 account for its sperm receptor activity. *Cell* **41**, 313.

26 Wassarman P.M. (1991) Cellular and molecular elements of mammalian fertilization. In *Mechanisms of Fertilization*. Ed. B. Dale, p. 305. Springer-Verlag, Berlin.

27 Bleil J.D., Greeve J.M. & Wassarman P.M. (1988) Identification of a secondary sperm receptor in the mouse egg zona pellucida: role in maintence and binding of acrosome reacted sperm. *Developmental Biology* **128**, 376.

28 Schickler M., Lira S.A., Kinloch R.A. & Wassarman P.M. (1992) A mouse oocyte-specific protein that binds to a region of mZP3 promoter responsible for oocyte-specific mZP3 gene expression. *Molecular and Cellular Biology* **12**, 120.

29 Liang L.F. & Dean J. (1993) Conservation of mammalian secondary sperm receptor genes enables the promoter of the human gene to function in mouse oocytes. *Developmental Biology* **156**, 399.

30 Whitaker M.J. & Patel R. (1990) Calcium and cell cycle control. *Development* **108**, 525.

31 Pines J. (1993) Cyclins and cyclin-dependent kinases: take your partners. *Trends in Biochemical Sciences* **18**, 195.

32 Channing C.P., Hillensjo T. & Schaerf F.W. (1978) Hormonal control of oocyte meiosis, ovulation and luteinization in mammals. *Clinical Endocrinology and Metabolism* **7**, 601.

33 Norbury C. & Nurse P. (1992) Animal cell cycle and their control. *Annual Review of Biochemistry* **61**, 441.

34 Choi T., Aoki F., Mori M., Yamashita M., Nagahama Y. & Kohomoto K. (1991) Activation of p34[cdc2] protein kinase activity in meiotic and mitotic cell cycles in mouse oocytes and embryos. *Development* **113**, 789.

35 Lorca T., Cruzalegul F.H., Fequet D., Cavadore J.C., Mery J., Means J. & Doree M. (1993) Calmodulin-dependent protein kinase II mediates inactivation of MPF and CSF upon fertilization of Xenopus eggs. *Nature* **366**, 270.

36 Pincus G. & Enzmann E.V. (1935) The comparative behaviour of mammalian eggs *in vivo* and *in vitro*. *Journal of Experimental Medicine* **62**, 655.

37 Edwards R.G. (1965) Maturation in vitro of human ovarian oocytes. *Lancet* **2**, 926.

38 De Smedt V., Crozet N. & Gall L. (1994) Morphological and functional changes accompanying the acquisition of meiotic competences in ovarian goat oocytes. *Journal of Experimental Zoology* **269**, 128.

39 de Vantéry C., Gavin A.C. Vassalli J.D. & Schorderet-Slatkine S. (1996) An accumulation of p34[cdc2] at the end of mouse oocyte growth correlates with the acquisition of meiotic competence. *Developmental Biology* **174**, 335.

40 Hampl A. & Eppig J.J. (1995) Analysis of the mechanism(s) of metaphase I arrest in maturing mouse oocytes. *Development* **121**, 925.

41 Downs S.M. (1995) Control of the resumption of meiotic maturation in mammalian oocytes. In *Gametes: The Oocyte*. Eds J.G. Grudzinskas & J.L. Yovich, p. 150. Cambridge University Press, Cambridge.

42 Tornell J. & Hillensjo T. (1993) Effect of cyclic AMP on the isolated human oocyte–cumulus complex. *Human Reproduction* **8**, 737.

43 Homa S.T. (1995) Calcium and meiotic maturation of the mammalian oocyte. *Molecular Reproduction and Development* **40**, 122.

44 Carroll J. & Swann K. (1992) Spontaneous cytoscolic calcium oscillations driven by Inositol Trisphosphate occur during *in vitro* maturation of mouse oocytes. *Journal of Biological Chemistry* **267**, 11196.

45 Kline D. & Kline J.T. (1992) Repetitive calcium transients and the role of calcium in exocytosis and cell cycle activation in the mouse egg. *Developmental Biology* **149**, 80.

46 Mattioli M., Barboni B. & Seren E. (1991) Luteinizing hormone inhibits potassium outward currents in swine granulosa cells by intracellular calcium mobilization. *Endocrinology* **129**, 2740.

47 Homa S.T., Carroll J. & Swann K. (1993) The role of calcium in mammalian oocyte maturation and egg activation. *Human Reproduction* **8**, 1274.

48 Kaufman M.L. & Homa S.T. (1993) Defining a role for calcium in the resumption and progression of meiosis in the pig oocyte. *Journal of Experimental Zoology* **265**, 69.

49 Tombes R.M., Simerly C., Borisy G. & Schatten S. (1992) Meiosis, egg activation and nuclear envelope breakdown are differentially reliant on Ca[2+], whereas germinal vesicle breakdown is Ca[2+] independent in the mouse oocyte. *Journal of Cell Biology* **117**, 799.

50 Griffin D.K. (1996) The incidence, origin and etiology of aneuploidy. *International Review of Cytology* **167**, 263.

51 Hassold T. & Sherman S. (1993) The origin of nondisjunction in humans. *Chromosomes Today* **11**, 313.

52 Fisher J.M., Harvey J.F., Morton N.E. & Jacobs P.A. (1995) Trisomy 18: studies of the parent and cell division of origin and the effect of aberrant recombination on non-disjunction. *American Journal of Human Genetics* **56**, 669.

53 Sherman S.L., Petersen M.B., Freemen S.B., Hersey J., Pettay D., Taft L., Frantzen M. *et al.* (1994) Non-disjunction of chromosome 21 in maternal meiosis. I. Evidence for a maternal-age dependent mechanism involving reduced recombination. *Human Molecular Genetics* **3**, 1529.

54 Henderson S.A. & Edwards R.G. (1968) Chiasma frequency and maternal age in mammals. *Nature* **218**, 22.

55 Hawley R.S., Frazier J.A. & Rasooly R. (1994) Separation anxiety: the etiology of non-disjunction in flies and people. *Human Molecular Genetics* **3**, 1521.

56 Eichenlaub-Ritter U., Chandley A.C. & Gosden R.G. (1988) The CBA mouse as a model for age-related aneuploidy in man: studies of oocyte maturation, spindle formation, and chromosome alignment during meiosis. *Chromosoma* **96**, 220.

57 Zenzes M.T., Wang P. & Casper R.F. (1995) Cigarette smoking may affect meiotic maturation of human oocytes. *Human Reproduction* **10**, 3213.

58 Trounson A. (1989) Fertilization and embryo culture. In *Clinical In Vitro Fertilization*, 2nd edn. Eds C. Wood & A. Trounson, p. 41. Springer-Verlag, Berlin.

59 Carroll J., Swann K., Whittingham D. & Whitaker M. (1994) Spatiotemporal dynamics of intracellular [CA²⁺]i oscillations during the growth and meiotic maturation of mouse oocytes. *Development* **120**, 3507.

60 Shiraishi K., Okada A., Shirakawa H., Nakanishi S., Mikoshiba K. & Miyazaki S (1995) Developmental chages in the distribution of the endoplasmic reticulum and inositol 1,4,5-triphosphate receptors and the spatial pattern of Ca²⁺ release during maturation of hamster oocytes. *Developmental Biology* **170**, 594.

61 Herbert M., Murdoch A.P. & Gillespie J.I. (1995) The thiol reagent thimerosal induces intracellular calcium oscillations in mature human oocytes. *Molecular Human Reproduction* **10**, 2183.

62 Perreault S.D., Barbee R.R. & Slott V.L. (1988) Importance of glutathione in the acquisition and maintenance of sperm nuclear decondensation activity in maturing hamster oocytes. *Developmental Biology* **125**, 181.

63 Yoshida M., Ishigaki K., Nagai T., Chikyu M. & Pursel V.G. (1993) Glutathione concentration during maturation and after fertilization in pig oocytes: relevance to the ability of oocytes to form male pronucleus. *Biology of Reproduction* **49**, 89.

64 Eppig J.J., Schroeder A.C. & O'Brien M.J. (1992) Developmental capacity of mouse oocytes matured in vitro: effects of gonadotropic stimulation, follicular origin and oocyte size. *Journal of Reproduction and Fertility* **95**, 119.

65 Huarte J., Belin D., Vassalli A., Strickland S. & Vassalli J.D. (1987) Meiotic maturation of mouse oocytes triggers the translation and polyadenilation of dormant tissue-type plasminogen activator mRNA. *Genes and Development* **1**, 1201.

66 Cohen J., Inge K.L., Suzman M. Wiker S. & Wright G. (1989) Videocinematography of fresh and cryopreserved embryos: a retrospective analysis of embryonic morphology and implantation. *Fertility and Sterility* **51**, 820.

67 Salustri A., Hascall V.C., Camaioni A. & Yanagishita M. (1993) Oocyte–granulosa cell interactions. In *The Ovary*. Eds E.Y. Adashi & P.C.K. Leung, p. 209. Raven Press. New York.

68 Le Guen P., Crozet N., Huneau D. & Gall L. (1989) Distribution and role of microfilaments during early events of sheep fertilization. *Gamete Research* **22**, 411.

69 Pickering S.J., Johnson M.H., Braude P.R. & Houliston E. (1988) Cytoskeletal organization in fresh, aged and spontaneously activated human oocytes. *Human Reproduction* **3**, 978.

70 Navara C.S., First N.L. & Schatten G. (1994) Microtubule organization in the cow during fertilization, polyspermy, parthenogenesis and nuclear transfer: the role of the sperm aster. *Developmental Biology* **162**, 29.

71 Pickering S.J., Braude P.R., Johnson M.H, Cant A. & Currie J. (1990) Transient cooling at room temperature can cause irreversible disruption of the meiotic spindle in the human oocyte. *Fertility and Sterility* **54**, 102.

72 Sathananthan A.H., Kola I., Osborne J., Trounson A., Ng S.C., Bongso A. & Ratnam S.S. (1991) Centrioles in the beginning of human development. *Proceedings of the National Academy of Sciences USA* **88**, 4806.

73 Kaneda H., Hayashi J.I., Takahama S., Taya C., Lindahl K.F. & Yonekawa H. (1995) Elimination of paternal mitochondrial DNA in intraspecific crosses during early mouse embryogenesis. *Proceedings of the National Academy of Sciences USA* **92**, 4542.

74 DeRooji D.G., Van Dissel-Emiliani F.M.F. & Van Pelt A.M.M. (1989) Regulation of spermatogonia proliferation. In *Regulation of Testicular Function Signalling Molecules and Cell–Cell Communication*. Eds B. Robaire & L.L. Ewing LL. *Annals of New York Academy of Sciences* **564**, 1140.

75 Hamilton D.W. & Waites G.M.H. (1990) Cellular and molecular events in spermiogenesis. Scientific basis of fertility regulation. *World Health Organization*, p. 334. Cambridge University Press, Cambridge.

76 Johnson M.D. (1991) Genes related to spermatogenesis: molecular and clinical aspects. *Seminars in Reproductive Endocrinology* **9**, 73.

77 Moore H.D.M. (1995) Post-testicular sperm maturation and transport in the excurrent ducts. In *Gametes: The Spermatozoon*. Eds J.G. Grudzinskas & J.L. Yovic, p. 140. Cambridge University Press, Cambridge.

78 Ariel M., Cedar H. & McCarrey J. (1994) Developmental changes in methylation of spermatogenesis-specific genes include reprogramming in the epididymis. *Nature Genetics* **7**, 59.

79 Yanagimachi R. (1970) The movement of golden hamster spermatozoa before and after capacitation. *Journal of Reproduction and Fertility* **23**, 193.

80 Benoff S. (1993) The role of cholesterol during capacitation of human spermatozoa. *Human Reproduction* **8**, 2001.

81 Benoff S., Cooper G.W., Hurley I., Napolitano B., Rosenfeld D.L., Scholl G.M. & Hershlag A. (1993) Human sperm fertilizing potential in vitro: differential expression of a head-specific mannose-ligand receptor. *Fertility and Sterility* **59**, 854.

464

82 Bielfeld P., Faridi A., Zaneveld L.J. & De Jonge C.J. (1994) The zona pellucida-induced acrosome reaction of human spermatozoa is mediated by protein kinases. *Fertility and Sterility* **61**, 536.

83 Green D.P.L. (1988) Sperm thrust and the problem of penetration. *Biological Reviews of Cambridge Philosophical Society* **63**, 79.

84 Foresta C., Mioni R., Rossato M., Varotto A. & Zorzi M. (1991) Evidence for the involvement of sperm angiotensin converting enzyme in fertilization. *International Journal of Andrology* **14**, 333.

85 Zaneveld L.J., De Jong C.J., Anderson R.A. & Mack S.R. (1991) Human sperm capacitation and the acrosome reaction. *Human Reproduction* **6**, 1265.

86 Wassarman P.M. (1987) The biology and chemistry of fertilization. *Science* **235**, 553.

87 Macek M.B. & Shur B.D. (1988) Protein–carbohydrate complementarity in mammalian gamete recognition. *Gamete Research* **20**, 93.

88 Miller D.J., Macek M.B. & Shur B.D. (1992) Complementarity between sperm surface β-1,4-galactosyltransferase and egg-coat ZP3 mediates sperm binding. *Nature* **357**, 589.

89 Bleil J.D. & Wassarman P.M. (1990) Identification of a ZP3-binding protein on acrosome intact mouse sperm by photoaffinity cross-linking. *Proceedings of the National Academy of Sciences USA* **87**, 5563.

90 Bookbinder L.H., Cheng A. & Bleil J.D. (1995) Tissue and species-specific expression of sp56, a mouse sperm fertilisation protein. *Science* **269**, 86.

91 Ramarao C.S., Myles D.G. & Primakoff P. (1994) Multiple roles for PH20 and fertilin in sperm–egg interactions. *Seminars in Developmental Biology* **5**, 265.

92 Blobel C.P., Wolsberg T.G., Turck C.W., Myles D.G., Primakoff P. & White J.M. (1992) A potential fusion peptide and an integrin ligan domain in a protein active in sperm–egg fusion. *Nature* **356**, 248.

93 Hagiwara S. & Jaffe L.A. (1979) Electrical properties of egg cell membranes. *Annual Review of Biophysics and Bioengineering* **8**, 385.

94 Whitaker M.J. & Steinhardt R.A. (1982) Ionic regulation of egg activation. *Quarterly Reviews of Biophysics* **15**, 593.

95 Taylor C.T., Lawrence Y.M., Kingsland C.R., Biljan M.M. & Cuthbertson K.S.R. (1993) Oscillations in intracellular free calcium induced by spermatozoa in human oocytes at fertilization. *Human Reproduction* **8**, 2174.

96 Igusa Y. & Miyazaki S. (1983) Effects of altered extracellular and intracellular calcium concentration on hyperpolarizing responses of hamster eggs. *Journal of Physiology* **340**, 611.

97 Swann K. & Ozil J.P. (1994) Dynamics of the calcium signal that triggers mammalian egg activation. *International Review of Cytology* **152**, 183.

98 Swann K. (1990) A cytosolic sperm factor stimulates repetitive calcium increases and mimics fertilisation in hamster eggs. *Development* **110**, 1295.

99 Parrington J., Swann K., Shevchenko P.I., Sesay A.K. & Lai F.A. (1996) Calcium oscillations in mammalian eggs triggered by a soluble sperm protein. *Nature* **379**, 364.

100 Fishel S., Timson J., Lisi F. & Rinaldi L. (1992) Evaluation of 225 patients undergoing sub-zonal insemination for the procurement of fertilization *in vitro*. *Fertility and Sterility* **57**, 840.

101 Sathananthan A.H., Trounson A., Freemann L. & Brady T. (1988) The effects of cooling oocytes. *Human Reproduction* **3**, 968.

102 Shabonowitz R.B. & O'Rand M.G. (1989) Characterization of the human zona pellucida from fertilized and unfertilized eggs. *Journal of Reproduction and Fertility* **82**, 151.

103 Moller C.C. & Wassarmann P.M. (1988) Characterization of a proteinase that cleaves zona pellucida glycoprotein ZP2 following activation of mouse eggs. *Developmental Biology* **132**, 103.

104 Sagata N., Watanabe N., Van de Woude G.F. & Ikawa Y. (1989) The *c-mos* proto-oncogene product is a cytostatic factor responsible for meiotic arrest in vertebrate eggs. *Nature* **342**, 512.

105 Weber M., Kubiak J.Z., Arlinghaus R.B., Pines J. & Maro B. (1991) *c-mos* proto-oncogene product is partly degraded after release from meiotic arrest and persists during interphase in mouse zygotes. *Developmental Biology* **148**, 393.

106 Kubiak J.Z. (1989) Mouse oocytes gradually develop the capacity for activation during the metaphase II arrest. *Developmental Biology* **136**, 537.

107 Tesarik J. & Testart J. (1989) Human sperm–egg interactions and their disorders: implications in the management of infertility. *Human Reproduction* **4**, 729.

108 Pieters M.H., Geraedts J.P., Dumoulin J.C., Evers J.L., Bras M., Kornips F.H. & Menheere P. (1989) Cytogenetic analysis of *in vitro* fertilization (IVF) failures. *Human Genetics* **81**, 367.

109 Jacobs P.A., Wilson C.M., Sprenkle J.A., Rosenhein N.B. & Migeon B.R. (1980) Mechanism of origin of complete hydatiform mole. *Nature* **286**, 714.

110 Surani M.A.H. & Barton S.C. (1983) Development of gynogenetic eggs in the mouse: implications for parthenogenetic embryos. *Science* **222**, 1034.

111 Strain L., Warner J.P., Johnson T. & Bonthorn D. (1995) A human parthenogenetic chimaera. *Nature Genetics* **11**, 164.

112 De Chiara T.M., Robertoson E.J. & Efstradiatis A. (1991) Parental imprinting of the mouse insulin-like growth factor II gene. *Cell* **64**, 849.

113 Barlow D.P., Stoger R., Hermann B.G., Saito K. & Scheifer N. (1991) The mouse insulin-like growth factor type-II receptor is imprinted and closely linked to the Tme locus. *Nature* **349**, 84.

114 Fishel S.B., Tesarik J. & Aslam I. (1996) Spermatid conception: a stage too early or a time too soon? *Human Reproduction* **11**, 1371.

115 Fishel S.B. & Symonds E.M. (1986) *In Vitro Fertilisation: Past, Present and Future*. IRL Press, Oxford.

116 Johnson M.H. & Marrow B. (1986) Time and space in the early mouse embryo. In *Experimental Approaches to Mammalian Embryonic Development*. Eds J. Rossant & R.A. Pedersen, p. 35. Cambridge University Press, Cambridge.

117 Veiga A., Calderon G., Barri P.N. & Coroleu B. (1987) Pregnancy after the replacement of a frozen-thawed embryo with less than 50% intact blastomeres. *Human Reproduction* **2**, 321.

118 Johnson M.H., Chrisholm J.C., Fleming T.P. & Houliston E. (1986) A role for cytoplasmic determinants in the early mouse embryo. *Journal of Embryology and Experimental Zoology* (Suppl.) **97**, 97.

119 Winkel G.K., Ferguson J.E., Takeichi M. & Nuccitelli R. (1990) Activation of protein kinase C trigger premature compaction in the 4-cell stage mouse embryo. *Developmental Biology* **138**, 1.

120 Sutherland A.E., Speed T.P. & Calarco P.G. (1990) Inner cell allocation in the mouse morula: the role of oriented division during fourth cleavage. *Developmental Biology* **137**, 13.

121 Dyce J., George M., Goodall H. & Fleming T.P. (1987) Do trophectoderm and ICM cells in the mouse blastocyst maintain discrete lineage? *Development* **100**, 685.

122 Hillman N., Sherman H. & Graham C.F. (1972) The effects of spatial arrangement of cell determination during mouse development. *Journal of Embryology and Experimental Morphology* **28**, 263.

123 Tesarik J., Kopecny V., Plachot M., Mandelbaum J., Da Lage C. & Flechon J.E. (1986) Nucleogenesis in the human embryo developing *in vitro*: ultrastructural and autoradiographic analysis. *Developmental Biology* **115**, 193.

124 Dale B., Gualtieri R., Talevi R., Tosti E., Santella L. & Elder K. (1991) Intercellular communication in the early human embryo. *Molecular Reproduction and Development* **29**, 22.

125 Braude P., Bolton V. & Moore S. (1988) Human gene expression first occurs between the four- and eight-cell stages of preimplantation development. *Nature* **332**, 459.

126 Schultz R.M. & Worrad D.M. (1995) Role of chromatin structure in zygotic gene activation in the mammalian embryo. *Seminars of Cell Biology* **6**, 201.

127 Renard J.P. (1996) Transcriptional activation of the embryonic genome. *Proceedings of the Development of the Human Egg Serono Symposium*, 13–15 September, Leeds, UK.

128 Zwingman T., Erickson R.P., Boyer T. & Ao A. (1993) Transcription of the sex-determining region genes *Sry* and *Zfy* in the mouse preimplantation embryo. *Proceedings of the National Academy of Sciences USA* **90**, 814.

129 Fishel S.B., Edwards R.G. & Evans C.J. (1984) Human chorionic gonadotropin secreted by preimplantation embryos cultured *in vitro*. *Science* **223**, 816.

130 Lopata A. & Hay D.L. (1989) The surplus human embryo: its potential for growth, blastulation, hatching, and human chorionic gonadatrophin production in culture. *Fertility and Sterility* **51**, 984.

131 Krumlauf R. (1993) Mouse Hox genetic functions. *Current Opinions in Genetics and Development* **3**, 621.

132 Paria B., Dey S.K. & Andrews G.K. (1992) Antisense *c-myc* effects on preimplantation mouse embryo development. *Proceedings of the National Academy of Sciences USA* **89**, 10051.

133 Austgulen R., Arntzen K.J., Vatten L.J., Kahn J. & Sunde A. (1995) Detection of cytokines (interleukin 1-6, transforming growth factor-beta) and soluble tumour necrosis factor receptors in embryo culture fluids during *in vitro* fertilization. *Human Reproduction* **10**, 171.

134 Hardy K., Handyside A.H. & Winston R.M. (1989) The human blastocyst: cell number, death and allocation during the preimplantation development *in vitro*. *Development* **107**, 597.

135 Overstrom E.W., Benos D.J. & Biggers J.D. (1989) Synthesis of Na+/K+ ATPase by the preimplantation rabbit blastocyst. *Journal of Reproduction and Fertility* **85**, 283.

136 Cohen J., Alikani M., Trowbridge J. & Rosenwaks Z. (1992) Implantation enhancement by selective assisted hatching using zona drilling of human embryos with poor prognosis. *Human Reproduction* **7**, 685.

137 Seshagiri P.B., Terasawa E. & Hearn J.P. (1994) The secretion of gonadotrophin-releasing hormone by peri-implantation embryos of the rhesus monkey: comparison with the secretion of chorionic gonadotrophin. *Human Reproduction* **9**, 1300.

138 Morin N. & Sullivan R. (1994) Expression of fibronectin and a fibronectin-binding molecule during preimplantation development in the mouse. *Human Reproduction* **9**, 894.

139 Charnock-Jones D.S., Sharkey A.M., Fenwick P. & Smith S.K. (1994) Leukaemia inhibitiory factor mRNA concentration peaks in human endometrium at the time of implantation and the blastocyst contains mRNA for the receptor at this time. *Journal of Reproduction and Fertility* **101**, 421.

140 Dor J., Rudak E., Rotmensch S., Levran D., Blankstein J., Lusky A., Nebel L. *et al.* (1988) The role of early post-implantation beta-HCG levels in the outcome of pregnancies following *in vitro* fertilization. *Human Reproduction* **3**, 663.

141 Check J.H., Weiss R.M. & Lurie D. (1992) Analysis of serum human chorionic gonadotrophin levels in normal singleton, multiple and abnormal pregnancies. *Human Reproduction* **7**, 1176.

142 Kadar N., Freedman M. & Zacher M. (1990) Further observations on the doubling time of human chorionic gonadotrophin in early asymptomatic pregnancies. *Fertility and Sterility* **54**, 783.

143 O'Neill C., Gidley-Baird A.A., Pike I.L., Porter R.N., Sinosich M.J. & Saunders D.M. (1985) Maternal blood platelet physiology and luteal-phase endocrinology as a means of monitoring pre- and postimplantation embryo viability following in vitro fertilization. *Journal of in Vitro Fertilization and Embryo Transfer* **2**, 87.

144 Cocchiara R., Di Trapani G., Azzolina A., Cittadini E. & Geraci D. (1986) Binding of human EPF to receptors on PMBC as a first signal of pregnancy immodulation. *Human Reproduction* **1**, 33.

145 Klentzeris L.D., Bulmer J.N., Lee T.C., Morrison L., Warren A. & Cooke I.D. (1991) Lectin binding of endometrium in women with unexplained infertility. *Fertility and Sterility* **56**, 660.

146 Can A., Teklioglu M. & Biberoglu K. (1991) Structure of premenstrual endometrium in HMG and HCG induced anovulatory women. *European Journal of Obstetrics, Gynaecology and Reproductive Biology* **42**, 119.

147 Wang J.D., Fu Y., Zhu P.D., Cheng J., Qiao G.M.,

466

Wang Y.Q. & Greene G.L. (1992) Immunohistochemical localization of progesterone receptor in human decidua of early pregnancy. *Human Reproduction* 7, 1123.

148 Anderson T.L. (1989) Biomolecular markers for the window of uterine receptivity. In *Blastocyst Implantation.* Ed. K. Yoshina, p. 214. Adams Publishing Group, Boston.

149 Tabibzadeh S. (1991) Ubiquitous expression of TNF-α/cachectin immunoreactivity in human endometrium. *American Journal of Reproductive Immunology* **26**, 1.

150 Tabibzadeh S., Sun X.Z., Kong Q.F., Kasnic G., Miller J. & Satyaswaroop P.G. (1993) Induction of a polarized micro-environment by human T cells and interferon-gamma in three-dimensional spheroid cultures of human endometrial epithelial cells. *Human Reproduction* **8**, 182.

151 Tabibzadeh S. (1994) Cytokines and the hypothalamic–pituitary–ovarian–endometrial axis. *Human Reproduction* **9**, 947.

152 Younis J.S., Mordel N., Ligovetzky G., Lewin A., Schenker J.G. & Laufer N. (1991) The effect of a prolonged artificial follicular phase on endometrial development in an oocyte donation program. *Journal of in Vitro Fertilization and Embryo Tansfer* **8**, 84.

153 Manners C.V. (1990) Endometrial assessment in a group of infertile women on stimulated cycles for IVF: immonuhistochemical findings. *Human Reproduction* **5**, 128.

154 Fernandez-Shaw S., Shorter S.C., Naish C.E., Barlow D.H. & Starkey P.M. (1992) Isolation and purification of human endometrial stromal and glandular cells using immunomagnetic microspheres. *Human Reproduction* **7**, 156.

155 Fay T.N. & Grudzinskas J.G. (1991) Human endometrial peptides: a review of their potential role in implantation and placentation. *Human Reproduction* **6**, 1311.

156 Kimber S.J. & Lindenberg S. (1990) Hormonal control of a carbohydrate epitope involved in implantation in mice. *Journal of Reproduction and Fertility* **89**, 13.

157 Earl U., Morrison L., Gay C. & Bulmer J.N. (1989) Proteinase and proteinase inhibitor localization in the human placenta. *International Journal of Gynaecological Pathology* **8**, 114.

158 Sadler T.W. (1992) Organogenesis and central nervous system development. In *Foetal Tissue Transplants in Medicine.* Ed. R.G. Edwards, p. 51. Cambridge University Press, Cambridge.

159 Whitaker M. (1996) Control of meiotic arrest. *Reviews of Reproduction* **2**, 132.

Fetal Nutrition and Growth

D.K. JAMES & T. STEPHENSON

Introduction

The importance of birthweight and its relationship to morbidity and survival into childhood has been known for some time [1]. However, more recently, interest has been generated over the relationships between fetal nutrition, growth and birthweight and long-term morbidity and mortality (the 'Barker hypothesis') [2,3].

The overview of this chapter is:
- Normal nutrition and growth in the fetus;
  - Biology of growth
  - Phases of growth
  - Determinants of growth
    Fetal
    Placental
    Maternal
- Abnormal or pathological nutrition and growth;
- Practical or clinical implications and applications.

In as far as is possible, the scientific background is presented for human studies. When animal data are used, this is specified.

Finally, for practical purposes we have considered fetal growth from the 9th week onwards, the fetal period.

Normal nutrition and growth

More extensive reviews of cell biology and growth are available elsewhere [4].

The cell cycle

Peptide growth factors (Table 18.1) are proteins which alter cell growth, differentiation, motility or division through interaction with cell-surface receptors on cells of the same type (autocrine activity), a dissimilar type (paracrine) or cells in a distant location (endocrine) [5]. Cells in G_0 (the resting phase of the cell cycle) can be stimulated by exposure to peptide growth factors (e.g. platelet-derived growth factor (PDGF), fibroblast growth factor (FGF)) to resume cell division by entering the G_1 (first gap) phase. To progress from G_1 to the S phase (cell irreversibly committed to DNA synthesis) may require other growth factors such as epidermal growth factor (EGF), insulin-like growth factor-1 (IGF1), and colony-stimulating factor. All growth factors act on cell-surface glycoprotein receptors and mediate their actions by increased specific RNA and protein synthesis leading to cell replication (or, in certain circumstances, inhibition of cell multiplication).

Table 18.1. Some peptide hormones and growth factors.

Peptide macromolecule	Number of amino acids	Molecular weight (kDa)	Gene on chromosome	Comments
Growth hormone	191	22	17	
Prolactin	198	23	6	Related to growth hormone and human placental lactogen
Insulin	51	6	11	Insulin is the major fetal growth hormone
IGF1	70	7.5	12	The somatomedins are mitogens and differentiating agents for all cells
IGF2	67	7.5	11	
EGF	53	6	4	Mitogens for epithelial and mesodermal cells
TGFα		7.5	2	Promote release of hCG and hPL from placenta. TGFα has 35% homology with EGF
TGFβ				Inhibitor of epithelial cell proliferation
TGF β_1		25	19	Promotes collagen synthesis
TGF β_2			1	
Platelet-derived growth factor		28–35		Mitogen for mesodermal cells
A chain			7	
B chain			22	
FGF				Mitogen for connective tissue cells and angiogenic for endothelial cells
Basic (bFGF)	146	16.5	5	
Acidic (aFGF)	140	15.5	4	

EGF: epidermal growth factor; FGF: fibroblast growth factor; IGF: insulin-like growth factor; TGF: transforming growth factor.

Intercellular control

At least three control mechanisms govern cell and tissue interactions in the embryo and fetus.

1 *Extracellular matrix molecules* (the scaffold which organizes groups of cells into discrete tissues) play a role in cell shape, division rate, cell migration and differentiation and are of two major classes:

    (a) Proteins such as collagen, fibronectin and laminin (which is abundant in basement membranes); tenascin, a molecule related to fibronectin, appears along cellular migration pathways (e.g. those of neural crest cells and palatal fusion) and is removed immediately after the appropriate cells have migrated;

    (b) Mucopolysaccharides such as hyaluronic acid (which creates a loose gel through which migrating cells can pass), heparin sulphate and keratin sulphate.

2 *Intercellular recognition molecules.* Cells recognize their anatomical position within a developing structure by recognition molecules which have been categorized into cell adhesion molecules (proteins which do not require calcium for their action) and cadherins (calcium-dependent glycoproteins). These systems can be so powerful that, *in vitro*, dispersed cells can assemble autonomously and reform tissues and in some primitive species complete embryos.

3 *Hormonal messengers and peptide growth factors.* Hormones were originally defined as chemicals which acted distant to their site of production. However, in addition to these endocrine (circulating) effects, more recent work has identified more local autocrine (acting on their own cell of production) and paracrine (acting on neighbouring cells) effects.

Fetal size and organ growth increase by a combination of cell hypertrophy and cell division [6]. Large mice have both more cells and larger cells than small mice but the relative contribution of each depends on the organ. In the lung, increased cell number accounts for 70% of the size difference, whereas in the liver, increased cell size and number contribute equally [7]. Programmed selective cell death (apoptosis) is as important as multiplication in the development of some organs (e.g. the separation of the digits and formation of the palate).

Major chromosomal anomalies usually result in smaller babies because of impaired cell division rather than cell growth, although abnormal placental function may also play a part. In aneuploidy, the placenta shares the abnormal fetal karyotype and may be grossly dysmorphic. Studies of mosaicism suggest that the degree of placental euploidy determines duration of intrauterine survival [8].

Phases of growth

Between conception and birth, 42 cell divisions occur, with only five more incremental cell divisions from birth to adult size. This, of course, excludes cell division to replace dead cells which continues throughout life in the skin and gut, for example. However, mitotic rate is not fixed throughout pregnancy [6]; rather, there are discrete phases of growth and development which serve different goals.

Embryogenesis (see also Chapter 17)

The embryonic period lasts from conception to 8 weeks and consists of:
1 Growth (cell multiplication and enlargement);
2 Cell differentiation (structural differentiation of a group of cells which form a specific tissue—histogenesis);
3 Organogenesis (tissues of more than one kind come together to develop organs);
4 Morphogenesis (development of shape).

This is the period of greatest susceptibility to teratogens, usually resulting in major morphological abnormalities; beyond the embryonic period, fetotoxins are more likely to impair fetal growth and development than produce structural changes.

Fetal period

This continues from the 9th week to term and involves both maturation of tissues and organs

formed during embryogenesis and continued growth at a more rapid rate than any other time in life. Differentiation is less sensitive to nutritional deficiencies than growth [6]. The human pregnancy is divided conveniently into trimesters.

First trimester

The first trimester includes the embryonic period (see Chapter 17). Growth occurs principally by increase in cell numbers and the fetal crown–rump length increases at approximately 1–1.5 mm/day.

Second trimester

Cell division continues at a slower rate but there is now increase in cell size too [6]. It is important to appreciate that there are a number of different ways of looking at growth rates. Fractional change per unit time is greatest for length and weight in the first trimester. However, the maximum absolute increment in any one week occurs at the 16th week for crown–rump length (15 mm/week) and at the 35th week for weight (200 g/week) [9]. Total length and weight increase steadily throughout gestation. These three different ways of looking at fetal growth are shown in Fig. 18.1 [10].

Third trimester

Cell division slows but increase in cell size continues. In the last trimester of human pregnancy, the fetus doubles in body weight and fat content increases from 3 to 16% (Fig. 18.2) [11]. Lipid accumulation is the major determinant of final weight and major influences on this are maternal nutrient availability and fetal insulin production.

Changes to abortion laws, and hence the greater availability of 'normal' early fetuses, and the advent of ultrasound imaging have provided a wealth of new data on fetal growth [12,13]. Early in the third trimester, estimated fetal weight gain is a straight line representing unrestricted growth. Maximum weight gain is 200 g/week in the 34th and 35th weeks. Subsequently, weekly weight gain is less; this is

469

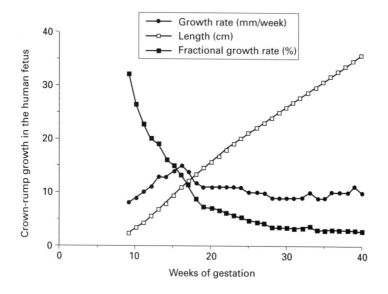

Fig. 18.1. Crown–rump growth. The open squares show total crown–rump length which increases steadily throughout gestation. The first-order growth velocity (increment per unit time, in this case per week) is maximal early in the second trimester. The fractional growth rate is expressed as a percentage (100 × increment per week/length at that age). Data from Milner [10].

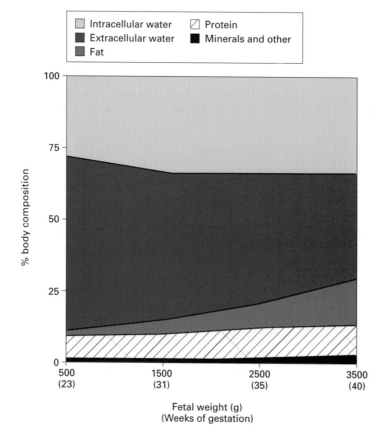

Fig. 18.2. Percentage body composition in relation to fetal weight and gestational age. From Dweck [11] with permission of the publisher.

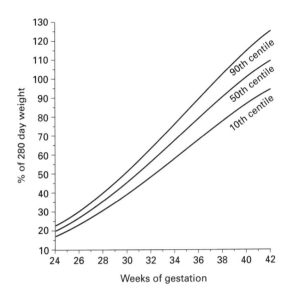

Fig. 18.3. Standard curve for fetal weight gain, expressed as a proportionality curve for percentage of term versus gestation. From Gardosi *et al.* [14] with the permission of the publisher.

postulated to be due to declining support by the uterine environment, since shortly after the baby is born weight gain is comparable to maximum gross intrauterine rates (200 g/week over each of the first 10 weeks). Most published weight growth curves are based on cross-sectional data and are typically sigmoid shaped, with a flattening of the curve towards and past term. However, the terminal flattening of the weight curve is less pronounced when gestational age is reliable and longitudinal weight charts can best be described as a curve with a weak sigmoid shape [9]. An example of a standard curve for fetal weight gain is shown in Fig. 18.3 [14].

In the final trimester of human pregnancy, the rate of organ maturation slows, a factor which allows the human infant to tolerate birth at earlier fractional gestations than any other mammal. Organ systems such as kidney, gut, pancreas and liver can function perfectly adequately from 0.7 of gestation onwards.

Individual organs

Brain

At birth, the brain is already 27% of the adult brain weight [15]. Most neurones in the cerebrum are formed at 10–18 weeks. This is the vulnerable period of cell multiplication, explaining why first trimester insults often result in microcephaly. Axon and dendrite growth comes later (see below). Glial cells start to form around 15 weeks and in the second half of pregnancy, hyperplasia of glial cells and growth of dendrites comprises the brain growth spurt [15] which continues into the second postnatal year. Fetal growth restriction before or after this brain growth spurt may have less lasting effects than insults during the growth spurt.

Liver

The liver is a relatively larger organ in the fetus than after birth, descending below the costal margin and well across the midline, and is therefore the main determinant of abdominal circumference. Tissues with the highest rate of protein turnover such as the liver may be most vulnerable to intrauterine growth retardation (IUGR) due to a decreased supply of amino acids restraining protein synthesis [16]. The fetal liver is the first organ obviously affected in IUGR (as stores of fat and glycogen are used up [17] and therefore head to abdomen ratio is a useful index of IUGR before brain growth is impaired.

Prenatal growth determinants: overview

Multiple gene loci contribute to fetal growth, and this genetic material (paternal, maternal and fetal) is predetermined. However, there is significant modulation during the fetal period by the environment (both immediate and distant) which is variable and mutable (Table 18.2) [10]. Hence the fetus may not grow to its genetic potential. Oncogenes are normal components of the genome and are expressed in a controlled pattern during embryogenesis and fetal development, often under the control of peptide growth

Table 18.2. Genetic and environmental contributions (%) to birthweight variation. From Milner [10].

Genetic	
Maternal genotype	20
Fetal genotype	16
Fetal sex	2
Total genetic contribution	38
Environmental	
General maternal environment	18
Immediate maternal environment	6
Maternal age and parity	8
Unknown environmental influences	30
Total environmental contribution	62

factors. Neoplasia only results when these genes are expressed inappropriately.

Paternal genome has little direct influence on size at birth (although obviously there are important indirect effects through the paternal contribution to 50% of the fetal genome and the fact than an X or Y chromosome from the father determines fetal sex), although it is a major influence on final adult height. In donkey–horse hybrids, the mule, born to a mare, is heavier than the hinny, whose mother is a donkey. In both hybrids, there is 50:50 paternal/maternal genetic material within the fetus but it is the maternal size (genotype and hence phenotype) which is the major influence on the size of the fetus at birth [18]. Similarly, in humans, birth weight is highly correlated in half-siblings who share the same mother but not between half-siblings who have a common father [18].

In Shire horse–Shetland pony crosses, the birthweight of hybrid foals from Shetland mares was typical of the smaller breed [19]. The hybrids from Shire mares weighed three times as much but were still lighter than the normal Shire birthweight. These classic experiments illustrate a growth-limiting effect of the smaller maternal genotype and an intrinsic limit on fetal growth set by the fetal genotype.

Embryo transfer experiments suggest that weight differences due to the genotype of the offspring arise early in embryogenesis. In contrast, phenotypic/genotypic growth restraint exerts its effect late in gestation [7]. In polytocous

species, individual birthweight is inversely related to litter size. However, in the mouse at midfetal stage, fetal size is determined solely by fetal genotype and the constraining influence of litter load/uterine size on fetal growth is only a function of late gestation. Similarly, experimental reduction of litter size *in utero* increases weight at term but not weight at 0.7 gestation. These data suggest uterine constraint of fetal growth occurs late and is due to total placentofetal mass reaching a critical level. Human twin pregnancies show a decline in fetal growth rate over the last 10 weeks, being the same size as singletons in the second trimester.

These issues are discussed further later in 'Maternal determinants' (see p. 482).

Fetal determinants

Fetal genome

At term, the male fetus weighs over 100 g more than the female (greater lean body mass and less fat), perhaps partly due to fetal testosterone production. By 8 weeks, Sertoli cells (produce Müllerian inhibitory factor) and Leydig cells (produce testosterone) are present and testosterone synthesis begins. In contrast to testes, ovaries have minimal capacity to synthesize sex steroids during intrauterine life. However, studies in mice show that the growth advantage of the XY embryo is present at the earliest stages of organogenesis, before endogenous gonadal hormone production could exert effects. These studies also suggest that it is the presence of the Y chromosome which confers a positive growth advantage rather than a growth restraint from two X chromosomes [7].

Parental imprinting of the fetal genome

In mice, paternal uniparental disomy for chromosome 11 results in newborn which are larger than normal but maternal disomy does not. In androgenetic mice (diploid but derived only from paternal chromosomes), the extraembryonic membranes develop well but early development of the embryo is poor, whereas the opposite is true in gynogenetic mice. Similarly, human triploid fetuses develop a large placenta if the extra genome is paternal but not if it is maternal. In humans, sporadic cases of Beckwith–Wiedemann syndrome (a syndrome characterized by fetal macrosomia) are associated with paternal, but not maternal, duplication of a gene on chromosome 11. Loci which map to this region include the genes for insulin and IGF2. There is a hypothesis that imprinting evolved because of the conflict of interests of maternal and paternal genes in relation to the transfer of nutrients from the mother to her offspring [20]. Essentially, the teleological argument, following the *selfish gene* notion, is that the paternal DNA is *'not concerned'* about possible ill effects of the pregnancy on the mother, since the father can choose a different mate next time, and therefore paternal genes maximize the *parasitic* nutritional drain of the fetus from the mother.

Fetal environment

Multiple pregnancy

That the fetus does not always reach genetic potential is shown powerfully by the fact that identical twins will on average be smaller than a singleton. Indeed, in polytocous mammals, position within uterus is also an important determinant of individual fetal size. The reason for this might be due to overcrowding or might have a haemodynamic explanation. The predominant view is that the haemodynamic explanation is more likely to be correct. Wigglesworth [21] elegantly demonstrated this in a ligation experiment which is summarized in Fig. 18.4. The fetuses at the middle of the non-ligated arterial arcade were heavier and on the side of the distally ligated arcade there was progressive diminution of fetal size in those further from the blood source.

Fetal hormones and growth factors

Oxygen and nutrients are necessary for fetal growth but the regulation of growth is governed by hormones and growth factors. These fetal peptides which control the environment are encoded by the fetal genome but transcription rates, and hence bioavailability, are determined presumably by a combination of the fetal genome and by the nutritional environment provided by the mother. These complex interactions emphasize the arbitrariness of dividing growth determinants neatly into genetic and environmental lists. Each growth factor may play various roles depending on gestation,

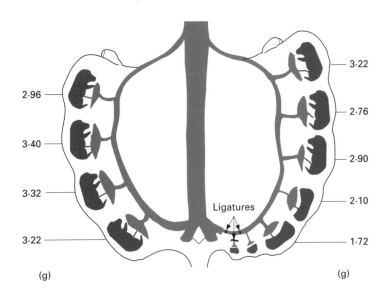

Fig. 18.4. Arterial blood supply of the rat uterus, showing the result observed on the 21st day of pregnancy, 5 days after the application of ligatures. The figures indicate the weights (g) of individual fetuses in a typical experiment. From Wigglesworth [21] with permission of the publisher.

receptors on the target tissue, the presence of other inhibitory or permissive growth factors, and the supply of oxygen, energy and nutrients [5]. Maternal and fetal peptide hormones do not cross the placenta in physiologically significant amounts and therefore the two endocrine systems undergo changes throughout the pregnancy largely independently of one another. For example, although thyrotrophin releasing hormone (TRH) crosses the placenta (and this has been used therapeutically to stimulate fetal lung surfactant production), TRH is not found in the maternal circulation in significant amounts, whereas thyroid-stimulating hormone (TSH) and thyroxine (T_4), which are, do not easily cross the placenta. In contrast, the small lipid-soluble steroid hormones (derived from cholesterol) do cross the placenta and the maternoplacental–fetal adrenal cortex unit must be considered together.

Corticosteroids

The fetal adrenal cortex accounts for 80% of the cortex at birth and interacts with the placenta to form the fetoplacental unit. The fetal adrenal has two unique functions:
1   To produce precursors for maternal oestrogen production rather than aldosterone and cortisol for the fetus. The fetal adrenal therefore contributes to the maintenance of pregnancy by ensuring the oestrogen surge in late pregnancy which leads to uterine growth and increased blood flow (and hence fetal growth).
2   To facilitate fetal organ enzyme maturation. The 20% of cortex at term made up of definitive adult type cortex produces cortisol and the rise in fetal plasma cortisol concentration matures the enzyme systems (e.g. in the lung, surfactant to prepare the neonate for independent respiration; in the liver, glycogen biosynthesis to prepare the neonate for separation from the continuous placental supply of nutrients).

Insulin

Insulin, an anabolic hormone which allows glucose to enter cells, is essential for fetal growth [22]. Euglycaemic pancreatectomized animals have lower circulating IGF1 levels, impaired growth, deficient muscle mass, and they lack adipose tissue. In the guinea-pig, fetal plasma insulin concentrations are closely related to fetal size. Insulin is an important regulator of fetal IGF secretion and the effects of insulin on fetal growth may be mediated by IGF1 release. Fetal hyperinsulinaemia is associated with macrosomia and increased IGF1.

Growth hormone

Growth hormone is the main regulator of IGF synthesis postnatally, but it has little effect on fetal growth [23]. Growth hormone reaches a greater plasma concentration than at any other time in life at 20 weeks. However, despite its abundance, growth hormone is not thought to be the major endocrine determinant of fetal weight gain because anencephalic fetuses have a relatively normal body weight, and umbilical cord growth hormone levels at delivery do not correlate with birthweight [24]. Birth length is reduced in congenital growth hormone deficiency [18]. Studies of growth hormone-deficient mice suggest relative pituitary independence of skeletal (only 14% reduction), brain and lung growth, whereas heart, liver and kidneys were undergrown. However, although organ growth varied, fetal serum IGF1 and IGF2 were decreased, suggesting therefore that actions of IGFs are organ specific or that insulin-like growth factor binding protein (IGFBP) expression is tissue specific and modulates local IGF activity [5].

Thyroid hormones

Late in gestation, there is a triiodothyronine (T_3) surge (due to rising fetal cortisol inducing fetal hepatic deiodinase and therefore increased peripheral monodeiodonation of T_4) which enhances fetal lung maturation. Fetal thyroid hormone is essential for normal maturation of bone and development of the brain and infants with congenital hypothyroidism are significantly shorter at birth, although there is no significant effect on birthweight [25].

Insulin-like growth factors

IGFs are single polypeptide chains which are similar to proinsulin [23]. IGFs stimulate cell multiplication and differentiation, are ubiquitous in all human fetal tissues (whereas m-RNA for proinsulin is found only in pancreatic islets), act on all fetal cell types, and can be detected in fetal blood from 13 weeks. The lowest concentrations of IGFs are found in fetal liver, which is the major source of circulating IGFs, 99% of which are bound to IGFBPs. The original somatomedin hypothesis was that the endocrine actions of growth hormone were mediated via IGF1 produced in the liver. However, it is now clear that locally produced IGF1 can induce tissue growth (paracrine role) under the control of a number of pituitary trophic hormones, including growth hormone, TSH and ACTH [26]. The action of growth factors is dependent on the ontogeny of receptors. IGF1 (similar to the insulin receptor) and IGF2 receptors are different and both are present in higher concentration in fetal life than in adult life.

Studies of mutant mice have shown that decreased IGF gene expression results in fetal growth retardation at mid-gestation [27]. Because IGFs facilitate progression through the cell cycle, this is probably due to a decreased number of mitotic divisions. In the human, cord IGF1 is directly related to birthweight [5] and cord IGF1 is lower in infants that are small for gestational age (SGA) in whom serial ultrasound scans demonstrate IUGR in the final trimester [24]. Cord IGFBP-1 (and maternal IGFBP-1) levels are inversely related to birthweight [5]. IGFBP-1 presumably inhibits IGF1, limiting bioavailability by preventing the interaction of IGF1 with its receptor. Animal studies support this regulatory hypothesis by showing that increased fetal serum IGFBP-1 is associated with growth retardation due to maternal starvation, steroid administration or uterine artery ligation. Increases in IGFBP-1 occur within 3 hours of decreased blood flow or fetal hypoxia [5].

Interventional experiments in animals support these observational studies. Treatment of rodents with IGF1 increases fetal growth. Infusion of IGF1 into pregnant ewes suppresses maternal insulin leading to greater availability of glucose to the placenta and increased placental amino acid uptake; infusion of IGF1 into the fetal lamb results in increased fetal protein anabolism and fetal glucose consumption [18]. Glucose availability to the fetus regulates fetal IGF1 in the sheep, possibly via fetal insulin, and both fetal IGF1 and IGF2 levels fall if nutrients are limited [18].

Other peptide growth factors

EGF and transforming growth factor-α (TGFα) are structurally related and are primarily epithelial and mesodermal cell mitogens but also promote differentiation in some cells. TGFα is widely detected in fetal rats in the second half of gestation and may serve as a general cell proliferation stimulator regulated by local growth factors for each tissue.

The TGFα family of peptides contains approximately 20 members [5]. In animal studies, TGFβ has a role in development of lung, kidney, heart and vascularization. In neonatal cells, TGFβ often inhibits cell proliferation. PDGF is stored in platelet granules and appears to have a role in vascular wall development. It is a potent mitogen for vascular smooth muscle cells and is chemotactic for white blood cells and smooth muscle cells. FGFs are also chemotactic for cells in the vascular wall and can elicit the formation of new blood vessels. Vascular endothelial growth factor (VEGF) is a major stimulus to angiogenesis and is induced by hypoxia. In the relatively hypoxic state of the fetus, VEGF is thought to be important for fetal and placental growth. Angiotensin II (A II) is now known to be a growth factor in addition to its well-documented direct cardiovascular effects. A II promotes vascular hypertrophy and interacts with other growth factors by inducing a rise in IGF1, up-regulating expression of TGFβ_1 genes and stimulating PDGF receptor synthesis.

Gestation specificity of growth factors

The gestation dependence of growth factor actions is shown by experiments in which removal of the submandibular glands of pregnant mice at 0.65 of gestation abolishes the usual rise in maternal EGF and results in reduced litter size and weight. Treatment with EGF reverses this but has no effect at 0.5 gestation, an age at which, paradoxically, EGF antibodies stimulate growth [5].

Tissue specificity of growth factors

Different varieties of PDGF and their receptors are expressed at different gestations in mice and yet all forms of PDGF stimulate *epithelial* cell growth and development [5]. All TGFβ act as inducers of *mesodermal* tissues.

Fetal metabolism

These interactions are discussed in more detail in the section on placental transfer. Fetal metabolic rate is relatively constant at widely differing glucose concentrations, indicating that there are important alternative substrates. Amino acid uptake is greater than needed for protein synthesis and certain amino acids act as reciprocal, alternative substrates for fetal energy requirements. During fetal starvation, fetal protein catabolism supplies amino acid substrates for gluconeogenesis and the fetus may be a net supplier to the placenta to ensure survival at the cost of impaired growth [28].

Placental determinants

Placental genome

The human placenta is derived entirely from tissue of fetal origin.

Placental environment

Placental structure

The trophoblast (the outer cell mass of the blastocyst) differentiates into an inner layer of mononucleated cells, the cytotrophoblast, and an outer multinucleated syncytiotrophoblast or syncytium. The placental villi are composed of an outer syncytial layer enclosing a cytotrophoblastic column and by the end of the 3rd week there is also a connective tissue core containing blood vessels (Fig. 18.5). By the 4th week this extra-embryonic circulation has made

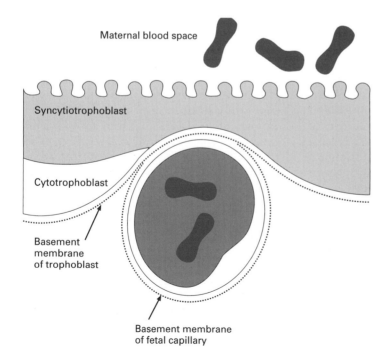

Maternal blood space

Syncytiotrophoblast

Cytotrophoblast

Basement membrane of trophoblast

Basement membrane of fetal capillary

Fig. 18.5. Schematic drawing of a villus within the mature human placenta. The cytotrophoblast does not normally intervene between fetal capillary and syncytiotrophoblast. Hence there is only one layer of trophoblast (haemomonochorial placenta) between fetal and maternal blood.

contact with the umbilical stalk vessels, connecting the placenta and embryo, and can supply nutrients to the embryo. Until that time, the embryo is nourished by diffusion from the uterine decidua [6]. The villi grow in size and complexity until term with a final diameter of 40 μm (a red cell is 7 μm). By the beginning of the 4th month, many of the cytotrophoblastic cells as well as some of the connective tissue disappears so that the placental barrier becomes much thinner (about 2 μm), the syncytium separated from the fetal capillary endothelium by only a basement membrane.

The fetal villi are bathed by about 150 ml of maternal blood in the intervillous spaces which is replenished three times per minute. Initially, the villi cover the entire surface of the chorion but by the 3rd month a specialized area of chorion becomes the human placenta, shaped as a single thick dish and attached to one-quarter of the uterine wall. There are approximately 20 cotyledons and the placenta weighs about 300 g, with a gross surface area of 3.4 m² at 28 weeks' gestation, when the fetus weighs 900 g. Although at term the placenta has doubled in weight to 600 g (and reached 20 cm in diameter and 3 cm in thickness, with a surface area of 11 m²) the placental to fetal weight ratio falls to 1:6. Each villus has a brush border with numerous microvilli (12×10^{12} microvilli per m²), increasing the actual area available for exchange still further.

Placental functions

The placenta combines in one organ many functions. It is a partial barrier to the transfer of cells from mother to fetus or vice versa, and hence provides an immunological and anti-infective fence; it acts as the fetal lung and kidney; it is the sole source of nutrition for the fetus from 6 weeks onwards; it is an important site of steroid and peptide hormone production; it grows rapidly early in gestation, adapting to the increasing metabolic requirements of the fetus and reaching maximum weight at 33 weeks though surface area and vascularity continue to develop thereafter; it becomes separated at birth and is expelled from the mother harmlessly, despite its extreme vascularity.

Determinants of placental transfer

General principles

Interruption of oxygen or nutrient delivery to the fetus has profound effects on fetal growth. However, in the normal pregnancy with a healthy placenta, data from the Dutch famine would suggest that severe deprivation is necessary before there is a substantial effect on human fetal growth. Interestingly, female fetuses exposed to maternal starvation in the first trimester subsequently gave birth, a generation later, to growth-retarded offspring despite a normal diet [18]. On the other hand, studies in normal pregnancies of malnourished women have shown that dietary supplementation increases birthweight [29]. Data from sheep suggest that periconceptional maternal nutrition may permanently reset later fetal growth, perhaps by reprogramming insulin or IGF resistance [18].

In a healthy pregnancy, the transfer of a substance from mother to fetus will depend on the following.

Vascular factors

1 Maternal uteroplacental blood flow. Uterine endometrial blood flow is the source of fetal nutrients. Oestrogens and progesterone have the synergistic effect of increasing uterine blood flow in experimental animals, possibly mediated via local endothelin-releasing factor (nitric oxide) or vasoactive intestinal peptide. PGI_2 may inhibit vasoconstictors such as A II, endothelin 1, neuropeptide Y and nicotine.
2 Fetal umbilical blood flow. The umbilical circulation is established by 6 weeks and adapts to fetal growth so that at term 40% of the fetal cardiac output reaches the placenta. The placental circulation has a low and fairly unchanging resistance and the fetus can only increase stroke volume slightly. Therefore the main determinant of fetal cardiac output is fetal heart rate. The cord vessels are not innervated and P_aO_2, P_aCO_2 and pH have little effect on the umbilical artery. Vasoconstriction may occur in response to angiotensin, vasopressin, catecholamines and prostaglandins.

3   The microscopic arrangement of the placental blood vessels (countercurrent in most primates [30,31]) and the insertion of the cord vessels (velamentous insertion and single umbilical artery both associated with decreased birth weight).

Placental factors

1   Surface area, both gross and functional (increased by convolutions and villi), and diffusion thickness.
2   Microscopic arrangement. In humans (Fig. 18.5), for example, no maternal layer of cells separates the maternal blood from fetal tissue so that the whole of the placenta is a fetal organ under the direction of fetal genes.
3   Placental metabolism.

Substrate factors

1   The concentration of the substance in the maternal circulation [32].
2   The mechanism of transfer across the placental cell membranes [33]; the transfer may be passive, facilitated or energy dependent or occur by pinocytosis (Table 18.3). Transfer may be influenced by the molecular weight, ionization, steric hindrance (e.g. conjugated bilirubin), lipid solubility and protein binding of the molecule being transferred. Lipid-soluble substances are usually transferred by diffusion down concentration gradients and, as rate of diffusion is so rapid, rate of transfer to the fetus depends on rate of supply or removal, so-called flow limited

transfer. For hydrophilic substances, diffusion occurs through notional water-filled pores in the syncytiotrophoblast, which restrict transfer according to molecular size and charge, and intercellular channels in the fetal capillary endothelium. The villus possesses the only epithelial syncytium which occurs in the human species and this limits the paracellular routes of transfer which are important in other membranes (see below). In-vitro studies show that the human placenta allows passage of water-soluble molecules (e.g. electrolytes, urea, many drugs and peptides) up to a molecular weight of 5000 [34]. Transport of some molecules is faster than can be explained by simple diffusion but does not require energy (carrier mediated, facilitated diffusion). Larger molecules are actively transported and macromolecules can only cross by endocytosis, both processes requiring energy. Endocytosis must be receptor mediated, since IgG crosses in significant amounts but smaller molecules such as insulin and thyroxine do not. Proteins produced within the fetus (e.g. α-fetoprotein) are at much lower concentration within maternal plasma but proteins produced by the placenta (e.g. placental lactogen) appear in the maternal blood in significant amounts.
3   The availability of appropriate fetal carrier proteins if required [35] and the relative affinities of fetal and maternal carriers (e.g. haemoglobin for oxygen).
4   The concentration in the blood feeding the fetal side of the placenta [36].

Table 18.3. Mechanisms of placental transfer.

Molecule	Mechanism
Water, urea	Paracellular diffusion, membrane limited
Oxygen, carbon dioxide	Transcellular diffusion, flow limited
Fatty acids, unconjugated bilirubin	Transcellular diffusion, flow limited
D-Glucose	Transcellular carrier mediated facilitated diffusion but no active transport
Na^+, K^+	Paracellular diffusion $\pm$ transcellular electrogenic active transport (varies with species)
Ca^{2+}	Transcellular carrier mediated, energy-dependent active transport
Amino acids	Transcellular carrier mediated, energy-dependent active transport
Iron, IgG, B_{12}	Transcellular receptor-mediated endocytosis
Fat-soluble vitamins	Transcellular passive diffusion
Water-soluble vitamins	Variable (p. 480–1)

Placental metabolism and transfer of individual nutrients

Glucose

Glucose is as constantly and readily available as oxygen in the maternal circulation. Glucose passes through the placenta at a faster rate than might be expected on the basis of simple diffusion alone, and certainly faster than many chemicals of similar structure and size, because there is a carrier system which binds glucose molecules selectively. It is the nature of facilitated transfer that it has a limit, that it can be saturated (although not at the physiological range of maternal blood sugar), and that it can also be reduced by competition with like chemicals. Given those characteristics, transfer will be determined by the maternal–fetal gradient, the blood flow on both sides and by the morphology of the placenta. Placental glucose carriers are insulin independent and therefore insulin can only affect glucose transfer indirectly by altering maternal or fetal arterial glucose concentrations [37].

As with oxygen, the placenta takes what glucose it needs [6,38], mostly from the fetal circulation [37]. In the guinea-pig and the lamb, the placenta consumes glucose at twice the rate of the fetal body [16,39]. In the growth-retarded guinea-pig, the placenta extracts even more glucose, whereas in the sheep, the fetal share increases [16].

In the sheep, glucose transport capacity increases eightfold in the second half of gestation [39], probably by an increase in the number of glucose transporter proteins per cell. Cordocentesis has shown a similar increase in the efficiency of glucose transport across the placenta with increasing gestation in the human pregnancy [39].

Amino acids

Amino acids provide half the fetal carbon requirement. The fetal proteins are formed from amino acids which cross the placenta but the concentrations in the maternal circulation are lower than those in the fetal blood, suggesting active transport by energy-dependent carriers. Different amino acids may compete for the same carrier. For example, the high phenylalanine levels in mothers with phenylketonuria may compete with tyrosine uptake, an amino acid required for neurotransmitter synthesis. A prolonged increase or decrease in maternal amino acid concentrations has been shown, in animal models, to result in a compensatory decrease or increase in placental transport. The mechanism of this feedback is unknown but is not insulin. During IUGR, as maternal supply falls, the placenta increases uptake of branched amino acids from the fetus but despite this adaptation, in SGA human fetuses studied by cordocentesis, a significant reduction in concentrations of most essential amino acids was found [40]. Alcohol and nicotine inhibit placental amino acid transfer [37].

The data for sheep reported by Lemons *et al.* [41] and Battaglia [39], show that the net flux does not mirror the fetal requirement for structure. The neutral amino acids, in particular, are transferred into the fetal circulation in excess of fetal requirement and are thought to be an energy source [31,39]. The acidic amino acids aspartate and glutamate do not appear to cross the placenta in significant amounts [42]. Glutamate, aspartate and serine produced by the fetal liver are taken up by the placenta which uses these amino acids to generate glutamine, asparagine and glycine respectively [37,39]. The basic amino acids appear to be transferred in amounts just sufficient for the needs of protein structure. The concept of essential (one that cannot be synthesized in the body) and non-essential nutrients is a relative one; endogenous production rates of so-called non-essential amino acids may not be adequate under adverse conditions and may then become rate limiting for fetal growth. Even an essential amino acid such as leucine has been shown to be metabolized within the placenta.

Lipids

Lipid transport across the placenta is quantitatively less than in rabbits and guinea-pigs [43] but significant cord differences have been shown [44] and the long aliphatic chains of these molecules represent an important carbon source. Two-thirds of the human brain is lipid and, at birth, head circumference is already three-quarters of the final adult value. Essential fatty acids (linoleic and linolenic), which cannot be synthesized by the fetus and must be obtained transplacentally, are important precursors for long-chain polyunsaturated fatty acids (important for neural membrane synthesis, particularly in the brain and retina [45] and for the ubiquitous eicosanoids. Fetal fatty acid composition varies with maternal diet [46], suggesting placental transport is non-selective.

Ketone bodies

Ketone bodies freely cross the placenta. The fetal brain can oxidise β-hydroxy-butyrate as an alternative energy source to glucose in early development [47,48].

Water

Water crosses the placenta by diffusion and filtration, following the balance of hydrostatic and osmotic pressures, either transversing the cells (transcellular) or running between the cells (paracellular) through notional pores. Studies in the term human pregnancy show a transfer rate for water of 3.6 litres/hour across the placenta and 150 ml/hour transferred between the fetus and the amniotic cavity. The term fetus accumulates water at a rate of 20 ml/day. Thus, the net transfer to the fetus is a very small fraction of the diffusional exchange [49,50]. If maternal osmotic pressure is lowered by infusion of hypotonic solutions, the fetus gains water [51]; if hypertonic solutions are infused, then the fetus shrivels a little.

Electrolytes and minerals

In the human haemochorial placenta, the main extracellular electrolytes sodium and chloride cross to the fetus easily by rapid diffusion along concentration gradients [52]. Placental transport of these and several other ions such as potassium, hydrogen, bicarbonate, iodide and sulphate are determined by diffusion and by electrochemical gradients established by co- and countertransport mechanisms, many linked to sodium pumps. As with water, the bidirectional fluxes are much greater than the net flux; the main exchange is probably via the paracellular route where presumably water and electrolytes move together as they do in serum. Water actually traversing the cells is thought to be solute free and sodium and chloride pass through only in relatively small amounts.

Calcium and phosphate

The growing fetus needs calcium. Despite the net flux to the fetus in all mammals studied, the maternal concentrations of total plasma calcium and ionized calcium have been *below* fetal levels. Both calcium and phosphate are transported by carrier-mediated energy-dependent mechanisms [53–55]. The calcium transporter is on the fetal surface of the placenta and is saturable, utilizes adenosine triphosphate (ATP) and is magnesium dependent. The phosphate transporter is on the maternal surface and sodium dependent [37]. There is some evidence that this active process is under the control of fetal 1,25 dehydroxycholecalciferol. This seems to be made in the maternal kidney and to be transferred across the placenta [56] and both the placenta and the fetal kidney have the capacity to convert it into its active form. By contrast, calcitonin and parathyroid hormone do not cross the placenta. The fetal parathyroid gland becomes active in early fetal life but it is unknown whether fetal parathormone or calcitonin directly affect placental calcium transport.

Iron

In late gestation, fetal iron concentrations are higher than maternal [37]. Maternal transferrin probably enters the placental cells by endocytosis.

Vitamins

By definition, these cannot be synthesized by human tissues and therefore they must reach the fetus by placental transfer. Fat-soluble vitamins (A, D, E, K) presumably flow by diffusion down concentration gradients. For many water-soluble vitamins, the fetal concentration is higher than the maternal, suggesting active transport (e.g. riboflavin, B_{12}). Vitamin B_{12} is bound to transcobalamin proteins which are produced by the placenta. There may also be metabolic interconversion of vitamins within the placenta. In the near-term human placenta, dehydroascorbic acid is taken up three to six times more readily than ascorbic acid (vitamin C) but is subsequently converted back by the fetus to ascorbate, to which the placenta is relatively impermeable. This has given rise to the concept of the placenta as a biochemical valve. The uptake of dehydroascorbic acid is inhibited by low sodium concentrations and high glucose concentrations, suggesting transfer using the glucose transporter or a specific sodium-dependent pathway.

Net maternal to fetal transfer of folic acid involves two steps. Circulating 5-methyltetrahydrofolate is captured by placental folate receptors on the maternally facing surface so that intervillous blood levels are three times higher than maternal blood. In the second step, folates are passively transferred to the fetal circulation along a downhill concentration.

Studies using the maternal facing membrane of human placental cells suggest that biotin (a coenzyme necessary for folic acid metabolism) and the water-soluble vitamin pantothenate share a sodium-dependent cotransport mechanism. Both placental biotin uptake and folate uptake are inhibited by alcohol. Vitamin B_6 (pyridoxine) transfer occurs by a different route but is also inhibited in the isolated human placenta by alcohol. There is passive transport of B_6 across the placenta (i.e. no concentration gradient between maternal and fetal sides) but placental concentration exceeded both maternal and fetal concentrations suggesting binding of the B_6 within the placenta.

Fetal excretion

Urea and creatinine are cleared by simple diffusion. Although uric acid is a larger molecule, this too crosses the placenta, although the mechanism is unknown. Unconjugated bilirubin crosses the placenta easily but not conjugated bilirubin.

Blood gases

The placenta itself has a high demand for O_2, up to 50% of the O_2 taken from the uterine circulation [37]. The transfer of oxygen does not appear to be limited by the diffusion characteristics of the barrier in a healthy pregnancy but is determined by uterine and umbilical blood flow and the O_2-carrying capacities of maternal and fetal blood. However, there is a wide margin of safety in healthy pregnancies and data from the sheep suggest uterine or umbilical blood flow must fall by more than 50% before O_2 delivery to the fetus is prejudiced [37]. Gaseous exchange in the placenta can be limited by the oxygen diffusing capacity in abnormal pregnancy. However, the diffusing capacity can increase by two-thirds in guinea-pig pregnancies retarded by maternal hypoxia through the adaptations of increased placental surface area, decreased diffusion distance, and increased fetal red-cell mass [16].

The partial pressure of oxygen in fetal blood leaving the placenta is relatively low. Nevertheless, because of the characteristics of the fetal haemoglobin oxygen dissociation curve and the relative polycythaemia of the fetus, the oxygen content is still high. At any value of Po_2 achieved in umbilical venous blood, delivery of oxygen to the fetus will depend on the haemoglobin flow rate (the product of umbilical blood flow and haemoglobin concentration) and the oxygen affinity of fetal haemoglobin (enhanced by lower 2,3-diphosphoglycerate binding of fetal haemoglobin). Fetal anaemia or fetal transfusion with adult red cells, or increased carboxyhaemoglobin due to smoking, decrease the margin of safety as they impair the O_2-carrying capacity of fetal blood.

Carbon dioxide also diffuses readily across the placental membranes and the diffusion capacity is some 20 times that of oxygen.

Placental hormones

The placenta synthesizes two hormones which are similar to pituitary growth hormone, human growth hormone variant (hGH-V or placental growth hormone [57]) and human placental lactogen (hPL or chorionic somatomammatrophin). Neither seem to be essential for successful pregnancy, since case reports have described viable outcomes in women with synthetic defects of both substances, but they may have a permissive action on fetal growth, just as fetal thyroxine does. hPL has anabolic actions on fetal tissues and stimulates insulin and IGF1 synthesis *in vitro* [23]. Fetoplacental steroid production becomes important from 8 weeks (see above).

Maternal determinants

Genetic and constitutional

The fetal genomic influences on fetal growth are discussed above. In this section the influence of the maternal genome will be considered.

In principle, the maternal genotype can act on the embryo in two ways. The first is by an early effect on the development of the oocyte and which is subsequently manifest in the zygote by a maternal cytoplasmic interaction with the paternal genome of the fertilizing sperm. There are very few examples of this influence in nature. Two such cytoplasmic effects which have been described in mice are hair-pin tail (Thp) and ovum mutant (Om). However, both of these are lethal mutations rather than genetic

abnormalities which can influence fetal growth [58,59].

The second way in which the maternal genotype can influence the fetus is in the general support of the fetus. This so-called uterine effect is not confined to local factors operating in the uterus. Most research has focused on the influence of maternal size on fetal growth. Classic studies using cross-breeding and embryo transfer techniques in many animal species have shown that, in addition to the intrinsic limit set to growth by the embryonic/fetal genotype, there is also a growth-limiting effect imposed by the genotype of a small mother (Table 18.4) [19,60–62]. The relative importance of the fetal genome versus other influences (including the maternal genome) on fetal growth is the subject of debate [63]. Recent studies into the control of fetal growth seem to suggest that the fetal genome regulates the growth in a predetermined pathway in which specific genes are switched on and off at specific stages of embryonic/fetal development and that the non-fetal genetic ('epigenetic') factors influence this normal genetic expression.

Presumably the maternal genetic modifiers of fetal growth operate through endocrine and physical mechanisms discussed below. It is

Table 18.4. The effect of maternal size on animal fetal birthweight.

Animal species	Maternal genotype	Mean fetal birthweight		Reference
		Large dam/mother	Small dam/mother	
Cross-breeding experiments				
Horse (kg) (*n* = 11)	Shire	71		[19]
	Hybrid	50	18	
	Shetland		20	
Cattle (kg) (*n* = 12)	South Devon	43		[60]
	Hybrid	33	26	
	Dexter		24	
Embryo transfer experiments				
Sheep (kg) (*n* = 15)	Border Leicester	6.4	5.0	[61]
	Welsh Mountain	4.6	3.6	
Mouse (g) (*n* = 291)	Large	1.7	1.6	[62]
	Small	1.3	1.4	

difficult, however, to distinguish the relative contribution of such factors, and furthermore, to rule out the possibility of pathological influences. The relationships between maternal height and weight and fetal growth illustrate these points.

There is a well-documented correlation both between maternal height and birthweight [64] and between maternal pre-pregnancy weight and birthweight [65]. Whilst some of this relationship is purely genetic [66], short- and long-term nutritional factors (and possibly other socio-economic factors) influence both the maternal height and weight and thus must independently affect fetal growth and size [67]. Furthermore, adult height is influenced by maternal birthweight and, overall, both mean birthweight and mean maternal height are increasing in successive generations [68].

As with maternal height and weight, genetic factors must play a part in producing the well-known differences in birthweight distribution between ethnic groups [69]. But as with height and weight, the relationship is confounded by the influence of nutritional and socio-economic factors [70]. Nevertheless, there have been studies which have tried to minimize the effects of these non-pathological factors. For example, Gardosi et al. [14] have developed a software programme which produces an adjustable birthweight standard for individual fetuses based on both fetal (sex and gestational age) and maternal characteristics (parity, height, weight at the beginning of pregnancy and ethnic group).

Nutritional

The potential influence of the maternal diet and level of nutrition on fetal growth has been recognized for many years. For example, in 1945 Wallace found that mature fetuses of ewes fed on a restricted diet for the last 8 weeks of gestation weighed only 57% of those from well-fed ewes [71]. Similar results have been reported in human studies on the effects of famines on previously well-nourished populations [72,73]. However, the relationship between maternal diet and fetal growth is not as straightforward as such studies would suggest.

There is a significant and positive correlation between maternal basal metabolic rate (BMR) and birthweight [74]. However, there is considerable individual variation in maternal BMR both at the beinning of and during apparently normal pregnancy. In a study of women in Cambridge, UK, Prentice et al. [75], using whole-body calorimetry, calculated the mean non-pregnant non-lactating BMR to be 6.1 MJ/d. During pregnancy they found that in some women the BMR nearly doubled whilst in others it fell by about 50% and only exceeded its pre-pregnancy values by the end of pregnancy. This work contributed to the recognition that some normal women in pregnancy were 'energy sparing' whilst others were' energy profligate' [76]. Other studies in different nationalities have shown similar group trends. For example, women from Sweden tend to be 'energy profligate' [74], whereas those from the Gambia are 'energy sparing' [77].

In summary, the relationship between substrate availability to the fetus and fetal growth is complex because of the varying maternal BMR. Furthermore, the maternal BMR below which substrate availability, and thus fetal growth, becomes pathological is not clear. Nevertheless, the role and importance of individual substrates in fetal growth is more clearly established and discussed already under 'Placental Determinants'.

Endocrine

The role of fetal growth factors, especially IGFs and IGFBPs, has been discussed above. However, evidence is now emerging that maternal IGFs play a role in the regulation of fetal growth.

IGFs or somatomedins are low molecular mass (7.5–7.7 kDa) polypeptides with various metabolic, mitogenic and differentiative properties [78,79]. After an early and transient fall, maternal plasma IGFs increase in pregnancy [80,81] with serum IGF1 levels in the third trimester being 2.5 times those in the first trimester [23]. Blood concentrations of placental growth hormone (GH), though not placental lactogen, correlate with IGF1 in the third trimester [82], suggesting an interdependence in production. The rapid fall in IGF concentration after delivery suggests that it is placental GH that directly stimulates IGF production [83]. Perfusion studies have suggested that this increase in IGFs is due to increased liver production [84]. An alternate explanation is that the IGF concentration increase is the result of an increase in IGFBP levels, analogous to the effect of thyroxine levels in pregnancy.

At term there is only a weak association between maternal and umbilical cord serum IGF1 levels and no significant relationship between maternal serum IGF1 levels and fetal birthweight [23]. In contrast, umbilical arterial and venous IGF1 levels are inversely related to birthweight [23]. This suggests that IGF production in the mother and the fetus is independent, with little significant passage across the placenta. The available evidence suggests that maternal IGF1 may promote placental growth and the transfer of nutrients to the fetus [85].

The serum concentration of IGFBP-1 rises rapidly to reach a peak at the end of the first trimester and thereafter remains at that plateau for the rest of the pregnancy [86]. The majority of this increase comes from decidualized endometrium [87]. One suggested function for this endometrial/decidual IGFBP-1 is to protect the endometrium from invasion by trophoblast by inhibition of IGF1 receptors in the placental membranes [88].

In early pregnancy, the concentration of IGFBP-1 is higher in extra-embryonic coelomic (EEC) fluid than in both amniotic fluid and maternal serum [23]. The origin of this EEC IGFBP-1 is unknown but could be decidualized endometrium. Another candidate is the chorion.

At delivery, maternal serum IGFBP-1 concentrations are inversely correlated with birthweight [85,86]. Circulating IGFBPs may inhibit the effects of IGF1 [89]. This leads to the speculation that increased levels of IGFBP-1 from the decidualized endometrium act to inhibit the trophic action of IGF1 on placental and secondarily fetal growth.

In contrast to IGFBP-1, the concentrations of IGFBP-2 and IGFBP-3 in the maternal serum decline through pregnancy [90]. The significance of these changes is unknown.

Physical and environmental

The role of exercise in pregnancy on fetal growth is much debated. The available evidence in the human supports the conclusion that moderate physical activity during pregnancy does not affect fetal growth in well-nourished mothers [91]. Most early studies looking at the level of physical work and fitness failed to show any significant relationship with newborn weight and size [92,93]. However, more recent studies have suggested that whilst most formal work has no effect on fetal growth, that involving moderate to severe exercise might have an influence [94]. Babies of jogging mothers are of normal weight [95,96]. There have been studies suggesting that babies born to women in training or physically fit are relatively heavier. For example, Erderly et al. [97] reported a study where the mean birthweight of babies of female athletes was higher than that of non-athletes; however, the mothers in that work were not matched for maternal size. When Erkola [98] reported a similar study, the placental weights were also significantly greater. Furthermore, that report suggested this finding was due to their greater circulating plasma volume and presumably uterine perfusion. Maternal plasma volume has been separately shown to correlate to birthweight [99], though part of this could be a reflection of the effect of maternal size.

Altitude is another factor which influences fetal growth. Birthweight distribution shifts downwards in a systematic way as altitude rises [100]. This effect has been compared to that of smoking, for in both circumstances relative placental weight is not reduced and similar placental histological changes are found [101].

There is a well-recognized tendency for subsequent babies to be heavier at birth. The underlying mechanisms for this effect of birth are not clear, though it has been suggested that the smaller size of the firstborn is a pathological effect representing fetal undergrowth [68].

Abnormal/pathological nutrition and growth

Much of the understanding of the determinants and control of fetal growth has come from instances where normal fetal growth is deranged.

Fetal and placental factors

Genetic

It has been estimated that over one-third of total birthweight variation is genetically determined (see Table 18.2). Thus, the true frequency of genetically determined fetal growth retardation is difficult to estimate.

Fetal growth is impaired in a high proportion of chromosomally abnormal fetuses [8]. For example, in Turner's syndrome and trisomies 21 and 13, birthweight is approximately 80% of normal [102]. The growth restriction with trisomy 18 and triploidy is even more pronounced.

Other examples of fetal undergrowth with congenital abnormality both genetic and non-genetic include the Russell Silver and Seckel syndromes (genetic syndromes with severe dwarfing a prominent feature) [103], anencephaly [104], osteogenesis imperfecta [105] and renal dysgenesis [102]. The Beckwith–Wiedemann syndrome (BWS) is an example of a genetic disorder associated with accelerated fetal growth [106]. The classical clinical stigmata are exomphalos, gigantism and macroglossia. Genetically, BWS is thought to be an autosomal dominant trait with varying expressivity and penetrance. The precise molecular abnormality and the resultant mechanism of fetal overgrowth is not yet clear.

Endocrine

Altered IGF1 and IGFBP-1 levels have been found in association with pre-eclamptic and idiopathic growth retardation. Specifically, IGFBP-1 levels have been consistently reported to be raised, whereas fetal IGF1 values have been found to be low [23]. It has been speculated that in the case of pre-eclamptic and idiopathic

growth retardation, the well-documented failure of trophoblastic invasion into the uterus [107] may result in inadequate uteroplacental blood flow which in turn will produce increased decidual IGFBP-1 production [23].

Fetal hyperinsulinaemia is accepted to be the cause of macrosomia in the fetus of a diabetic mother, which in turn is directly related to the quality of maternal glucose homeostatis [108]. However, fetal hyperinsulinaemia secondary to maternal hyperglycaemia may inhibit fetal hepatic synthesis and secretion of IGFBP-1. Reduced IGFBP-1 would allow the unrestricted action of IGF1 on fetal tissue growth which might also be an important contributor to macrosomia [23].

Placental disease

The relationship between fetal weight and placental weight is complex, since weight and size are poor reflections of function and adaptations may have occurred during pregnancy. Experimental reduction of endometrial caruncles before pregnancy in sheep to reduce placental mass results in fewer cotyledons but each may be larger [109]. Maternal smoking in pregnancy may cause an increase in placental weight despite a lower birthweight [110]. Most growth-retarded fetuses have a higher fetal to placental weight ratio [111], suggesting that the growth-restricted fetus adapts in some way to improve placental transfer or uptake when the placenta is small [102].

Specific abnormalities of the placenta which have been associated with fetal growth retardation, include single umbilical artery [111], placental chorioangiomas [112], the twin–twin transfusion syndrome [102] and circumvallate placenta [113]. Recurrent placental abruption, especially in the first and second trimesters, is associated with fetal growth retardation [114], whereas placenta praevia appears to have no association with growth pathology [115].

Physical

Physical restriction of space has been a reported cause of growth retardation in animals and humans for many years [116,117]. The lower birthweight in multiple pregnancies is often cited as the best example of this phenomenon. Whilst it is undoubtedly a real occurrence, some of the growth retardation seen in multiple pregnancies may be a reflection of placental factors such as the twin–twin transfusion syndrome. Similarly, fetal growth retardation reported in women with congenital uterine abnormalities may be a reflection of physical and/or vascular factors.

Infection

Rubella is the classic example of a fetal infection causing growth retardation [118]. About 30% of fetuses with cytomegalovirus are growth retarded [119]. The underlying reasons for this association are not known. Growth retardation as a result of other intrauterine viral and bacterial infections is less extensively documented [102].

Maternal and environmental factors

Endocrine

Maternal diabetes is the best example of an endocrine disorder which is associated with pathological fetal growth and has been discussed above.

Nutrition

There have been many studies relating to the effects of reduced maternal nutritional intake and fetal growth retardation. They are well reviewed by Rush [120]. The main conclusions from these studies are, firstly, that during famines mean birthweight can be reduced by as much as 550 g. Secondly, it is only in such severely malnourished women that dietary supplementation, principally in the form of calories, will produce any significant improvement in fetal growth.

It is assumed that the lower birthweights reported in association with socio-economic deprivation and frequent pregnancies are due to nutritional factors. However, other confounding influences such as smoking and genetic factors may apply.

Maternal illness

The relationship between pre-eclampsia and fetal growth retardation is well described and discussed above under fetal and placental factors. However, it is now debated whether pre-eclampsia is a single disease entity at all, perhaps being better considered as a syndrome with different underlying aetiologies.

There are a number of definite maternal diseases which can restrict fetal growth. Maternal hypertension may not have any influence on fetal growth itself unless pre-eclampsia supervenes [102,121]. It is not clear what factors operate to induce pre-eclampsia in women with pre-existing hypertension. However, the failure of trophoblast invasion in the late first and early second trimester appears to be a critical part of the underlying pathophysiology. Fetal growth retardation has been reported to be found in over 50% of women with cyanotic heart disease compared to under 10% in women with acyanotic disease [122]. Maternal chest diseases (e.g. asthma, cystic fibrosis, bronchiectasis, kyphoscoliosis) have been reported to reduce fetal growth but only in severe cases with marked respiratory compromise [102,123]. Chronic renal disease is associated with growth retardation in about one quarter of cases [124]. This effect is most pronounced in patients with hypertension, elevated serum creatinines and proteinuria.

A number of different pathophysiological processes (especially nutritional and vascular) probably operate to produce the effect on growth. Collagen disorders, including systemic lupus erythematosus, produce growth retardation [125]. Whilst some effects may be mediated through renal compromise and the effect of immunosuppressive drugs, a direct effect producing decidual bed vasculitis is possible [102]. There is doubt whether maternal anaemia in itself produces growth retardation, since there may be confounding nutritional factors. Nevertheless, sickle cell disease and its variants do carry a risk of fetal undergrowth due to impaired uteroplacental blood supply [126].

Physical and environmental

The effects of altitude on fetal birthweight and their similarity to the effects of smoking have been discussed above.

High-dose irradiation is known to cause fetal growth retardation; however, this is a very rare cause in clinical practice [127].

Chemical

Therapeutically administered drugs which have been reported to cause growth retardation are listed in Table 18.5 [102]. However, it must be stressed that the evidence of this effect in humans is not always strong.

Maternal heroin addiction is well established as a cause of fetal growth retardation. This effect appears to persist even when allowance is made for confounding factors such as maternal nutrition [128]. The mechanism whereby this effect is mediated is unclear.

Maternal smoking has been consistently shown to be associated with smaller birthweight for many years. Most studies show that mothers who smoke will deliver babies who are, on average, 200–300 g lighter that their non-smoking peers [129]. The studies showing reduced birthweight and crown–rump length but no effect on ponderal index would support the view that smoking results in decreased growth potential rather than impaired fetal nutrition [130]. The effects of smoking are synergistic with other factors with pathological effects on fetal growth. The mechanisms by which smoking can produce these effects include nicotine-induced uterine vasoconstriction, carbon monoxide-induced reduction in oxygen diffusion across the placenta, and cyanide inactivation of cytochrome oxidase and

Table 18.5. Therapeutic drugs reported to produce fetal growth retardation. From Wigglesworth [102].

Folate antagonists (aminopterin, methotrexate)
Antiepileptics (trimethadione)
Anticogulants (warfarin)
Immunosuppressants (cyclophosphamide, azathiaprine)
Cytotoxics (many examples including cyclosporin)

carbonic anhydrase systems with the fetus [102].

Growth retardation is a prominent feature of the fetal alcohol syndrome. The severity of growth restriction is related to the quantity of alcohol consumed. Growth generally is affected by consumption in excess of 40 ml (4 units) per day [131]. It is not clear whether the effect of alcohol is mediated by the alcohol itself, by its metabolite acetaldehyde or through uteroplacental vascular impairment.

Clinical implications and applications in pregnancy

Screening for pathological fetal growth

Clearly a number of epidemiological factors (e.g. fetal gender, birth order, socioeconomic status, maternal height and weight, ethnic group and interpregnancy interval) are associated with an increased risk of a fetus being small for gestational age (SGA), i.e. that birthweight falls below a given centile for the population (e.g. 3rd, 5th or 10th). Several workers have used these associations to try and predict the fetus that will be SGA. For example, Galbraith et al. [132] in a study of 8030 pregnancies, claimed a positive predictive value of their risk scoring system of 9.8% and a false negative rate of 2.3% (sensitivity, 69.1%; specificity, 67.1%). Such risk scores have not been widely implemented; they are cumbersome to use, they have a poor predictive value, and they do not always predict the fetus that is pathologically undergrown (as opposed to the constitutionally or genetically small fetus).

In practice, obstetricians identify pregnancies at risk of pathological fetal growth on the basis of identification of individual risk factors (e.g. previous growth retardation, recurrent bleeding during pregnancy, multiple pregnancy, specific maternal medical diseases, maternal drug or alcohol abuse). They then measure the fetal growth in such pregnancies serially, using ultrasound to identify which fetuses actually develop pathological fetal growth. Ironically, whilst maternal smoking is arguably the most common risk factor for fetal growth retardation, the habit is too widespread to make it a practical proposition to perform serial ultrasonic growth scans for all pregnant women who smoke. Furthermore, by itself it is a poor predictor of the fetus being severely small for dates.

Biochemical screening for pregnancies at risk of fetal growth retardation at present is confined to the use of the maternal serum alphafetoprotein concentration at about 16 weeks. When such values are raised in the absence of fetal abnormality, the pregnancy carries an increased risk of fetal undergrowth later in pregnancy [133]. Other biochemical tests, largely discarded over the past 20 years, perhaps warrant a further examination as predictors of fetal growth failure before it becomes clinically or ultrasonically apparent. Assays of human placental lactogen, oestriol and Schwangerschaftsprotein-1 all have a sensitivity and positive predictive value for a fetus being SGA of 30–50% [134]. Indeed, in the future, biochemical screening using IGF1 and IGFBP-1 may be a reality.

Clinical screening in the form of inspection and palpation have been reported to have a sensitivity of 44%, a specificity of 88% and a positive predictive value of 29% in predicting the fetus that is SGA [135]. Measurement of symphysial–fundal length is only slightly better with sensitivities between 62 and 86%, specificities between 79 and 89%, and positive predicative values between 18 and 79% [135,136]. More accurate results have come from studies in high-risk pregnancies [136].

A number of studies have been undertaken to assess the effectiveness of fetal ultrasound measurements on one, or at most, two occasions during pregnancy to screen for the fetus that is SGA. The results are difficult to compare because the studies are not identical in design, equipment used or personnel performing the examinations. The sensitivities vary from 43 to 94%, the specificities from 84 to 92%, and the positive predictive values from 20 to 70% [135]. These figures are not dissimilar from the ranges reported for serial symphysial–fundal length

measurements (see above). Indeed, in a comparative study in the same group of women, there was no difference between a single measurement of abdominal circumference performed in the last trimester and such clinical measurements [137]. It may be that use of customized fetal growth charts may improve the predictive value of single or double scans in screening the low risk population [14] and an example is provided in Fig. 18.6.

The ability of Doppler ultrasound to predict the fetus at risk of growth retardation has been studied using recordings from both the uteroplacental and fetal circulations. Whilst there have been some encouraging reports from small studies, convincing evidence of the value of such screening methods from large studies of normal or low-risk pregnancies is awaited [138].

Finally, it must be stressed that a fundamental problem besetting such screening methods is that they more commonly set out to predict the fetus that is SGA rather than identifying the fetus that is pathologically undergrown. Not all pathologically grown fetuses will be SGA and not all fetuses that are small for gestational age are pathologically undergrown and at risk of the associated complications such as perinatal asphyxia, necrotizing enterocolitis, neurodevelopmental disability.

Measurement of fetal growth with ultrasound

Fetal measurement with ultrasound remains the best method by which pathological fetal growth is monitored and identified in high-risk pregnancies. A variety of fetal parameters can be recorded, but the abdominal circumference is the single most effective measurement for monitoring fetal growth and predicting fetal size. Inclusion of other parameters such as head size and femur length may actually distort the prediction of size, especially in pathologically growing fetuses. Thus, the fetus that is pathologically undergrown may have a degree of pre-

Fig. 18.6. *Opposite.* (a) Customized growth chart for 'Mrs Big', showing the weight percentiles of two previous babies. The fetal weight based on an antenatal scan at 35 weeks is also shown. (b) Customized chart for 'Mrs Small'. The centiles are different for the same weight data, as the norm for fetal growth is lower after adjustment for this pregnancy's characteristics. From Gardosi *et al.* [14] with the permission of the publishers.

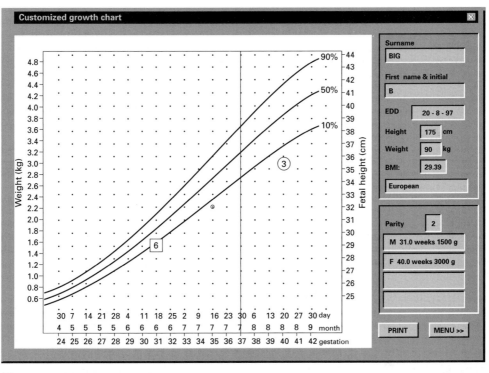

(a)

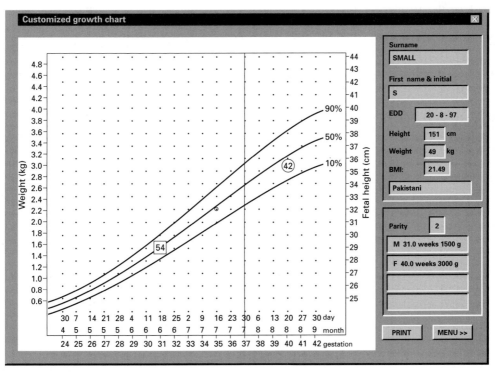

(b)

servation of head growth (head sparing) which will lead to an overestimation of fetal size if that parameter is included in the fetal weight estimation. Conversely, the fetus that is macrosomic (as opposed to genetically large) may have a relatively normal head size and thus fetal weight estimation using several parameters may result in an underestimation. Nevertheless, even if only abdominal circumference measurements are used, prediction of fetal weight is associated with an error of 10–15% [136,137]. Serial fetal measurements and plotting growth trajectories are better than single recordings in diagnosing pathological fetal growth. Again, in this area of monitoring fetal growth the use of customized growth charts may represent a significant advance [14].

Interventions with pathological fetal growth

Macrosomia

In practical terms, the main occasion when this is encountered is in the infant of a diabetic mother. However, it is also recognized that fetuses with identical growth profiles (excessively large abdominal circumference but normal head circumference) can be found in women without evidence of impaired glucose tolerance. Whether such macrosomic fetuses have the same risks and should be managed in the same way as macrosomic infants of diabetic mothers is currently being addressed.

Macrosomic infants to diabetic mothers (assuming fetal abnormality has been excluded earlier in pregnancy) are principally at risk of intrauterine fetal death and traumatic delivery especially shoulder dystocia [139]. Such fetuses, therefore, are monitored during pregnancy with biophysical methods in the same way as fetuses that are SGA. However, it is recognized that there is a higher false-negative rate with such methods in these cases, presumably because the fetal risk may not be solely related to the hypoxic insult [140].

The risk of traumatic delivery is approached empirically. Many units, however, have guidelines which involve elective caesarean section if the estimated fetal weight is in excess of 4.0–4.5 kg [139].

Growth retardation

Careful counselling is necessary when a fetus is suspected to be small. It is clear there are limitations in our ability to identify the fetus that is small for gestational age and also pathologically undergrown. This is especially important when more than one professional is involved in the mother's care so that confusion and unnecessary anxiety are avoided.

Where pathological growth is suspected, further evaluation is necessary both to confirm the diagnosis and to establish the cause. The first requirement is to confirm that the fetus is normal. This is necessary even if there was a preceding 'routine normality' scan at 18–20 weeks. Further ultrasonic documentation of growth may be helpful in distinguishing the genetic/constitutionally small fetus (whose growth should follow the normal growth trajectories) from the pathologically growing fetus (whose growth, especially of the abdomen, should fall away from the expected trajectories). Because of the errors associated with ultrasound measurements, it is advisable to ensure that the intervals between growth scans are not less than 2 weeks [136]. Placental biopsy (for rapid karyotyping) or fetal blood sampling (for karyotyping and viral studies) are being performed increasingly [138]. However, these procedures are not without risk and there are no clear guidelines as to when they are appropriate.

Specific management depends on cause. In the case of fetal abnormality, this will depend on the diagnosis, the prognosis, the gestational age and the parents' wishes. In the case of a viral infection, the prognosis is not always easy to predict, because it is difficult to detect which organs are affected before birth and subtle neuronal damage may not be recognized until later in infancy. In the case of other causes, such as uteroplacental vascular disease (with or without pre-eclampsia), recurrent bleeding or idiopathic growth retardation, in the fetus that is normal and has no viral disease, the current approach to management can be considered under four headings.

General measures

Women who smoke and drink should be advised to discontinue these habits as they are synergistic with many causes of growth retardation. There is no evidence that bed rest improves the prognosis for fetal growth retardation [138].

Assessment of fetal well-being

Ultrasound can be used to identify and assess the well-being of the fetus when growth retardation is suspected. Abnormalities of both umbilical artery Doppler recordings [137] and the biophysical profile score [141] are known to predict the risk of adverse outcome in such fetuses. Many obstetricians use these characteristics in combination to monitor the fetal condition and alongside assessment of maternal complications and gestational age they form the basis of decisions to deliver the fetus [142]. Evidence is now emerging from randomized trials to show that the use of these ultrasound parameters in clinical practice improves fetal outcome, at least in the short term [143]. The use of both Doppler and recordings of regional blood flow within the growth retarded fetus and fetal blood gas analysis for management of such cases should still be regarded as areas for research [138].

Specific treatments

A variety of specific treatments have been tried to improve or ameliorate pathological fetal growth. These include aspirin, β-sympathomimetics, Solcoseryl (a hemodialysate containing no protein or antigens derived from calf blood which has been reported to have effects on fetal metabolism and maternal circulation in an experimental setting), allyloestrenol (a synthetic progesterone which experimentally has improved maternal uterine blood supply by either an α-blockage or by an antiplatelet action), hyperalimentation, and hyperoxygentation [138]. At present, there is no evidence that any of these methods should be introduced into clinical practice.

Delivery

The timing and method of delivery of the fetus with growth retardation is dependent on a number of factors, including the diagnosis, the prognosis, the gestational age and maternal complications. These decisions may be relatively easy if there is a lethal fetal abnormality. When the fetus is normal, however, the decisions are not as straightforward, mainly because the necessary prospective randomized controlled studies with long-term follow-up into childhood have not been performed. A number of unanswered questions remain, therefore. For example, where a fetus is recognized to have a chronic hypoxic problem in progress (with worsening growth retardation and abnormal umbilical artery Doppler recordings), there is a management dilemma of whether to deliver early to reduce the risks of continuing asphyxia or to wait with ongoing monitoring for evidence of acute-on-chronic hypoxia (with the biophysical profile) to avoid the complications of premature delivery [142].

Finally, when vaginal delivery is undertaken with a growth-retarded fetus, there is an increased risk of intrapartum hypoxia and continuous fetal heart rate monitoring and intermittent pH testing, are necessary, though it must be admitted that such a monitoring strategy for labour is a far from perfect method of assessing fetal health.

Outcomes

Short-term growth, morbidity and mortality

Small for gestational age babies are at increased risk of hypothermia, hypoglycaemia, polycythaemia, pulmonary haemorrhage, infection, encephalopathy [144] and necrotizing enterocolitis [145] compared with appropriate for gestational age (AGA) babies of similar gestation. Neonatal morbidity and mortality is increased in SGA babies compared with AGA babies of the same gestation [146]. Looked at another way, a 30-week SGA infant weighing 1000 g will have only a slightly lower risk of mortality to a 27-week AGA infant weighing 1000 g. Low birthweight seems to be the most powerful predictor of mortality and largely outweighs the advantages of greater maturity. This contrasts with morbidity in survivors, in whom gestation seems to be a more powerful predictor of outcome. If both of the above examples survive, the 27-week infant is more likely to have long-term handicaps. Although there are demonstrable differences in the EEG and central conduction velocities of the brain of SGA infants at term, periventricular haemorrhage and infarction are not increased in SGA infants [147].

Preterm SGA infants have more fat and less muscle at the expected date of delivery (EDD) than their AGA term counterparts, which may reflect the limitations of enteral and total parenteral nutrition (TPN) for preterm infants rather than any fundamental fetal biology [5].

Later growth

A cohort of infants with birthweights more than 2 SD below the mean and followed for 4 years were still smaller than AGA babies; only 8% were above the 50th centile and one-third were still below the 3rd centile [148]. Infants whose growth failure started after 34 weeks [149] or were disproportionate at birth [150] (late-onset, asymmetrical IUGR) were most likely to have normal weight, length and head circumference at 4 years. Most of this catch-up growth occurred in the first year. Compared with these studies from 20 years ago, a more recent cohort provides some reassurance [151]. Eighty-seven per cent of SGA infants (defined as below –2 SD for length or weight at birth in this study) were within the normal range by 2 years, most of the catch-up occurring in the first few months. Part of the catch-up represents simple regression towards the mean [152]. However, at final adult height, as a group they remained on average smaller than their peers (mean final height was –0.7 SD). The remaining 13% remained below –2 SD throughout childhood, with a mean final height of –1.8 SD. The improvement compared with the older studies may be because of better postnatal nutrition of the SGA infant. This cohort study is consistent with reports from a selected population of children attending growth clinics who were IUGR and remained

small beyond the age of 4 years [153]. Ultimately, they had an adult height deficit of about 8.5 cm compared with genetic potential (parental target height).

A recent study of infants born to smokers suggested significant catch-up in weight by 6 months of age. Compared to non-smokers, the infants of smokers were lighter by an average of 88–247 g at birth, depending on number of cigarettes smoked. By 6 months, the mean deficit varied from 9 to 64 g, a maximum of 1% of bodyweight [154].

Later mortality and morbidity

Infants born SGA are at increased risk of sudden infant death syndrome in the first year of life. Infants born SGA because of maternal smoking are at increased risk of respiratory problems in early childhood.

Neurodevelopmental sequelae

Major neurodevelopmental disability is more likely if growth impairment is associated with chromosomal anomaly, congenital malformation or first trimester insult. Moreover, the increased risk of complications in the newborn period (see above) also increases the risk of long-term handicaps, including cerebral palsy, in survivors. Morbidity in SGA infants is determined largely by gestation, but term infants with birthweights below the 3rd centile have an excess of serious neuromotor impairments and cognitive deficits on follow-up [155,156]. Although the overall outcome of SGA infants may be similar to their AGA peers of comparable gestation, the type of impairments at follow-up are different. Minor disabilities such as clumsiness, learning difficulties and behaviour disturbance are commoner in term SGA infants [146]. Cognitive testing at 4 years was related to the duration of impaired intrauterine head growth [157].

Disease in adulthood

Recent retrospective epidemiological studies by Barker and his colleagues have suggested that a range of degenerative diseases of older age have their origins in fetal life. Infants small at birth, particularly if the placenta was large and the infant remained small at 1 year, seem to be at greatest risk from these later cardiovascular and metabolic derangements [2,3,158]. Clearly, more prospective studies are required, but the inference is that there are critical windows of time in fetal life when nutrition or other environmental influences can modify our genetic predisposition to disease half a century later [159].

Summary/conclusions

Fetal growth is controlled by genetic (maternal and fetal) and environmental (maternal and external) factors. There are many determinants of fetal growth which are not yet identified. Given this wide range of underlying determinants of fetal growth, it is not surprising that there are many mechanisms by which fetal growth can be compromised.

The clinical application of this knowledge in screening, diagnosis and management is limited for two principal reasons. Firstly, the distinction between genetically/constitutionally small and pathologically small is not always possible or easy. Secondly, even when pathological growth is correctly identified in a pregnancy, there are no data to use as guidance for making decisions relating to the timing of delivery. There are very few therapeutic measures to prevent or ameliorate pathological fetal growth.

There are recent more detailed reviews of fetal development and physiology [10,42].

Acknowledgement We are grateful to Mrs Lynda Straw and Mrs Sue Shepherd for secretarial help.

References

1 Stewart A. (1989) Fetal growth: Mortality and morbidity. In *Fetal Growth*. Eds F. Sharp, R.B. Fraser & R.D.G. Milner, p. 403. RCOG Publications, London.
2 Barker D.J.P., Bull A.R., Osmond C. & Simmond S.J. (1990) Fetal and placental size and risk of hypertension in adult life. *British Medical Journal* 301, 259.
3 Barker D.J.P., Osmond C., Simmonds S.J. & Wield G.A. (1993) The relation of small head circumference at birth to death from cardiovascular disease in adult life. *British Medical Journal* 306, 422.
4 Akeson R. (1993) Cell interaction with the microenvironment. In *Perinatal and Pediatric Pathophysiol-ogy: A Clinical Perspective.* Eds. P. Gluckman & M. Hyman, p. 60. Edward Arnold, London.
5 Price W. & Stiles A. (1994) Determinants of fetal and neonatal growth. *Current Opinion in Pediatrics* 6, 135.
6 Luke B. (1994) Nutritional influences on fetal growth. *Clinical Obstetrics and Gynecology* 37, 538.
7 Snow M. (1989) Effect of genome on size at birth. In *Fetal Growth*. Eds F. Sharp, R. Milner & R. Fraser, p. 3. Royal College of Obstetricians and Gynaecologists, London.
8 Droste S. (1992) Fetal growth in aneuploid conditions. *Clinical Obstetrics and Gynecology* 35, 119.
9 Persson P. (1989) Fetal growth curves. In *Fetal Growth*. Eds F. Sharp, R. Milner & R. Fraser, p. 13. Royal College of Obstetricians and Gynaecologists, London.
10 Milner R. (1993) Prenatal growth control. In *Perinatal and Pediatric Pathophysiology: A Clinical Perspective*. Eds P. Gluckman & M. Heymann, p. 162. Edward Arnold, London.
11 Dweck H. (1975) Feeding the prematurely born infant. *Clinics in Perinatology* 2, 183.
12 Waldenstrom U., Axelsson O. & Nilsson S. (1992) Ultrasonic dating of pregnancies: Effect on incidence of SGA diagnosis — A randomised controlled trial. *Early Human Development* 30, 75.
13 Gardosi J. (1992) Customised antenatal growth charts. *Lancet* 339, 283.
14 Gardosi J., Mongelli M., Wilcox M. & Chang A. (1995) An adjustable fetal weight standard. *Ultrasound in Obstetrics and Gynecology* 6, 168.
15 Dobbing J. & Sands J. (1979) Comparative aspects of the brain-growth spurt. *Early Human Development* 311, 79.
16 Carter A. (1993) Current topic: Restriction of placental and fetal growth in the guinea-pig. *Placenta* 14, 125.
17 Shelley H. & Basset J. (1975) Control of carbohydrate metabolism in the fetus and the newborn. *British Medical Bulletin* 31, 37.
18 Gluckman P. & Harding J.E. (1994) Nutritional and hormonal regulation of fetal growth: Evolving concepts. *Acta Paediatrica* (Suppl.) 399, 60.
19 Walton A. & Hammond J. (1954) The maternal effects on growth and conformation in Shire horse–Shetland pony crosses. *Proceedings of the Royal Society*, Series B 125, 311.
20 Moore T. & Haig D. (1991) Genomic imprinting in mammalian development: A parental tug-of-war. *Trends in Genetics* 7, 45.
21 Wigglesworth J.S. (1964) Experimental growth retardation in the foetal rat. *Journal of Pathology and Bacteriology* 88, 1.
22 Fowden A. (1989) The endocrine regulation of fetal metabolism and growth. In *Advances in Fetal Physiology: Reviews in Honor of G.C. Liggins*. Eds P. Gluckman, B. Johnston & P. Nathanielsz, p. 229. Perinatology Press, Ithaca, N.Y.
23 Wang H. & Chard T. (1991) The role of insulin-like growth factor-1 and insulin-like growth factor binding protein-1 in the control of human fetal growth. *Journal of Endocrinology* 132, 11.

494

24 Spencer J., Chang T., Jones J., Robson S. & Preece M. (1995) Third trimester fetal growth and umbilical venous blood concentrations of IGF-1, IGFBP-1, and growth hormone at term. *Archives of Disease in Childhood* **73**, F87.

25 Virtanen M. (1988) Manifestations of congenital hypothyroidism during the first week of life. *European Journal of Paediatrics* **147**, 270.

26 Underwood L., D'Ercole A., Clemmons D. & Wyk J.V. (1986) Paracrine regulation of somatomedins. *Clinics in Endocrinology and Metabolism* **13**, 59.

27 Baker J., Liu J., Robertson E. & Etstratiadis A. (1993) Role of insulin like growth factors in embryonic and postnatal growth. *Cell* **75**, 73.

28 Bassett J. (1986) Nutrition of the conceptus: aspects of its regulation. *Proceedings of the Nutrition Society*, **45**, 1.

29 Prentice A.M. (1991) Can maternal dietary supplements help in preventing infant malnutrition? *Acta Paediatrica* (Suppl.) **374**, 67.

30 Faber J. & Thornburg K. (1983) *Placental Physiology*. Raven Press, New York.

31 Battaglia G.C. & Meschia G. (1986) *An Introduction to Fetal Physiology*. Academic Press, New York.

32 Faber J.J. & Hart F.M. (1966) The rabbit placenta as an organ of diffusional exchange. Comparison with other species by dimensional analysis. *Circulation Research* **19**, 816.

33 Sibley C.P. & Boyd R.D.H. (1988) Control of transfer across the mataure placenta. *Oxford Reviews of Reproductive Biology* **10**, 382.

34 Schneider H. (1991) The role of the placenta in nutrition of the human fetus. *American Journal of Obstetrics and Gynecology* **164**, 967.

35 Stephenson T.J., Stammers J.P. & Hull D. (1993) Placental transfer of free fatty acids: Importance of fetal albumin concentration and acid-base status. *Journal of Developmental Physiology* **63**, 273.

36 Stephenson T.J., Stammers J.P. & Hull D. (1991) Effects of altering umbilical flow and umbilical free fatty acid concentration on transfer of free fatty acids across the rabbit placenta. *Journal of Developmental Physiology* **15**, 221.

37 Harding J. (1993) Placental physiology. In *Perinatal and Pediatric Pathophysiology: A Clinical Perspective*. Eds P. Gluckman & M. Heymann, p. 136. Edward Arnold, London.

38 Battaglia G.C. & Meschia G. (1988) Fetal nutrition. *Annual Review of Nutrition* **8**, 43.

39 Battaglia F. (1992) Metabolic aspects of fetal and neonatal growth. *Early Human Development* **29**, 99.

40 Cetin L., Corbetta C., Sereni L., Marconi A., Bozzetti P., Pardi G. & Battaglia F. (1990) Umbilical amino acid concentrations in normal and growth retarded fetuses sampled in utero by cordocentesis. *American Journal of Obstetrics and Gynecology* **162**, 253.

41 Lemons J., Vargas P. & Delaney J. (1981) Infant of the diabetic mother: Review of 225 cases. *Obstetrics and Gynaecology* **57**, 187.

42 Pipkin F.B., Hull D. & Stephenson T. (1994) Fetal physiology. In *Marshall's Physiology of Reproduction*. Ed. G. Lamming, p. 767. Chapman Hall, London.

43 Hendrickse W., Stammers J.P. & Hull D. (1985) The transfer of free fatty acids across the human placenta. *British Journal of Obstetrics and Gynaecology* **92**, 945.

44 Elphick M.C., Hull D. & Sanders, R.R. (1976) Concentrations of free fatty acids in maternal and umbilical cord blood during elective cesarean section. *British Journal of Obstetrics and Gynaecology* **83**, 539.

45 Leaf A.A., Leighfield M.J., Costeloe K.L. & Crawford M.A. (1992) Long chain polyunsaturated fatty acids and fetal growth. *Early Human Development* **30**, 183.

46 Stammers J.P., Hull D., Abraham R. & McFayden I.R. (1989) High arachidonic acid levels in the cord blood of infants of mothers on vegetarian diets. *British Journal of Nutrition* **61**, 89.

47 Adam P.A.J., Raiha N., Rahiala E.L. & Kemenomaki M. (1975) Oxidation of glucose and D-B-OH Butyrate by the early human fetal brain. *Acta Paediatrica Scandinavica* **64**, 17.

48 Patel M.S., Johnson C.A., Rajan R. & Own O.E. (1975) The metabolism of ketone bodies in developing human brain: Development of ketone-body-utilising enzymes and ketone bodies as precursors of lipid synthesis. *Journal of Neurochemistry* **25**, 906.

49 Hytten F.E. & Leitch I. (1971) *The Physiology of Human Pregnancy*. Blackwell Scientific Publications, Oxford.

50 Hytten F.E. (1979) Nutrition in pregnancy. *Postgraduate Medical Journal* **55**, 295.

51 Tarnow-Mordi W., Shaw J., Liu D., Gardener D. & Flynn F. (1981) Iatrogenic hyponatraemia of the newborn due to maternal fluid overload: A prospective study. *British Medical Journal* **283**, 636.

52 Canning J. & Boyd R. (1984) Mineral and water exchange between mother and fetus. In *Fetal Physiology and Medicine*. Eds R. Beard & P. Nathanielsz, p. 481. Marcel Dekker, New York.

53 Care A. & Ross R. (1984) Fetal calcium homeostasis. *Journal of Developmental Physiology* **6**, 59.

54 Lajeunesse D. & Brunette N. (1988) Sodium gradient-dependent phosphate transport in placental brush border membrane vesicles. *Placenta* **9**, 117.

55 Stulc J. (1988) Is there control of solute transfer at placental level? *Placenta* **9**, 19.

56 Clements M.R. (1988) Vitamin D supply to the rat fetus and neonate. *Journal of Clinical Investigation* **81**, 7768.

57 Evain-Brion D., Alsat E., Igout A., Frankenne F. & Hennen G. (1994) Placental growth hormone variant: assay and clinical aspects. *Acta Paediatrica Scandinavica* (Suppl.) **399**, 49.

58 Johnson D.R. (1974) Hair-pin tail: A case of post-reduction gene action in the mouse egg? *Genetics* **76**, 795.

59 Wagasuki N.A. (1974) A genetically determined incompatability system between spermatozoa and eggs leading to embryonic death in mice. *Journal of Reproductive Fertility* **41**, 85.

60 Joubert D.M. & Hammond J. (1954) Maternal effect on birthweight in South Devon x Dexter cattle crosses. *Nature* **174**, 540.

61 Hunter G.L. (1956) The maternal influence on size in sheep. *Journal of Agricultural Science* **48**, 36.

62 Brumby P.J. (1960) The influence of the maternal environment on growth in mice. *Heredity* **14**, 1.

63 Robson E.B. (1981) Human birth weight: Natural selection and genetics. In *The Biology of Normal Human Growth*. Eds M. Ritzen, A. Peria, K. Hall, A. Larsson, A. Zetterberg & R. Zetterstrom, p. 183. Raven Press, New York.

64 Witter F.R. & Luke B. (1991) The effect of maternal height on birthweight and birth length. *Early Human Development* **25**, 181.

65 Eastman N.J. & Jackson, E. (1968) Weight relationships in pregnancy. *Clinical Obstetrics and Gynecology* **35**, 119.

66 Polani P.E. (1974) Chromsomal and other genetic influences on birthweight variation. In *Size at Birth*, Ciba Foundation Symposium 27. Eds K. Elliott & J. Knight, p. 127. Elsevier, Amsterdam.

67 Mascie-Taylor C.G. (1991) Biosocial influences on stature: A review. *Journal of Biosocial Science* **23**, 113.

68 Alberman E.D. (1989) Fetal undergrowth: Epidemiology. In *Fetal Growth*. Eds F. Sharp, R.B. Fraser & R.D.G. Milner, p. 175. RCOG Publications, London.

69 Ounsted M. & Ounsted C. (1973) On fetal growth rate. *Clinics in Developmental Medicine* **46**, 182.

70 Hoffman H.J., Stark C.R., Lundin F.E. & Ashbrook J.D. (1974) Analysis of birth weight, gestational age and fetal viability. *Obstetrics and Gynecology Survey* **29**, 651.

71 Wallace L.R. (1945) The effect of diet on fetal development. *Journal of Physiology* **104**, 34.

72 Antonov A.V. (1947) Children born during the siege of Leningrad in 1942. *Journal of Pediatrics* **30**, 250.

73 Smith C.A. (1947) The effect of wartime starvation in Holland upon pregnancy and its product. *American Journal of Obstetrics and Gynecology* **53**, 599.

74 Forsum E., Sadurskis A. & Wager J. (1988) Resting metabolic rate and body composition of healthy Swedish women during pregnancy. *American Journal of Clinical Nutrition* **47**, 942.

75 Prentice A.M., Goldberg G.R., Murgatroyd P.R., Davies H.L. & Scott W. (1989) Energy sparing adaptations in human pregnancy assessed by whole body calorimetry. *British Journal of Nutrition* **65**, 5.

76 Davies H.L., Prentice A.M., Coward W.A., Goldber G.R., Black A.E., Murgatroyd P.R., Scott W. *et al.* (1988) Individual variation in the energy cost of pregnancy: Doubly labelled water method. *Proceedings of the Nutrition Society* **47**, 45.

77 Lawrence M., Lawrence F., Coward W.A., Cole T.J. & Whitehead R.G. (1987) Energy requirements of pregnancy in The Gambia. *Lancet* **ii**, p. 1072.

78 Humbel R.E. (1990) Insulin-like growth factors I and II. *European Journal of Biochemistry* **190**, 445.

79 Sara V.R. & Hall K. (1990) Insulin growth factors and their binding proteins. *Physiology Review* **70**, 591.

80 Wilson D.M., Bennett A., Adamson G.D., Nagashima J., Liu F., Denatale M.L., Hintz R.L. *et al.* (1982) Somatomedins in pregnancy: A cross-sectional study of insulin-like growth factors I and II and somatomedin peptide content in normal human pregnancies. *Journal of Clinical Endrocinology Metabolism* **55**, 858.

81 Gargosky S.E., Moyse K.J., Walton P.E., Owens J.A., Robinson J.S. & Owens P.C. (1990) Circulating levels of insulin-like growth factors increase and the molecular forms of their serum binding proteins change with human pregnancy. *Biochemical Biophysical Research Communication* **170**, 1157.

82 Caufriez A., Frankenne F., Englert Y., Goldstein J., Contraine F., Hennen G. & Copinschi G. (1990) Placental growth hormone as a potential regulator of maternal IGF-U during human pregnancy. *American Journal of Physiology* **258**, E1014.

83 Frankenne F., Closset J., Gomez F., Scippo M.L., Smal J. & Henne G. (1988) The physiology of growth hormones (GHs) in pregnant women and partial characterisation of the placental GH variant. *Journal of Clinical Endorcinology and Metabolism* **66**, 1171.

84 Shwander J.C., Hauri C., Zapf J. & Froesch E.R. (1983) Synthesis and secretion of insulin-like growth factor and its binding protein by the perfused rat liver: Dependence on growth hormone status. *Endocrinology* **113**, 297.

85 Hall K., Hansson U., Lundin G., Luthman M., Persson B., Povoa G., Stangenberg M. *et al.* (1986) Serum levels of somatomedins and somotomedin-binding protein in pregnant women with type I or gestational diabetes and their infants. *Journal of Clinical Endocrinology and Metabolism* **63**, 1300.

86 Wang H.S., Lim J., English J., Irvine L. & Chard T. (1991) The concentration of insulin-like growth factor-I (IGF-I) and insulin-like growth factor-binding protein-I (IGFBP-I) in human cord serum at delivery: relation to fetal weight. *Journal of Endocrinology* **129**, 459.

87 Rutanen E.-M., Menabawey M., Isaka K., Bohn, H., Chard, T. & Grudzinskas J.G. (1986) Synthesis of placental protein 12 by decidua from early pregnancy. *Journal of Clinical Endocrinology and Metabolism* **63**, 675.

88 Pekonen F., Suikkari A.M., Makinen T. & Rutanen E.M. (1988) Different insulin-like growth factors binding species in human placenta and ecidua. *Journal of Clinical Endocrinology and Metabolism* **67**, 1250.

89 Cascieri M.A., Saperstein R., Hayes N.S., Green B.G., Chicchi G.G., Applebaum J. & Bayne M.L. (1988) Serum half-life and biological activity of mutants of human insulin-like growth factor-I which do not bind to serum binding protein. *Endocrinology* **123**, 373.

90 Giudice L.C., Farrell E.M., Pham H., Lamson G. & Rosenfeld R.G. (1990) Insulin-like growth factor binding proteins in maternal serum throughout gestation and in puerperium: Effects of a pregnancy-associated serum protease activity. *Journal of Clinical Endocrinology and Metabolism* **71**, 806.

91 Revelli A., Durando A. & Massobrio M. (1992) Exercise and pregnancy: A review of maternal and fetal effects. *Obstetrics and Gynecology Survey* **47**, 355.

92 Soiva K., Salvi A. & Gronroos M. (1964) Physical working capacity during pregnancy and effect of physical work tests on fetal heart rate. *Annals of Chir Gynaecology* **53**, 187.

496

93 Pommerance J.J., Gluck L. & Lynch V.A. (1974) Physical fitness in pregnancy: its effect on pregnancy outcome. *American Journal of Obstetrics and Gynaecology* **119**, 867.

94 Spinollo A., Capuyzo E., Baltaro F., Piazza G., Nicola S. & Iasei A. (1996) The effect of work activity in pregnancy on the risk of fetal growth retardation. *Acta Obstetrica et Gynaecologia Scandinavica* **75**, 531.

95 Dressendorfer R.H. (1978) Physical training during pregnancy and lactation. *Physiology Sportsmedicine* **6**, 74.

96 Korcok M. (1981) Pregnant jogger: What a record! *Journal of the American Medical Association* **246**, 201.

97 Erderly G.J. (1962) Gynecological survey of female athletes. *Journal of Sports Medicine and Physical Fitness* **2**, 174.

98 Erkola R. (1976) The physical work capacity of the expectant mother and its effect on pregnancy, labor and the newborn. *International Journal of Obstetrics and Gynecology* **14**, 153.

99 Pirani B.B.K., Campbell D.M. & MacGillivray I. (1973) Plasma volume in normal first pregnancy. *British Journal of Obstetrics and Gynaecology* **80**, 894.

100 Grahn D. & Kratchman J. (1965) Variation in neonatal death rate and birthweight in the US and possible relations to environmental radiation, geology and altitude. *American Journal of Human Genetics* **15**, 329.

101 Meyer M.B. (1977) Effects of maternal smoking and altitude on birth weight and gestation. In *The Epidemiology of Prematurity*. Eds D.W. Reed & F.W. Stanley, p. 81. Baltimore: Urban and Schwarzenberg.

102 Wigglesworth J.S. (1989) Aetiology of fetal undergrowth. In *Fetal Growth*. Eds F. Sharp, R.B. Fraser & R.D.G. Milner, p. 185. RCOG Publications, London.

103 Smith D.W. (1982) *Recognisable Patterns of Human Malformation*, 3rd edn. W.B. Saunders. Philadelphia.

104 Honnenbier W.J. & Swaab D.F. (1973) The influence of anencephaly on intrauterine growth of the fetus and placenta and upon gestation length. *Journal of Obstetrics and Gynaecology of the British Commonwealth* **80**, 577.

105 Elias S., Simpson J.L. & Griffin L.P. (1978) Intrauterine growth retardation in osteogenesis imperfecta. *Journal of the American Medical Association* **239**, 12.

106 Engstrom W., Lindham S. & Schofield P. (1988) Wiedemann–Beckwith syndrome. *European Journal of Pediatrics* **147**, 450.

107 Fox H. (1986) Pathology of the placenta. *Clinical Obstetrics and Gynaecology* **13**, 501.

108 Fallucca F. & Gargiulo P. (1985) Amniotic fluid insulin, C peptide concentration and fetal morbidity in infants of diabetic mother. *American Journal of Obstetrics and Gynaecology* **153**, 534.

109 Robinson J.S., Kingston E.J. & Joens C.T. (1979) Studies on experimental growth retardation in sheep: The effect of removal of emdometrial caruncles on fetal size and metabolism. *Journal of Dec Physiology* **1**, 379.

110 Naeye R.L. (1978) Effects of maternal cigarette smoking on the fetus and placenta. *British Journal of Obstetrics and Gynaecology* **85**, 732.

111 Thompson A.M., Billewicz W.Z. & Hytten F.E. (1969) The weight of the placenta in relation to birthweight. *Journal of Obstetrics and Gynaecology of the British Commonwealth* **76**, 865.

112 Bryan E.M. & Kohler H.G. (1974) The missing umbilical artery. *Archives of Disease in Childhood* **49**, 844.

113 Fox H. (1981) Placental malfunction as a factor in intrauterine growth retardation. In *Fetal Growth Retardation*. Eds F.A. Van Assche & W.B. Robertson, p. 117. Churchill Livingstone, Edinburgh.

114 Federick J. & Adelstein P. (1978) Factors associated with low birth weight of infants delivered at term. *British Journal of Obstetrics and Gynaecology* **85**, 1.

115 Gabert H.A. (1971) Placental praevia and fetal growth. *Obstetrics and Gynecology* **38**, 403.

116 McKeown T. & Record R.G. (1953) The influence of placental size on foetal growth in man with special reference to multiple pregnancy. *Journal of Endocrinology* **9**, 418.

117 Eckstein P., McKeown T. & Record R.G. (1955) Variation in placental weight according to litter size in the guinea pig. *Journal of Endocrinology* **12**, 108.

118 Alford C.A. (1976) Rubella. In *Infectious Diseases of the Fetus and Newborn Infant*. Eds J.S. Remington & J.O. Klein, p. 71. W.B. Saunders, Philadelphia.

119 McCracken G.H., Shinefield H.R., Cobb K., Rausen A.R., Dische M.R. & Eichenwald H.F. (1969) Congenital cytomegalic inclusion disease. *American Journal of Disease in Childhood* **117**, 522.

120 Rush D. (1989) Effects of changes in maternal energy and protein intake during pregnancy, with special reference to fetal growth. In *Fetal Growth*. Eds F. Sharp, R.B. Fraser & R.D.G. Milner, p. 203. RCOG Publications, London.

121 Boyd P.A. & Scott A. (1985) Quantitative studies on human placentas associated with pre-eclampsia, essential hypertension and intrauterine growth retardation. *British Journal of Obstetrics and Gynaecology* **92**, 714.

122 Shime J., Mocarski E.J.M., Hastings D., Webb G.D. & McLaughlin P.R. (1987) Congenital heart disease in pregnancy: Short and long term complications. *American Journal of Obstetrics and Gynecology* **156**, 313.

123 Greenberger P.A. & Patterson R. (1983) Beclomethasone diproprionate for several asthma during pregnancy. *Annals of Internal Medicine* **98**, 478.

124 Katz A.I., Davison J.M., Hayslett J.P., Singson E. & Lindheimer M.D. (1980) Pregnancy in women with kidney disease. *Kidney International* **18**, 192.

125 Carlson D.E. (1988) Maternal diseases associated with intrauterine growth retardation. *Seminars in Perinatology* **12**, 17.

126 Powers D.R., Sandhu M., Niland-Weiss J., Johnson C., Bruce S. & Manning P.R. (1986) Pregnancy in sickle cell disease. *Obstetrics and Gynecology* **67**, 217.

127 Kierse M. (1981) Aetiology of fetal growth retardation. In *Fetal Growth Retardation*. Eds F.A. Van

Assche & W.B. Robertson, p. 37. Churchill Livingstone, Edinburgh.

128 Naeye R.L., Blanc W., Leblanc W. & Khatamee M.A. (1973) Fetal complications of maternal heroin addiction: abnormal growth, infections and episodes of stress. *Journal of Pediatrics* **83**, 1055.

129 Pirani B.B. (1978) Smoking during pregnancy. *Obstetrics and Gynecology Survey* **33**, 1.

130 Miller H.C. & Hussein K. (1964) Maternal smoking and fetal growth in full term infants. *Pediatric Research* **8**, 960.

131 Quellette E.M., Rosett H.L., Rosman N.P. & Weiner L. (1977) Adverse effects on offspring of maternal alcohol abuse during pregnancy. *New England Journal of Medicine* **297**, 528.

132 Galbraith R.S., Karchman E.J. & Piercy W.A. (1979) The clinical prediction of intrauterine growth retardation. *American Journal of Obstetrics and Gynecology* **133**, 281.

133 Evans J. & Stokes I.M. (1984) Outcome of pregnancies associated with raised serum and normal amniotic fluid AFP concentrations. *British Medical Journal* **288**, 1494.

134 Chard T. & Howell R.J.S. (1989) Detection of fetal growth retardation by biochemical tests. In *Fetal Growth*. Eds F. Sharp, R.B. Fraser & R.D.G. Milner, p. 263. RCOG Publications, London.

135 Villar J. & Belizan J.M. (1983) The evaluation of the methods used in the diagnosis of intrauterine growth retardation. *Obstetrics and Gynecology Survey* **41**, 187.

136 Whittle M.J. (1987) An overview of fetal monitoring. *Baillère's Clinical Obstetrics and Gynaecology* **1**, 203.

137 Campbell S. (1989) The detection of intrauterine growth retardation. In *Fetal Growth*. Eds F. Sharp, R.B. Fraser & R.D.G. Milner, p. 251. RCOG Publications, London.

138 James D. (1990) Diagnosis and management of fetal growth retardation. *Archives of Disease in Childhood* **65**, 390.

139 Landon M.B. & Gabbe S.G. (1994) Diabetes mellitus. In *High Risk Pregnancy: Management Options*. Eds. D. James, P. Steer, C. Weiner & B. Gonik, p. 277. W.B. Saunders, London.

140 Johnson J.M., Lange I.R., Harman C.R., Torchia, M.G. & Manning F.A. (1988) Biophysical profile scoring in the management of the diabetic pregnancy. *Obstetrics and Gynecology* **72**, 841.

141 Manning F.A., Monticoglou S., Harman C.R., Morrison I. & Lange I.R. (1987) Antepartum fetal risk assessment: The role of the biophysical profile score. *Clinical Obstetrics and Gynecology* **1**, 55.

142 James D.K., Parker M.J. & Smoleniec J. (1992) Comprehensive fetal assessment with three ultrasound characteristics. *American Journal of Obstetrics and Gynecology* **166**, 1486.

143 Alfirevic Z. & Neilson J.P. (1995) Doppler ultrasonography in high-risk pregnancies: Systematic review with meta-analysis. *American Journal of Obstetrics and Gynecology* **172**, 1379.

144 Adamson S., Alessandri L., Badawi N., Burton P., Pemberton P. & Stanley F. (1995) Predictors of neonatal encephalopathy in full term infants. *British Medical Journal* **311**, 598.

145 Hackett G., Campbell S., Gamsu H., Cohen-Overbeek T. & Pearce J. (1987) Doppler studies in the growth retarded fetus and prediction of neonatal necrotising enterocolitis, haemorrhage, and neonatal morbidity. *British Medical Journal* **294**, 13.

146 Chiswick M. (1985) Intrauterine growth retardation. *British Medical Journal* **291**, 845.

147 Levene M. (1989) Neonatal management of the SGA infant. In *Fetal Growth*. Eds F. Sharp, R. Milner & R. Fraser, p. 393. Royal College of Obstetricians and Gynaecologists, London.

148 Fitzhardinge P. & Steven E. (1972) The small-for-date infant: Later growth patterns. *Pediatrics* **49**, 671.

149 Fancourt R., Campbell S., Harvey D. & Norman A. (1976) Follow-up study of small for dates babies. *British Medical Journal* **272**, 1421.

150 Ounsted M., Moar V.A. & Scott A. (1985) Children of deviant birthweight: The influence of genetic and other factors on size at seven years. *Acta Paediatrica Scandinavica* **74**, 707.

151 Albertsson-Wikland K. & Karlberg J. (1994) Natural growth in children born small for gestational age with and without catch-up growth. *Acta Paediatrica Scandinavica* (Suppl.) **399**, 64.

152 Cole T. (1995) Conditional reference charts to assess weight gain in British infants. *Archives of Disease in Childhood* **73**, 8.

153 Chaussain J., Colle M. & Ducret J. (1994) Adult height in children with prepubertal short stature secondary to intrauterine growth retardation. *Acta Paediatrica* (Suppl.) **399**, 72.

154 Conter V., Cortinovis I., Rogari P. & Riva L. (1995) Weight growth in infants born to mothers who smoked during pregnancy. *British Medical Journal* **310**, 768.

155 Fitzhardinge P. & Steven E. (1972) The small-for-date infant: Neurological and intellectual sequelae patterns. *Pediatrics* **50**, 50.

156 Rantakallio P. (1985) A 14 year follow-up of children with normal and abnormal birth weight for their gestational age: A population study. *Acta Paediatrica Scandinavica* **74**, 62.

157 Harvey D., Prince J., Bunton J., Parkinson C. & Campbell S. (1982) Abilities of children who were SGA babies. *Pediatrics* **69**, 296.

158 Robinson R.J. (1992) Is the child the father of the man? *British Medical Journal* **304**, 789.

159 Barker D.J.P. (1995) Fetal origins of coronary heart disease. *British Medical Journal* **311**, 171.

Index